Pseudomonas

BIOTRANSFORMATIONS, PATHOGENESIS, AND EVOLVING BIOTECHNOLOGY

Pseudomonas

BIOTRANSFORMATIONS, PATHOGENESIS, AND EVOLVING BIOTECHNOLOGY

Edited by

Simon Silver
Department of Microbiology and Immunology
The University of Illinois College of Medicine
Chicago, Illinois

Ananda M. Chakrabarty
Department of Microbiology and Immunology
The University of Illinois College of Medicine
Chicago, Illinois

Barbara Iglewski
Department of Microbiology and Immunology
The University of Rochester
Rochester, New York

Samuel Kaplan
Department of Microbiology and Immunology
The University of Texas Medical School
Houston, Texas

AMERICAN SOCIETY FOR MICROBIOLOGY
Washington, D.C.

Library of Congress Cataloging-in-Publication Data

Pseudomonas : biotransformations, pathogenesis, and evolving
  biotechnology / edited by Simon Silver . . . [et al.].
      p.   cm.
    Based on a symposium held in Chicago, Ill., in July, 1989;
  sponsored by the American Society for Microbiology.
    1. Pseudomonas—Congresses.   I. Silver, S. (Simon)   II. American
  Society for Microbiology.
    [DNLM: 1. Pseudomonas—congresses.   QW 131 P9743 1989]
  QR82.P78P78 1990
  589.9′5—dc20

ISBN 1-55581-019-5

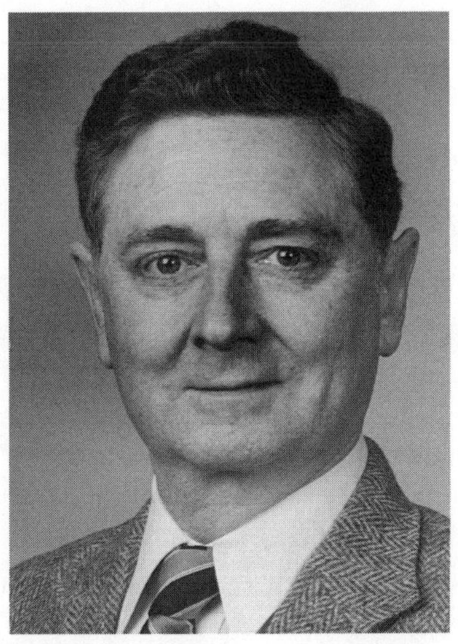

Irving P. Crawford, a major contributor to understanding of the metabolism and molecular biology of *Pseudomonas* and a gentle and warm human being, died on 8 October 1989. At the time of the *Pseudomonas* Symposium in July, Irv was unaware of the cancer that was to rapidly spread and take his life. He was full of enthusiasm for future experimental work and protein evolution. He was in need of another visit to the western suburbs of Chicago to enrich his orchid collection, which, together with his family (Irv and Edna married while he was at Washington University and they have two grown sons), science, Japanese culture, and the performance of chamber music, occupied his life.

Irv obtained both his B.A. and M.D. at Stanford University. Then, following brief postdoctorate stints with Arthur Kornberg at Washington University (two years of virology at the Walter Reed Army Institute of Research in Washington) and with Charles Yanofsky at Stanford, he accepted an academic position at Western Reserve Medical School in Cleveland, Ohio. Six years later he moved to the Scripps Clinic and Research Foundation in La Jolla, California, and 12 years afterwards he accepted the chairmanship of the Department of Microbiology at the University of Iowa in Iowa City. During his 12 years there, Irv recruited and built a vibrant, intellectually active department. In addition to his more than 100 publications (which attest to his intellectual curiosity and enthusiasm for microbial science, not chasing fashion and fame), Irv served on many editorial boards, study sections, and professional committees. His sound, quiet wisdom was sought and appreciated by his many friends. His much too early death at age 58, while full of enthusiasm and joy of life, impoverishes all of us.

Contents

I. PATHOGENESIS

II. PLANT-BACTERIAL INTERACTIONS

III. BIOTRANSFORMATIONS

IV. PLASMIDS, VECTORS, GENE MAPPING, AND CLONING

V. CELL ENVELOPE AND TRANSPORT

VI. HONORARY PSEUDOMONADS

Contributors

Douglas H. Anderson • Department of Biochemistry, Purdue University, West Lafayette, Indiana 47907   (16)*

W. Arnold • Faculty of Biology, Department of Genetics, University of Bielefeld, Postbox 8640, D-4800 Bielefeld 1, Federal Republic of Germany (10)

Frederick M. Ausubel • Department of Genetics, Harvard Medical School, and Department of Molecular Biology, Massachusetts General Hospital, Boston, Massachusetts 02114 (9)

Michael Bagdasarian • Department of Microbiology, Michigan State University and Michigan Biotechnology Institute, 3900 Collins Road, Lansing, Michigan 48909 (23)

Mira M. Bagdasarian • Department of Microbiology, Michigan State University and Michigan Biotechnology Institute, 3900 Collins Road, Lansing, Michigan 48909 (23)

Michael J. Beach • Department of Biochemistry, Purdue University, West Lafayette, Indiana 47907 (16)

Allan Berry • Bio-Products Division, Eastman Kodak Company, Rochester, New York 14652-3615 (2)

Robert A. Bever • Department of Microbiology and Immunology, University of Rochester School of Medicine and Dentistry, Rochester, New York 14642 (4)

W. Bitter • Department of Molecular Cell Biology and Institute of Molecular Biology, University of Utrecht, Padualaan 8, 3584 CH Utrecht, The Netherlands (7)

Christian Böcker • Institut für Pflanzenphysiologie und Mikrobiologie der Freien Universität Berlin, D-1000 Berlin 33, Federal Republic of Germany (38)

Françoise Brunel • European Patent Office, Erhardtstrasse 27, D-8000 Munich, Federal Republic of Germany (17, 24)

Gayle Burns • Department of Biochemistry and Molecular Biology, The University of Oklahoma Health Sciences Center, P.O. Box 26901, Oklahoma City, Oklahoma 73190 (19)

---

* Parentheses indicate corresponding chapter in this volume.

A. Byrne • Department of Microbiology, University of Massachusetts, Amherst, Massachusetts 01003   (27)

Carlos Cervantes • Instituto de Investigationes Quimico-Biologicas, Universidad Michoacana, 58240 Morelia, Michoacan, Mexico   (34)

Ananda M. Chakrabarty • Department of Microbiology and Immunology, University of Illinois College of Medicine, Chicago, Illinois 60612   (2)

Ming Chang • Department of Microbiology, University of Iowa, Iowa City, Iowa 52242   (28)

A. K. Chatterjee • Department of Plant Pathology, University of Missouri, 108 Waters Hall, Columbia, Missouri 65211   (6)

S. Chauhan • Department of Microbiology and Biocatalysis Research Group, The University of Iowa, Iowa City, Iowa 52242   (13)

Nathalie Chevalier • Unit of Molecular Biology, International Institute of Cellular and Molecular Pathology, 75 Avenue Hippocrate, 1200 Brussels, Belgium   (24)

Irving P. Crawford • Department of Microbiology, University of Iowa, Iowa City, Iowa 52242 (deceased)   (28)

Matthew D. Davies • Department of Biochemistry, University of Illinois, Urbana, Illinois 61801   (11)

Keith R. Davis • Department of Molecular Biology, Massachusetts General Hospital, Boston, Massachusetts 02114   (9)

John Davison • Transgene s.a., Rue de Molsheim 11, 67000 Strasbourg, France   (17, 24)

James D. DeVault • Department of Microbiology and Immunology, University of Illinois College of Medicine, Chicago, Illinois 60612   (2)

S. Dharmsthiti • Department of Genetics and Developmental Biology, Monash University, Clayton, Victoria 3168, Australia   (26)

Xinnian Dong • Department of Molecular Biology, Massachusetts General Hospital, Boston, Massachusetts 02114   (9)

Günther Eberz • Institut für Pflanzenphysiologie und Mikrobiologie der Freien Universität Berlin, D-1000 Berlin 33, Federal Republic of Germany   (38)

Gerrit Eggink • Laboratory of Biochemistry, Groningen Biotechnology Center, Nijenborgh 16, 9747 AG Groningen, The Netherlands   (15)

Thomas Eitinger • Institut für Pflanzenphysiologie und Mikrobiologie der Freien Universität Berlin, D-1000 Berlin 33, Federal Republic of Germany   (38)

David W. Essar • Department of Microbiology, University of Iowa, Iowa City, Iowa 52242   **(28)**

A. Ferrante • Department of Microbiology, University of Massachusetts, Amherst, Massachusetts 01003   **(27)**

JoAnne L. Flynn • Scripps Research Institute, La Jolla, California 92037   **(3)**

R. D. Frederick • Department of Plant Pathology, University of California, Berkeley, California 94720   **(8)**

Bärbel Friedrich • Institut für Pflanzenphysiologie und Mikrobiologie der Freien Universität Berlin, D-1000 Berlin 33, Federal Republic of Germany   **(38)**

Kensuke Furukawa • Department of Agricultural Chemistry, Kyushu University, Fukuoka 812, Japan   **(12)**

Marc Galimand • Mikrobiologisches Institut, Eidgenössische Technische Hochschule, CH-8092 Zurich, Switzerland   **(29)**

Marianne Gamper • Mikrobiologisches Institut, Eidgenössische Technische Hochschule, CH-8092 Zurich, Switzerland   **(29)**

D. T. Gibson • Department of Microbiology and Biocatalysis Research Group, The University of Iowa, Iowa City, Iowa 52242   **(13)**

John F. Gill, Jr. • Protein Chemistry Division, Boehringer Mannheim Diagnostics, 9115 Hague Road, Indianapolis, Indiana 46250   **(16)**

Joanna B. Goldberg • Channing Laboratory, Brigham and Women's Hospital, Boston, Massachusetts 02115   **(3)**

Leslie A. Gregg • Department of Biology, Yale University, New Haven, Connecticut 06511   **(22)**

C. Grimm • Department of Plant Pathology, University of California, Berkeley, California 94720   **(8)**

Pablo Guevara • Department of Genetics, Harvard Medical School, and Department of Molecular Biology, Massachusetts General Hospital, Boston, Massachusetts 02114   **(9)**

Dieter Haas • Mikrobiologisches Institut, Eidgenössische Technische Hochschule, CH-8092 Zurich, Switzerland   **(29)**

R. E. W. Hancock • University of British Columbia, Vancouver, British Columbia, Canada V6T 1W5   **(31)**

K. Hatter • Department of Biochemistry and Molecular Biology, The University of Oklahoma Health Sciences Center, P.O. Box 26901, Oklahoma City, Oklahoma 73190   **(19)**

E. Hatziloukas • Institute of Molecular Biology and Biotechnology, Foundation for Research and Technology-Hellas, Heraklion, Crete, Greece (8)

Nobuki Hayase • Biotechnology Laboratory, Kobe Steel Ltd., Tsukuba, Ibaraki 305, Japan (12)

B. W. Holloway • Department of Genetics and Developmental Biology, Monash University, Clayton, Victoria 3168, Australia (26)

Tadao Horiuchi • Faculty of Pharmaceutical Sciences, Kyushu University, Fukuoka 812, Japan (11)

Karin Horstmann • Institut für Pflanzenphysiologie und Mikrobiologie der Freien Universität Berlin, D-1000 Berlin 33, Federal Republic of Germany (38)

John Houghton • Department of Biology, Yale University, New Haven, Connecticut 06511 (22)

Barbara H. Iglewski • Department of Microbiology and Immunology, University of Rochester School of Medicine and Dentistry, Rochester, New York 14642 (4)

Sachiye Inouye • Department of Biochemistry, Yamaguchi University School of Medicine, Ube, Yamaguchi 755, Japan (14)

C. Johnson • Department of Genetics and Developmental Biology, Monash University, Clayton, Victoria 3168, Australia (26)

Tuajuanda C. Jordan-Starck • Department of Pharmacology and Cell Biophysics, University of Cincinnati College of Medicine, Cincinnati, Ohio 45267 (16)

Makoto Kageyama • Mitsubishi Kasei Institute of Life Sciences, 11, Minami-ooya, Machida-shi, Tokyo 194, Japan (33)

Kone Kaniga • Unit of Molecular Biology, International Institute of Cellular and Molecular Pathology, 75 Avenue Hippocrate, 1200 Brussels, Belgium (24)

Samuel Kaplan • Department of Microbiology, The University of Texas Medical School at Houston, 6431 Fannin, P.O. Box 20708, Houston, Texas 77225 (37)

D. Kapp • Faculty of Biology, Department of Genetics, University of Bielefeld, Postbox 8640, D-4800 Bielefeld 1, Federal Republic of Germany (10)

Junichi Kato • Department of Microbiology and Immunology, University of Illinois College of Medicine, Chicago, Illinois 60612 (2)

A. Kearney • Department of Genetics and Developmental Biology, Monash University, Clayton, Victoria 3168, Australia (26)

M. Keller • Faculty of Biology, Department of Genetics, University of Bielefeld, Postbox 8640, D-4800 Bielefeld 1, Federal Republic of Germany (10)

Kazuhide Kimbara • Department of Microbiology and Immunology, University of Illinois College of Medicine, Chicago, Illinois 60612 (2)

Kiyoyuki Kitano • Department of Microbiology and Immunology, University of Illinois College of Medicine, Chicago, Illinois 60612 (2)

Hans-Joachim Knackmuss • Institut für Mikrobiologie der Universität Stuttgart, Azenbergstrasse 18, D-7000 Stuttgart 1, Federal Republic of Germany (20)

Mieko Kobayashi • Mitsubishi Kasei Institute of Life Sciences, 11, Minami-ooya, Machida-shi, Tokyo 194, Japan (33)

Hideo Koga • Faculty of Pharmaceutical Sciences, Kyushu University, Fukuoka 812, Japan (11)

Menno Kok • Laboratory of Biochemistry, Groningen Biotechnology Center, Nijenborgh 16, 9747 AG Groningen, The Netherlands (15)

Tyler A. Kokjohn • Department of Biochemistry and The Program in Molecular Biology, Loyola University of Chicago, Maywood, Illinois 60153 (25)

Christiane Kortlüke • Institut für Pflanzenphysiologie und Mikrobiologie der Freien Universität Berlin, D-1000 Berlin 33, Federal Republic of Germany (38)

M. Koster • Department of Molecular Cell Biology and Institute of Molecular Biology, University of Utrecht, Padualaan 8, 3584 CH Utrecht, The Netherlands (7)

V. Krishnapillai • Department of Genetics and Developmental Biology, Monash University, Clayton, Victoria 3168, Australia (26)

J. Leong • Department of Molecular Cell Biology and Institute of Molecular Biology, University of Utrecht, Padualaan 8, 3584 CH Utrecht, The Netherlands (7)

T. G. Lessie • Department of Microbiology, University of Massachusetts, Amherst, Massachusetts 01003 (27)

K. T. Madhusudhan • Department of Biochemistry and Molecular Biology, The University of Oklahoma Health Sciences Center, P.O. Box 26901, Oklahoma City, Oklahoma 73190 (19)

N. L. Martin • University of British Columbia, Vancouver, British Columbia, Canada V6T 1W5 (31)

J. D. Marugg • Department of Molecular Cell Biology and Institute of Molecular Biology, University of Utrecht, Padualaan 8, 3584 CH Utrecht, The Netherlands (7)

Hidenori Matsui • Mitsubishi Kasei Institute of Life Sciences, 11, Minami-ooya, Machida-shi, Tokyo 194, Japan (33)

Thomas B. May • Department of Microbiology and Immunology, University of Illinois College of Medicine, Chicago, Illinois 60612 (2)

Robert V. Miller • Department of Biochemistry and The Program in Molecular Biology, Loyola University of Chicago, Maywood, Illinois 60153 (25)

Dallice Mills • Department of Botany and Plant Pathology, Oregon State University, Corvallis, Oregon 97331 (5)

M. N. Mindrinos • Department of Plant Pathology, University of California, Berkeley, California 94720 (8)

Michael Mindrinos • Department of Molecular Biology, Massachusetts General Hospital, Boston, Massachusetts 02114 (9)

Tapan K. Misra • Department of Microbiology and Immunology, University of Illinois College of Medicine, Chicago, Illinois 60612 (2)

Victor Morales • Department of Microbiology, Michigan State University and Michigan Biotechnology Institute, 3900 Collins Road, Lansing, Michigan 48909 (23)

A. F. Morgan • Department of Genetics and Developmental Biology, Monash University, Clayton, Victoria 3168, Australia (26)

Pradip Mukhopadhyay • Crop Protection Department, Monsanto Agricultural Company, St. Louis, Missouri 63198 (5)

P. Müller • Department of Biology/Botany, Philipps University Marburg, Karl-von-Frisch Strasse, D-3550 Marburg, Federal Republic of Germany (10)

Atsushi Nakazawa • Department of Biochemistry, Yamaguchi University School of Medicine, Ube, Yamaguchi 755, Japan (14)

Teruko Nakazawa • Department of Microbiology, Yamaguchi University School of Medicine, Ube, Yamaguchi 755, Japan (14)

Ellen L. Neidle • Department of Microbiology, University of Illinois, 407 South Goodwin Avenue, Urbana, Illinois 61801 (22)

J. B. Neilands • Biochemistry Department, University of California, Berkeley, California (36)

K. Niehaus • Faculty of Biology, Department of Genetics, University of Bielefeld, Postbox 8640, D-4800 Bielefeld 1, Federal Republic of Germany (10)

Hiroshi Nikaido • Department of Microbiology and Immunology, University of California, Berkeley, California 94720   **(30)**

R. O. Nordeen • Department of Plant Pathology, University of Missouri, 108 Waters Hall, Columbia, Missouri 65211   **(6)**

Dennis E. Ohman • Department of Microbiology and Immunology, University of Tennessee, and VA Medical Center, Memphis, Tennessee 38163   **(3)**

L. Nicholas Ornston • Department of Biology, Yale University, New Haven, Connecticut 06511   **(22)**

Rachel M. Ostroff • Department of Microbiology and Immunology, University of Colorado Health Sciences Center, Denver, Colorado 80262   **(1)**

N. J. Panopoulos • Department of Plant Pathology, University of California, Berkeley, California 94720   **(8)**

William Paranchych • Department of Microbiology, University of Alberta, Edmonton, Alberta, Canada T6G 2E9   **(32)**

Brittan L. Pasloske • Department of Microbiology, University of Alberta, Edmonton, Alberta, Canada T6G 2E9   **(32)**

John M. Pemberton • Department of Microbiology, University of Queensland, St. Lucia, Queensland 4067, Australia   **(35)**

Robert J. Penfold • Department of Microbiology, University of Queensland, St. Lucia, Queensland 4067, Australia   **(35)**

Angelika Phanopoulos • Unit of Molecular Biology, International Institute of Cellular and Molecular Pathology, 75 Avenue Hippocrate, 1200 Brussels, Belgium   **(17)**

Dietmar H. Pieper • Gesellschaft für Strahlen- und Umweltforschung, Ingolstädter Landstrasse 1, D-8042 Neuherberg, Federal Republic of Germany   **(20)**

Arthur E. Pritchard • Department of Microbiology and Immunology, University of Colorado Health Sciences Center, Denver, Colorado 80262   **(1)**

A. Pühler • Faculty of Biology, Department of Genetics, University of Bielefeld, Postbox 8640, D-4800 Bielefeld 1, Federal Republic of Germany   **(10)**

J. Quandt • Faculty of Biology, Department of Genetics, University of Bielefeld, Postbox 8640, D-4800 Bielefeld 1, Federal Republic of Germany   **(10)**

L. G. Rahme • Department of Plant Pathology, University of California, Berkeley, California 94720   **(8)**

E. Ratnaningsih • Department of Genetics and Developmental Biology, Monash University, Clayton, Victoria 3168, Australia   **(26)**

Victor W. Rodwell • Department of Biochemistry, Purdue University, West Lafayette, Indiana 47907   (16)

Detlef Römermann • Institut für Pflanzenphysiologie und Mikrobiologie der Freien Universität Berlin, D-1000 Berlin 33, Federal Republic of Germany   (38)

Siddhartha Roychoudhury • Department of Microbiology and Immunology, University of Illinois College of Medicine, Chicago, Illinois 60612   (2)

Lynn Rust • Department of Microbiology and Immunology, University of Rochester School of Medicine and Dentistry, Rochester, New York 14642   (4)

R. Saffery • Department of Genetics and Developmental Biology, Monash University, Clayton, Victoria 3168, Australia   (26)

Yumiko Sano • Mitsubishi Kasei Institute of Life Sciences, 11, Minamiooya, Machida-shi, Tokyo 194, Japan   (33)

Parimi A. Sastry • Department of Microbiology, University of Alberta, Edmonton, Alberta, Canada T6G 2E9   (32)

Gary S. Sayler • Department of Microbiology and The Program in Ecology, University of Tennessee, Knoxville, Tennessee 37932   (25)

Mark A. Schell • Department of Microbiology, University of Georgia, Athens, Georgia 30602   (18)

David S. Scher • Boehringer Ingelheim Pharmaceuticals, Ridgefield, Connecticut 06877   (16)

Michael Schlömann • Department of Biology, Yale University, New Haven, Connecticut 06511   (20)

M. Schmidt • Faculty of Biology, Department of Genetics, University of Bielefeld, Postbox 8640, D-4800 Bielefeld 1, Federal Republic of Germany   (10)

Eric J. Schott • Department of Molecular Biology, Massachusetts General Hospital, Boston, Massachusetts 02114   (9)

Edward Schwartz • Institut für Pflanzenphysiologie und Mikrobiologie der Freien Universität Berlin, D-1000 Berlin 33, Federal Republic of Germany   (38)

Dean Shinabarger • Department of Microbiology and Immunology, University of Illinois College of Medicine, Chicago, Illinois 60612   (2)

R. J. Siehnel • University of British Columbia, Vancouver, British Columbia, Canada V6T 1W5   (31)

Joke Sijtsema • Laboratory of Biochemistry, Groningen Biotechnology Center, Nijenborgh 16, 9747 AG Groningen, The Netherlands   (15)

Simon Silver • Department of Microbiology and Immunology, University of Illinois College of Medicine, Chicago, Illinois 60680   **(34)**

M. Sinclair • Department of Genetics and Developmental Biology, Monash University, Clayton, Victoria 3168, Australia   **(26)**

Stephen G. Sligar • Department of Biochemistry, University of Illinois, Urbana, Illinois 61801   **(11)**

J. R. Sokatch • Department of Biochemistry and Molecular Biology, The University of Oklahoma Health Sciences Center, P.O. Box 26901, Oklahoma City, Oklahoma 73190   **(19)**

G. Somlyai • Department of Plant Pathology, University of Missouri, 108 Waters Hall, Columbia, Missouri 65211   **(6)**

J. C. Spain • U.S. Air Force Engineering and Services Laboratory, Tyndall Air Force Base, Florida 32403   **(21)**

D. Strom • Department of Genetics and Developmental Biology, Monash University, Clayton, Victoria 3168, Australia   **(26)**

Antonius Suwanto • Department of Microbiology, The University of Texas Medical School at Houston, 6431 Fannin, P.O. Box 20708, Houston, Texas 77225   **(37)**

Kazunari Taira • Fermentation Research Institute, Agency of Industrial Science and Technology, Tsukuba Science City, Ibaraki 305, Japan   **(12)**

Andrea Tran-Betcke • Institut für Pflanzenphysiologie und Mikrobiologie der Freien Universität Berlin, D-1000 Berlin 33, Federal Republic of Germany   **(38)**

Joaquim Trias • Department of Microbiology and Immunology, University of California, Berkeley, California 94720   **(30)**

Michael L. Vasil • Department of Microbiology and Immunology, University of Colorado Health Sciences Center, Denver, Colorado 80262   **(1)**

Yuli Wang • Department of Biochemistry, Purdue University, West Lafayette, Indiana 47907   **(16)**

Ute Warnecke • Institut für Pflanzenphysiologie und Mikrobiologie der Freien Universität Berlin, D-1000 Berlin 33, Federal Republic of Germany   **(38)**

Jürgen Warrelmann • Institut für Pflanzenphysiologie und Mikrobiologie der Freien Universität Berlin, D-1000 Berlin 33, Federal Republic of Germany   **(38)**

P. J. Weisbeek • Department of Molecular Cell Biology and Institute of Molecular Biology, University of Utrecht, Padualaan 8, 3584 CH Utrecht, The Netherlands   **(7)**

W. M. Weng • Faculty of Biology, Department of Genetics, University of

Bielefeld, Postbox 8640, D-4800 Bielefeld 1, Federal Republic of Germany   **(10)**

Bernard Witholt • Laboratory of Biochemistry, Groningen Biotechnology Center, Nijenborgh 16, 9747 AG Groningen, The Netherlands   **(15)**

M. S. Wood • Department of Microbiology, University of Massachusetts, Amherst, Massachusetts 01003   **(27)**

C. Zhang • Department of Genetics and Developmental Biology, Monash University, Clayton, Victoria 3168, Australia   **(26)**

Nicolette A. Zielinski • Department of Microbiology and Immunology, University of Illinois College of Medicine, Chicago, Illinois 60612   **(2)**

Axel Zimmermann • Mikrobiologisches Institut, Eidgenössische Technische Hochschule, CH-8092 Zurich, Switzerland   **(29)**

G. J. Zylstra • Department of Microbiology and Biocatalysis Research Group, The University of Iowa, Iowa City, Iowa 52242   **(13)**

Preface

This monograph originated with the papers presented at the second of a series of international symposia on the molecular biology of *Pseudomonas*. The first of these meetings was held in 1986 in Geneva, Switzerland, and the second in Chicago, Ill., in July, 1989. The Chicago symposium, involving 335 experts in the field, was sponsored by the American Society for Microbiology and organized by A. M. Chakrabarty, I. C. Gunsalus, B. Iglewski, S. Kaplan, T. Nakazawa, S. Silver, K. N. Timmis, and B. Witholt. The ASM organization of the meeting was carried out ably by Caroline Polk and Richard Bray. The efforts at the University of Illinois were coordinated competently and enthusiastically by Bernadette Gillard and Marian Lawrence.

As understanding of the biology of these important organisms and their complex metabolism increases rapidly from year to year, the need for international gatherings such as those in Geneva and Chicago grows also. A decision was made that a third symposium would be held near Lake Como, Italy, under the auspices of the University of Milan, probably in 1992.

The science of *Pseudomonas* has reached a maturity that speaks for itself through the papers in this book. The field continues to expand. Molecular biology is having an impact on understanding of metabolic biotransformations in *Pseudomonas*, its mechanisms of pathogenicity (in both humans and plants), and its use in the exciting world of biotechnology. As research blossoms into new discoveries, we will continue to enjoy this fascinating organism for years to come.

Acknowledgments

Argonne National Laboratory
Boehringer Mannheim Company
Cystic Fibrosis Foundation
Eastman Kodak Company
Eli Lilly and Company
Fischer Scientific
General Electric
GIBCO
Hoffmann-La Roche
Kelco
National Institutes of Health
National Science Foundation
University of Illinois
U.S. Air Force
U.S. Department of Energy
U.S. Environmental Protection Agency

These companies, foundations, and government agencies contributed substantially to the costs of the *Pseudomonas* symposium and therefore to the assembly of this monograph.

Introduction

There has been an explosion of new and important information about the genus *Pseudomonas*—not only in terms of its ability to cause disease in plants and animals, including humans, and its well-known ability to act as scavengers in nature, resulting in the biodegradation and removal of a large number of natural and synthetic compounds, but also for its usefulness as a system to study metabolic pathways and gene structure and expression. Because of the diversity of the genus and its close relationship to a number of other bacteria which are grouped under different genera, some accommodation had to be made to bring a unified picture and a general theme out of the heterogeneity of the pseudomonads and their close neighbors. These other organisms, some of whose features so closely resemble those of *Pseudomonas*, are therefore included at the end under the title Honorary Pseudomonads.

Within *Pseudomonas*, various topics are grouped under common headings. For example, papers dealing with virulence factors targeted towards humans or animals, or the processes and molecular mechanisms by which *Pseudomonas* spp. cause animal diseases, are grouped under Pathogenesis. This is not fully satisfactory, however, since *Pseudomonas* is also a phytopathogen, causing diseases in plants. Furthermore, many metabolic features of *Pseudomonas* are alternatively beneficial for plants, such as the production of siderophores that inhibit fungal growth and prevent ice nucleation. Such beneficial activities are also apparent in *Rhizobium* spp., which enhance plant growth through symbiotic association by forming nitrogen-fixing nodules in plants. These specialized characteristics are therefore grouped under a common heading, Plant-Bacterial Interactions. It is important to point out here that pseudomonads play many critical roles in interacting with plants, and the first few isolates for which permission was sought from the Environmental Protection Agency for field testing of recombinant DNA microorganisms are *Pseudomonas* species.

Pseudomonads are, however, best known for their extreme nutritional versatility and their ability to produce interesting industrial products from simple, frequently cheap carbon sources. A substantial number of articles dealing with bioconversion of natural or synthetic compounds, roles of specific enzymes in catalyzing such reactions, and the genetic and molecular basis of such dissimilations are grouped in the section Biotransformations. Studies of *Pseudomonas* pathogenesis and plant-bacterial interactions typically have employed highly sophisticated techniques including cloning of genes, the specific substitution of nucleotides in the genes by site-directed mutagenesis, and studies of the gene products by X-ray crystallography and physicochemical analysis. Similarly, bioconversion studies have dealt with the most modern physical and molecular techniques and original concepts about the mechanisms of enzymatic reactions, the regulation of gene expression, and the molecular aspects of DNA-protein interactions.

Bioconversion studies necessarily involve an understanding of the genetic organizations in various pseudomonads, the development of genetic and molecular tools such as expression vectors and efficient systems of transpositional mutagenesis, newer methods of gene mapping, etc. A number of articles dealing with such topics have been included in the section Plasmids, Vectors, Gene Mapping, and Cloning. Such articles illustrate the extensive amount of information presently available on various technical developments applicable to pseudomonads and related bacterial genera.

Finally, the metabolic activities of pseudomonads, and for that matter, all other microorganisms, depend on the structural integrity and the defined specificity of the cellular outer layers which control the entry of various important nutrients and exclude harmful toxic compounds. Cell envelope and transport has been an active area of research for decades, and a wealth of information is presently available on the mechanistics of cellular transport and permeation. This is a particularly fruitful area to study in pseudomonads, since many members of the genus are well known for their ability to resist the entry of foreign molecules, such as antibiotics, by regulating the sizes of their porins or by producing extracellular gel matrix. Articles reporting exciting results on this topic have been incorporated under the heading Cell Envelope and Transport.

All in all, the editors feel that the present treatise is a true reflection of the extraordinary amount of available information on the diverse aspects of the important group of organisms known as the pseudomonads. Since pseudomonads are basically soil- and waterborne organisms capable of carrying out functions important to humankind, they have been subject to biochemical, biophysical, genetic, and molecular studies and have also been the focal point in recent legal cases involving their application in open environments. It is apparent that important information is continually being generated and will continue to grow in the future. The next few years should see major progress in understanding of this broad group of saprophytic microorganisms which we call collectively *Pseudomonas*.

A. M. Chakrabarty
S. Silver

Part I

PATHOGENESIS

Chapter 1

Molecular Biology of Exotoxin A and Phospholipase C of *Pseudomonas aeruginosa*

Michael L. Vasil, Arthur E. Pritchard, and Rachel M. Ostroff

Of the abundant extracellular products of *Pseudomonas aeruginosa* which are thought to contribute to the virulence of this opportunistic pathogen (Liu, 1974), our attention for the past several years has focused on the biochemistry and molecular biology of exotoxin A (ETA) and phospholipase C (PLC). Both extracellular products are protein enzymes which have been shown to be toxic to animals at the microgram or submicrogram level (Berk et al., 1987; Iglewski and Kabat, 1975). ETA is an ADP-ribosyltransferase toxin which inhibits protein synthesis in eucaryotic cells (Iglewski and Kabat, 1975). PLC is capable of preferentially degrading phospholipids which are plentiful in eucaryotic cells (Berka and Vasil, 1982) but uncommon in procaryotic cell membranes. Additionally, one of the substrate products of PLC (diacylglycerol) can have toxic effects on the whole animal by inducing the production of potent substances (e.g., arachidonic acid metabolites and protein kinase C) which are known to alter eucaryotic cell metabolism and incite inflammatory responses (Besterman et al., 1986).

Although, in general, the regulation of expression and the physical properties of these enzyme-toxins are quite distinct, there are some interesting parallels in several facets of their molecular biology. In this report we will discuss these similarities and differences with respect to (i) genetic organization, (ii) regulation of synthesis, and (iii) structure-function relationships.

GENETIC ORGANIZATION

One question we wished to address once the ETA structural gene (*toxA*) was cloned was: did multiple copies of the gene account for the variable amounts of ETA produced by different strains? Using probes derived from *toxA* and sur-

Michael L. Vasil, Arthur E. Pritchard, and Rachel M. Ostroff • Department of Microbiology and Immunology, University of Colorado Health Sciences Center, Denver, Colorado 80262.

rounding sequences, we examined a large number of clinical, laboratory, and environmental isolates of *P. aeruginosa* by Southern DNA-DNA hybridization blots. Every strain examined thus far (>400), including ones from North America, Australia, Africa, and Europe, has only one or no copy of *toxA* per genome. The positions of restriction endonuclease sites within *toxA* and 4 to 5 kilobases (kb) 3' to the *toxA* termination codon were remarkably well conserved (Vasil et al., 1986; Vasil et al., 1987). In contrast, the positions of restriction endonuclease sites 5' to *toxA* were highly variable from strain to strain. This 5' region was so variable from strain to strain that we and others have been able to use this variability as a sensitive and specific epidemiological marker to distinguish strains of *P. aeruginosa* that cannot be distinguished by conventional methods such as pyocin typing and serotyping (Ogle et al., 1987; Ogle et al., 1988; Pasloske et al., 1988; Vasil et al., 1987). Although the restriction sites in this 5' region are exceptionally variable from strain to strain, they do not appear to change at a discernible high frequency within a given strain even when it is grown in different conditions or it is treated with mutagenic agents. For example, we examined a large number of laboratory-derived mutants of strain PAO1 and did not observe the restriction pattern in this region to change in any of these mutants (Ogle et al., 1987; Vasil et al., 1986). The stability of the region 5' to *toxA* within a single strain grown in vitro is a desirable feature for epidemiological studies because it allows reproducible identification of different isolates of the same strain by its unique restriction endonuclease pattern, but this stable nature makes it difficult to examine the mechanisms of how the variability was ultimately generated.

It was considered that this variability might be seen surrounding other genes in *P. aeruginosa*. However, in contrast to the variability 5' to the ETA gene, the restriction endonuclease sites within the PLC structural gene (*plcS*) and on both sides flanking this gene were very well conserved (Vasil et al., 1986; Vasil et al., 1987). Recently, using transverse-pulse field gel electrophoresis and Southern blotting with other probes derived from other *P. aeruginosa* genes (e.g., elastase [*lasB*], alginate [*algD*], ETA regulatory [*toxR*], and two PLC [*plcS, plcN*] genes), we have found that *toxA* is the most variable in terms of the size of the restriction fragment it is associated with in different strains (R. Fick, V. Shortridge, M. Pato, and M. Vasil, *Abstr. Annu. Meet. Am. Soc. Microbiol. 1989*, D145, p. 106). Thus, this variability seems to be due to more than random base changes resulting in restriction polymorphisms that are generally observed in intergeneic coding sequences. It is more likely that this variability is due to significant localized rearrangements in the DNA structure in this region. Alternatively, it is possible that *toxA* could be in different locations in the chromosome in different strains. Localized rearrangements as well as alternative locations of *toxA* in different strains could certainly make a major contribution to the remarkable variability which has been described above. The region 5' to *toxA* also might play a role in the regulation of ETA expression.

To address these questions more precisely, we selected three different strains of *P. aeruginosa* and cloned the region of DNA 5' to *toxA*. A diagrammatic representation of the DNA sequences of this region in these strains is shown in Fig. 1. Strain PA103 is the natural hyper-toxin-producing strain from which we

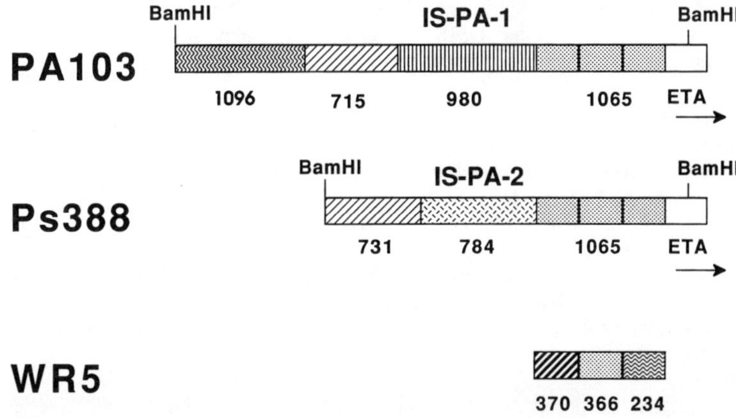

FIGURE 1. Diagrammatic representation of the mosaic pattern of genetic organization 5′ to the ETA gene in three strains of *P. aeruginosa*. Sections with identical patterns are highly homologous (>95%), while regions with different patterns do not show any significant homology by computer analysis of the DNA sequences in these regions. The arrow indicates the direction of transcription of the ETA gene. The numbers are distances in base pairs, derived from DNA sequence analysis, between the sections of DNA in this region 5′ to *toxA*. WR5 lacks *toxA* sequences but carries a 366-bp fragment which is highly homologous with a fragment in PA103 and Ps388 that is located just upstream of *toxA* in these strains. The fragments flanking this 366-bp fragment in WR5 are not homologous with any other fragment shown in this diagram.

originally cloned *toxA* (Gray et al., 1984; Vasil et al., 1986). Ps388 is a clinical isolate which produces a minute amount of ETA and which has a distinct restriction pattern in the region 5′ to *toxA* in comparison with that of PA103 (Gray et al., 1984; Vasil et al., 1986). WR5 is a member of a small, but not uncommon, class of strains which do not have any DNA that hybridizes with *toxA* but which have sequences that hybridize with a probe which covers 746 base pairs (bp) 5′ to the initiation codon of *toxA* in strain PA103 (Vasil et al., 1986). As shown in this diagram, the 1-kb region 5′ to *toxA* in both PA103 and Ps388 is remarkably well conserved. Only minor single-base changes are found in this region. These results are also consistent with those observed by others for strain PAO1 (Chen et al., 1987). They found that sequences immediately 5′ to the ETA gene (~250 bp) in both PA103 and PAO1 were well conserved with only minor base changes.

Because there are no substantial differences in the region 250 bp upstream of *toxA* in strains which carry this gene, the hypervariability cannot be significantly related to this segment of DNA. In contrast, a little more than 1 kb upstream from the start of the ETA gene the sequences from PA103 and Ps388 dramatically diverge. The sequences in PA103 and Ps388 from approximately 1 kb to almost 2 kb do not share detectable homology (A. E. Pritchard and M. L. Vasil, submitted for publication). These regions are designated IS-PA-1 and IS-PA-2 for the nonhomologous regions from PA103 and Ps388, respectively (Fig. 1). Then, just as noteworthy as the disappearance of the homology between PA103 and Ps388, homology reappears again after the IS-PA sequences. Although we do not have sequence data for Ps388 beyond the left-hand *Bam*HI site, using Southern

TABLE 1

Characteristic IS-PA elements of *P. aeruginosa*

Characteristic	Reference
Sizes are approximately 700 to 1,000 bp. The IS-PA elements are similar in size to those of described insertion sequences.	Calos and Miller, 1980
Five-base-pair direct repeats at each end indicate possible duplication of target sequence.	Bartlet and Silverman, 1989
G+C content of IS-PA elements (50%) is distinct from usual *P. aeruginosa* G+C percentage (67%).	Pritchard and Vasil, submitted
Found only in some strains of *P. aeruginosa*. Many strains have been found which lack both IS-PA-1 and IS-PA-2.	Pritchard and Vasil, submitted
IS-PA-1 is found in more than one copy in some strains. The second copy found in some strains is not tandem with the copy near *toxA*.	Pritchard and Vasil, submitted
Exhibit an integration site preference: 1 kb from 5′ end of *toxA*.	Bartlet and Silverman, 1989; Quirk et al., 1989; Pritchard and Vasil, submitted

hybridization analysis we have found that probes from the 1,096-bp region in PA103 do not hybridize with the genome of Ps388. Thus, it appears that there is another nonhomologous region besides the IS-PA-1 and IS-PA-2.

It is likely that this mosaic pattern makes a considerable contribution to the hypervariability in restriction sites in this region of the *P. aeruginosa* chromosome. The question then arises, how is this mosaic pattern generated? From analysis of the IS-PA sequences and additional Southern hybridization experiments using probes derived from the nonhomologous and homologous regions, there is strong circumstantial evidence that these nonhomologous regions are insertion sequences (IS) (Pritchard and Vasil, submitted). The properties of these IS-PA regions, which are like those of IS elements in other procaryotic organisms, are described in Table 1.

Thus, although we can account for at least some of the hypervariability 5′ to *toxA*, there are some new questions which have yet to be answered. It is still not known whether *toxA* is located in different regions of the chromosome in different strains and whether these IS-like elements play a role in the expression of ETA. We have found recently, using transverse-pulse field electrophoresis, that *toxA* in two strains of *P. aeruginosa*, PAT and PAK, is within 7 min of two genes, *argF* and *algD*, which have been mapped at 34 min on the *P. aeruginosa* chromosome. This is considerably distal to the map location of *toxA* in strain PAO1, which is approximately at 65 min on the recalibrated linkage map (Hanne et al., 1983; O'Hoy and Krishnapillai, 1987; V. Shortridge and M. L. Vasil, unpublished observations). Thus, the hypervariability flanking *toxA* may be a consequence of the presence of different IS-PA elements as well as a different location of *toxA* in some strains.

Because the IS-PA elements are more than 1 kb upstream from the start of the ETA gene, it would seem to be unlikely that they would have any effect on expression of ETA. However, in recent years enhancerlike sequences which can affect the expression of genes more than 1 kb away (Reitzer and Magasanik, 1986) have been found in procaryotic organisms.

Although some IS elements have been described in *P. aeruginosa*, they are relatively uncommonly found in this species in comparison with other pseudomonads such as *Pseudomonas cepacia* (Holloway and Morgan, 1986; Lessie and Gaffney, 1986). Further study of the IS-PA elements may provide a clue in understanding the evolution of pseudomonads. For example, it would be interesting to know if the IS-PA elements are found in other *Pseudomonas* species, particularly because the ETA gene is not (Vasil et al., 1986). In this regard, it is notable that the G+C content of the IS-PA elements (50%) is considerably lower that the usual G+C content of most *Pseudomonas* species (65 to 67%). Although we have found that these elements are also located in other parts of the chromosome in some strains, they seem to have a preference for the 5' region of *toxA*. There are IS elements in procaryotic organisms (including *Pseudomonas*) and movable introns in T-even bacteriophage which demonstrate site preferences for integration (Bartlet and Silverman, 1989; Quirk et al., 1989). However, direct proof that these IS-PA sequences are indeed IS elements must await demonstration that they can move from one replicon to another.

Because the production of hemolysin and PLC activity in different strains of *P. aeruginosa* was as variable as ETA production (Berka and Vasil, 1982), we examined a relatively large number (>100) of strains by Southern blot using a gene-specific DNA fragment as a probe. There is only one copy of the hemolytic PLC gene per genome in each strain. We did not find any strains which failed to hybridize with the PLC-specific probe, nor did we find any significant restriction fragment length polymorphisms associated with or flanking this gene. These observations therefore are a notable contrast to those relating to the variability of restriction sites 5' to the ETA gene (Vasil et al., 1986; Vasil et al., 1987).

It is worthwhile to note that the hemolytic PLC gene is not always stable. Recently, we were able to clone a gene encoding hemolysin and PLC activity from *P. cepacia* by using a PLC-specific probe from *P. aeruginosa*. A number of hemolytic and nonhemolytic strains of *P. cepacia* were then examined using a gene-specific probe derived from the cloned hemolytic PLC gene of *P. cepacia*. In striking contrast to the consistent patterns observed with the *P. aeruginosa* gene as described above, hypervariability was observed in the genetic organization of the PLC gene of *P. cepacia*. With Southern hybridization analysis, each strain of *P. cepacia* had a distinct restriction pattern with the *P. cepacia* gene-specific probe, and multiple hybridizing fragments were seen with each strain. Even nonhemolytic strains carried multiple restriction fragments which hybridized with the probe (J. L. Kuhns and M. L. Vasil, submitted for publication). The reason for this extreme variability in expression and hybridization patterns with PLC in *P. cepacia* is not clear at present, but it may be related to the relatively large number of distinct IS elements (>15) in *P. cepacia*. These IS elements inactivate a gene by insertion or activate gene expression by providing regulatory sequences (e.g., promoters) to an otherwise inactive gene (Lessie and Gaffney, 1986).

Further sequencing and molecular analysis of the genes encoding PLC and ETA in *P. aeruginosa* revealed additional differences in their genetic organization. Sequencing data revealed a strong rho-independent transcriptional terminator immediately after the translation termination codon of *toxA* (Gray et al., 1984). These data and subsequent data from other laboratories indicate that *toxA* is in a monocistronic operon (Frank and Iglewski, 1988; Grant and Vasil, 1986; Gray et al., 1984; Lory, 1986). The structural gene for the hemolytic PLC (*plcS*) of *P. aeruginosa*, however, was found to be part of a somewhat unusual polycistronic operon that contains three genes (Pritchard and Vasil, 1986; Shen et al., 1987). The unusual aspect of this operon is that the two genes designated *plcR1* and *plcR2*, which are downstream of *plcS*, are overlapping and in the same reading frame. The larger gene, *plcR1*, has a sequence which encodes a canonical-type signal sequence for secretion, while the smaller gene, *plcR2*, does not have this feature (Shen et al., 1987). It is possible that the larger product is secreted to the periplasmic space, outer membrane, or extracellular spaces while the smaller product remains in the cytoplasm. The possible function of these genes will be discussed below.

REGULATION

The production of ETA and PLC is regulated by environmental conditions. When iron is limiting, ETA production is elevated (Bjorn et al., 1978), while when P_i is limiting, PLC production is likewise increased (Pritchard and Vasil, 1986). Early studies indicated that there are several genes which are likely to play a role in the regulation of ETA or PLC (Gray et al., 1981, 1982; Gray and Vasil, 1981; Ohman et al., 1980). More recently, we and others using molecular techniques have found that *toxA* and *plcS* are regulated by iron and P_i at the level of transcription (Frank and Iglewski, 1988; Grant and Vasil, 1986; Hindahl et al., 1987; Lory, 1986; Pritchard and Vasil, 1986). Additionally, positive regulatory genes for ETA and PLC have been cloned and characterized (Filloux et al., 1988; Hedstrom et al., 1986). However, in spite of these significant studies it is not clear how iron, P_i, and other environmental conditions regulate ETA or PLC synthesis. Some recent observations from our laboratory may provide clues to this complex problem.

fur in *Escherichia coli* encodes an iron-binding repressor. If iron is bound to the product encoded by *fur*, this complex can then bind to a consensus sequence near the promoter of iron-regulated genes, thereby halting transcription of the regulated gene (Bragg and Neilands, 1987). The *fur* product without iron does not efficiently bind the consensus sequence. Recently, data have been presented suggesting that there may be a *fur* analog which is involved in the regulation of diphtheria toxin by iron in *Corynebacterium diphtheriae* (Tai and Holmes, 1988). Because ETA synthesis is sensitive to iron concentrations in a manner similar to diphtheria toxin synthesis, we examined the effect of *fur* on ETA synthesis. When a *toxA-lacZ* operon fusion was integrated into the chromosome of a *P. aeruginosa* strain, β-galactosidase production was regulated by iron in a manner similar to ETA production. When we introduced multiple copies of the *fur* gene into this strain and grew it under iron-limiting conditions, β-galactosidase synthesis and

ETA synthesis were not derepressible (R. W. Prince and M. L. Vasil, manuscript in preparation). These and other data suggest that there is a site in *P. aeruginosa* to which the product of *fur* can bind to affect the transcription of *toxA*. This site could be near *toxA* or near another gene which regulates expression of *toxA*. A corollary to this hypothesis would be that there is a *fur* analog in *P. aeruginosa*. Thus, there may be negative as well as positive regulatory elements which play a role in the complex mechanisms governing the synthesis of ETA.

As described above, there are three genes in the hemolytic PLC operon. We do not know the function of the *plcR* genes. Recently, we found that a *P. aeruginosa* mutant constructed by gene replacement techniques which carries a deletion in the *plcR* genes, but not the PLC structural gene, was 1,000-fold less virulent than the wild-type strain in the mouse thermal injury model of *Pseudomonas* infection (Ostroff et al., 1989). While studying the expression of the hemolytic PLC gene and *plcR* using a T7 expression system in *E. coli*, it was seen that one or both of the *plcR* products altered the charge but not the apparent molecular weight of the hemolytic PLC. In the presence of the *plcR* product the hemolytic PLC was substantially more negatively charged (A. I. Vasil and M. L. Vasil, unpublished observations). We have not yet been able to express the *plcR1* and *plcR2* products separately because, as mentioned above, they are overlapping and in the same reading frame. Therefore, we are not yet certain whether one or both of these products are responsible for the charge modification of the PLC. The *plcR* products do not appear to bind to the PLC. Although at present we do not know what the nature of the modification is, it is tempting to speculate. Because there is no detectable change in the molecular weight, as determined by sodium dodecyl sulfate-polyacrylamide gel electrophoresis, of the PLC with or without the *plcR* products, the modification does not appear to be related to cleavage of a signal sequence. Recently, it has been reported that mammalian PLC enzymes are phosphorylated by protein kinase C (Rhee et al., 1989). The function of the phosphorylation of the mammalian PLC is not clear, but it has been proposed that it is regulatory in nature. Because P_i is associated with the regulation of PLC synthesis and synthesis of the *plcR* product in *P. aeruginosa*, we have hypothesized that one or both of the *plcR* products are a protein kinase which phosphorylates the hemolytic PLC. Phosphorylation of the hemolytic PLC would explain the unusual charge difference described above. It will be of interest to examine whether the hemolytic PLC is phosphorylated by one of the *plcR* products or whether the charge modification is due to other mechanisms. It will also be of interest to determine whether the *plcR* products can modify other proteins in *P. aeruginosa* and how such a modification might affect the expression of virulence in this opportunistic pathogen. Only a limited number of specific protein kinases have been described in procaryotic organisms as compared with eucaryotic organisms (Cozzone, 1988).

STRUCTURE-FUNCTION RELATIONSHIPS

The A-B model of structure-function relationships of many bacterial toxins including ETA is well known (Douglas and Collier, 1987; Eidels et al., 1983;

Guidi-Rontani and Collier, 1987). There is a domain designated B which is required for binding to a receptor on the target eucaryotic cell, and there is a domain designated A which is responsible for the enzymatic activity of the toxin. Sometimes an additional domain may be necessary for transport of the enzymatic domain into the eucaryotic cell. Our laboratory is now directly studying the structure-function relationships of ETA. Excellent work on this subject has been done by Douglas and Collier (1987) and Guidi-Rontani and Collier (1987), and therefore this subject will not be discussed further in this report.

In contrast to bacterial toxins like ETA, the structure-function relationships of hemolytic or cytolytic toxins have not usually been thought of in terms of the A-B model described above. However, hemolysins have been divided into two classes based on their mechanisms of action. There are those that function by forming pores in eucaryotic cell membranes (e.g., *E. coli* α-hemolysin or α-toxin of *Staphylococcus aureus*) and those which can degrade the phospholipids in the eucaryotic cell membrane by an enzymatic mechanism (e.g., PLC). One problem with this classification, however, is that not all bacterial PLC enzymes are hemolytic or cytolytic. Recent studies from our laboratory and others may provide some insight as to why only certain kinds of these enzymes are hemolytic while others are not.

Using gene replacement methods, we constructed a mutant strain of *P. aeruginosa* which carries a deletion of the entire *plcS* gene and a portion of the *plcR* gene (Ostroff and Vasil, 1987; Ostroff et al., 1989). Somewhat surprisingly, this mutant still produced an extracellular PLC activity. The synthesis of the PLC activity in the mutant is regulated by P_i-like synthesis of the hemolytic PLC activity as in the wild-type strain (Pritchard and Vasil, 1986). However, concentrated culture supernatants from the deletion mutant which synthesizes this PLC activity do not have any hemolytic activity, in contrast to culture supernatants from the wild-type strain, which have both PLC activity and hemolytic activity. These data indicate that there is a gene in *P. aeruginosa* which encodes an extracellular hemolytic PLC and another gene which encodes a nonhemolytic PLC. Because these enzymes appeared to be similar in several respects, we decided to examine whether there was any possible DNA homology between the genes encoding these enzymes. Using a gene-specific probe derived from the hemolytic PLC gene (*plcS*) in Southern hybridization analysis of the genome of the deletion mutant described above, we found that there was a restriction endonuclease fragment in this mutant which hybridized with the probe only under conditions of low stringency (R. M. Ostroff, A. I. Vasil, and M. L. Vasil, submitted for publication). These data suggest that the hemolytic PLC gene and the nonhemolytic PLC gene share significant DNA homology. Using the hemolytic PLC gene as a probe, we were then able to clone a DNA fragment from the deletion mutant which carries the gene encoding the nonhemolytic PLC. Using a T7 expression system in *E. coli*, we have found that this DNA fragment encodes a 77-kilodalton protein which has PLC activity but no hemolytic activity (R. M. Ostroff and M. L. Vasil, submitted). We have recently sequenced the gene encoding the nonhemolytic PLC and found that there is significant DNA as well as amino acid homology between these hemolytic and nonhemolytic en-

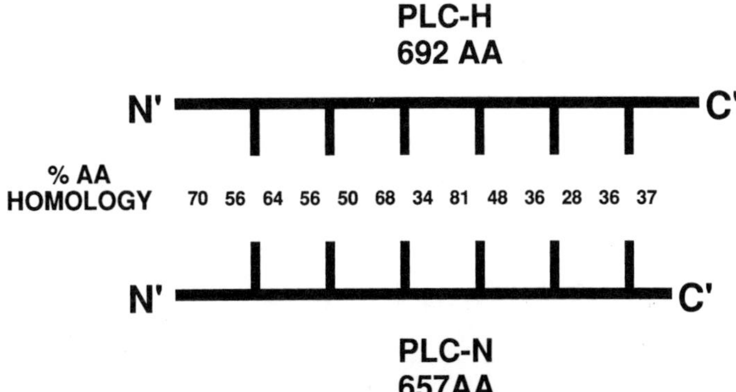

FIGURE 2. Diagrammatic representation of the percent amino acid (AA) homology between the mature form (i.e., without the signal sequence) of the hemolytic PLC (PLC-H) and the mature form of the nonhemolytic PLC (PLC-N). Values given represent the percent homology for a 50-amino-acid window. Homology is defined as identity or only a conservative change in an amino acid.

zymes. They are also very similar in molecular size. The molecular mass from the deduced amino acid sequence of the mature nonhemolytic PLC is 73.5 kilodaltons, while the molecular mass of the mature hemolytic PLC is 78.4 kilodaltons (Pritchard and Vasil, 1986). Figure 2 shows that there are two domains or regions of these enzymes which are strikingly similar, a region at the amino terminus (70%) and a region near the middle (81%) of these enzymes. Further analysis of the regions of relatively high homology and low homology may aid in understanding why one PLC is hemolytic and the other one is not.

One model for the differences in the *P. aeruginosa* PLC enzymes comes from a molecular analysis of the cereolysin of *Bacillus cereus* (Gilmore et al., 1989). These studies revealed that there are two components, A and B, which are necessary for its hemolytic property. The hemolysin is the product of two tandem genes in this organism, one which encodes a phosphatidylcholine-specific PLC activity and another which encodes a sphingomyelinase C activity. Neither of these products is hemolytic by itself, but the combination of the two enzymatic activities results in lysis of erythrocytes. The structural differences between phosphatidylcholine and sphingomyelin are shown in Fig. 3. We found that the hemolytic PLC produced from the cloned gene in *E. coli* or in culture supernatants of the wild-type *P. aeruginosa* strain was active on both substrates, while the nonhemolytic PLC produced from the cloned gene in *E. coli* or in culture supernatants from the *P. aeruginosa* deletion mutant was only active on phosphatidylcholine. Because the same moiety of both substrates (i.e., phosphoryl-choline, seen in the shaded portion in Fig. 3) is cleaved from the phospholipids by the hemolytic and nonhemolytic PLCs (see Fig. 3), it is possible that there is a domain of the hemolytic PLC which is necessary for recognition of the sphingosine moiety of the molecule. This domain would be lacking in the nonhemolytic PLC. Alternatively, other factors may also be significant such as arrangement of these phospholipids in the membrane of eucaryotic cells. Whatever the reason for

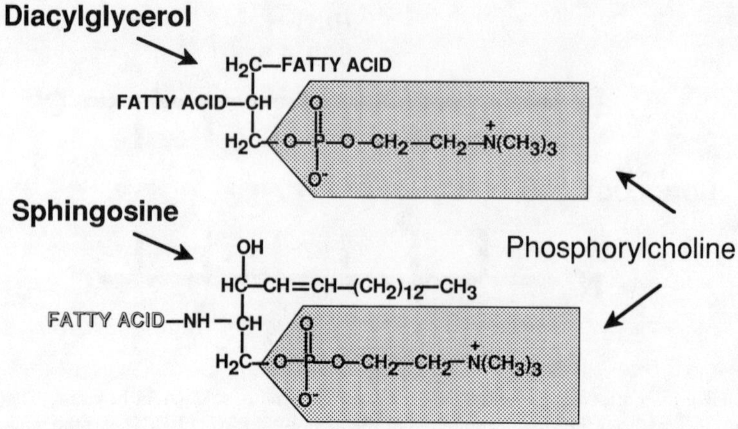

FIGURE 3. Structure of the phosphatidylcholine (top) and sphingomyelin (bottom). The hemolytic PLC can degrade both substrates, while the nonhemolytic PLC can only degrade phosphatidylcholine. The shadowed fatty acid in the sphingomyelin molecule is not part of the sphingosine moiety.

the ability of one PLC to be hemolytic while another one is not, it is clear that the interaction of hemolytic or cytolytic toxins with eucaryotic cells is considerably more complex than previously appreciated.

ACKNOWLEDGMENTS. M.L.V. thanks those who have passed through his laboratory and made important contributions to this research, including Randy Berka, Connie Chamberlain, Chris Grant, Greg Gray, Debra Krieg, Janet Kuhns, John Ogle, Rob Prince, Dee Shortridge, and Adriana Vasil.

Research reported here was supported by Public Health Service grant AI 15940 from the National Institute of Allergy and Infectious Diseases and by Student Traineeships and Research Fellowships from the Cystic Fibrosis Foundation. Support for travel to the *Pseudomonas*—1989 symposium was made possible by the Cystic Fibrosis Foundation.

LITERATURE CITED

Bartlet, D. H., and M. Silverman. 1989. Nucleotide sequence of IS*492*, a novel insertion sequence causing variation in extracellular polysaccharide production in the marine bacterium *Pseudomonas atlantica*. *J. Bacteriol.* **171:**1763–1766.

Berk, R. S., D. Brown, I. Coutinho, and D. Meyers. 1987. In vivo studies with two phospholipase C fractions from *Pseudomonas aeruginosa*. *Infect. Immun.* **55:**1728–1730.

Berka, R. M., and M. L. Vasil. 1982. Phospholipase C (heat-labile hemolysin) of *Pseudomonas aeruginosa*: purification and preliminary characterization. *J. Bacteriol.* **152:**239–245.

Besterman, J. M., V. Duronio, and P. Cuatrecasas. 1986. Rapid formation of diacylglycerol from phosphatidylcholine: a pathway for generation of a second messenger. *Proc. Natl. Acad. Sci. USA* **83:**6785–6789.

Bjorn, M., B. H. Iglewski, J. Sadoff, and M. L. Vasil. 1978. Effect of iron on yields of exotoxin A in cultures of *Pseudomonas aeruginosa* PA103. *Infect. Immun.* **19:**785–791.

Bragg, A., and J. B. Neilands. 1987. Molecular mechanisms of regulation of siderophore-mediated iron assimilation. *Microbiol. Rev.* **51:**509–518.

Calos, M. P., and J. H. Miller. 1980. Transposable elements. *Cell* **20:**579–595.

Chen, S., E. M. Jordan, R. B. Wilson, R. K. Draper, and R. C. Clowes. 1987. Transcription and expression of the exotoxin A gene of *Pseudomonas aeruginosa*. *J. Gen. Microbiol.* **133:**3081–3091.

Cozzone, A. J. 1988. Protein phosphorylation in prokaryotes. *Annu. Rev. Microbiol.* **42:**97–125.

Douglas, C. M., and R. J. Collier. 1987. Exotoxin A of *Pseudomonas aeruginosa*: substitution of glutamic acid 553 with aspartic acid drastically reduces toxicity and enzymatic activity. *J. Bacteriol.* **169**:4967–4971.

Eidels, L., R. L. Proia, and D. A. Hart. 1983. Membrane receptors for bacterial toxins. *Microbiol. Rev.* **47**:596–620.

Filloux, A., M. Bally, C. Soscia, M. Murgier, and A. Lazdunski. 1988. Phosphate regulation in *Pseudomonas aeruginosa*: cloning of the alkaline phosphatase gene and identification of *phoB* and *phoR*-like genes. *Mol. Gen. Genet.* **212**:510–513.

Frank, D. W., and B. H. Iglewski. 1988. Kinetics of *toxA* and *regA* mRNA accumulation in *Pseudomonas aeruginosa*. *J. Bacteriol.* **170**:1112–1119.

Gilmore, M. S., A. L. Cruz-Rodz, M. Leimeister-Wächter, J. Kreft, and W. Goebel. 1989. A *Bacillus cereus* cytolytic determinant, cereolysin AB, which comprises the phospholipase C and sphingo-myelinase genes: nucleotide sequence and genetic linkage. *J. Bacteriol.* **171**:744–753.

Grant, C. C. R., and M. L. Vasil. 1986. Analysis of transcription of the exotoxin A gene of *Pseudomonas aeruginosa*. *J. Bacteriol.* **168**:1112–1119.

Gray, G. L., R. M. Berka, and M. L. Vasil. 1981. A *Pseudomonas aeruginosa* mutant non-derepressible for orthophosphate-regulated proteins. *J. Bacteriol.* **147**:675–678.

Gray, G. L., R. M. Berka, and M. L. Vasil. 1982. Phospholipase C regulatory mutation of *Pseudomonas aeruginosa* that results in constitutive synthesis of several phosphate-repressible proteins. *J. Bacteriol.* **150**:1221–1226.

Gray, G. L., D. Smith, J. Baldridge, R. Harkins, M. L. Vasil, E. Chen, and H. Heyneker. 1984. Cloning, nucleotide sequence, and expression in *Escherichia coli* of the exotoxin A structural gene of *Pseudomonas aeruginosa*. *Proc. Natl. Acad. Sci. USA* **81**:2645–2649.

Gray, G. L., and M. L. Vasil. 1981. Isolation and characterization of toxin-deficient mutants of *Pseudomonas aeruginosa*. *J. Bacteriol.* **147**:275–281.

Guidi-Rontani, C., and R. J. Collier. 1987. Exotoxin A of *Pseudomonas aeruginosa*: evidence that domain I functions in receptor binding. *Mol. Microbiol.* **1**:67–72.

Hanne, L., T. Howe, and B. Iglewski. 1983. Locus of the *Pseudomonas* toxin A gene. *J. Bacteriol.* **154**:383–386.

Hedstrom, R. C., C. R. Funk, J. B. Kaper, O. R. Pavlovskis, and D. R. Galloway. 1986. Cloning of a gene involved in regulation of exotoxin A expression in *Pseudomonas aeruginosa*. *Infect. Immun.* **51**:37–42.

Hindahl, M. S., D. W. Frank, and B. H. Iglewski. 1987. Molecular studies of a positive regulator of toxin A synthesis in *Pseudomonas aeruginosa*. *Antibiot. Chemother.* (Basel) **39**:279–289.

Holloway, B. W., and A. F. Morgan. 1986. Genome organization in *Pseudomonas*. *Annu. Rev. Microbiol.* **40**:79–106.

Iglewski, B. H., and D. Kabat. 1975. NAD-dependent inhibition of protein synthesis by *Pseudomonas aeruginosa* toxin. *Proc. Natl. Acad. Sci. USA* **72**:2284–2288.

Lessie, T. G., and T. Gaffney. 1986. Catabolic potential of *Pseudomonas cepacia*, p. 439–481. *In* J. R. Sokatch (ed.), *The Biology of Pseudomonas*. Academic Press, Inc., San Diego, Calif.

Liu, P. V. 1974. Extracellular toxins of *Pseudomonas aeruginosa*. *J. Infect. Dis.* **130**(Suppl.):S94–S99.

Lory, S. 1986. Effect of iron on accumulation of exotoxin A-specific mRNA in *Pseudomonas aeruginosa*. *J. Bacteriol.* **168**:1451–1456.

Ogle, J. L., J. M. Janda, D. E. Woods, and M. L. Vasil. 1987. Characterization and use of a DNA probe as an epidemiological marker for *Pseudomonas aeruginosa*. *J. Infect. Dis.* **155**:119–126.

Ogle, J. W., L. B. Reller, and M. L. Vasil. 1988. Development of resistance in *Pseudomonas aeruginosa* to imipenem, norfloxacin, and ciprofloxacin during therapy: proof provided by typing with a DNA probe. *J. Infect. Dis.* **157**:743–748.

Ohman, D. E., J. C. Sadoff, and B. H. Iglewski. 1980. Toxin-deficient mutants of *Pseudomonas aeruginosa* PA103: isolation and characterization. *Infect. Immun.* **28**:899–908.

O'Hoy, K., and V. Krishnapillai. 1987. Recalibration of the *Pseudomonas aeruginosa* strain PAO chromosome map in time units using high-frequency-of-recombination donors. *Genetics* **115**:611–618.

Ostroff, R. M., and M. L. Vasil. 1987. Identification of a new phospholipase C activity by analysis of an insertional mutation in the hemolytic phospholipase C structural gene of *Pseudomonas aeruginosa*. *J. Bacteriol.* **169**:4597–4601.

Ostroff, R. M., B. Wretlind, and M. L. Vasil. 1989. Mutations in the hemolytic-phospholipase C operon result in decreased virulence of *Pseudomonas aeruginosa* PAO1 grown under phosphate-limiting conditions. *Infect. Immun.* **57**:1369–1373.

Pasloske, B. L., M. Joffe, Q. Sun, K. Volpel, W. Parynchych, D. P. Speert, and F. Eftekhar. 1988. Serial isolates of *Pseudomonas aeruginosa* from a patient with cystic fibrosis have identical pilin sequences. *Infect. Immun.* **56**:665–672.

Pritchard, A. E., and M. L. Vasil. 1986. Nucleotide sequence and expression of a phosphate-regulated gene encoding a secreted hemolysin of *Pseudomonas aeruginosa*. *J. Bacteriol.* **167**:291–298.

Quirk, S. M., D. Bell-Pederson, and M. Belfort. 1989. Intron mobility in T-even phages: high frequency inheritance of group I introns promoted by intron open reading frames. *Cell* **56**:455–465.

Reitzer, L. J., and B. Magasanik. 1986. Transcription of *glnA* in *E. coli* is stimulated by activator bound to sites far from the promoter. *Cell* **45**:785–792.

Rhee, S. G., P. G. Suh, S. H. Ryu, and S. Y. Lee. 1989. Studies of inositol phospholipid-specific phospholipase C. *Science* **244**:546–550.

Shen, B., P. C. Tai, A. E. Pritchard, and M. L. Vasil. 1987. Nucleotide sequences and expression in *Escherichia coli* of the in-phase overlapping *Pseudomonas aeruginosa plcR* genes. *J. Bacteriol.* **169**:4602–4607.

Tai, S. S., and R. K. Holmes. 1988. Iron regulation of the cloned diphtheria toxin promoter in *Escherichia coli*. *Infect. Immun.* **56**:2430–2436.

Vasil, M. L., C. Chamberlain, and C. C. R. Grant. 1986. Molecular studies of *Pseudomonas* exotoxin A gene. *Infect. Immun.* **52**:538–548.

Vasil, M. L., J. W. Ogle, C. C. R. Grant, and A. I. Vasil. 1987. Recombinant DNA approaches to the study of the regulation of virulence factors and epidemiology of *Pseudomonas aeruginosa*. *Antibiot. Chemother.* (Basel) **39**:264–278.

Chapter 2

Molecular Genetics of Alginate Biosynthesis in *Pseudomonas aeruginosa*

Nicolette A. Zielinski, James D. DeVault, Siddhartha Roychoudhury,
Thomas B. May, Kazuhide Kimbara, Junichi Kato,
Dean Shinabarger, Kiyoyuki Kitano, Alan Berry, Tapan K. Misra,
and A. M. Chakrabarty

Pseudomonas aeruginosa is an opportunistic pathogen responsible for a wide range of infections, one of the most debilitating being chronic pulmonary infection in cystic fibrosis (CF) patients. The pathogenicity of *P. aeruginosa* in the CF lung is attributed in part to the synthesis of the exopolysaccharide alginate by the bacterium. Nonmucoid strains of *P. aeruginosa* initially colonize the upper respiratory tract of CF patients (Høiby, 1974). However, mucoid alginate-producing variants appear with prolonged infection and eventually predominate in the CF lung (Høiby, 1974). The alginate produced by these mucoid strains of *P. aeruginosa* compounds the problems related to the hyperviscous bronchial secretions of CF patients. Alginate-producing strains of *P. aeruginosa* are almost exclusively associated with respiratory tract infections that accompany CF (Govan, 1988). Alginate appears to protect *P. aeruginosa* by shielding it from host immune defense mechanisms (Høiby, 1974; Govan, 1988) and antibiotic therapy (Govan and Fyfe, 1978), and possibly enables it to adhere more effectively to respiratory tract tissues (Woods et al., 1980). Once established in the CF lung, these mucoid strains tend to persist and parallel the progressive clinical deterioration of the patient (Pitcher-Wilmott et al., 1982).

CF is the most common fatal genetic disease among the Caucasian population, affecting approximately 1 per 2,000 newborns (Davis and di Sant' Agnese, 1980) with a carrier frequency of 4 to 5% (Govan, 1988). The median age of

Nicolette A. Zielinski, James D. DeVault, Siddhartha Roychoudhury, Thomas B. May, Kazuhide Kimbara, Junichi Kato, Dean Shinabarger, Kiyoyuki Kitano, Tapan K. Misra, and A. M. Chakrabarty • Department of Microbiology and Immunology, University of Illinois College of Medicine, Chicago, Illinois 60612. *Alan Berry* • Bio-Products Division, Eastman Kodak Company, Rochester, New York 14652-3615.

survival of patients with CF has dramatically increased over the past 2 decades from less than 10 years to more than 30 years (Goodchild and Dodge, 1985). This progress has occurred primarily through improved nutritional support and aggressive management (e.g., antibiotic therapy) of acute pulmonary infections (Goodchild and Dodge, 1985). The CF gene, which resides on chromosome 7, has recently been cloned and sequenced (Rommens et al., 1989; Riordan et al., 1989). The primary defect is a result of an altered chloride channel. This change appears to be responsible for the various pathological expressions of the disease (Kerem et al., 1989).

MICROBIOLOGY OF BRONCHIAL SECRETIONS

The basic alteration in the bronchial/pulmonary environment of the CF lung causing increased secretion of hyperviscous mucus favors bacterial colonization by *Staphylococcus aureus*, *Haemophilus influenzae*, and *P. aeruginosa* (Reynolds et al., 1975). Prolonged antibiotic therapy and the increasing life expectancy of CF patients may influence the prevalence of all of these organisms in the lung flora (Goodchild and Dodge, 1985).

P. aeruginosa is found in patients with moderate and severe pulmonary disease, being the sole pathogen found in sputum in the most advanced stages of the disease (Govan, 1988). *P. aeruginosa* is particularly resistant to even the most aggressive chemotherapy (Govan, 1988) and has been found to colonize the lungs of from 50% (Kulczycki et al., 1978) to 90% (Luray-Cuasay et al., 1976) of all CF patients. It has been shown that the severity of the lung infection is directly correlated to the presence of mucoid strains (Govan, 1988). It is interesting that *P. aeruginosa* infections are rarely observed elsewhere in nature, including tissues outside the respiratory tract of CF patients as well as the lungs of patients suffering from other pulmonary diseases (Høiby, 1974). In addition, the mucoid *P. aeruginosa* isolates revert at a high frequency to a nonmucoid form upon serial transfer in the laboratory (Govan, 1975).

PATHOGENICITY OF MUCOID *P. AERUGINOSA*

The environment of the CF lung is unique in its capacity to induce alginate production by *P. aeruginosa* (Høiby, 1974). However, the factors which contribute to this unusual host-pathogen interaction have not yet been determined. Currently there is no effective combination of therapies which completely eradicates alginate-producing *P. aeruginosa* from the CF lung environment. The development of new compounds effective in preventing alginate synthesis represents a major step towards reaching this goal. Such inhibitors of alginate synthesis have potential clinical applications in that elimination of the alginate capsule might render *P. aeruginosa* more susceptible to both antibiotic therapy and the host's immune system. Our laboratory is involved in an extensive study of the alginate biosynthetic pathway in *P. aeruginosa* in an effort to identify (i) nontoxic compounds that inhibit alginate synthesis by inhibiting the enzymes directly involved in the pathway and (ii) factors unique to the CF lung environment that trigger expression of the genes involved in alginate biosynthesis. This report reviews the progress made in understanding the genetics and regulation of alginate biosynthesis in *P. aeruginosa*.

BIOCHEMISTRY OF ALGINATE SYNTHESIS

Alginate is a linear copolymer consisting of β-1,4-linked D-mannuronic acid and variable amounts of its C-5 epimer L-guluronic acid (Evans and Linker, 1973). This exopolysaccharide is used commercially as a gelling agent and thickener to stabilize foods, medicines, and industrial products (Gacesa, 1988). Alginate is produced by several bacterial species, the most widely known being *Azotobacter vinelandii* (Gorin and Spencer, 1966) and *P. aeruginosa* (Linker and Jones, 1964). Bacterial alginates differ from algal alginate in that the former contain *O*-acetyl groups (Evans and Linker, 1973). The viscosity level of alginate, as determined by the mannuronate/guluronate ratio, may play a role in the pathogenesis of mucoid *P. aeruginosa* in the CF respiratory tract (Reynolds et al., 1975).

The alginate biosynthetic pathway in *P. aeruginosa* (Fig. 1, top) was first proposed based on work with the marine brown alga *Fucus gardneri* (Lin and Hassid, 1966a, 1966b) and the bacterium *A. vinelandii* (Pindar and Bucke, 1975). In *F. gardneri*, the pathway is proposed to proceed from mannose through GDP-mannose to form GDP-mannuronic acid and GDP-guluronic acid, and finally to alginate after polymerization of mannuronate and guluronate residues (Lin and Hassid, 1966a). A similar pathway appears to operate in *A. vinelandii* and *P. aeruginosa*, with the initial alginate precursor being fructose 6-phosphate (Banerjee et al., 1985) which is obtained from the cell's carbohydrate pool via the Entner-Doudoroff pathway (Lynn and Sokatch, 1984). However, the epimerization of mannuronate to guluronate occurs at the polymer level in *A. vinelandii*, while the stage at which this conversion occurs in *P. aeruginosa* is unknown. The finding that the activity levels of the enzymes proposed to be involved in alginate synthesis correspond to the level of alginate production in *A. vinelandii* cultured under different conditions (Evans and Linker, 1973) substantiated the putative pathway.

Piggott et al. (1981) first detected activity of several enzymes involved in the alginate biosynthetic pathway (phosphomannose isomerase [PMI], GDP-mannose pyrophosphorylase [GMP], and GDP-mannose dehydrogenase [GMD]) in mucoid, alginate-producing *P. aeruginosa*. Activities of the enzymes were either absent or greatly reduced in nonmucoid strains. These results were consistent with those of Pugashetti et al. (1983), who observed that GMD activity was present in cell extracts of mucoid *P. aeruginosa* strains but not in extracts of nonmucoid strains. In addition, Padgett and Phibbs (1986) detected consistently higher levels of phosphomannomutase (PMM) activity in mucoid strains. Our laboratory (Sá-Correia et al., 1987) has demonstrated that the first four enzymatic activities are present in mucoid *P. aeruginosa* and that the levels of the first three

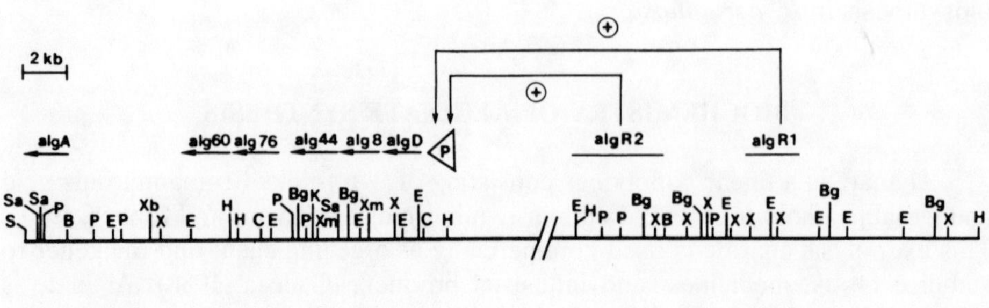

FIGURE 1. (Top) Pathway of alginate synthesis in *P. aeruginosa*. Abbreviations: F6P, fructose 6-phosphate; M6P, mannose 6-phosphate; M1P, mannose 1-phosphate; GDPM, GDP-mannose; GMA, GDP-mannuronic acid; PMI, phosphomannose isomerase; PMM, phosphomannomutase; GMP, GDP-mannose pyrophosphorylase; GMD, GDP-mannose dehydrogenase. The remaining steps of alginate synthesis are polymerization, epimerization, acetylation, and export. The *algA* gene encodes a bifunctional PMI-GMP enzyme, while *algD* encodes GMD. (Bottom) Restriction nuclease site map showing the alginate gene cluster at 34 min on the *P. aeruginosa* chromosome and the *algR* genes (located at 10 min). The direction of transcription of the alginate gene cluster was established by Wang et al. (1987). The *algR1* and *algR2* gene products act as positive regulators of the *algD* promoter (Deretic et al., 1987b). Abbreviations of restriction sites: B, *Bam*HI; Bg, *Bgl*II; C, *Cla*I; E, *Eco*RI; H, *Hin*dIII; K, *Kpn*I; P, *Pst*I; S, *Sst*I; Sa, *Sal*I; X, *Xho*I; Xb, *Xba*I; and Xm, *Xma*I. The chromosome map of *P. aeruginosa* was recently recalibrated (O'Hoy and Krishnapillai, 1987). Thus the map locations of *alg* genes reported in this article, 10, 34, and 67 min, correspond to the previously reported map locations of 19, 45, and 95 min, respectively.

enzymes are low even in heavily mucoid strains. The subsequent steps of alginate biosynthesis, which include polymerization, acetylation, export, and epimerization, are not as well characterized.

MOLECULAR BIOLOGY AND ENZYMOLOGY OF ALGINATE SYNTHESIS IN *P. AERUGINOSA*

It was imperative to isolate a stable mucoid (alginate-producing) strain of *P. aeruginosa* before a genetic analysis of alginate biosynthesis could begin. A stable alginate-producing (Alg⁺) strain, designated 8830, was isolated following ethyl methanesulfonate mutagenesis of a spontaneous nonmucoid revertant (strain 8822) of the original CF isolate (strain 8821) (Darzins and Chakrabarty, 1984). This stable mucoid strain, 8830, was subjected to further ethyl methanesulfonate mutagenesis to obtain several alginate-negative (Alg⁻) mutants. A cosmid clone bank (constructed from 8830) was then screened for recombinant plasmids that restored the mucoid phenotype to nonmucoid mutants (Darzins and Chakrabarty, 1984). Genetic analyses determined that most of the Alg⁻ mutants could be divided into seven groups on the basis of complementation by various recombinant plasmids (Darzins et al., 1985b). Six of the seven groups form a cluster at 34 min on the *P. aeruginosa* chromosome (Darzins et al., 1985b). This region is transcribed from *argF* to *algA* (Wang et al., 1987). To alleviate the inherently low activities of alginate biosynthetic enzymes in *P. aeruginosa*, the *P. aeruginosa* genes involved in alginate biosynthesis were cloned (Darzins et al., 1985a; Gill et al., 1986; Sá-Correia et al., 1987; Wang et al., 1987) into broad-host-range controlled-expression vectors (Bagdasarian et al., 1983). This allowed the overexpression of the *alg* genes to provide sufficient amounts of the corresponding gene products for subsequent purification, characterization, and inhibitor studies.

The first reaction of the alginate biosynthetic pathway in *P. aeruginosa* is the conversion of fructose 6-phosphate to mannose 6-phosphate (Fig. 1, top; Table 1). Darzins et al. (1985a) showed that a 2.0-kilobase (kb) *Bam*HI-*Sst*I fragment could complement an *Escherichia coli manA* mutant (that lacked PMI activity and as a result was deficient in capsular polysaccharide synthesis). Introduction of this fragment into the *P. aeruginosa alg-43* mutant restored the mucoid phenotype and increased PMI activity 10- to 25-fold (Darzins et al., 1985a; Gill et al., 1986). The functional identification of this gene product was achieved by overexpressing the gene present in the *Bam*HI-*Sst*I fragment in both *E. coli* and *P. aeruginosa* using the broad-host-range expression vector pMMB22, which places the fragment directly under control of the *tac* promoter (Gill et al., 1986). The 2.0-kb fragment contains the *algA* gene that encodes a 56,000-M_r polypeptide on sodium dodecyl sulfate-polyacrylamide gels (Gill et al., 1986).

Overexpression of *algA* leads not only to an increase in PMI specific activity, but also to an increase in the levels of PMM and GMP activity (Sá-Correia et al., 1987). The level of GMD remained unchanged. Ion-exchange chromatography of cell extracts revealed that PMI and GMP activities eluted in the same peak, while PMM eluted earlier in the gradient (Sá-Correia et al., 1987). Overexpression of *algA* in an *E. coli* strain which had no detectable PMI or GMP activity resulted in the appearance of both enzymatic activities in cell extracts. In combination, these results suggested either that *algA* encoded a bifunctional protein or that *algA* induced GMP activity in both *E. coli* and *P. aeruginosa*. The *algA* gene product has been purified, and the N-terminal amino acid sequence has been found to match with that predicted from the DNA sequence analysis, confirming that this protein is the *algA* gene product. Throughout the purification scheme of hydrophobic interaction, affinity, ion-exchange, and gel filtration chromatography, PMI and GMP activities copurified (Berry et al., 1988). In addition, we have cloned a defective *algA* gene containing a point mutation which reduces only the GMP activity by 50%, resulting in the loss of the mucoid phenotype (Berry et al., 1988). These results strongly suggest that the *algA* gene encodes a 53-kilodalton bifunctional protein having both PMI and GMP activities. We are analyzing *algA* mutants that lack either PMI or GMP activity in an effort to determine whether independent domains exist for each activity.

The conversion of mannose 6-phosphate to mannose 1-phosphate (Fig. 1, top; Table 1) is catalyzed by PMM. PMM was shown to be a separate protein from PMI/GMP (Sá-Correia et al., 1987). To clone the gene(s) involved in PMM

TABLE 1
Enzymes involved in alginate biosynthesis

Biosynthetic enzyme	Substrate	Product	Subunit mol wt	Native mol wt	Protein hyper-production achieved	Purity	Nucleotide sequence	Verification of nucleotide sequence by N-terminal amino acid sequencing
PMI/GMP	Fructose 6-phosphate (PMI) Mannose 1-phosphate (GMP)	Mannose 6-phosphate (PMI) GDP-mannose (GMP)	53,000		+	>90%	+	+
PMM	Mannose 6-phosphate	Mannose 1-phosphate	52,000		+		+	−
GMD	GDP-mannose	GDP-mannuronic acid	48,000	290,000	+	>95%	+	+
GDP-mannuronic acid-binding protein	GDP-mannuronic acid	GDP-mannuronic acid reversibly bound to protein?		<10,000	−		−	−

expression, we used a strategy based on the fact that overexpression of the *algA* gene not only leads to elevated levels of its product PMI/GMP, but also results in a concomitant increase in PMM activity (Berry et al., 1988). A *P. aeruginosa* mutant deficient in PMM activity was identified by introducing and overexpressing the *algA* gene in all of the available Alg⁻ mutants of *P. aeruginosa*. One mutant, 8858, exhibited high levels of PMI/GMP upon *algA* hyperexpression as expected but showed no concomitant increase in PMM. This suggested that mutant 8858 harbored a mutation either in the PMM structural gene or in the gene(s) responsible for PMM induction in response to elevated PMI activity. Strain 8858 was used as a recipient to screen a cosmid clone bank of strain 8830 for a fragment that would complement the PMM deficiency. One recombinant plasmid, pAB8, restored alginate synthesis to mutant strain 8858. The level of alginate produced by strain 8858(pAB8) was comparable to that observed for the mucoid parent strain 8830. Subcloning of DNA fragments from within the 26-kb cloned insert in pAB8 localized the PMM activity to a 2.6-kb *Hin*dIII-*Sst*I fragment (plasmid pNZ15). The analogous DNA fragment was cloned from the mutant strain 8858, thus allowing comparison of the wild-type and mutant sequences. The cloned insert in pNZ15 encodes one polypeptide having an approximate subunit molecular mass of 52,000 as determined using the T7 RNA polymerase/plasmid promoter system. We have further subcloned the fragment contained within pNZ15, using exonuclease III (from the *Hin*dIII end), to a 1.6-kb fragment which restores alginate production in strain 8858 and results in elevated levels of PMM activity in 8858. The location of the *pmm* gene on the *P. aeruginosa* chromosome has not yet been determined. Genetic analyses suggested that it is not contained in either the alginate biosynthetic gene cluster at 34 min or the regulatory gene cluster at 10 min on the *P. aeruginosa* chromosome.

The fourth step leading to the formation of GDP-mannuronic acid is catalyzed by GMD (Fig. 1, top; Table 1), which is encoded by the *algD* gene (Deretic et al., 1987a). GMD is of particular interest for two reasons: (i) its expression is subject to positive regulation by the products of at least two other genes, *algR1* and *algR2*, and (ii) the reaction catalyzed by GMD favors the formation of GDP-mannuronic acid, which is not known to be an intermediate in any pathway in *P. aeruginosa* other than that for alginate synthesis. These two facts suggest that the reaction catalyzed by GMD is the point at which the cell commits its precursors to alginate synthesis.

Purification of GMD (Roychoudhury et al., 1989) was facilitated by overexpressing *algD* from the *tac* promoter. GMD activity corresponds with the appearance of a 48-kilodalton polypeptide on a sodium dodecyl sulfate-polyacrylamide gel. The native enzyme appears to exist as a hexamer (M_r 290,000 as estimated by gel filtration) (Roychoudhury et al., 1989). GMD is highly specific for its natural substrate GDP-mannose (apparent K_m, 15 μM). Inhibition studies indicated that the guanosine moiety binds the enzyme to make the mannose moiety accessible to the enzyme (Roychoudhury et al., 1989). ATP was found to inhibit GMD activity. Interestingly, the amino acid sequence of GMD (predicted from DNA sequence and confirmed by N-terminal amino acid sequencing) was found to share homology with the ATP-binding consensus sequences of several

ATP-binding proteins (Higgins et al., 1986). GMD activity was also sensitive to sulfhydryl modifying agents, suggesting a possible involvement of cysteine residue(s) in the reaction. The amino acid sequence around the Cys-268 residue of GMD showed homology with regions around catalytically active cysteine residues of two other four-electron transfer dehydrogenases (UDP-glucose dehydrogenase from bovine liver and histidinol dehydrogenase from *E. coli*) (Feingold and Franzen, 1981), suggesting that Cys-268 might be involved in the catalytic site. We are subjecting the *algD* gene to site-directed mutagenesis to identify the amino acids involved in substrate binding, cofactor (NAD^+) binding, or catalytic activity of the enzyme. Also, we are isolating sufficient enzyme for crystallization of GMD.

The product of the GMD reaction, GDP-mannuronic acid, was proposed to serve as the direct donor of mannuronate moieties in the alginate polymer of *P. aeruginosa* (Fig. 1, top; Roychoudhury et al., 1989). Our current model, based upon analogy with alginate synthesis in *A. vinelandii* (Pindar and Bucke, 1975), is that polymannuronate is the first product of polymerization. It is possible that mannuronate residues are sequentially linked to a C_{55}-isoprenoid lipid carrier present in the cytoplasmic membrane, are partially *O*-acetylated, and are then released for transport to the cell exterior in a fashion similar to the synthesis of other cell wall polymers (Sutherland, 1979). *A. vinelandii* produces an extracellular C-5 epimerase which acts to convert some nonacetylated mannuronate to guluronate residues (Haug and Larsen, 1971; Sutherland, 1979). The putative *P. aeruginosa* epimerase gene has been cloned, but the protein product has not yet been characterized or localized to a specific site in the cell (C. Chitnis and D. E. Ohman, *Abstr. Annu. Meet. Am. Soc. Microbiol. 1988*, D48, p. 79).

We have identified a particulate membrane fraction from the mucoid, alginate-producing *P. aeruginosa* strain 8821 which promotes an Mg^{2+}-dependent incorporation of ^3H- or ^{14}C-labeled GDP-mannuronic acid into an ethanol-insoluble material. A membrane fraction from the nonmucoid revertant strain 8822 was devoid of this activity. The ethanol-precipitable material comigrated with GDP-mannuronic acid upon paper chromatography. Incubation of the membrane in assay buffer (lacking substrate) either at 42°C for 1 h or in the presence of 500 mM NaCl at 4°C for 15 min released a small (<10-kilodalton) membrane component which retained activity. Incubation of the reaction mixture with 100 mM EDTA or 500 mM NaCl reversed incorporation. These results suggest that binding of GDP-mannuronic acid to a small membrane component is the initial polymerization event.

REGULATION OF ALGINATE SYNTHESIS

A pivotal step in alginate biosynthesis is the activation of the *algD* gene in mucoid, alginate-producing *P. aeruginosa*. GMD catalyzes the oxidation of GDP-mannose to form GDP-mannuronic acid (the putative alginate polymerization precursor) and therefore is a likely point of regulation. RNA transcript analysis revealed that the *algD* gene is transcriptionally activated in mucoid *P.*

TABLE 2
Auxiliary factors involved in regulation of alginate biosynthesis

Gene	Nucleotide sequence	Protein hyperproduction	Subunit mol wt	Target
algR1	+	−	28,000	*algD* promoter
algR2	+	+	18,000	*algD* promoter
algR3	+	+	33,000	NK[a]
gyrA	−	−	NK	*algD* promoter
rpoN	−	−	54,000	*algD* and *algR1* promoter

[a] NK, Not known.

aeruginosa (Deretic et al., 1987a). DNA sequence analysis revealed a significant number of direct and inverted repeats extending 110 base pairs upstream of the *algD* transcriptional start site (Deretic et al., 1987b), including a sequence showing identity with *E. coli* activator and repressor binding sites (Deretic et al., 1987c). These results suggested a potential involvement of some *trans*-acting auxiliary factor(s) in the transcriptional activation of the *algD* promoter. An *algD-xylE* fusion vector (pVD2X) was constructed to investigate this possibility, thereby allowing *algD* transcription to be measured as catechol 2,3-dioxygenase activity (Deretic et al., 1987a).

Two mutations outside the *algD* gene have been identified which abolish *algD* activation (Deretic et al., 1987b; DeVault et al., 1989). The two mutations (designated *alg-22* and *alg-52*, corresponding respectively to mutant strains 8852 and 8882) have been shown to be complemented by two distinct loci, *algR1* and *algR2*, respectively (Fig. 1, bottom; Table 2) (DeVault et al., 1989). Deletion analysis and subsequent DNA sequencing in this laboratory have localized the complementation ability of *algR2* to a 747-base-pair fragment (Kato et al., 1989). The ability to complement the *alg-22* mutant has been localized to an 813-base-pair fragment (Deretic et al., 1989). A computer-assisted homology search revealed that the *algR1* gene product has significant functional amino acid homology with a class of regulatory proteins responsive to environmental stimuli (DeVault et al., 1989). Among those proteins showing homology with *algR1* was the *E. coli ompR* gene (Deretic et al., 1989). OmpR transcriptionally regulates the expression of two outer membrane porin genes in *E. coli* (*ompC* and *ompF*) in response to medium osmolarity (Nikaido, 1979; Norioka et al., 1986). We found that *algD* was highly activated in response to increased concentrations of either KCl or NaCl. This was an interesting finding since the CF lung is rich in Na^+, Cl^-, and K^+ ions (as reviewed by Berry et al., 1988). Also, *algD* activation is observed when *P. aeruginosa* is starved for either phosphate or nitrogen (DeVault et al., 1989) or grown in the presence of a membrane-perturbing, dehydrating agent such as ethanol (J. D. DeVault, K. Kimbara, and A. M. Chakrabarty, submitted for publication).

OmpR is able to activate *algD* in *E. coli* in response to medium osmolarity. Interestingly, there appears to be a functional interchangeability between *ompR*, *algR1*, and *algR2* in the osmolarity-induced activation of the *algD* promoter in *E.*

coli (DeVault et al., 1989; Kato et al., in press). Of particular consequence is the osmolarity-induced, synergistic effect seen when both *algR1* and *algR2* are present in the *ompR E. coli* strains harboring pVD2X. Such cooperativity between transcriptional activators is not unprecedented (Stibitz et al., 1988). Further studies remain to determine the significance of this cooperativity. Despite the fact that the *algR2* gene product appears to directly interact with the *algD* promoter in *E. coli*, DNA sequence analysis of the *algR2* coding region (which predicts a polypeptide of 160 amino acids) shows no homology with any known DNA-binding proteins.

Sequence analysis of the *algD* and *algR1* promoter regions shows a striking degree of homology throughout the entire 170-base-pair upstream region (DeVault et al., 1989). Therefore, it was not surprising that an *algR1-xylE* fusion vector, introduced into *E. coli* and subjected to a high-osmotic growth environment, showed a significant level of activation (Kimbara and Chakrabarty, 1989). Analysis of RNA transcript formation of the *algR1* and *algR2* from wild-type and mutant strains of *P. aeruginosa* demonstrated that *algR1* transcription is dependent on the *algR1* gene product. In fact, the *algR1* gene appears to be both positively as well as negatively regulated. This observation is reminiscent of the regulatory mechanisms controlling *E. coli lysR* transcription (Stragier and Patte, 1983). Also, we have shown that a functional alternative *rpoN* sigma factor (sigma-54) is required for *algD* and *algR1* transcription (Kimbara and Chakrabarty, 1989).

The regulation of alginate biosynthesis by *P. aeruginosa* appears to involve a fine tuning of several factors. The *algR1* and *algR2* genes are intimately involved in the *trans*-activation of both *algR1* and *algD*. Their involvement in the transcriptional regulation of other alginate genes remains to be determined, as does the involvement of other regulatory loci. We have demonstrated that osmotically induced activation of *algD* in *E. coli*, as well as environmentally induced activation of *algD* in *P. aeruginosa*, is sensitive to DNA gyrase subunit A inhibitors (nalidixic acid and ciprofloxacin hydrochloride) as well as being nonresponsive in the putative gyrase A mutant PAO1 derivative PAO515, suggesting an active role of DNA supercoiling in regulating alginate synthesis (Berry et al., 1989; DeVault et al., submitted).

Alginate-producing strains of three other *Pseudomonas* species (*P. fluorescens, P. putida,* and *P. mendocina*) have been isolated in vitro by growth on subinhibitory concentrations of carbenicillin (Hacking et al., 1983). Also, certain phytopathogenic *Pseudomonas* species produce alginate both in planta and in vitro (Fett et al., 1986). These observations suggest that many species of *Pseudomonas* harbor genes involved in alginate biosynthesis, but that they are not normally expressed. Since many of the *P. aeruginosa* alginate genes had been cloned, it was possible to examine genomic DNA from various *Pseudomonas* species and phylogenetically related organisms for sequences homologous to the *P. aeruginosa alg* genes. Southern hybridization studies using *algA, pmm, algD,* and *algR1* as probes showed some degree of homology with several *Pseudomonas* species belonging to *Pseudomonas* RNA homology group I. Some probes also hybridized with *Azotobacter, Azomonas,* and *Serpens* species (A. M. Fialho,

N. A. Zielinski, W. F. Fett, A. M. Chakrabarty, and A. Berry, *Appl. Environ. Microbiol.*, in press).

CONCLUSION

Continuing studies with the cloned alginate genes will be useful for understanding the details of both the alginate biosynthetic pathway and the regulatory mechanisms that govern alginate gene expression. A fundamental knowledge of these mechanisms governing alginate synthesis in *P. aeruginosa* will be required to develop nontoxic inhibitors targeted specifically to the alginate biosynthetic pathway in *P. aeruginosa*.

ACKNOWLEDGMENTS. This work was supported by Public Health Service grants AI-16790 (to A.M.C.) and AI-07890 (to A.B.) from the National Institutes of Health, and in part by grant Z061 9-1 from the Cystic Fibrosis Foundation. N.A.Z. is partly supported by a predoctoral grant from the Cystic Fibrosis Foundation. T.B.M. is supported by grant F0719 C-1 from the Cystic Fibrosis Foundation. K. Kimbara is supported by a fellowship from the Toyobo Biotechnology Foundation. K. Kitano is on leave from and is supported by Komatsu Ltd.

We especially thank Lula Johnson for typing the many revisions of this manuscript.

LITERATURE CITED

Bagdasarian, M., E. Amann, R. Lurz, B. Ruckert, and M. Bagdasarian. 1983. Activity of the hybrid *trp-lac* (*tac*) promoter of *Escherichia coli* in *Pseudomonas putida*. Construction of broad-host range, controlled-expression vectors. *Gene* **26**:273–282.

Banerjee, P. C., R. I. Vanags, A. M. Chakrabarty, and P. K. Maitra. 1985. Fructose-1,6-bisphosphate aldolase activity is essential for synthesis of alginate from glucose by *Pseudomonas aeruginosa*. *J. Bacteriol.* **165**:458–460.

Berry, A., J. D. DeVault, and A. M. Chakrabarty. 1989. High osmolarity is a signal for enhanced *algD* transcription in mucoid and nonmucoid *Pseudomonas aeruginosa* strains. *J. Bacteriol.* **171**:2312–2317.

Berry, A., J. D. DeVault, S. Roychoudhury, N. A. Zielinski, T. B. May, E. C. Wynn, R. K. Rothmel, A. Fialho, M. Hussein, V. Krylov, and A. M. Chakrabarty. 1988. *Pseudomonas aeruginosa* infection in cystic fibrosis: molecular approaches to a medical problem. *CHIMICAoggi* **9**:13–19.

Darzins, A., and A. M. Chakrabarty. 1984. Cloning of genes controlling alginate biosynthesis from a mucoid cystic fibrosis isolate of *Pseudomonas aeruginosa*. *J. Bacteriol.* **159**:9–18.

Darzins, A., L. L. Nixon, R. I. Vanags, and A. M. Chakrabarty. 1985a. Cloning of *Escherichia coli* and *Pseudomonas aeruginosa* phosphomannose isomerase genes and their expression in alginate-negative mutants of *Pseudomonas aeruginosa*. *J. Bacteriol.* **161**:249–257.

Darzins, A., S.-K. Wang, R. I. Vanags, and A. M. Chakrabarty. 1985b. Clustering of mutations affecting alginic acid biosynthesis in mucoid *Pseudomonas aeruginosa*. *J. Bacteriol.* **164**:516–524.

Davis, P. B., and P. A. di Sant' Agnese. 1980. A review. Cystic fibrosis at forty—quo vadis? *Pediatr. Res.* **14**:83–87.

Deretic, V., R. Dikshit, W. M. Konyecsni, A. M. Chakrabarty, and T. Misra. 1989. The *algR* gene, which regulates mucoidy in *Pseudomonas aeruginosa*, belongs to a class of environmentally responsive genes. *J. Bacteriol.* **171**:1278–1283.

Deretic, V., J. F. Gill, and A. M. Chakrabarty. 1987a. Gene *algD* coding for GDP-mannose dehydrogenase is transcriptionally activated in mucoid *Pseudomonas aeruginosa*. *J. Bacteriol.* **169**:351–358.

Deretic, V., J. F. Gill, and A. M. Chakrabarty. 1987b. *Pseudomonas aeruginosa* infections in cystic fibrosis: nucleotide sequence and transcriptional regulation of the *algD* gene. *Nucleic Acids Res.* **15**:4567–4581.

Deretic, V., J. F. Gill, and A. M. Chakrabarty. 1987c. Alginate biosynthesis: a model system for gene regulation and function in *Pseudomonas aeruginosa. Bio/Technology* **5:**469–477.

DeVault, J. D., A. Berry, T. K. Misra, A. Darzins, and A. M. Chakrabarty. 1989. Environmental sensory signals and microbial pathogenesis: *Pseudomonas aeruginosa* infection in cystic fibrosis. *Bio/Technology* **7:**352–357.

Evans, L. R., and A. Linker. 1973. Production and characterization of the slime polysaccharide of *Pseudomonas aeruginosa. J. Bacteriol.* **116:**915–924.

Feingold, D. S., and J. S. Franzen. 1981. Pyridine nucleotide-linked four-electron transfer dehydrogenases. *Trends Biochem. Sci.* **6:**103–105.

Fett, W. F., S. F. Osman, M. L. Fishman, and T. S. Siebles III. 1986. Alginate production by plant-pathogenic pseudomonads. *Appl. Environ. Microbiol.* **52:**466–473.

Gacesa, P. 1988. Enzymatic modification of polysaccharides. *CHIMICAoggi* **4:**23–27.

Gill, J. F., V. Deretic, and A. M. Chakrabarty. 1986. Overproduction and assay of *Pseudomonas aeruginosa* phosphomannose isomerase. *J. Bacteriol.* **167:**611–615.

Goodchild, M. C., and J. A. Dodge (ed.). 1985. *Cystic Fibrosis. Manual of Diagnosis and Management.* Bailliere Tindall, London.

Gorin, P. A. J., and J. F. T. Spencer. 1966. Exocellular alginic acid from *Azotobacter vinelandii. Can. J. Chem.* **44:**993–998.

Govan, J. R. W. 1975. Mucoid strains of *Pseudomonas aeruginosa*: the influence of culture medium on the stability of mucus production. *J. Med. Microbiol.* **8:**513–522.

Govan, J. R. W. 1988. Alginate biosynthesis and other unusual characteristics associated with the pathogenesis of *Pseudomonas aeruginosa* in cystic fibrosis, p. 67–96. *In* E. Griffith, W. Donachie, and J. Stephan (ed.), *Bacterial Infections of Respiratory and Gastrointestinal Mucosae.* IRL Press, Oxford.

Govan, J. R. W., and J. Fyfe. 1978. Mucoid *Pseudomonas aeruginosa* and cystic fibrosis: resistance of the mucoid form to carbenicillin, flucloxacillin and tobramycin and the isolation of mucoid variants *in vitro. J. Antimicrob. Chemother.* **4:**233–240.

Hacking, A. J., I. W. F. Taylor, T. R. Jarman, and J. R. W. Govan. 1983. Alginate biosynthesis by *Pseudomonas mendocina. J. Gen. Microbiol.* **129:**3473–3480.

Haug, A., and B. Larsen. 1971. Biosynthesis of alginate. II. Polymannuronic acid C-5 epimerase from *Azotobacter vinelandii. Carbohydr. Res.* **17:**297–308.

Higgins, C. F., I. D. Hines, G. P. Salmond, D. R. Gill, J. A. Donnie, I. J. Evans, I. B. Holland, L. Gray, S. D. Buckel, A. W. Bell, and M. A. Hermodson. 1986. A family of related ATP-binding subunits coupled to many distinct biological processes in bacteria. *Nature* (London) **323:**448–450.

Høiby, N. 1974. *Pseudomonas aeruginosa* infection in cystic fibrosis. Relationship between mucoid strains of *Pseudomonas aeruginosa* and the humoral immune response. *Acta Pathol. Microbiol. Scand. Sect. B* **82:**551–558.

Kato, J., L. Chu, K. Kitano, J. D. DeVault, K. Kimbara, A. M. Chakrabarty, and T. K. Misra. 1989. Nucleotide sequence of a regulatory region controlling alginate synthesis in *Pseudomonas aeruginosa*: characterization of the *algR2* gene. *Gene* **84:**31–38.

Kerem, B.-S., J. M. Rommens, J. A. Buchanan, D. Markiewicz, T. K. Cox, A. Chakravarti, M. Buchwald, and L.-C. Tsui. 1989. Identification of the cystic fibrosis gene: genetic analysis. *Science* **245:**1073–1080.

Kimbara, K., and A. M. Chakrabarty. 1989. Control of alginate synthesis in *Pseudomonas aeruginosa*: regulation of the *algR1* gene. *Biochem. Biophys. Res. Commun.* **164:**601–608.

Kulczycki, L. L., T. M. Murphy, and J. A. Bellanti. 1978. *Pseudomonas* colonization in cystic fibrosis. *J. Am. Med. Assoc.* **240:**30–34.

Larsen, B., and A. Haug. 1971. Biosynthesis of alginate. III. Tritium incorporation with polymannuronic acid C-5-epimerase from *Azotobacter vinelandii. Carbohydr. Res.* **20:**225–232.

Lin, T. Y., and W. Z. Hassid. 1966a. Isolation of guanosine diphosphate uronic acids from a marine brown alga, *Fucus gardneri* silva. *J. Biol. Chem.* **241:**3283–3293.

Lin, T. Y., and W. Z. Hassid. 1966b. Pathway of alginic acid synthesis in the marine brown alga *Fucus gardneri* silva. *J. Biol. Chem.* **241:**5284–5297.

Linker, A., and R. S. Jones. 1964. A polysaccharide resembling alginic acid from *Pseudomonas* micro-organism. *Nature* (London) **204:**187–188.

Luray-Cuasay, L. R., K. R. Kundy, and N. H. Huang. 1976. *Pseudomonas* carrier rates of patients with cystic fibrosis and of members of their families. *J. Pediatr.* **89**:23–26.

Lynn, A. R., and J. R. Sokatch. 1984. Incorporation of isotope from specifically labeled glucose into alginates of *Pseudomonas aeruginosa* and *Azotobacter vinelandii*. *J. Bacteriol.* **158**:1161–1162.

Nikaido, H. 1979. Nonspecific transport through the outer membrane, p. 361–407. *In* M. Inouye (ed.), *Bacterial Outer Membranes: Biogenesis and Functions*. John Wiley and Sons, Inc., New York.

Norioka, S., G. Ramakrishnan, K. Ikenak, and M. Inouye. 1986. Interaction of a transcriptional activator, OmpR, with reciprocally osmoregulated genes, *ompF* and *ompC*, of *Escherichia coli*. *J. Biol. Chem.* **261**:17113–17119.

O'Hoy, K., and V. Krishnipillai. 1987. Recalibration of the *Pseudomonas aeruginosa* genome strain PAO chromosome map in time units using high-frequence-of-recombination donors. *Genetics* **115**:611–618.

Padgett, P. J., and P. V. Phibbs. 1986. Phosphomannomutase activity in wild-type and alginate-producing strains of *Pseudomonas aeruginosa*. *Curr. Microbiol.* **14**:187–192.

Piggott, M. H., I. W. Sutherland, and T. R. Jarman. 1981. Enzymes involved in the biosynthesis of alginate by *Pseudomonas aeruginosa*. *Eur. J. Appl. Microbiol. Biotechnol.* **13**:179–183.

Pindar, D. F., and C. Bucke. 1975. The biosynthesis of alginic acid by *Azotobacter vinelandii*. *Biochem. J.* **152**:617–622.

Pitcher-Wilmott, R. W., R. J. Levinsky, I. Gordon, M. W. Turner, and D. J. Mathew. 1982. *Pseudomonas* infection, allergy, and cystic fibrosis. *Arch. Dis. Child.* **57**:582–586.

Pugashetti, B. K., L. Vadas, H. S. Prihar, and D. S. Feingold. 1983. GDP-mannose dehydrogenase and biosynthesis of alginate-like polysaccharide in a mucoid strain of *Pseudomonas aeruginosa*. *J. Bacteriol.* **153**:1107–1110.

Reynolds, H. Y., A. S. Levine, R. E. Wood, C. H. Zierdt, D. C. Dale, and J. E. Pennington. 1975. *Pseudomonas aeruginosa* infections: persisting problems and current research to find new therapies. *Ann. Intern. Med.* **82**:819–832.

Riordan, J. R., J. M. Rommens, B. Kerem, N. Alon, R. Rozmahel, Z. Grzelezak, J. Zielenski, S. Lok, N. Plavsic, J.-L. Chou, M. L. Drumm, M. C. Iannuzzi, F. S. Collins, and L.-C. Tsui. 1989. Identification of the cystic fibrosis gene: cloning and characterization of complementary DNA. *Science* **245**:1066–1073.

Rommens, J. M., M. C. Iannuzzi, B.-S. Kerem, M. L. Drumm, G. Melmer, M. Dean, R. Rozmahel, J. L. Cole, D. Kennedy, N. Hidaka, M. Zsiga, M. Buchwald, J. R. Riordan, L.-C. Tsui, and F. S. Collins. 1989. Identification of the cystic fibrosis gene: chromosome walking and jumping. *Science* **245**:1059–1065.

Roychoudhury, S., T. B. May, J. F. Gill, S. K. Singh, D. S. Feingold, and A. M. Chakrabarty. 1989. Purification and characterization of guanosine diphospho-D-mannose dehydrogenase. *J. Biol. Chem.* **264**:9380–9385.

Sá-Correia, I., A. Darzins, S.-K. Wang, A. Berry, and A. M. Chakrabarty. 1987. Alginate biosynthetic enzymes in mucoid and nonmucoid *Pseudomonas aeruginosa*: overproduction of phosphomannose isomerase, phosphomannomutase, and GDP-mannose pyrophosphorylase by overexpression of the phosphomannose isomerase (*pmi*) gene. *J. Bacteriol.* **169**:3224–3231.

Stibitz, S., A. A. Weiss, and S. Falkow. 1988. Genetic analysis of a region of the *Bordetella pertussis* chromosome encoding filamentous hemagglutinin and the pleiotropic regulatory locus *vir*. *J. Bacteriol.* **170**:2904–2913.

Stragier, P., and J. C. Patte. 1983. Regulation of diaminopimelate decarboxylase synthesis in *Escherichia coli*. III. Nucleotide sequence and regulation of the *lysR* gene. *J. Mol. Biol.* **168**:333–350.

Sutherland, I. W. 1979. Microbial exopolysaccharides: control of synthesis and acetylation, p. 1–34. *In* R. C. W. Berkeley, G. W. Gooday, and D. C. Ellwood (ed.), *Microbial Polysaccharides and Polysaccharases*. Academic Press, Inc. (London) Ltd., London.

Wang, S.-K., I. Sá-Correia, A. Darzins, and A. M. Chakrabarty. 1987. Characterization of the *Pseudomonas aeruginosa* alginate (*alg*) gene region II. *J. Gen. Microbiol.* **133**:2303–2317.

Woods, D. E., J. A. Bass, W. G. Johnson, Jr., and D. C. Straus. 1980. Role of adherence in the pathogenesis of *Pseudomonas aeruginosa* infection in patients with cystic fibrosis. *Infect. Immun.* **30**:694–699.

Chapter 3

Molecular Analysis of the Genetic Switch Activating Alginate Production

Dennis E. Ohman, Joanna B. Goldberg, and JoAnne L. Flynn

PSEUDOMONAS INFECTION IN CYSTIC FIBROSIS

Pseudomonas aeruginosa is a very adaptable bacterial saprophyte and is nearly ubiquitous in the environment. It is also the only *Pseudomonas* species with great potential to cause a variety of severe and lethal opportunistic infections. Currently, chronic pulmonary infection of patients with cystic fibrosis (CF) is a major cause of disease by this organism (George, 1987; Wood et al., 1976). CF is an inherited, autosomal-recessive disease affecting exocrine gland function. Oversecretion of pulmonary mucus leads to respiratory congestion and marked susceptibility to bronchopulmonary disease, the leading cause of morbidity and mortality among these patients (George, 1987; Wood et al., 1976). The susceptibility of CF patients to bacterial infection is probably due to a breakdown in nonspecific host defenses in the pulmonary tract that is a consequence of the excess mucus. Infections with *Staphylococcus aureus* and *Haemophilus influenzae* can now be treated effectively with oral antibiotics. In contrast, *P. aeruginosa* is intractable even to treatment with aggressive intravenous therapy with the most potent antipseudomonal agents (Hoiby, 1974). The incidence of *P. aeruginosa* colonization in CF patients is high, 60 to 90% (George, 1987; Wood et al., 1976).

ALGINATE PRODUCTION AND PATHOGENESIS

The striking feature peculiar to the *P. aeruginosa* strains infecting CF patients is their mucoid colony morphology. This feature is due to the production of copious amounts of alginate, a viscous exopolysaccharide. Alginate is an acetylated linear polymer composed of D-mannuronic acid and L-guluronic acid.

Dennis E. Ohman • Department of Microbiology and Immunology, University of Tennessee, and VA Medical Center, Memphis, Tennessee 38163. *Joanna B. Goldberg* • Channing Laboratory, Brigham and Women's Hospital, Boston, Massachusetts 02115. *JoAnne L. Flynn* • Scripps Research Institute, La Jolla, California 92037.

Although about 80% of the *P. aeruginosa* isolates from CF patients are mucoid, only about 1% of clinical *P. aeruginosa* isolates from other types of infections are mucoid (Doggett et al., 1966). The role of alginate in pathogenesis is complex and appears to confer antiphagocytic properties (Baltimore and Mitchell, 1982; Schwarzmann and Boring, 1971) and an adherence mechanism (Marcus and Baker, 1985; Ramphal and Pier, 1985) upon the organisms. Autopsies show that mucoid *P. aeruginosa* forms adherent microcolonies in the lung (Govan and Harris, 1986). Alginate does not firmly adhere to the organisms but is released in large quantities into the respiratory environment. Because alginate is very viscous in aqueous solution, it probably contributes to the high viscosity of the bronchial secretions in the CF lung, resulting in obstruction of small airways, interference with mucociliary airway clearance, and impaired movement of phagocytes (Govan and Harris, 1986). The mucoid organisms may be more adapted to a chronic infection because they secrete lower levels of proteases, which would otherwise cause extensive lung damage and an acute infection (Ohman and Chakrabarty, 1982). Also, *P. aeruginosa* can utilize the respiratory secretions of the CF lung to support rapid growth and alginate biosynthesis (Ohman and Chakrabarty, 1982); thus, the mucus-congested CF respiratory tract provides *P. aeruginosa* with a nutritionally rich environment favorable to colonization.

ALGINATE SWITCHING OCCURS AT *algS*

The initial colonization of the CF upper respiratory tract appears to be with a nonmucoid strain and is often asymptomatic (Govan and Harris, 1986). This usually precedes the emergence of mucoid variants of the original strain and is followed by chronic infection and a poor prognosis for the patient (George, 1987; Govan and Harris, 1986). In the laboratory, the alginate-producing (Alg$^+$) phenotype is somewhat unstable, and nonmucoid (Alg$^-$) revertants are commonly seen. Genetic mapping experiments have shown that the switching between Alg$^+$ and Alg$^-$ is due to a genetic change in one region of the chromosome (Flynn and Ohman, 1988a; Fyfe and Govan, 1980, 1981; MacGeorge et al., 1986; Ohman and Chakrabarty, 1981) located at about 68 min on the 75-min chromosomal linkage map (O'Hoy and Krishnapillai, 1987). This was originally referred to as the *muc* locus (Fyfe and Govan, 1980). We have been characterizing the genes in this region and refer to the genetic switch involved in alginate conversion as *algS* and a closely linked *trans*-active gene as *algT* (Flynn and Ohman, 1988a) (Fig. 1). Two other regions contain genes involved in the regulation of alginate production. *algR* (Deretic et al., 1987; Deretic et al., 1989) at 9 min and *algB* (Goldberg and Ohman, 1984, 1987) at 13 min, both of which are required for high-level alginate production. Most of the alginate biosynthetic genes appear to be located in a large gene cluster at 34 min (Darzins et al., 1985; Deretic et al., 1987) (Fig. 1).

CLONING OF *algT* AND *algS*

We refer to the alginate switch as *algS*(On) or *algS*(Off), depending on whether alginate production genes are active or inactive. The *algS*(On) and

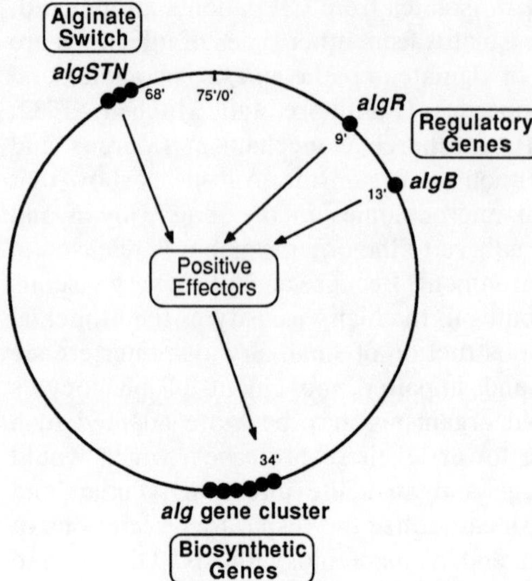

FIGURE 1. Relative locations of the alginate (*alg*) genes on the revised (O'Hoy and Krishnapillai, 1987) 75-min linkage map of the chromosome of *P. aeruginosa*.

algS(Off) alleles are apparently different at the DNA sequence level because an *algS*(On) donor strain (i.e., carrying a sex factor plasmid) mating with an *algS*(Off) strain forms Alg$^+$ recombinants after selection for recombination near 68 min. In our initial efforts to clone *algS*(On), genomic banks of the Alg$^+$ CF isolate FRD1 were constructed in *Escherichia coli* by using IncP1 broad-host-range cosmid cloning vectors (Friedman et al., 1982) and then conjugally transferred to *algS*(Off) strains. However, *trans* complementation of the nonmucoid phenotype to Alg$^+$ was never observed, suggesting that *algS* was *cis* acting. An Alg$^-$ mutant was isolated with a mutation in a newly recognized gene called *algT*, which also mapped at ~68 min (Flynn and Ohman, 1988a). We identified a clone called pJF15 (containing 7.6 kilobases of *P. aeruginosa* DNA) that complemented the *algT* mutation, thus restoring the Alg$^+$ phenotype (Fig. 2A). No *trans*-active alginate gene from the 68-min region of the chromosome had been previously reported. The physical location of *algT* on pJF15 was determined by construction of deletion (Fig. 2B) and transposon insertion (Fig. 2C) derivatives of the original clone in combination with *algT* complementation tests. Partial DNA sequence analysis (data not shown) suggests that the direction of *algT* transcription is as indicated in Fig. 2.

Although pJF15 could complement an *algT* mutation, it could not complement the *algS*(Off) allele (Flynn and Ohman, 1988a). However, certain Tn*501*-containing derivatives of pJF15 did partially complement the *algS*(Off) allele, and the Alg$^+$ phenotype was restored. This finding suggested that pJF15 also carried *algS*(On). The Tn*501* insertions in pJF15 that allowed the clone to activate alginate production were in a region approximately 1 kilobase upstream of *algT* (Fig. 2D). This observation suggested that pJF15 also contained *algS*(On). The locus identified by the transposon insertions was termed *algN* to signify its apparent role as a negative regulator that prevented *trans* complementation by

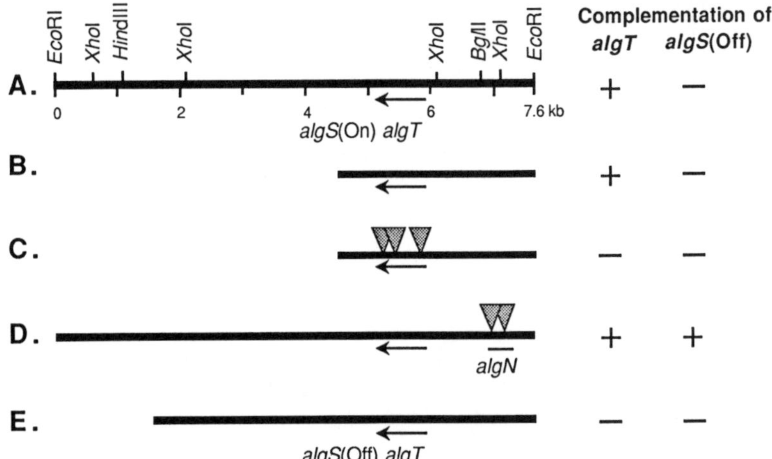

FIGURE 2. (A) Partial restriction map of *P. aeruginosa* DNA in pJF15. The arrow shows the location of *algT* and direction of its transcription. pJF15 can complement *algT* mutations but not *algS*(Off) alleles. (B) Subclone of pJF15 that still complements *algT*. (C) Positions of Tn*501* insertions that block complementation of *algT* mutations (triangles). (D) Positions of Tn*501* insertions in *algN* that allow pJF15 to complement the chromosomal *algS*(Off) allele (triangles). (E) Schematic showing that a clone containing *algS*(Off)*T* does not complement an *algT* mutation. kb, Kilobases.

algS(On)*T*. Whether *algN* encodes a protein or is a *cis*-active site, and how it affects *algT* expression, is under investigation.

CONSTRUCTION OF *algT* MUTANTS BY GENE REPLACEMENT

We have developed an efficient method for gene replacement whereby fragments of *P. aeruginosa* DNA on recombinant plasmids can be used to replace chromosomal alleles (Ohman et al., 1985). Gene replacement has allowed us to construct a variety of genetically defined mutants of *P. aeruginosa*. We used a method called transduction-mediated gene replacement to construct *algT*-null mutants. Derivatives of pJF15 with *algT*::Tn*501* were transferred to *P. aeruginosa* PAO1, a replicative host for the generalized transducing phage F116L (Fig. 3A). The lysates obtained were used to transduce plasmid fragments into Alg$^+$ strains of FRD, and recombinants were obtained by selection for the mercury resistance marker on Tn*501*. The *algT*::Tn*501* mutants obtained displayed a nonmucoid phenotype, and no alginate could be detected in culture supernatants of these strains. These mutants were complemented to the Alg$^+$ phenotype by pJF15, indicating that any potential polar effects of the transposon insertion in the chromosome did not affect the ability of pJF15 to complement the Alg$^-$ phenotype (Flynn and Ohman, 1988a).

DEMONSTRATION OF CLONED *algS*(ON) BY GENE REPLACEMENT

As described above, pJF15 cannot complement *algS*(Off) strains, but derivatives of pJF15 with an *algN*::Tn*501* allele do activate alginate production in *trans*

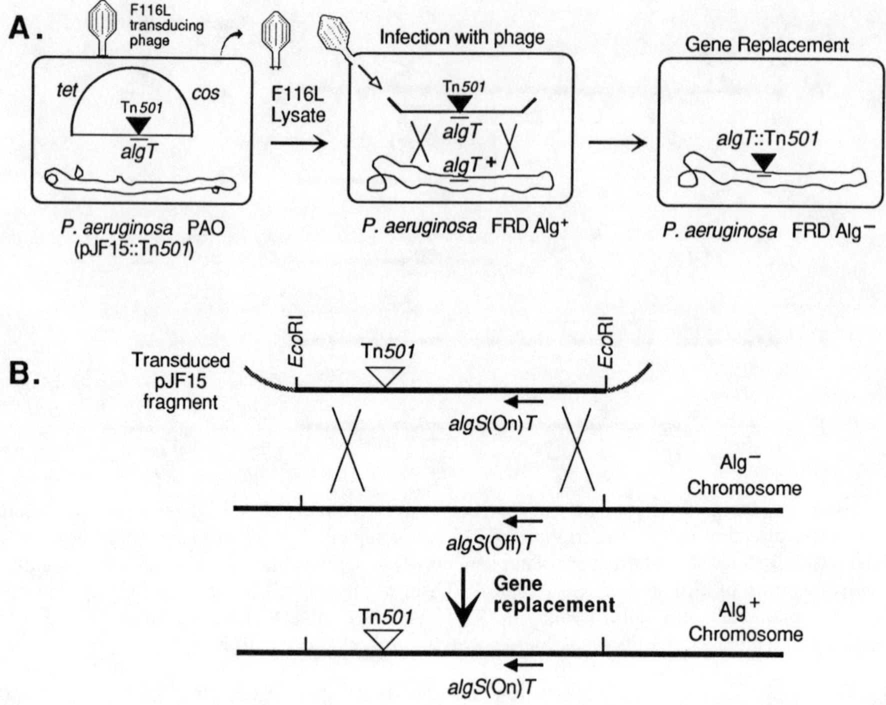

FIGURE 3. (A) Method for phage-mediated gene replacement used to construct *algT*::Tn*501* mutants. Such Alg− mutants display an Alg+ phenotype when they contain pJF15. (B) Demonstration of the presence of *algS*(On) on pJF15, using gene replacement into an *algS*(Off) strain. Tn*501* (encoding mercury resistance) was used as an adjacent selectable marker.

in *algS*(Off) strains. This finding suggested that pJF15 contained the *algS*(On) allele, and the gene replacement technique was used to verify this. A Tn*501* insertion on pJF15 downstream of *algT* was used as an adjacent selectable marker. When DNA from this pJF15::Tn*501* replaced homologous chromosomal DNA, *algS*(Off) was replaced with the transduced *algS*(On)-containing fragment, and restoration of the Alg+ phenotype was frequently observed (Fig. 3B). Thus, pJF15 contained *algS*(On), *algT*, and *algN*. We also confirmed the chromosomal map location of the *algSTN* cluster. The transposon thus placed in the chromosome next to *algS* was used as a marker in mapping experiments, which showed that pJF15 DNA originated from the region of the chromosome near *hisI* at ~68 min (Flynn and Ohman, 1988a).

algS CONTROLS *algT* EXPRESSION

The above-described method of placing a Tn*501* insertion in the chromosome of *P. aeruginosa* next to *algS*(On) was also used to place Tn*501* adjacent to *algS*(Off) (Flynn and Ohman, 1988b). This permitted the cloning of DNA containing the *algS*(Off) allele by selection for the mercury resistance marker of the transposon. In contrast to clones containing *algS*(On)*T*, clones containing *algS*(Off)*T* cannot complement *algT* mutations (Fig. 2E). Thus, *algS* controls the expression of *algT* (Flynn and Ohman, 1988b). Physical comparisons of DNA fragments containing *algS*(On) and *algS*(Off) by restriction analyses have not demonstrated any gross difference between these two clones. This finding suggests that the genetic change from *algS*(On) to *algS*(Off) does not involve a large deletion, insertion, or major inversion of DNA. We are now sequencing this DNA containing *algS*(On) and *algS*(Off) to determine the nature of the alginate switch at *algS*.

We are also studying the mechanism that causes the genetic change from *algS*(Off) to *algS*(On) and vice versa. We have shown that the switching that takes place at *algS* during alginate conversion is independent of the *recA* gene product, indicating that it is not dependent on normal homologous recombination mechanisms in the cell (Ohman et al., 1985). If genetic rearrangement takes place at *algS*, then there is likely to be a site-specific recombinase that catalyzes this event. Although alginate conversion may be a random event, there may be environmental factors (found in the CF lung) that enhance alginate conversion or stimulate expression of genes directly involved in alginate production. There is now evidence that another alginate regulatory gene, *algR*, at 9 min may be responsive to environmental stimuli (Deretic et al., 1989; DeVault et al., 1989).

EVOLUTION OF ALGINATE GENE REGULATION

The regulation of the alginate biosynthetic pathway in *P. aeruginosa* is multigenic and appears to be relatively complex, which suggests that this system has a long evolutionary history. Distant from the alginate biosynthetic gene cluster are the three regulatory regions, *algB*, *algR*, and *algSTN*. The gene products of *algB* and *algR* are required for efficient expression of alginate biosynthetic genes. The genetic switch *algS* appears to initiate alginate gene activation. *algS* acts in *cis* to control the expression of the *trans*-active gene *algT*. Preliminary data indicate that *algT* expression is required for transcriptional activation of the biosynthetic gene cluster (data not shown). In addition to the positive regulatory gene *algT*, the alginate switch region contains a negative regulatory element, *algN*. Elucidation of this complex genetic switching mechanism and the role of the *algT* protein in alginate gene regulation is in progress and should lead to a better understanding of this multigenic regulatory system.

Alginate is secreted in copious amounts (e.g., ~2 mg/ml in culture supernatants), thus channeling much of the available carbon and energy sources toward its production. It is not surprising that alginate biosynthesis would be tightly regulated. Activation of alginate secretion at *algS* may be a rare and spontaneous event that occurs in any population of *P. aeruginosa*. However, when production of alginate is advantageous to the organism (such as in the CF respiratory tract), the rare mucoid cells in the population become predominant because of their selective advantage. When alginate production is no longer advantageous, the instability of the Alg$^+$ phenotype (controlled by the genetic switch *algS*) allows the nonmucoid population to quickly become predominant as a result of the ability to conserve carbon and energy resources. Environmental factors may also play a role in the frequency of alginate conversion.

It is unlikely that this complex regulatory scheme to activate alginate production evolved solely as a pathogenic mechanism specific for the infection of CF patients. *P. aeruginosa* normally dwells in the soil environment, and alginate conversion may have evolved to protect the bacterial population from destruction due to attack by bacteriophages or bacteriocins or from desiccation during periods of dryness. However, *P. aeruginosa* is a remarkable opportunistic pathogen and has adapted the alginate conversion system to promote debilitating and life-threatening pulmonary infections of CF patients. Our continued efforts to understand alginate gene regulation in *P. aeruginosa* may lead to treatments that could turn off alginate production by the organisms resident in the CF lung, thus improving the longevity and quality of life for these patients.

ACKNOWLEDGMENTS. This work was supported by Public Health Service grant AI-19146 from the National Institute of Allergy and Infectious Diseases and by a grant from the Cystic Fibrosis Foundation.

LITERATURE CITED

Baltimore, R. S., and M. Mitchell. 1982. Immunologic investigations of mucoid strains of *Pseudomonas aeruginosa*: comparison of susceptibility to opsonic antibody in mucoid and nonmucoid strains. *J. Infect. Dis.* **141**:238–247.

Darzins, A., S.-K. Wang, R. I. Vanags, and A. M. Chakrabarty. 1985. Clustering of mutations affecting alginic acid biosynthesis in mucoid *Pseudomonas aeruginosa*. *J. Bacteriol.* **164**:516–524.

Deretic, V., R. Dikshit, M. Konyecsni, A. M. Chakrabarty, and T. K. Misra. 1989. The *algR* gene, which regulates mucoidy in *Pseudomonas aeruginosa*, belongs to a class of environmentally responsive genes. *J. Bacteriol.* **171**:1278–1283.

Deretic, V., J. F. Gill, and A. M. Chakrabarty. 1987. Gene *algD* coding for GDPmannose dehydrogenase is transcriptionally activated in mucoid *Pseudomonas aeruginosa*. *J. Bacteriol.* **169**:351–358.

DeVault, J. D., A. Berry, T. K. Misra, A. Darzins, and A. M. Chakrabarty. 1989. Environmental sensory signals and microbial pathogenesis: *Pseudomonas aeruginosa* infection in cystic fibrosis. *Bio/Technology* **7**:352–357.

Doggett, R. G., G. M. Harrison, R. N. Stillwell, and E. S. Wallis. 1966. An atypical *Pseudomonas aeruginosa* associated with cystic fibrosis of the pancreas. *J. Pediatr.* **68**:215–221.

Flynn, J. L., and D. E. Ohman. 1988a. Cloning genes from mucoid *Pseudomonas aeruginosa* which control spontaneous conversion to the alginate producing phenotype. *J. Bacteriol.* **170**:1452–1460.

Flynn, J. L., and D. E. Ohman. 1988b. Use of gene replacement cosmid vector for cloning alginate conversion genes from mucoid and nonmucoid *Pseudomonas aeruginosa* strains: *algS* controls expression of *algT*. *J. Bacteriol.* **170**:3228–3236.

Friedman, A. M., S. R. Long, S. E. Brown, W. J. Buikema, and F. M. Ausubel. 1982. Construction of a broad host range cosmid cloning vector and its use in the genetic analysis of *Rhizobium* mutants. *Gene* **18**:289–296.

Fyfe, J. A. M., and J. R. W. Govan. 1980. Alginate synthesis in mucoid *Pseudomonas aeruginosa*: a chromosomal locus involved in control. *J. Gen. Microbiol.* **119**:443–450.

Fyfe, J. A. M., and J. R. W. Govan. 1981. A revised chromosomal location for *muc*: a locus involved in the control of alginate production by mucoid *Pseudomonas aeruginosa*. *Soc. Gen. Microbiol. Q.* **8**:250–251.

George, R. H. 1987. *Pseudomonas* infection in cystic fibrosis. *Arch. Dis. Child.* **62**:438–439.

Goldberg, J. B., and D. E. Ohman. 1984. Cloning and expression in *Pseudomonas aeruginosa* of a gene involved in the production of alginate. *J. Bacteriol.* **158**:1115–1121.

Goldberg, J. B., and D. E. Ohman. 1987. Construction and characterization of *algB* mutants of *Pseudomonas aeruginosa*: role of *algB* in high-level production of alginate. *J. Bacteriol.* **169:** 1593–1602.

Govan, J. R. W., and G. S. Harris. 1986. *Pseudomonas aeruginosa* and cystic fibrosis: unusual bacterial adaptation and pathogenesis. *Microbiol. Sci.* **3:**302–308.

Hoiby, N. 1974. *Pseudomonas aeruginosa* infection in cystic fibrosis: relationship between mucoid strains of *Pseudomonas aeruginosa* and the humoral immune response. *Acta Pathol. Microbiol. Scand.* **82:**551–558.

MacGeorge, J., V. Korolik, A. F. Morgan, V. Ashe, and B. Holloway. 1986. Transfer of a chromosomal locus responsible for mucoid colony morphology in *Pseudomonas aeruginosa* isolated from cystic fibrosis patients to *P. aeruginosa* PAO. *J. Med. Microbiol.* **21:**331–336.

Marcus, H., and N. R. Baker. 1985. Quantitation of adherence of mucoid and nonmucoid *Pseudomonas aeruginosa* to hamster tracheal epithelium. *Infect. Immun.* **47:**723–729.

Ohman, D. E., and A. M. Chakrabarty. 1981. Genetic mapping of chromosomal determinants for the production of the exopolysaccharide alginate in a *Pseudomonas aeruginosa* cystic fibrosis isolate. *Infect. Immun.* **33:**142–148.

Ohman, D. E., and A. M. Chakrabarty. 1982. Utilization of human respiratory secretions by mucoid *Pseudomonas aeruginosa* of cystic fibrosis origin. *Infect. Immun.* **37:**662–669.

Ohman, D. E., M. A. West, J. L. Flynn, and J. B. Goldberg. 1985. Method for gene replacement in *Pseudomonas aeruginosa* used in construction of *recA* mutants: *recA*-independent instability of alginate production. *J. Bacteriol.* **162:**1068–1074.

O'Hoy, K., and V. Krishnapillai. 1987. Recalibration of the *Pseudomonas aeruginosa* strain PAO chromosome map in time units using high-frequency-of-recombination donors. *Genetics* **115:** 611–618.

Ramphal, R., and G. B. Pier. 1985. Role of *Pseudomonas aeruginosa* mucoid exopolysaccharide in adherence to tracheal cells. *Infect. Immun.* **41:**345–351.

Schwarzmann, S., and J. R. Boring III. 1971. Antiphagocytic effect of slime from a mucoid strain of *Pseudomonas aeruginosa*. *Infect. Immun.* **3:**762–767.

Wood, R. E., T. F. Boat, and C. F. Doershuk. 1976. Cystic fibrosis: state of the art. *Am. Rev. Respir. Dis.* **113:**833–878.

Chapter 4

Molecular Analysis of *Pseudomonas aeruginosa* Elastase

Barbara H. Iglewski, Lynn Rust, and Robert A. Bever

Pseudomonas aeruginosa produces a number of extracellular proteins that are thought to be involved in the pathogenesis of *P. aeruginosa* infections (Liu, 1974; Nicas and Iglewski, 1985). One such protein is elastase. This metalloproteinase degrades a number of biologically important proteins including elastin (Morihara, 1964), collagen (Heck et al., 1986), complement components (Schultz and Miller, 1974), human immunoglobulin (Doring et al., 1981), and serum α_1-proteinase inhibitor (Morihara et al., 1979). Evidence that elastase plays a role in the pathogenesis of *P. aeruginosa* includes the enhancement of *P. aeruginosa* growth in burned skin by elastase (Cicmanec and Holden, 1979), decreased virulence of an elastase mutant (Nicas and Iglewski, 1985), and the production of antielastase antibody during infection by *P. aeruginosa* (Homma et al., 1975). Recently the elastase structural gene has been cloned (Schad et al., 1987) and sequenced (Bever and Iglewski, 1988) and the protein has been crystallized and its structure has been solved (D. McKay, personal communication). Analysis of these data has provided considerable information on the structure, function, processing, and secretion of elastase. The availability of the cloned elastase gene has also permitted us to begin studies on the regulation of elastase expression.

STRUCTURE AND FUNCTION OF ELASTASE

Synthesis, Processing, and Excretion of Elastase

The elastase structural gene (*lasB*) was cloned from a cosmid library prepared using DNA from *P. aeruginosa* PAO (Schad et al., 1987). The clone (pRF1) directed the synthesis of active elastase in *Escherichia coli* and hybridized to an oligonucleotide probe corresponding to the amino acid sequence of the amino

Barbara H. Iglewski, Lynn Rust, and Robert A. Bever ● Department of Microbiology and Immunology, University of Rochester School of Medicine and Dentistry, Rochester, New York 14642.

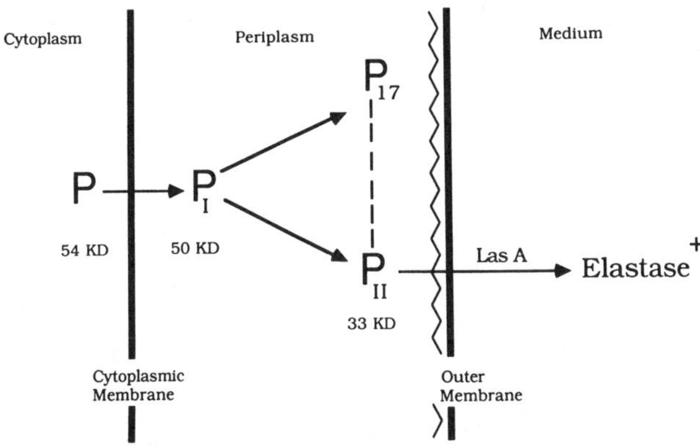

FIGURE 1. Model of processing of elastase in *P. aeruginosa*. P_I, Preproelastase; P_I and P_{II}, proelastase. The *lasA* protein is thought to reside on or in the outer membrane. (From Iglewski, 1989.)

terminus of purified elastase which we had previously determined using Edman degradation (Schad et al., 1987). The sequence of the DNA inclusive of the *lasB* gene contained an open reading frame of 1,491 nucleotides. This open reading frame would code for a 497-amino-acid protein of molecular mass 53.6 kilodaltons (kDa) (Bever and Iglewski, 1988), whereas extracellular elastase has a molecular mass of 33 kDa (Morihara and Isuzuki, 1975). From the deduced amino acid sequence of the *lasB* gene, we located the amino terminus of the mature extracellular elastase at amino acid 199. There was perfect agreement from amino acids 199 to 239 between the sequence derived by Edman degradation and the amino acid sequence deduced from the DNA sequence. We confirmed the existence of this large 53.6-kDa precursor by using a cell-free transcription-translation system. This precursor was named preproelastase (Bever and Iglewski, 1988) (Fig. 1).

The amino-terminal region of the preproelastase contains a putative signal sequence which was similar to others from procaryotes. Interestingly, there are four possible cleavage sites (Ala-Ala) within this leader peptide: amino acids 20–21, 23–24, 36–37, and 48–49. While it is possible that the leader peptide is cleaved from the preproelastase in several steps, cell fractionation studies (Kessler and Saffrin, 1988) and our data using the cell-free transcription-translation system suggest that a single cleavage occurs between amino acids 36 and 37, giving rise to a proelastase of 50 kDa. Kessler and Saffrin (1988) have further shown that the 50-kDa proelastase is cleaved into two proteins (33 and 17 kDa) in the periplasm of *P. aeruginosa*. These two proteins are noncovalently associated and as such are enzymatically inactive (Kessler and Saffrin, 1988). This suggests that the function of the 17-kDa propeptide is to block the enzymatic activity of elastase in order to protect other periplasmic proteins from proteolytic destruction. Proteinases produced by *Bacillus amyloliquefaciens*, *Bacillus subtilis*, and *Serratia* spp. (Nakahama et al., 1986; Vasnatha et al., 1984; Wells et al., 1983) also have propeptides between their signal sequences and the mature (extracellular) proteinase which presumably block the proteolytic activity of the cell-associated proteinase. These are removed upon secretion, giving rise to an enzymatically active extracellular proteinase. In the case of *P. aeruginosa* elastase, transport of the 33-kDa elastase across the outer membrane (thereby separating it from the 17-kDa propeptide) is not sufficient in itself to yield a fully enzymatically active elastase.

A mutant (*lasA1*) was isolated which produces wild-type levels of a 33-kDa extracellular elastase which has greatly reduced elastolytic activity (Ohman et al., 1980). The *lasA1* mutation was mapped at 75 min on the PAO1 chromosome (Howe et al., 1983). The *lasA* gene is distinct from the elastase structural gene (*lasB*). We have cloned and sequenced the *lasA* gene (Schad and Iglewski, 1988; Schad et al., 1987). Analysis of the *lasA* gene sequence showed an open reading frame which codes for a 41-kDa protein. The *lasA* promoter did not function in *E. coli*; however, when *lasA* was expressed in *E. coli* under the PT-7 promoter, a 40-kDa protein was detected. The LasA protein was localized to the outer membrane of *E. coli* and shown to activate the elastolytic activity of the extracellular elastase produced by the *P. aeruginosa lasA* mutant, PAO-E64 (Schad and Iglewski, 1988). The LasA protein has also been localized to the outer membrane in *P. aeruginosa* (J. M. Rose, S. J. Cryz, Jr., and D. E. Ohman, *Abstr. Annu. Meet. Am. Soc. Microbiol. 1989*, abstr. no. B234, p. 69). Although the exact mechanism whereby LasA activates elastase is not known, Rose et al. have suggested that the LasA protein is involved in correctly forming the disulfide bonds in elastase. Further, we have shown that deletion of six amino acids from the carboxy terminus of elastase, which includes the fourth cysteine, yields an enzymatically inactive elastase (Bever and Iglewski, 1988).

Structure and Function of Extracellular Elastase

Extracellular elastase contains 299 amino acids. It is a neutral metalloproteinase which contains one zinc and one calcium (Morihara and Isuzuki, 1975). While considerable homology was found between the amino acid sequence of elastase and those of other procaryotic metalloproteinases, the greatest homology was with thermolysin. The overall homology between thermolysin and extracellular elastase was 28%. The area of greatest homology (48%) encompassed positions 138 to 182 of thermolysin and 136 to 180 of elastase. This region spans the active site cleft of thermolysin, which includes the three zinc ligands at His-142, His-146, and Glu-166; the active-site Glu-143 (considered essential for catalysis); and the three amino acids Tyr-157, His-231, and Asp-226, which are thought to compose the substrate-binding region of thermolysin (Holmes and Matthews, 1982; Matthews et al., 1974). All of these amino acids are conserved in elastase. Based on these homologies, we predicted the zinc ligands of *P. aeruginosa* elastase to be His-140, His-144, and Glu-164 and the active site to be Glu-141. We also predicted that substrate binding should occur with Tyr-155, His-233, and Asp-221 (Bever and Iglewski, 1988) (Fig. 2).

Elastase has recently been crystallized, and its three-dimensional structure has been solved at 1.6 Å (0.16 nm) resolution (McKay, personal communication). The overall tertiary structures of elastase and thermolysin are very similar, both

		ELASTASE	THERMOLYSIN
ZINC LIGANDS		His-140 His-144 Glu-164	His-142 His-146 Glu-166
ACTIVE CENTER		Glu-141	Glu-143
SUBSTRATE BINDING		Tyr-155 His-223 Asp-221	Tyr-157 His-231 Asp-226

FIGURE 2. Comparison of critical amino acids in the active site of elastase and thermolysin.

having an upper and a lower domain separated by a cleft. The amino acids predicted to bind zinc, the active center His-223, and the substrate-binding amino acids are all located at the inner surface of the elastase cleft. The major difference between these two enzymes is that the substrate-binding cleft is more open in elastase than in thermolysin. Presumably, this accounts for the differences in substrate specificity and reactivity exhibited by elastase as compared to thermolysin. Other differences between elastase and thermolysin include the presence of four cysteines in elastase at positions 30, 58, 270, and 297, whereas thermolysin has no cysteines. The crystalline model shows that in elastase the cysteines form disulfide bonds with their nearest neighbor (e.g., Cys-30–Cys-58). In addition, thermolysin has four calcium-binding sites, whereas elastase has only one. The structure and function of thermolysin have been extensively studied using the purified protein, but to our knowledge the gene coding for thermolysin has not been cloned. The availability of the cloned *lasB* gene will permit us to directly test the role of various amino acids in substrate binding and catalysis.

REGULATION OF ELASTASE PRODUCTION

Elastase is not produced constitutively. While there is considerable variation in the maximum amount of elastase produced by different strains of *P. aeruginosa*, most strains (>90%) produce some elastase. Extracellular elastase appears during late log phase, and there is an inverse relationship between growth rate and elastase yields which correlates with the proton motive forces (Whooley et al., 1983). Higher yields of elastase are achieved by increasing the pH of the growth medium (Whooley and McLaughlin, 1983). Elastase yields are decreased by increasing the concentration of iron, ammonium chloride, or certain carbon sources such as glucose (Bjorn et al., 1979; Kessler and Safrin, 1983; Whooley et al., 1983). Extracellular elastase activity is also decreased by adding certain antibiotics to the growth medium, even when the amount of drug added is 10% or less of that required to inhibit bacterial growth (Grimwood et al., 1989; Shibl and Al-Sowaygh, 1980). Given the complex posttranslational modifications elastase undergoes, it is not possible to determine the level at which these environmental stimuli (or inhibitors) act by examining extracellular yields or activity of elastase. Therefore, we have utilized the cloned *lasB* gene to study the regulation of elastase expression in *P. aeruginosa*.

The *lasB* clone (Bever and Iglewski, 1988) contained several hundred nucleotides upstream of the translational start site. We used S1 nuclease analysis to determine whether the *lasB* promoter was located within this region. A single start of transcription was identified at 139 base pairs upstream of the translational start site (L. Rust, V. Deretic, D. G. Storey, A. Sinai, and B. H. Iglewski, manuscript in preparation).

To study the regulation of elastase synthesis, we constructed a gene fusion utilizing a promoterless reporter gene coding for β-galactosidase. β-Galactosidase was chosen as an indicator since it requires no posttranslational modification and is active in the cytoplasm. The *lacZ* gene was fused in frame with 388 base pairs of *P. aeruginosa* DNA. In this construct, expression of β-galactosidase is under the control of the *lasB* promoter, ribosome binding site, and ATG start codon.

The *lasB* promoter and ribosome binding site are both functional in *E. coli*. However, much less β-galactosidase was produced in *E. coli* containing the *lasB-lacZ* fusion than in *P. aeruginosa*. Using identical growth conditions and correcting for plasmid copy number, we estimate that the *lasB* promoter is 0.1% as active in *E. coli* as in *P. aeruginosa*. This suggests that *P. aeruginosa* (but not *E. coli*) contains one or more factors which positively affect *lasB* gene expression.

Yields of elastase are inversely proportional to the concentration of iron in the growth medium (Bjorn et al., 1979). We examined the effect of iron on production of the LasB-LacZ fusion protein. Increasing the concentration of Fe^{3+} ion in the growth medium from 0.05 to 2 μg/ml reduced the amount of LasB-LacZ fusion protein by over 70%. In contrast, the amount of LasB-LacZ fusion protein produced in *E. coli* MC1061 was not significantly reduced when the cells were grown in the presence of increasing concentrations of Fe^{3+} ion, nor did depletion of iron from the growth medium increase the expression of *lasB* in *E. coli*. Elastase production may be negatively regulated by iron in *P. aeruginosa* at the level of either transcription or translation. The expression of the LasB-LacZ fusion protein was examined over the growth cycle of *P. aeruginosa* in medium containing 0.05 μg of Fe^{3+} (low iron) or 10 μg of Fe^{3+} (high iron) per ml. In both cultures, β-galactosidase activity was first detectable at 5 to 6 h of growth, which corresponded to early stationary phase. In high-iron medium, β-galactosidase activity continued to increase until 7 to 8 h, after which it remained constant. A different pattern was seen when PAO1 containing the *lasB-lacZ* fusion was grown in low-iron medium. For the first 7 h, β-galactosidase activity increased in parallel with the high-iron cultures. Beginning at 8 h, a second burst of *lasB* expression was seen in the low-iron cultures which continued through late log phase (10 h). The first phase of *lasB* expression is independent of the iron concentration of the growth medium, whereas the second phase is negatively regulated by iron (Rust et al., in preparation). This biphasic pattern of *lasB* expression is identical to what we have observed for exotoxin A expression in *P. aeruginosa* (Frank and Iglewski, 1988; Frank et al., 1989; Hindahl et al., 1987). The exotoxin A gene has but a single promoter (Grant and Vasil, 1986) which is positively regulated by the *regA* gene (Hedstrom et al., 1986). The *regA* gene has two promoters, P1 and P2 (Frank et al., 1989). Transcription from P1 occurs in early log phase and is independent of iron regulation, whereas transcription from P2 occurs during mid- to late log phase and is completely inhibited by increasing the iron concentration in the growth medium (Frank et al., 1989). The similarity of expression of *lasB* and *toxA*, together with the reduced activity of the *lasB* promoter in *E. coli*, strongly suggests that *lasB* is positively regulated in *trans* by a second gene in *P. aeruginosa*. We have begun to search for this hypothetical *P. aeruginosa* gene.

SUMMARY

The cloning and sequencing of the *lasB* gene (Bever and Iglewski, 1988; Holmes and Matthews, 1982), together with the recent solution of the crystal structure of elastase, have contributed greatly to our knowledge of the structure and function of this metallo-endopeptidase. Use of site-directed mutagenesis will permit us to substantiate the relative importance of specific amino acids in substrate specificity and their contributions to enzyme catalysis. Characterization of the *lasB* gene (Bever and Iglewski, 1988; Schad et al., 1987) and cell fractionation studies (Kessler and Safrin, 1983) have provided information on the complex posttranslational modifications elastase undergoes as it is excreted from *P. aeruginosa*. The interaction of at least six gene products appears to be involved in processing and transport of elastase from the cytoplasm to the external environment. Isolation and characterization of these genes and their products should contribute much to our understanding of protein secretion and excretion by gram-negative bacteria. Finally, elastase expression is highly regulated. Initial studies employing a gene fusion between *lasB* and *lacZ* indicate that *lasB* is under both positive and negative regulation.

ACKNOWLEDGMENTS. We thank D. G. Storey and A. Sinai for the *lasB-lacZ* gene fusion and V. Deretic for the S1 mapping of *lasB*.

This work was supported by a grant from the Cystic Fibrosis Foundation and by Public Health Service grant AI25669 from the National Institutes of Health.

LITERATURE CITED

Bever, R. A., and B. H. Iglewski. 1988. Molecular characterization and nucleotide sequence of the *Pseudomonas aeruginosa* elastase structural gene. *J. Bacteriol.* **170:**4309–4314.

Bjorn, M. J., P. A. Sokol, and B. H. Iglewski. 1979. Influence of iron on yields of extracellular products of *Pseudomonas aeruginosa*. *J. Bacteriol.* **138:**193–200.

Cicmanec, J. F., and I. A. Holden. 1979. Growth of *Pseudomonas aeruginosa* in normal and burned skin extract: role of extracellular proteases. *Infect. Immun.* **25:**477–483.

Doring, G., H. J. Obernesser, and K. Botzenhart. 1981. Extracellular toxin of *Pseudomonas aeruginosa*. II. Effect of two proteases on human immunoglobulins IgG, IgA and secretory IgA. *Zentralbl. Bakteriol. Mikrobiol. Hyg. 1 Abt. Orig. Reihe A* **249:**89–98.

Frank, D. W., and B. H. Iglewski. 1988. Kinetics of *toxA* and *regA* mRNA accumulation in *Pseudomonas aeruginosa*. *J. Bacteriol.* **170:**4477–4483.

Frank, D. W., D. G. Story, M. S. Hindahl, and B. H. Iglewski. 1989. Differential regulation by iron of *regA* and *toxA* transcript accumulation in *Pseudomonas aeruginosa*. *J. Bacteriol.* **171:**5304–5313.

Grant, C. C. R., and M. L. Vasil. 1986. Analysis of transcription of the exotoxin A gene of *Pseudomonas aeruginosa*. *J. Bacteriol.* **168:**1112–1119.

Grimwood, K., M. To, H. R. Rabin, and D. E. Woods. 1989. Inhibition of *Pseudomonas aeruginosa* exoenzyme expression by subinhibitory antibiotic concentrations. *Antimicrob. Agents Chemother.* 33:41–47.

Heck, L. W., K. Morihara, W. B. McRae, and E. J. Miller. 1986. Specific cleavage of human type III and IV collagens by *Pseudomonas aeruginosa* elastase. *Infect. Immun.* 51:115–118.

Hedstrom, R. C., C. R. Funtz, J. B. Kaper, O. R. Pavlovskio, and D. R. Calloway. 1986. Cloning of a gene involved in regulation of exotoxin A expression in *Pseudomonas aeruginosa*. *Infect. Immun.* 51:37–42.

Hindahl, M. S., D. W. Frank, and B. H. Iglewski. 1987. Molecular studies of a positive regulator of toxin A synthesis in *Pseudomonas aeruginosa*. *Antibiot. Chemother.* 39:279–289.

Holmes, M. A., and B. W. Matthews. 1982. Structure of thermolysin refined at 1.6 angstrom resolution. *J. Mol. Biol.* 160:623–639.

Homma, J. V., T. Tomiyama, H. Sano, Y. Hirao, and K. Sakui. 1975. Passive hemagglutination reaction test using formalinized sheep erythrocytes treated with tannic acid and coated with protease or elastase from *Pseudomonas aeruginosa*. *Jpn. J. Exp. Med.* 45:361–365.

Howe, T., R. B. Wretlind, and B. H. Iglewski. 1983. Comparison of two methods of genetic exchange in determination of the genetic locus of the structural gene for *Pseudomonas aeruginosa*. *J. Bacteriol.* 156:58–61.

Iglewski, B. H. 1989. Probing *Pseudomonas aeruginosa*, an opportunistic pathogen. *ASM News* 55:303–308.

Kessler, E., and M. Safrin. 1983. Comparative effect of ammonium and sodium salts on growth of *Pseudomonas aeruginosa* and on protease (elastase) production. *FEMS Microbiol. Lett.* 20:87–90.

Kessler, E., and M. Safrin. 1988. Synthesis, processing and transport of *Pseudomonas aeruginosa* elastase. *J. Bacteriol.* 170:5241–5247.

Liu, P. V. 1974. Extracellular toxins of *Pseudomonas aeruginosa*. *J. Infect. Dis.* 130:S94–S99.

Matthews, B. W., L. H. Weaver, and W. R. Kester. 1974. The conformation of thermolysin. *J. Biol. Chem.* 249:8030–8044.

Morihara, K. 1964. Production of elastase and proteinase by *Pseudomonas aeruginosa*. *J. Bacteriol.* 88:745–757.

Morihara, K., and H. Isuzuki. 1975. *Pseudomonas aeruginosa* elastase: affinity chromatography and some properties as a metallo-neutral proteinase. *Agric. Biol. Chem.* 39:1123–1128.

Morihara, K., H. Isuzuki, and K. Oda. 1979. Protease and elastase of *Pseudomonas aeruginosa*: inactivation of plasma α_1-proteinase inhibitor. *Infect. Immun.* 24:188–193.

Nakahama, K., K. Yoshimura, R. Marumoto, M. Kikuchi, I. S. Lee, T. Hase, and H. Matsubara. 1986. Cloning and sequencing of Serratia protease gene. *Nucleic Acids Res.* 14:5843–5855.

Nicas, T. I., and B. H. Iglewski. 1985. The contribution of exoproducts to virulence of *Pseudomonas aeruginosa*. *Can. J. Microbiol.* 31:387–392.

Ohman, D. E., S. J. Cryz, and B. H. Iglewski. 1980. Isolation and characterization of a *Pseudomonas aeruginosa* PAO mutant that produces altered elastase. *J. Bacteriol.* 142:836–842.

Schad, P. A., R. A. Bever, T. I. Nicas, F. Leduc, L. F. Homme, and B. H. Iglewski. 1987. Cloning and characterization of elastase genes from *Pseudomonas aeruginosa*. *J. Bacteriol.* 169:2691–2696.

Schad, P. A., and B. H. Iglewski. 1988. Nucleotide sequence and expression in *Escherichia coli* of the *Pseudomonas aeruginosa* lasA gene. *J. Bacteriol.* 170:2784–2789.

Schultz, D. R., and K. D. Miller. 1974. Elastase of *Pseudomonas aeruginosa*: inactivation of complement components and complement derived chemotactic and phagocytic factors. *Infect. Immun.* 10:128–135.

Shibl, A. M., and I. A. Al-Sowaygh. 1980. Antibiotic inhibition of protease production by *Pseudomonas aeruginosa*. *J. Med. Microbiol.* 13:345–349.

Vasnatha, N., L. Thompson, C. Rhodes, C. Banner, J. Nagle, and D. Filpula. 1984. Genes for alkaline protease and neutral protease from *Bacillus amyloliquefaciens* contain a large open reading frame between the regions coding for signal sequence and mature protein. *J. Bacteriol.* 159:811–819.

Wells, J. A., E. Farrari, D. J. Henner, D. A. Estell, and E. Y. Chen. 1983. Cloning sequencing and secretion of *Bacillus amyloliquefaciens* subtilisin in *Bacillus subtilis*. *Nucleic Acids Res.* 11:7911–7925.

Whooley, M. A., and A. J. McLaughlin. 1983. The proton motive force in *Pseudomonas aeruginosa* and its relationship to exoprotease production. *J. Gen. Microbiol.* **129:**989–996.
Whooley, M. A., J. A. O'Callahan, and A. J. McLaughlin. 1983. Effect of substrate on the regulation of exoprotease production by *Pseudomonas aeruginosa* ATCC 10145. *J. Gen. Microbiol.* **129:** 981–988.

Part II

PLANT-BACTERIAL INTERACTIONS

Organization of the *hrpM* Locus of *Pseudomonas syringae* pv. *syringae* and Its Potential Function in Pathogenesis[†]

Dallice Mills and Pradip Mukhopadhyay

The *Pseudomonas* group of phytopathogenic bacteria consists of approximately 40 pathovars that are distinguished by their host range, pathogenesis, the disease symptoms elicited in their host plants, and biochemical properties (Young et al., 1978). Bacterial brown spot disease of bean (*Phaseolus vulgaris* L.) is caused by *Pseudomonas syringae* pv. *syringae* and was first described by Burkholder (1930). The disease symptoms on leaves are characterized by necrotic, brown lesions that occasionally have chlorotic margins (Patel et al., 1964), and the leaves frequently bend or pucker at the point of inoculation. In pod assays, strains of *P. syringae* pv. *syringae* from diverse sources produced either water-soaked lesions or brown, necrotic, sunken lesions (Saad and Hagedorn, 1971). Although first described about 60 years ago, bacterial brown spot disease was not a serious problem until its discovery in the 1960s in Wisconsin (Patel et al., 1964). Today it is present in other bean-producing states and can be introduced through use of contaminated seed (Hoitink et al., 1968).

The development of molecular genetic tools for analysis of medically important pseudomonads has immensely benefited similar studies of phytopathogenic pseudomonads. Major advances have been realized in the identification and cloning of genes that appear to specifically function in pathogenesis of host plants. However, the mechanism by which products of many of these genes function in susceptible hosts remains an enigma. Studies of the molecular genetics of toxin production among the phytopathogenic pseudomonads (A. K. Chatterjee, G. Somlyai, and R. O. Nordeen, this volume; Morgan and Chatterjee, 1985; Xu and Gross, 1988a, 1988b) are providing insight into the evolution of mechanisms

---

[†] Oregon State Agricultural Experiment Station technical paper no. 8970.

Dallice Mills • Department of Botany and Plant Pathology, Oregon State University, Corvallis, Oregon 97331.   ***Pradip Mukhopadhyay*** • Crop Protection Department, Monsanto Agricultural Company, St. Louis, Missouri 63198.

that contribute to the overall virulence of these pathogens. However, a large number of genes have been cloned by functional complementation of homologous mutant genes about which little is known except that their products are required to incite disease in susceptible hosts. As the molecular genetics of plant pathogenic bacteria have rapidly evolved, the methodology and progress have been the subjects of several timely reviews (Chatterjee and Vidaver, 1986; Daniels et al., 1988; Keen and Staskawicz, 1988; Mills, 1985; Panopoulos and Peet, 1985).

The approaches and strategies used to clone the pathogenicity locus described in this chapter, which has been designated *hrpM*, were generally used in other laboratories (see, for example, Chatterjee et al., this volume, and Panopoulos and co-workers [Mindrinos et al., this volume]) to clone genes from various phytopathogenic pseudomonads. The organization, nucleotide sequence, and speculation about the function of this locus are also discussed.

TAGGING PATHOGENICITY GENES BY TRANSPOSON MUTAGENESIS

Notable among advances that led to the rapid cloning of pathogenicity determinants among pseudomonads was the development of a selection of plasmids referred to as suicide plasmids because of their inability to replicate in the recipient cells. These plasmids contain antibiotic resistance-encoding transposable elements for general use in transposon mutagenesis (reviewed by Mills [1985]). They are maintained in *Escherichia coli* strains and may be introduced into recipient pseudomonads by conjugation with relatively high frequencies. Transposable element Tn*5*, which encodes resistance to kanamycin (Km^r) and transposes randomly with high efficiency in *Pseudomonas* spp., thereby providing large numbers of Tn*5*-containing colonies for mutational analysis from a single experiment, has been widely used for general mutagenesis.

A procedure used to mutagenize *P. syringae* pv. *syringae* is presented in Fig. 1. The mating between *E. coli* SM10(pSUP1011) (Km^r chloramphenicol resistant [Cm^r]) and *P. syringae* pv. *syringae* PS9020 (streptomycin resistant [Sm^r]) is performed on dry 3% agar (LB medium), using a 1:2 donor/recipient ratio. Medium containing streptomycin and kanamycin is used to counterselect *E. coli* and permit growth of Tn*5*-containing transconjugants, which are then screened for properties unique to *Pseudomonas* spp. (fluorescence on King medium B and failure to grow at 37°C). Prototrophic Km^r Sm^r colonies are bioassayed on a susceptible bean cultivar to identify colonies with altered pathogenicity. The pathogenicity-deficient mutants identified in our studies (Anderson and Mills, 1985) were obtained after toothpick inoculation of young primary leaves of the susceptible bean cultivar Red Mexican UI-36.

PROPERTIES OF PATHOGENICITY MUTANTS

Typically, foliar pathogens incite disease symptoms 3 to 6 days after inoculation of susceptible plants. Resistant plants or nonhost plants exhibit a rapid

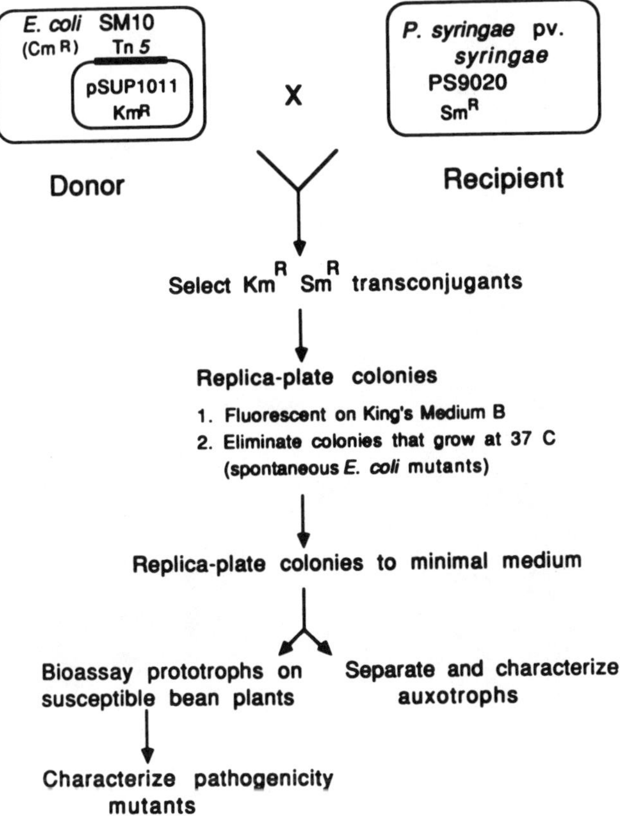

FIGURE 1. Scheme for transposon mutagenesis of phytopathogenic pseudomonads. The construction and genetic properties of the donor strain, SM10, and of suicide vector pSUP1011 have been previously described (Simon et al., 1983); they represent one of several delivery systems available for use with phytopathogenic pseudomonads (reviewed by Mills [1985]).

hypersensitive reaction (HR) that is characterized by localized host cell death and necrosis at the site of inoculation. The HR frequently occurs within 24 h of inoculation and is thought to be a generalized form of plant resistance to pathogens (Klement, 1982). Transposon insertion into some pathogenicity genes has produced pleiotropic effects in which the abilities to incite both disease in susceptible hosts and the HR in nonhosts are lost. The acronym Hrp was chosen by Lindgren et al. (1986) to describe this phenotype, which is exemplified by PS9021 (Niepold et al., 1985; Fig. 2). The locus affected in PS9021 has been designated *hrpM* (Mukhopadhyay et al., 1988b). PS9021 also exhibits a mucoidal colony morphology, whereas the parental strain has firm, smooth colonies. The growth of PS9021::Tn5 is unaffected in liquid complete or minimal salts medium (not shown); however, the strain is unable to grow in susceptible bean cultivars (Bertoni and Mills, 1987; Fig. 3), and cessation of growth is rapid, which could explain the Hrp phenotype, as it is generally acknowledged that a period of growth is required to elicit the HR (Klement, 1982).

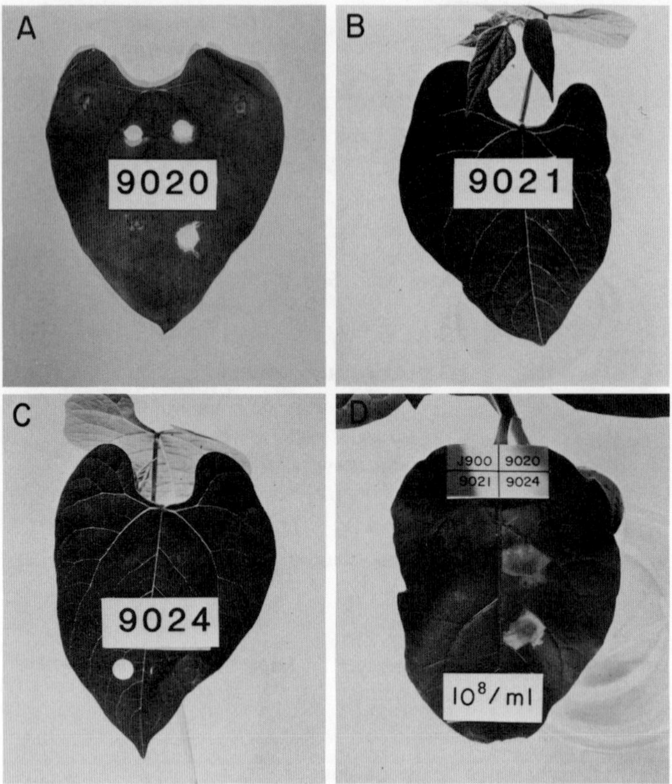

FIGURE 2. Pathogenicity mutants that express the Hrp and Dsg phenotypes. (A) Disease symptoms incited by parental strain PS9020 on susceptible bean cultivar Eagle; (B and C) leaves inoculated at similar sites with PS9021::Tn5 and PS9024::Tn5; (D) the HR in tobacco elicited by pathogenic bacterial brown spot strains J900 and PS9020 and nonpathogenic strain PS9024::Tn5 (Dsg) and the inability of PS9021::Tn5 (Hrp) to elicit the HR.

Some mutations only abolish the ability to incite disease in susceptible plants without affecting the ability to elicit the HR in nonhosts. The phenotype of PS9024 is of this type (Fig. 2), which is referred to as Dsg (disease-specific genes).

MOLECULAR ANALYSIS OF THE *hrpM* LOCUS

The intact Tn5 element can be readily cloned from any mutant strain by digesting total cellular DNA with *Eco*RI, which does not cut within Tn5, ligating the fragments into a vector such as pBR325, and using the ligation mixture to transform *E. coli*. Cells that express resistance to kanamycin usually have the *Eco*RI fragment of interest, which is verified by restriction analysis and Southern hybridization with a probe made from Tn5. The fragment can also be radiolabeled and used to probe a genomic library that is usually constructed in a cosmid vector so as to identify clones that contain homologous wild-type DNA. These cosmid

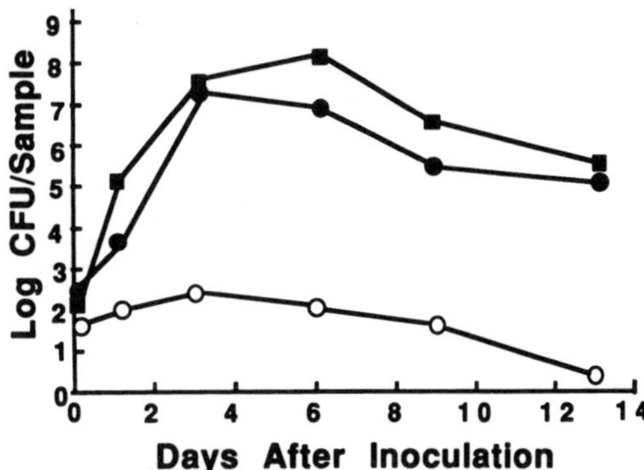

FIGURE 3. Growth kinetics of bacterial brown spot strains in susceptible cultivar Eagle. Symbols: ■, J900; ●, PS9020; ○, PS9021::Tn5.

clones are then used to verify the causal relationship between Tn5 insertion and the mutant phenotype by genetic complementation.

This general approach is frequently used to clone and characterize pathogenicity mutants and was used to obtain the cosmid clone that complements PS9021 (Niepold et al., 1985). All mutant phenotypes (Hrp and mucoidal colony morphology) were complemented by introducing an 8.5-kilobase-pair (kb) *Hin*dIII-*Xho*I fragment from the cosmid clone, pOSU3101. Sequences within a 3.9-kb *Hin*dIII fragment from the 8.5-kb fragment were shown to be colinear with the Tn5-containing mutant *Eco*RI fragment. Using Tn5 site-directed mutagenesis, single Tn5 insertions were obtained and mapped throughout the 8.5-kb fragment. Each of these was then introduced into the wild-type strain PS9020 by gene replacement techniques, also referred to as marker exchange mutagenesis, to generate a series of single-site mutants. That each mutant resulted from double homologous recombination and insertion of Tn5 into the bacterial genome was verified by Southern blot analysis using Tn5 as a probe.

Thus, reverse genetics can provide an estimate of the size and organization of sequences within a cloned region that are essential for expression of a particular phenotype. Transposons that contain promoterless reporter genes, such as Tn3-Spice (Lindgren et al., 1989) or Tn3HoHo1 (Stachel et al., 1985a), can also provide information about the location of the promoter and the direction of transcription of the mutated gene.

Tn5 insertions within the 3.9-kb *Hin*dIII fragment produced the Hrp phenotype (Mills et al., 1985), and promoter activity was detected in subclones from the left end of this fragment (Fig. 4). The nucleotide sequence of the *Hin*dIII fragment (Mukhopadhyay et al., 1988b) revealed an *E. coli*-like consensus promoter sequence in this region, which is upstream of two open reading frames, ORF1 and ORF2. The −10 region of this promoter overlaps the translation initiation codon ATG of ORF1, and no promoter activity was detected immediately upstream of this region. A putative 40-kilodalton polypeptide could be encoded by ORF1, but a second ATG codon located 405 nucleotides downstream and in frame with the translational stop codon may be the correct translation initiation codon and would encode a 28-kilodalton polypeptide. The tryptophan monooxygenase gene, a

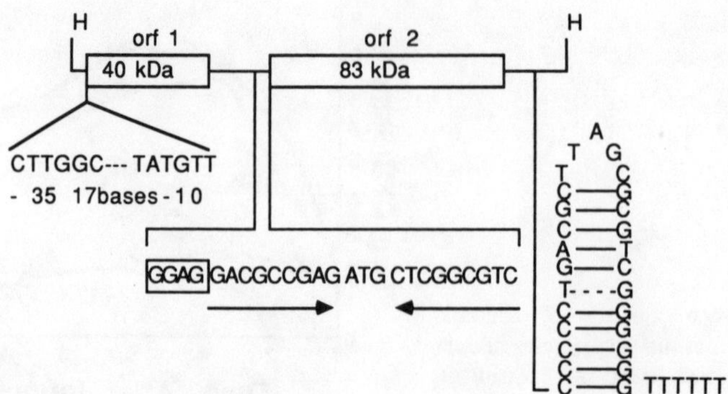

FIGURE 4. The *hrpM* locus of *P. syringae* pv. *syringae*. The organization of ORF1 and ORF2 is depicted (not drawn to scale), with the *E. coli*-like promoter consensus sequence upstream of ORF1, the translational initiation codon for ORF2, and a transcriptional terminator consensus sequence (after Mukhopadhyay et al. [1988a]). kDa, Kilodaltons.

virulence factor of *P. syringae* pv. *savastanoi*, has been shown to be transcribed from an *E. coli*-like promoter located approximately 400 nucleotides upstream of the translation initiation site (T. Gaffney, personal communication).

The translation initiation codon ATG of ORF2 is located 205 nucleotides downstream of the translational stop codon of ORF1. Thirteen nucleotides upstream of this ATG codon is a consensus ribosome-binding site, GGAGGA, the last two bases of which extend into a 9-base-pair repeated sequence (Fig. 4). This repeated sequence forms a perfect palindrome, with the ATG codon located at the apex, and suggests that expression of ORF2 is controlled at the translational level. The features of a consensus transcription terminator are located 175 nucleotides downstream of ORF2 (Mukhopadhyay et al., 1988a, 1988b). The sequencing data indicate that ORF1 and ORF2 are components of a polycistronic operon. The Tn*5* mutation in PS9021 maps within ORF2, but Tn*5* mutations in either ORF produce the Hrp phenotype.

PROPERTIES OF THE PUTATIVE POLYPEPTIDES ENCODED BY ORF1 AND ORF2

A search for amino acid homology with proteins in the GenBank and European Molecular Biology Laboratory data bases failed to identify proteins for which extensive homology could be demonstrated for either of the putative polypeptides encoded by the *hrpM* locus. However, ORF1 has approximately 40 to 45% amino acid identity with the histone H1 genes from rainbow trout, chicken, and *Xenopus laevis* and with other histone genes, suggesting that ORF1 may encode a DNA-binding protein. The identity is primarily near the carboxy terminus of ORF1, which shows an interesting nine-amino-acid motif that is repeated eight times (Fig. 5). The significance of this amino acid repeat is unclear at this time, but work in progress is focused on determining whether these repeated amino acids fold into fingerlike complexes that interact with DNA. It is interesting to speculate that if this is a DNA-binding protein, it may function in regulating the expression of ORF2, perhaps by binding at or near the palindrome at the projected translation initiation codon (Fig. 4).

The distribution of hydrophilic and hydrophobic amino acids was determined for ORF2 by using several computer programs to obtain insight regarding its function. This ORF encodes a protein that has membrane-spanning helices characteristic of transmembrane proteins such as rhodopsin (Mukhopadhyay et al., 1988b). Since mutations in this gene result in altered colony morphology, this protein may reside in the periplasmic membrane.

SPECULATION ON THE FUNCTION OF THE *hrpM* GENE

Transposon mutagenesis has been very successfully used in many recent studies to identify pathogenicity genes in phytopathogenic pseudomonads. Ascertaining a function for any cloned pathogenicity genes that lack homology with previously characterized, cloned genes is extremely challenging. However, clue of a possible function of the *hrpM* gene has emerged by exhaustively testing *hrpM* strains for physiological and biochemical parameters that may have been altered.

The *hrpM* mutants may be routinely cultured on King medium B or on a minimal salts medium, but unlike the parental strain and other pathogenicity mutants in our collection, they fail to grow on these media when the nutrients are diluted 20-fold (P. Mukhopadhyay and D. Mills, unpublished data). However, growth resumes if only the nitrogen source is amended to the normal concentration. By using several nitrogen sources, including amino acids and organic nitrogenous compounds that are synthesized by the host bean plant, experiments were initiated to ascertain whether *hrpM* controls uptake and assimilation of plant-synthesized nitrogenous compounds.

During growth in culture media containing ammonium chloride as the nitrogen source, the uptake of the ammonium ion through diffusion or a general permease system may be sufficient to account for growth of *hrpM* mutants and the parental strain. The availability of nitrogenous compounds varies in planta, depending on growth conditions of the plant and whether the bean plant is fixing nitrogen, and specific permeases may be required by these bacterial pathogens for uptake and subsequent assimilation of plant-synthesized nitrogenous compounds. It is conceivable that the *hrpM* gene product is a permease for plant-synthesized nitrogenous compounds, which would explain the rapid cessation of growth by *hrpM* mutants in susceptible host plants. Recent work (Mukhopadhyay and Mills, unpublished results) has revealed that glutamine, a constituent of plant xylem and a factor in repression of nitrogen uptake in *E. coli*, inhibits growth of the mutant strain and, to a lesser extent, the parental wild-type strain, fueling speculation that *hrpM* is involved in nitrogen uptake. Other alternative functions for *hrpM* should not be discounted, however, as it is entirely possible that the inability of *hrpM* mutants to grow in 20-fold-diluted culture media is yet another manifestation of the pleiotropic effect of this mutation. As previously noted, *hrpM* mutants are

ORF1

```
AAG CTT GGC GTT GCT CCT CTG ACC AGT ATG TTC CTG TTC GGC GCC AAC CAG CCT TCG CGT GTG CCT AAC TAC CGT CGT GAA CTG CAC GAT 90
            MET Phe Leu Phe Gly Ala Asn Gln Pro Ser Arg Val Pro Asn Tyr Arg Arg Glu Leu His Asp

TCC AGC GGT CTG TCG ATT CAG GCG GCC AAC GGT GAG TGG CTG TGG CGT CCG CTG AAC AAC CCT AAA CAT CTG TCC ATC AGC AGC TTC TCG 180
Ser Ser Gly Leu Ser Ile Gln Ala Ala Asn Gly Glu Trp Leu Trp Arg Pro Leu Asn Asn Pro Lys His Leu Ser Ile Ser Ser Phe Ser

GTC GAG AAC CCG CGT GGT TTC GGT CTG CTG CAA CGT GGC CGC GAC TTC AGC CAG TAC GAA GAC CTG GAT GAC CGC TAC GAC AAG CGT CCA 270
Val Glu Asn Pro Arg Gly Phe Gly Leu Leu Gln Arg Gly Arg Asp Phe Ser Gln Tyr Glu Asp Leu Asp Asp Arg Tyr Asp Lys Arg Pro

AGT GCC TGG ATC GAG CCG AAG GGC GAT TGG GGT AAA GGG ACT GTC GAG CTG GTC GAA ATT CCG ACT GCC GAC GAG ACC AAC GAC AAC ATC 360
Ser Ala Trp Ile Glu Pro Lys Gly Asp Trp Gly Lys Gly Thr Val Glu Leu Val Glu Ile Pro Thr Ala Asp Glu Thr Asn Asp Asn Ile
                                                                      orf
GTA GCT TAC TGG AAG CCT GAA ACG CTG GCC GAG CCT GGT CAG GAA ATG GCG TTC GAC TAC CGT CTG CAC TGG ACC ATG CAG GAA AAC TCG 450
Val Ala Tyr Trp Lys Pro Glu Thr Leu Ala Glu Pro Gly Gln Glu MET Ala Phe Asp Tyr Arg Leu His Trp Thr MET Gln Glu Asn Ser
                                                              ──▶
ATT CAC TCG CCG GAT CTG GGC TGG GTC AAG CAG ACT CAA CGC TCC ATC GGT GAC GTG CGT CAG TCC AAC CTG ATC CGT CAG CCG GAC GGC 540
Ile His Ser Pro Asp Leu Gly Trp Val Lys Gln Thr Gln Arg Ser Ile Gly Asp Val Arg Gln Ser Asn Leu Ile Arg Gln Pro Asp Gly

AGC CTT GCC TTC CTG GTC GAC TTC GTG GGC CCG GTG CTG GCC GCA CTG CCG GAA GAC AAG ACC ATT CGC AGC CAG GTG ACC ACT GAC GAC 630
Ser Leu Ala Phe Leu Val Asp Phe Val Gly Pro Val Leu Ala Ala Leu Pro Glu Asp Lys Thr Ile Arg Ser Gln Val Thr Thr Asp Asp

AAC GTC GAG CTG GTG GAA AAC AAC CTG CGC TAC AAC CCG GTC ACC AAA GGT TAC CGC CTG ACC CTG CGT GTC AAG GTC AAG GAT TCC AGC 720
Asn Val Glu Leu Val Glu Asn Asn Leu Arg Tyr Asn Pro Val Thr Lys Gly Tyr Arg Leu Thr Leu Arg Val Lys Val Lys⌈Asp Ser Ser
                                                                                                        −  ⊝  ⊝
AAG CCG ACC GAA ATG CGC GCC TAC CTG TTG CGT GAA ATC CCT GCC GAA CCG GGC AAG GAA CCT GCG CTG CTC GTG GCT GAC AAA GCC GAA 810
Lys Pro Thr Glu MET Arg⌋Ala Tyr Leu Leu Arg Glu Ile Pro Ala⌈Glu Pro Gly Lys⌋Glu Pro Ala Leu Leu Val Ala Asp Lys Ala⌈Glu
 +  P  ⊝  ⊝  ⊝  +                              −  ⊝  ⊝  +                                          −
GAG AAG AAG GCT GCC GCG AAG GAA GCT GCC AAG CCG GCA GTC TCC AAG GAG TCC GCC AAC GAC CAG GTA GAA ATC GCC AAG GCC GAC GCA 900
Glu Lys Lys Ala Ala Ala Lys⌋Glu Ala Ala Lys Pro Ala Val Ser Lys⌋Glu Ser Ala Asn Asp Gln Val⌈Glu Ile Ala Lys Ala Asp Ala
 ⊝  •  +  A  ⊝  ⊝  +   −  ⊝  ⊝  +  P  ⊝  ⊝  ⊝  +                          −  ⊝  ⊝  +  A  ⊝  ⊝
CCC AAG CCG GAA GCT GCC AAG CCT GAG ACT GCC AAG TCC GAA GCT GGC AAG GCT GAC GCA GCC AAA GGC AAA GGC GAA GTC GCC AAG GCC 990
Pro Lys⌋Pro⌈Glu Ala Ala Lys Pro Glu Thr Ala Lys⌋Ser⌈Glu Ala Gly Lys Ala Asp Ala Ala Lys⌋Gly Lys Gly⌈Glu Val Ala Lys Ala
 ⊝  +   −  ⊝  ⊝  +  P  ⊝  ⊝  ⊝  +   −  ⊝  ⊝  +  A  ⊝  ⊝  ⊝  +                  −  ⊝  ⊝  +  A
GAT GCA GGC AAA GCC GAC GCA TCC AAG GCT GAA GCA GCC AAG GAT AAG GAC GGT AAG GAA ATT CAG CAG CCT GAA ACC GAG GCA GCA CCC 1080
Asp Ala Gly Lys⌋Ala Asp Ala Ser Lys Ala⌈Glu Ala Ala Lys Asp Lys Asp Gly Lys⌋Glu Ile Gln Gln Pro Glu Thr Glu Ala Ala Pro
 ⊝  ⊝  ⊝  +              −  ⊝  ⊝  +  •  •  •  •  +
ACC CAT CCG GAA CCG GCC AAG ACG TTG CAA GTC ATG ACC GAG ACC TGG AGC TAT CAG TTG CCG AGC GAT GAG TAA TTC TCT ACC GGT GCC 1170
Thr His Pro Glu Pro Ala Lys Thr Leu Gln Val MET Thr Glu Thr Trp Ser Tyr Gln Leu Pro Ser Asp Glu END
```

mucoidal when grown on certain agar media, a property that might adversely affect the activity of membrane-associated enzymes such as permease.

That the *hrpM* product may function as a signal transducer molecule analogous to the *virA* gene product from *Agrobacterium tumefaciens* (Stachel et al., 1985b, 1986; reviewed by Daniels et al. [1988]) should not be overlooked. The *virA* gene product is localized to the membrane of *A. tumefaciens* and responds to a plant-synthesized phenolic compound, acetosyringone. When activated, it acts as a signal transducer and induces expression of *virG*, which in turn regulates expression of other virulence genes. Whether *hrpM* has a similar role remains to be determined. However, virulence determinants cloned from phytopathogenic pseudomonads have recently been shown to have homology with genes that constitute these two gene component systems (N. Panopoulos, personal communication; M. N. Mindrinos, L. G. Rahme, C. Frederick, E. Hatziloukas, R. Grimm, and N. J. Panopoulos, this volume), and expression of certain pathogenicity genes may be similarly regulated.

STABLE CLONING VECTORS FOR EXPRESSION OF PATHOGENICITY GENES

During the course of these studies and through discussions with other colleagues (personal communications), it has become very apparent that the broad-host-range cosmids and other plasmids that have been derived from RK2 (Ditta et al., 1985) and routinely used to express genes in *Pseudomonas* spp. are frequently very unstable in pathovars of *P. syringae*. Plasmids chosen for expression of cloned pathogenicity genes during in planta growth of bacteria must be stable for a minimum of 4 to 7 days, the period of time required for symptom development in many plant diseases.

To eliminate problems of plasmid instability in the absence of drug selection, an expression vector system was developed (Mukhopadhyay et al., 1990) that is based on the origin of replication and stability gene(s) of pOSU900, a cryptic 80-kb plasmid indigenous to strain J900 (Fig. 3). A high-copy-number *Pseudomonas-E. coli* shuttle vector, designated pOSU223, was constructed with an exogenous *Pseudomonas fluorescens* siderophore promoter cloned upstream of several cloning sites plus antibiotic resistance markers for selection. This vector can be transformed into *P. syringae* pathovars and *P. fluorescens* with high efficiency (ca. 10^6 transformants per μg of DNA), and it is stable during growth of strain PS9020 in planta over a 14-day period without adversely affecting the growth of

---

Figure 5. The repeating amino acid motif within ORF1. The consensus amino acid sequence is Glu-X-X-Lys-Pro/Ala-X-X-X-Lys, where X can be one of several amino acids that are frequently small and carry a neutral charge. A second in-frame ATG translation initiation codon at position 405 is identified as an ORF (see text for discussion). Symbols: +, positively charged amino acid; −, negatively charged amino acid; ⊙, small, usually neutral amino acid; •, amino acid that is inconsistent with the consensus sequence.

the bacteria. Furthermore, efficient transformation of pseudomonads was observed (10^3 to 10^5 transformants per μg of DNA) when large (>20 kb) fragments were cloned into it.

We have established that the *hrpM* gene product is not required for growth in minimal culture medium but is required for growth of bacteria in planta. Using this vector system to overexpress the antisense strand of *hrpM*, we have effectively produced the HrpM phenotype in the parental, pathogenic strain, PS9020 (P. Mukhopadhyay and D. Mills, manuscript in preparation). This phenotype can be reversed by reducing the concentration of antisense *hrpM* RNA. Furthermore, overexpression of *hrpM* can result in a more aggressive or virulent strain on bean or, conversely, lethality. The ability to transiently regulate the level of *hrpM* gene expression should greatly facilitate future studies of the function of this locus and possibly of other pathogenicity genes in the phytopathogenic pseudomonads.

ACKNOWLEDGMENTS. This research was supported by U.S. Department of Agriculture Science and Education Administration grant 85-CRCR-1-1771 from the Competitive Research Grants Office and grant MB8315689 from the National Science Foundation and the Oregon State Agricultural Experiment Station.

LITERATURE CITED

Anderson, D. M., and D. Mills. 1985. The use of transposon mutagenesis in the isolation of nutritional and virulence mutants in two pathovars of *Pseudomonas syringae*. *Phytopathology* **75**:104–108.

Bertoni, G., and D. Mills. 1987. A simple method to monitor growth of bacterial populations in leaf tissue. *Phytopathology* **77**:832–835.

Burkholder, W. H. 1930. The bacterial diseases of the bean: a comparative study. *Cornell Univ. Agric. Exp. Station Mem.* **127**.

Chatterjee, A. K., and A. K. Vidaver. 1986. Genetics of pathogenicity factors: application to phytopathogenic bacteria. *Adv. Plant Pathol.* **4**:1–218.

Daniels, M. J., J. M. Dow, and A. E. Osbourn. 1988. Molecular genetics of pathogenicity in phytopathogenic bacteria. *Annu. Rev. Phytopathol.* **26**:285–312.

Ditta, G., T. Schmidhauser, E. Yakebson, P. Lu, X.-W. Liang, D. R. Finlay, D. Guiney, and D. R. Helinski. 1985. Plasmids related to the broad host range vector, pRK290, useful for gene cloning and for monitoring gene expression. *Plasmid* **13**:149–153.

Hoitink, H. A. J., D. J. Hagedorn, and E. McCoy. 1968. Survival, transmission, and taxonomy of *Pseudomonas syringae* van Hall, the causal organism of bacterial brown spot of bean (*Phaseolus vulgaris* L.) *Can. J. Microbiol.* **14**:437–441.

Keen, N. T., and B. Staskawicz. 1988. Host range determinants in plant pathogens and symbionts. *Annu. Rev. Microbiol.* **42**:421–440.

Klement, Z. 1982. Hypersensitivity, p. 149–177. *In* M. S. Mount and G. H. Lacy (ed.), *Phytopathogenic Procaryotes*, vol. 2. Academic Press, Inc., New York.

Lindgren, P. B., R. Frederick, A. G. Govindarajan, N. J. Panopoulos, B. J. Staskawicz, and S. E. Lindow. 1989. An ice nucleation reporter gene system: identification of inducible pathogenicity genes in *Pseudomonas syringae* pv. *phaseolicola*. *EMBO J.* **8**:1291–1301.

Lindgren, P. B., R. C. Peet, and N. J. Panopoulos. 1986. Gene cluster of *Pseudomonas syringae* pv. "*phaseolicola*" controls pathogenicity of bean plants and hypersensitivity on nonhost plants. *J. Bacteriol.* **168**:512–522.

Mills, D. 1985. Transposon mutagenesis and its potential for studying virulence genes in plant pathogens. *Annu. Rev. Phytopathol.* **23**:381–419.

Mills, D., F. Niepold, and M. Zuber. 1985. Cloned sequence controlling colony morphology and pathogenesis of *Pseudomonas syringae* pv. *syringae*, p. 97–102. *In* I. Sussex, A. Ellingboe, M. Crouch, and R. Malmberg (ed.), *Plant Cell/Cell Interactions*. Cold Spring Harbor Laboratory, Cold Spring Harbor, N.Y.

Morgan, M. K., and A. K. Chatterjee. 1985. Isolation and characterization of Tn*5* insertion mutants of *Pseudomonas syringae* pv. *syringae* altered in the production of the peptide phytotoxin syringotoxin. *J. Bacteriol.* **164:**14–18.

Mukhopadhyay, P., M. Mukhopadhyay, and D. Mills. 1990. Construction of a stable shuttle vector for high-frequency transformation in *Pseudomonas syringae* pv. *syringae*. *J. Bacteriol.* **172:**477–480.

Mukhopadhyay, P., M. Mukhopadhyay, J. Williams, Y. Zhao, and D. Mills. 1988a. Pathogenicity genes of *Pseudomonas syringae*, p. 247–252. *In* R. Palacios and D. P. S. Verma (ed.), *Molecular Genetics of Plant-Microbe Interactions.* APS Press, St. Paul, Minn.

Mukhopadhyay, P., J. Williams, and D. Mills. 1988b. Molecular analysis of a pathogenicity locus in *Pseudomonas syringae* pv. *syringae*. *J. Bacteriol.* **170:**5479–5488.

Niepold, F., D. Anderson, and D. Mills. 1985. Cloning determinants of pathogenesis from *Pseudomonas syringae* pathovar *syringae*. *Proc. Natl. Acad. Sci. USA* **82:**406–410.

Panopoulos, N., and R. Peet. 1985. The molecular genetics of plant pathogenic bacteria and their plasmids. *Annu. Rev. Phytopathol.* **23:**381–419.

Patel, P. N., J. C. Walker, D. J. Hagedorn, C. D. Garcia, and M. Teliz-Ortiz. 1964. Bacterial brown spot of bean in central Wisconsin. *Plant Dis. Rep.* **48:**335–337.

Saad, S. M., and D. J. Hagedorn. 1971. Improved techniques for initiation of bacterial brown spot of bean in the greenhouse. *Phytopathology* **61:**1310–1311.

Simon, R., U. Priefer, and A. Puhler. 1983. A broad host range mobilization system for in vitro genetic engineering: transposon mutagenesis in gram-negative bacteria. *Bio/Technology* **1:**784–791.

Stachel, S. E., G. An, C. Flores, and E. W. Nester. 1985a. A Tn*3-lacZ* transposon for the random generation of β-galactosidase gene fusions: application to the analysis of gene expression in *Agrobacterium. EMBO J.* **4:**891–898.

Stachel, S. E., E. Messens, M. van Montague, and P. Zambryski. 1985b. Identification of the signal molecules produced by wounded plant cells that activate T-DNA transfer in *Agrobacterium tumefaciens. Nature* (London) **318:**624–629.

Stachel, S. E., E. W. Nester, P. C. Zambryski. 1986. *VirA* and *virG* control the plant-induced activation of the T-DNA transfer process of *Agrobacterium tumefaciens. Cell* **46:**325–333.

Xu, G.-W., and D. Gross. 1988a. Evaluation of the role of syringomycin in plant pathogenesis by using Tn*5* mutants of *Pseudomonas syringae* pv. *syringae* defective in syringomycin production. *Appl. Environ. Microbiol.* **54:**1345–1353.

Xu, G.-W., and D. Gross. 1988b. Physical and functional analysis of the *syrA* and *syrB* genes involved in syringomycin production by *Pseudomonas syringae* pv. *syringae*. *J. Bacteriol.* **170:**5680–5688.

Young, J. M., D. W. Dye, J. F. Bradbury, C. G. Panagopoulos, and C. F. Robbs. 1978. A proposed nomenclature and classification for plant pathogenic bacteria. *N.Z. Agric. Res.* **21:**153–177.

Chapter 6

Molecular Cloning and Expression of Syringotoxin (*syt*) Genes of *Pseudomonas syringae* pv. *syringae*

A. K. Chatterjee, G. Somlyai, and R. O. Nordeen

Pseudomonas syringae pathovars cause diseases in a wide variety of plants worldwide (Gross and Cody, 1985). Most of these bacteria produce metabolites that by virtue of their toxicity to plant cells (i.e., by eliciting chlorosis or necrosis) contribute to the development of disease symptoms. Examples of such phytotoxic substances include phaseolotoxin, coronatine, tabtoxin, tagetitoxin, syringotoxin (ST), and syringomycin (SR) (Mitchell, 1981). SR is produced by a variety of *P. syringae* pv. *syringae* strains regardless of host range, whereas ST is produced by strains isolated from *Citrus* spp. These two phytotoxins are similar in several respects, including mode of action (Surico and DeVay, 1982), susceptibility to inactivation by basic solutions (Gonzalez et al., 1981), and broad spectrum of activity (Backman and DeVay, 1971; DeVay et al., 1978). Both of these toxins inhibit the growth of the fungus *Geotrichum candidum*, and this property is exploited in a bioassay.

Structural investigations of SR indicate that this compound is a cyclic hexapeptide consisting of arginine, phenylalanine, serine, diaminobutyric acid (Zhang and Takemoto, 1987), and dehydroaminobutyric acid in a 2:1:1:1:1 molar ratio. The fatty acid 3-hydroxydodecanoic acid is also a component of the toxin (D. Gross, personal communication). ST appears to contain a pentapeptide of serine, threonine, glycine, ornithine, and possibly diaminobutyric acid (Gross et al., 1977; see also Morgan and Chatterjee, 1988). Despite the differences in peptide composition, an overall structural similarity is predicted to account for properties that the toxins have in common.

Synthesis of these toxins is believed to be nonribosomal as in *Bacillus* spp., in which peptide antibiotics are produced on high-molecular-weight multienzyme

---

A. K. Chatterjee, G. Somlyai, and R. O. Nordeen • Department of Plant Pathology, University of Missouri, 108 Waters Hall, Columbia, Missouri 65211.

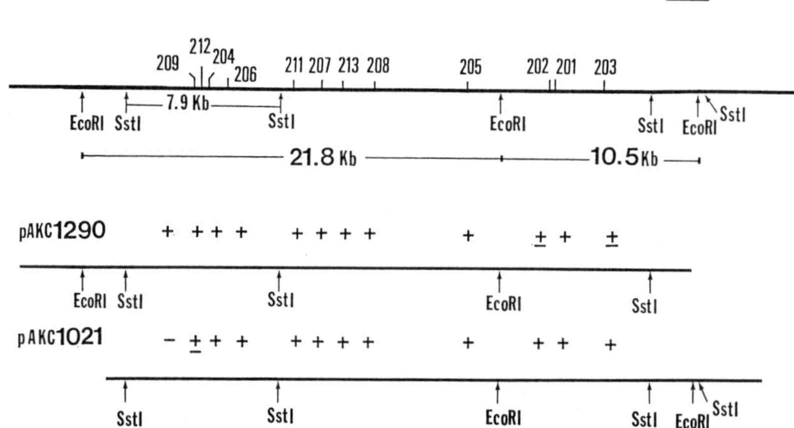

FIGURE 1. Restriction map of plasmids complementing ST⁻ mutants. Locations of Tn5 insertions in ST⁻ mutants are shown above the uppermost bold line. Complementation of ST⁻ mutants with pAKC1290 and pAKC1021 is indicated above the two lower lines. +, +/−, or − indicate the inhibition, slight inhibition, or no inhibition, respectively, of *G. candidum* growth with the agar bioassay (Morgan and Chatterjee, 1988).

complexes (Kleinkauf and von Dohren, 1983). Structural considerations imply that in the biosynthesis of these toxins, enzymatic steps would be required for amino acid activation and epimerization, elongation of the peptide chain and cyclization, as well as synthesis and addition of the fatty acid molecule. Moreover, the toxins would have to be exported out of the cell, although structural characteristics of the molecules may determine this step.

Initial efforts to elucidate the organization of ST (*syt*) and SR (*syr*) genes focused on identifying whether these genes are plasmid borne or located on the chromosome. The *syr* genes have a chromosomal location, which is probably true for *syt* genes as well (Currier and Morgan, 1983). Subsequent analysis indicated clustering of the toxin genes. For example, in strain B457, which produces ST, 13 Tn5 insertions in Tox⁻ mutants were in a 10.5- or 21.8-kilobase (kb) *Eco*RI DNA fragment (Morgan and Chatterjee, 1985, 1988). Furthermore, nine of these insertions were localized on a 19.2-kb *Sst*I fragment (Fig. 1).

Analysis of proteins produced in the wild-type strain B457 by sodium dodecyl sulfate-polyacrylamide gel electrophoresis revealed the presence of large-molecular-mass protein species of approximately 470 and 435 kilodaltons (ST1 and ST2, respectively) (Morgan and Chatterjee, 1988). Changes in the occurrence of ST1 and ST2 and the appearance of truncated forms of these proteins in the Tn5 insertion mutants indicated a polarity in the expression of the genes specifying ST1 and ST2.

We should note that SR strains also produce large-molecular-mass proteins presumed to be associated with toxin synthesis. Evidence for this was the finding that Tn5 insertions into the *syrB* gene caused a Tox⁻ phenotype and concomitantly abolished the synthesis of a 350-kilodalton protein (Xu and Gross, 1988).

The clustering of Tn5 insertions within about 32 kb of DNA and the apparent polar effect of the insertions on the formation of ST1 and ST2 were consistent with a single large transcriptional unit specifying two translational products. However, a finding with SR⁻ mutants (Xu and Gross, 1988) revealed that SyrB, presumed to be a component of the 350-kilodalton protein, was encoded by a 3.1-kb DNA segment. The apparent paradox presented by this finding, i.e., the detection of a relatively small transcriptional unit contributing to the formation of a large protein, can be reconciled by invoking the assembly of several gene products leading to protein complexes represented by ST1 and ST2. In this report, we provide genetic evidence supporting this model. In addition, our data suggest that the expression of some of the ST genes may account for the stimulation of toxin synthesis in the presence of iron.

ISOLATION OF GENETIC REGIONS FOR ST PRODUCTION

For a detailed analysis of genes involved in ST biosynthesis, we isolated the DNA segments from the wild-type strain B452. A library was constructed in the cosmid pSF6 (Selvaraj et al., 1984), and the individual plasmids were transferred to ST⁻ mutants in triparental matings (Ditta et al., 1980). Restoration of toxin production was detected by using the *Geotrichum* bioassay (Gross et al., 1977). Of approximately 600 plasmids tested, 7 complemented ME203, ME207, or ME209. The ME203 and ME209 mutants have Tn5 insertions located at the extreme ends of the 21.8- and 10.5-kb *Eco*RI fragments (Fig. 1). Two plasmids, pAKC1021 and pAKC1290, together appeared to complement all 12 Tox⁻ mutants derived from Tn5 insertions in these fragments. There is good agreement in the location of restriction sites on these two plasmids and on the DNA flanking the Tn5 insertions in the Tox⁻ mutants (Fig. 1). These data demonstrate that the 21.8- and 10.5-kb *Eco*RI fragments are contiguous on the B452 genome and that pAKC1021 and pAKC1290 have about 29 kb of DNA in common.

Kinetics of toxin production and the occurrence of ST1 and ST2 were examined in ME209 carrying pAKC1290. ME209 carrying pAKC1290 produced toxin levels comparable to those of the wild-type parent. In addition, as in the wild-type strain, B457, toxin production was detected in ME209 carrying pAKC1290 with onset of stationary growth phase. Sodium dodecyl sulfate-polyacrylamide gel electrophoresis analysis of ME209 harboring pAKC1290 indicated that this plasmid allowed accumulation of proteins that comigrated with ST1 and ST2. ME209 carrying pAKC1021 did not allow the accumulation of these proteins. This observation and the fact that pAKC1021 does not complement the Tox⁻ phenotype of ME209 further demonstrate that the left edge of the insert DNA in pAKC1290 (Fig. 1) is required in ST production. pAKC1021 is missing about 6 kb of DNA that is found at the left edge of the pAKC1290 insert, whereas pAKC1290 is missing about 4.5 kb of DNA found at the right edge of the insert in pAKC1021. These findings suggest that approximately 32 kb of B452 DNA contained in pAKC1290 and pAKC1021 is involved in ST production.

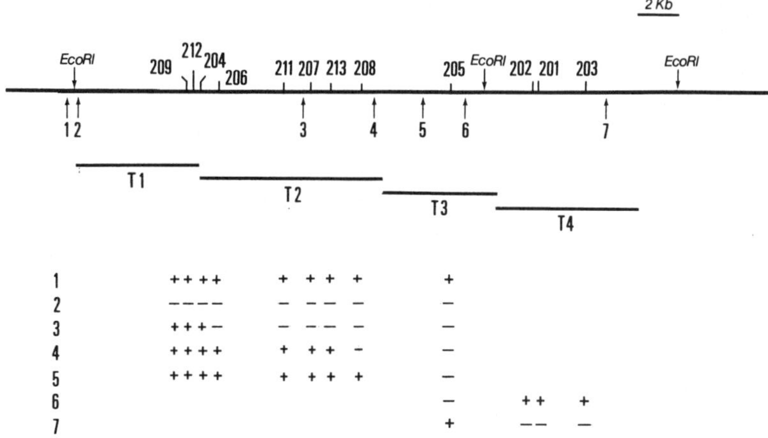

FIGURE 2. Proposed organization of transcriptional units involved in ST synthesis. Numbers 1 to 5 indicate Tn*3*HoHo insertions in pAKC1290; numbers 6 and 7 indicate Tn*3*HoHo insertions in pAKC1021. Arrows indicate the positions of these insertions. T1 through T4 represent the proposed transcriptional units based on the complementation pattern of plasmids with Tn*3*HoHo insertions. Only the relevant data are included. The *Geotrichum* bioassay used in the complementation studies was performed as previously described (Morgan and Chatterjee, 1988).

EVIDENCE FOR TRANSCRIPTIONAL UNITS

Complementation analysis with pAKC1021, pAKC1225, and pAKC1290 and characterization of *lacZ*-Tn*3*HoHo fusions (Stachel et al., 1985) of pAKC1021 and pAKC120 were conducted to identify transcriptional units. The complementation data with pAKC1290 and pAKC1021 (Fig. 2) suggest the presence of two transcriptional units. The start site of one transcriptional unit (T1) could be approximately 2 kb to the left of the 7.9-kb *Sst*I fragment. The second transcriptional unit (T2) may begin about 6.5 kb to the right of the proposed T1 starting point.

Evidence for an additional transcriptional unit is provided by the following results. pAKC1225 complemented 4 of the 12 Tn*5* mutants. Three of these mutants, ME201, ME202, and ME203, were caused by Tn*5* insertions in the 10.5-kb *Eco*RI fragment. The fourth mutant was due to a Tn*5* insertion in the right edge of the 21.8-kb *Eco*RI fragment (Fig. 1). pAKC1225 contains DNA extending no more than 5 kb to the left of the 10.5-kb *Eco*RI fragment. These results suggest that at least one transcriptional unit is in the segment of DNA from 5 kb to the left of and including the 10.5-kb *Eco*RI fragment (Fig. 2).

To confirm the presence of these transcriptional units and to delineate others, Tn*3*HoHo mutagenesis of pAKC1021 and pAKC1290 was performed. Over 200 Tn*3*HoHo insertions were obtained with pAKC1021, and over 100 insertions were obtained with pAKC1290. Insertions to the left of the 21.8-kb *Eco*RI DNA fragment (e.g., insertion 1, Fig. 2) and those to the right of the 10.5-kb *Eco*RI DNA fragment had no effect on the complementation of the Tox⁻ mutants, again revealing the limits of the DNA segment essential for ST synthesis. Insertions into the proposed T1 and T2 regions of pAKC1290 (Fig. 2) yielded high levels of β-galactosidase activity. Furthermore, fusions in the T2 region of pAKC1021 (presumed to lack the promoter region of T1) still yielded high β-galactosidase levels, supporting the presence of two transcriptional units. Insertion 6 (Fig. 2) in pAKC1021 complemented ME201, ME202, and ME203 but did not complement ME205. In contrast, insertion 7 complemented ME205 but did not complement ME201, ME202, and ME203. These findings indicate two separate transcriptional units (T3 and T4) within this region. We should note that insertions 3, 4, and 5 show a polar effect on the complementation of mutations in the DNA segment spanning T2 and T3 (Fig. 2). One explanation for this finding could be that the gene products must interact to allow toxin synthesis.

EXPRESSION OF *syt* GENES

Two classes of Tn*3*HoHo fusions in pAKC1021 and pAKC1290 were observed with respect to the levels of β-galactosidase activity. The first class of Tn*3*HoHo fusions yielded about 200 to 500 β-galactosidase units (Miller, 1972) even when the iron concentration in the medium was as low as 1 μM. Some of these fusions (e.g., those in the T3 region depicted in Fig. 2) are suspected of being in genes that may be regulated by iron. We should point out that iron has been shown to influence toxin production (Gross, 1985), accumulation of ST1 and ST2 (Morgan and Chatterjee, 1988), and expression of *syrB* (Gross, personal communication). The second class of fusions yielded low levels of β-galactosidase activity regardless of the iron concentration in the medium used. These fusions are probably in genes that are constitutively expressed and are not regulated by iron.

In summary, a large contiguous stretch of DNA of about 32 kb is required for ST synthesis in *P. syringae* pv. *syringae* B457. The latest findings with ST and SR genes implicate multimeric protein complexes in ST synthesis. The several gene products presumed to be encoded by this large stretch of DNA could be necessary for the synthesis of the toxin components, their polymerization, and possibly their export.

ACKNOWLEDGMENTS. This investigation was supported by the Food for the 21st Century program of the University of Missouri.

We much appreciate the assistance of J. L. McEvoy and H. Murata with preparation of the manuscript. We thank D. Gross for sharing with us unpublished observations on syringomycin genes.

LITERATURE CITED

Backman, P. A., and J. E. DeVay. 1971. Studies on the mode of action and biogenesis of the phytotoxin syringomycin. *Physiol. Plant Pathol.* **1**:215–233.

Currier, T. C., and M. K. Morgan. 1983. Plasmids of *Pseudomonas syringae*: no evidence of a role in toxin production or pathogenicity. *Can. J. Microbiol.* **29**:84–89.

DeVay, J. E., C. F. Gonzalez, and R. J. Wakeman. 1978. Comparison of the biocidal activities of syringomycin and syringotoxin and the characterization of isolates of *Pseudomonas syringae* from citrus hosts, p. 643–650. *In* Station de Pathologie Vegetale et Phytobacteriologie (ed.), *Proceedings of the IVth International Conference on Plant Pathogenic Bacteria*. Institut National de la Recherche Agronomique, Angers, France.

Ditta, G., S. Stanfield, D. Corbin, and D. R. Helinski. 1980. Broad host range DNA cloning system for gram-negative bacteria: construction of a gene bank of *Rhizobium meliloti. Proc. Natl. Acad. Sci. USA* **77:**7347–7351.

Gonzalez, C. F., J. E. DeVay, and R. J. Wakeman. 1981. Syringotoxin: a phytotoxin unique to citrus isolates of *Pseudomonas syringae. Physiol. Plant Pathol.* **18:**41–50.

Gross, D. C. 1985. Regulation of syringomycin synthesis in *Pseudomonas syringae* pv. *syringae* and defined conditions for its production. *J. Appl. Bacteriol.* **56:**167–174.

Gross, D. C., and Y. S. Cody. 1985. Mechanisms of plant pathogenesis by *Pseudomonas* species. *Can. J. Microbiol.* **31:**403–410.

Gross, D. C., J. E. DeVay, and E. H. Stadtman. 1977. Chemical properties of syringomycin and syringotoxin: toxigenic peptides produced by *Pseudomonas syringae. J. Appl. Bacteriol.* **43:** 453–463.

Kleinkauf, H., and H. von Dohren. 1983. Peptides, p. 95–145. *In* L. C. Vining (ed.), *Biochemistry and Genetic Regulation of Commercially Important Antibiotics*. Addison-Wesley Publishing Co., Reading, Mass.

Miller, J. H. 1972. *Experiments in Molecular Genetics*. Cold Spring Harbor Laboratory, Cold Spring Harbor, N.Y.

Mitchell, R. E. 1981. Structure: bacterial, p. 259–293. *In* R. D. Durbin (ed.), *Toxins in Plant Disease*. Academic Press, Inc., Orlando, Fla.

Morgan, M. K., and A. K. Chatterjee. 1985. Isolation and characterization of Tn*5* insertion mutants of *Pseudomonas syringae* pv. *syringae* altered in the production of the peptide phytotoxin syringotoxin. *J. Bacteriol.* **164:**14–18.

Morgan, M. K., and A. K. Chatterjee. 1988. Genetic organization and regulation of proteins associated with production of syringotoxin by *Pseudomonas syringae* pv. *syringae. J. Bacteriol.* **170:** 5689–5697.

Selvaraj, G., Y. C. Fong, and V. N. Iyer. 1984. A portable DNA sequence carrying the cohesive site (*cos*) of bacteriophage λ and the *mob* (mobilization) region of the broad-host-range plasmid RK2· a module for the construction of new cosmids. *Gene* **32:**235–241.

Stachel, S. E., G. An, C. Flores, and E. W. Nester. 1985. A Tn*3 lacZ* transposon for the random generation of β-galactosidase gene fusions: application to the analysis of gene expression in *Agrobacterium. EMBO J.* **4:**891–898.

Surico, G., and J. E. DeVay. 1982. Effect of syringomycin and syringotoxin produced by *Pseudomonas syringae* pv. *syringae* on structure and function of mitochondria isolated from holcus spot resistant and susceptible maize lines. *Physiol. Plant Pathol.* **21:**39–53.

Xu, G.-W., and D. C. Gross. 1988. Physical and functional analyses of the *syrA* and *syrB* genes involved in syringomycin production by *Pseudomonas syringae* pv. *syringae. J. Bacteriol.* **170:** 5680–5688.

Zhang, L., and J. Y. Takemoto. 1987. Effects of *Pseudomonas syringae* phytotoxin, syringomycin, on plasma membrane functions of *Rhodotorula pilimanae. Phytopathology* **77:**297–303.

Chapter 7

Genetics of Iron Uptake in Plant Growth-Promoting *Pseudomonas putida* WCS358

P. J. Weisbeek, W. Bitter, J. Leong, M. Koster, and J. D. Marugg

The genus *Pseudomonas* comprises a vast group of bacteria that are found in a variety of natural environments (soils, fresh water, and seawater) and in many different associations with plants and animals. Their ecological diversity is a reflection of their simple nutritional requirements and ability to metabolize a wide range of organic compounds. The fluorescent pseudomonads, including the species *P. aeruginosa*, *P. fluorescens*, *P. putida*, and *P. syringae*, constitute a major group among rhizosphere microorganisms. They produce and excrete a yellow-green, fluorescent, water-soluble pigment that has a very high affinity for ferric iron and functions as an iron transport agent (siderophore) (Neilands, 1984). They also produce a variety of other secondary metabolites, some of which are antibiotics; others may act as phytotoxins or as plant growth hormones (Gross and Cody, 1985; Leisinger and Margraff, 1979).

From many investigations in recent years, it has become clear that fluorescent pseudomonads play an important role in the protection of plants against deleterious microorganisms (Burr and Caesor, 1984). Because of the production of siderophores and antibiotics, many rhizosphere pseudomonads are antagonistic to phytopathogenic fungi and bacteria. It has been proposed that these siderophores promote plant growth by depriving deleterious rhizosphere microorganisms of iron, thereby inhibiting their growth (Leong, 1986; Schippers et al., 1987). Harmful, nonparasitic microorganisms increase with increasing cropping frequencies and thereby decrease crop yield. Certain beneficial fluorescent pseudomonads can reverse this effect by inhibiting the growth of these deleterious microorganisms in the rhizosphere.

Beneficial fluorescent *Pseudomonas* spp. strains have been isolated from potato roots on the basis of their ability to inhibit a variety of pathogenic and

---

P. J. Weisbeek, W. Bitter, J. Leong, M. Koster, and J. D. Marugg • Department of Molecular Cell Biology and Institute of Molecular Biology, University of Utrecht, Padualaan 8, 3584 CH Utrecht, The Netherlands.

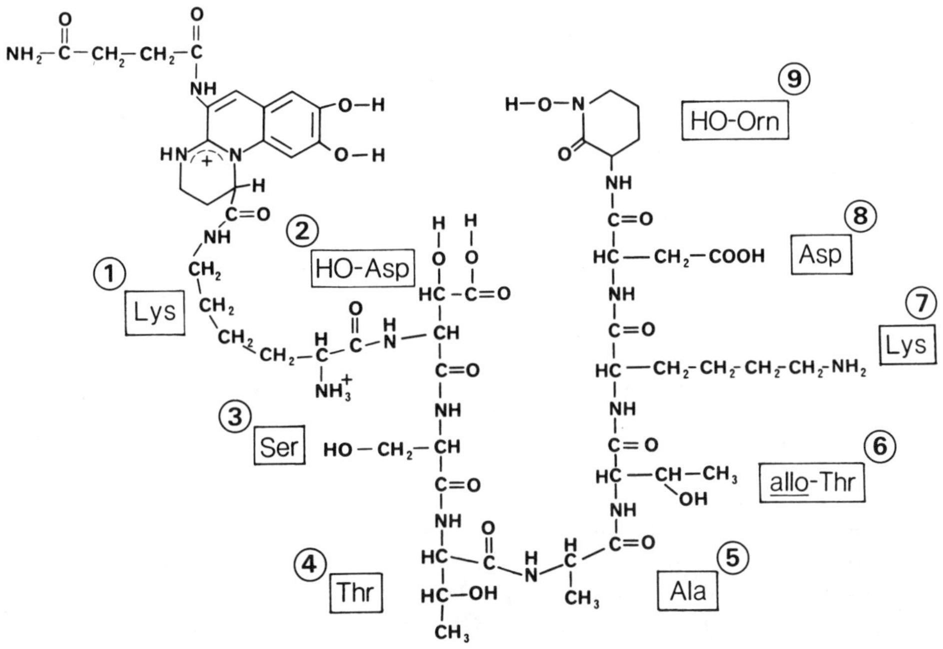

1 Lys
2 HO-Asp
3 Ser
4 Thr
5 Ala
6 allo-Thr
7 Lys
8 Asp
9 HO-Orn

FIGURE 1. Proposed chemical structure of pseudobactin 358, the siderophore of *P. putida* WCS358.

saprophytic rhizosphere fungi and bacteria (e.g., *Fusarium tabacinum, Rhizoctonia solani, Erwinia carotovora,* and *Streptomyces scabies*). This chapter describes the use of molecular genetic techniques to study siderophore biosynthesis and high-affinity Fe(III) assimilation in the selected isolates *P. fluorescens* WCS374 and *P. putida* WCS358.

PSEUDOBACTIN 358

Structure

The production of yellow-green, fluorescent siderophores is characteristic of the fluorescent pseudomonads. These siderophores are produced only when cells are grown under iron-limited conditions, and they display strong affinity for ferric ion. The chemical structures of several siderophores produced by fluorescent pseudomonads have been reviewed (Leong, 1986). The structure of pseudobactin 358, the siderophore produced by *P. putida* WCS358, has recently been elucidated (G. A. J. M. van der Hofstad, personal communication) and is given in Fig. 1. In the nonapeptide, the α-hydroxyaspartic acid and the ω-*N*-hydroxyornithine constitute, together with the *o*-dihydroxy aromatic group derived from the quinoline derivative, the three bidentate Fe(III)-chelating groups. The structure of pseudobactin 358 strongly resembles those of the other fluorescent siderophores (Leong, 1986).

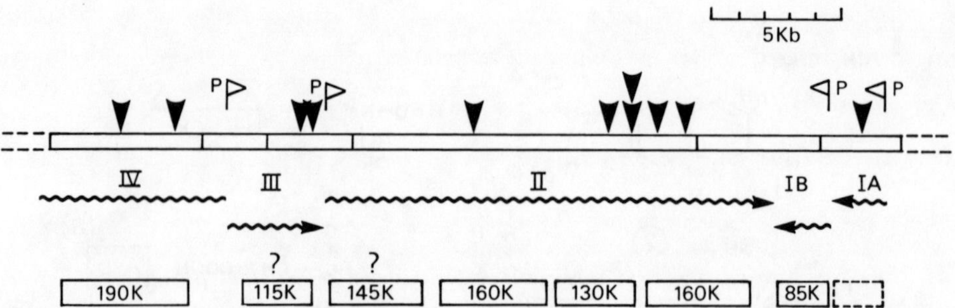

FIGURE 2. Genetic organization of cluster A. Locations and orientations of the transcriptional units (IA, IB, II, III, IV) are indicated by wavy lines. Arrowheads on the *Eco*RI restriction map represent Tn*5* insertions in the siderophore-defective mutants. Flags with the letter P represent possible promoter regions. The proposed locations and sizes of the polypeptide products are indicated by the boxes at the bottom. The size of the protein represented by the broken-line box is unknown.

These structural differences in fluorescent siderophores are believed to be important in iron uptake, since outer membrane receptor proteins for ferric siderophores appear to recognize specific features of the ferric siderophore. Pseudobactin 358 could be utilized by only a few of several hundred rhizosphere fluorescent pseudomonads that were tested.

Organization of Pseudobactin 358 Biosynthetic Genes

Genes required for the biosynthesis of yellow-green, fluorescent pseudobactin 358 were identified by complementing nonfluorescent transposon Tn*5* mutants of strain WCS358 defective in the biosynthesis of pseudobactin 358 with a gene bank of DNA from strain WCS358 maintained in *Escherichia coli*. Approximately 15 genes distributed over five gene clusters were identified in this manner (Marugg et al., 1985). This minimum number of genes seems reasonable, considering the structural complexity of pseudobactin 358 and the fact that only a fraction of the nonfluorescent mutants could be complemented. In a similar way, Moores et al. (1984) identified a minimum of 12 genes arranged in four clusters that were required for biosynthesis of pseudobactin, the native siderophore of plant growth-promoting *Pseudomonas* sp. strain B10.

The transcriptional organization and iron-regulated expression of a major gene cluster (cluster A) in strain WCS358 were analyzed in more detail (Fig. 2). Mapping of the Tn*5* integration sites of 11 siderophore-defective mutants, together with complementation analysis, demonstrates that at least a region of 33.5 kilobase pairs (kb) is required for biosynthesis of the siderophore. At least five transcriptional units are present in this region (IA, IB, II, III, and IV; Fig. 2), some of which are relatively large (Marugg et al., 1988). The polypeptides that were encoded by these transcriptional units were determined by analysis of *E. coli* minicells. The sizes of the encoded polypeptides shown in Fig. 2 are minimal ones.

With the exception of the 85-kilodalton protein, which is probably the outer membrane receptor protein for ferric pseudobactin 358 (see below), the biosynthetic functions of genes in this cluster are not known. However, three mutants in this region synthesized altered nonfluorescent siderophores that contained the complete wild-type peptide (van der Hofstad, personal communication). These results, together with the overall structure of the siderophore, i.e., a short peptide chain attached to a fluorescing group, suggest a biosynthetic pathway in which the biosynthesis of the fluorescing group is preceded by the enzymatic synthesis of the peptide part and the possibility that specific mutants in cluster A are defective in certain steps of the synthesis of the hydroxyquinoline derivative.

Regulation

Pseudobactin 358 is produced only under iron-limiting conditions. Under these conditions, certain outer membrane proteins are also expressed specifically (de Weger et al., 1986). By RNA-RNA hybridization, it was found that the expression of specific genes within cluster A is regulated by Fe(III) at the transcriptional level. This effect of Fe(III) can be mediated via a regulatory protein (activator or repressor) that allows initiation of transcription strictly under iron-limited conditions. This implies that the promoter or operator regions of the respective genes contain specific features that are recognized by such a regulatory protein in the presence or absence of iron. Since the positions and direction of transcription of four transcriptional units in cluster A have been determined, the promoter regions on the DNA were localized as depicted in Fig. 2.

These promoter regions were analyzed in broad-host-range promoter probe vectors by constructing transcriptional fusions with the structural genes for β-galactosidase (*lacZ*) and catechol-2,3-dioxygenase (*xylE*). The promoter region of transcriptional unit III was localized to a 189-base-pair (bp) *Hae*III-*Bam*HI fragment; this promoter caused the synthesis of β-galactosidase or catechol-2,3-dioxygenase in *P. putida* WCS358 only when cells were grown under iron-limited conditions. This finding confirms that regulation by iron occurs at the transcriptional level. This promoter and other iron-regulated siderophore promoters are not expressed in *E. coli*. The nucleotide sequence of the promoter on the 189-bp *Hae*III-*Bam*HI fragment present within a 0.4-kb *Hind*III-*Bam*HI fragment was determined (Fig. 3). By nuclease S1 mapping, the transcriptional start site was mapped within this fragment, which showed that the necessary information for iron-regulated expression is present within 73 bp upstream of the transcription start site. Deletion analysis revealed that the region from −73 to −67 is required for proper promoter functioning. This region may be involved in recognition or binding of a regulatory protein(s) at the siderophore promoter. We are using this and other iron-regulated promoter fusions to identify iron regulatory genes in strain WCS358.

IRON UPTAKE AND FERRIC SIDEROPHORE RECEPTORS

The inability of *P. fluorescens* WCS374 to transport Fe(III) via pseudobactin 358 was exploited to identify a gene coding for the 90-kilodalton outer membrane

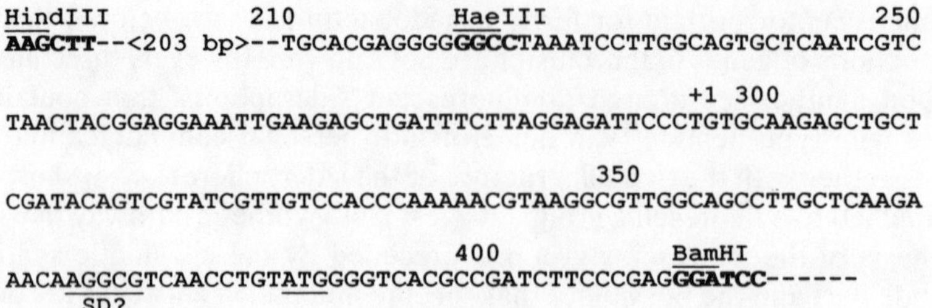

FIGURE 3. Nucleotide sequence of the promoter region present on a 0.4-kb *Hind*III-*Bam*HI fragment. The sequence is numbered from the *Hind*III site. The sequence between nucleotides 7 and 210 is not shown. The transcription initiation site is indicated. The putative Shine-Dalgarno (SD) sequence and ATG start codon are underlined.

receptor protein for ferric pseudobactin 358. By mobilization of a gene bank of DNA from strain WCS358 to strain WCS374, a unique cosmid clone, pMR, was identified that made strain WCS374 competent to utilize pseudobactin 358. The essential genetic information of pMR was localized by subcloning to a 5.3-kb *Bgl*II fragment (pAK21-pAK22) (Fig. 4). Transposon Tn5 mutagenesis limited the functional gene to a region of approximately 2.5 kb, consistent with the observed molecular size of the receptor protein (Fig. 4). The gene is flanked on both sides by pseudobactin 358 biosynthetic genes and is on a separate transcriptional unit (Fig. 5). Strain WCS374 harboring the putative receptor gene was able to transport Fe(III) via pseudobactin 358, whereas strain WCS374 carrying pMR derivatives with Tn5 in the receptor gene were not (Fig. 6).

Only the 90- and 92-kilodalton proteins of cell envelopes isolated from Fe(III)-limited cells of strain WCS358 reacted in immunoblots with antiserum raised against these two proteins (Fig. 7, lanes 2 and 9). The antiserum also cross-reacted with a 91-kilodalton protein present in cell envelopes isolated from Fe(III)-limited cells of strain WCS374 (lane 1). A new protein, which comigrated with the WCS358 protein of 90 kilodaltons, was expressed only in cell envelopes of WCS374 cells that harbored cosmid pMR (lane 3) or its derivatives (lanes 6 and 7) and that were grown under iron limitation along with the endogenous 91-kilodalton protein. Under iron-sufficient conditions, the 90-kilodalton (and the 91-kilodalton) protein was not observed. This result indicates that the mechanisms of iron regulation in the two strains are very similar or even identical. In cell envelopes of strain WCS374 harboring the mutagenized pMR derivatives 36 and 47, the 90-kilodalton protein disappeared (Fig. 7, lanes 4 and 5). Together with the fact that these cells were no longer able to transport Fe(III) via pseudobactin 358 (Fig. 6), this finding demonstrates that the 90-kilodalton protein is responsible for pseudobactin 358-specific iron assimilation.

The DNA sequence of this receptor gene has been determined; the mature protein consists of 772 amino acids (86.01 kilodaltons), with a signal sequence of 47 amino acids, which is extremely long for procaryotes. The receptor protein shares strong homology with four regions of TonB-dependent receptor proteins of *E. coli*, including BtuB (Heller and Kadner, 1985), FecA (Pressler et al., 1988),

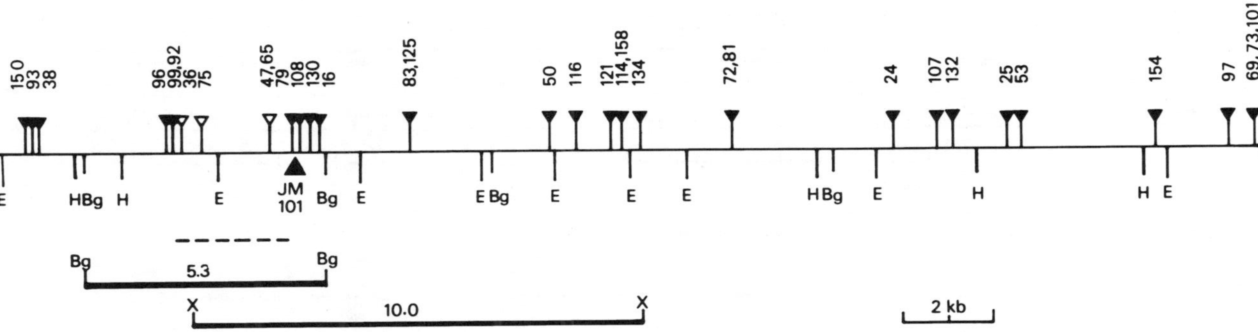

FIGURE 4. Locations of Tn*5* insertions on the insert of cosmid pMR. Symbols: ▽, Tn*5* insertions that cause a loss of the ability to make WCS374 cells competent for pseudobactin 358 utilization; ▼, Tn*5* insertions that do not affect pseudobactin 358 utilization by WCS374 cells; – – –, DNA region required for utilization of pseudobactin 358. Positions of the 5.3-kb *Bgl*II and the 10.0-kb *Xho*I fragments are indicated. The latter fragment does not make strain WCS374 competent to use pseudobactin 358. The location of the genomic Tn*5* insertion of the siderophore-defective mutant JM101 is indicated by the large triangle. Abbreviations for restriction enzymes: E, *Eco*RI; H, *Hin*dIII; B, *Bam*HI; Bg, *Bgl*II; X, *Xho*I.

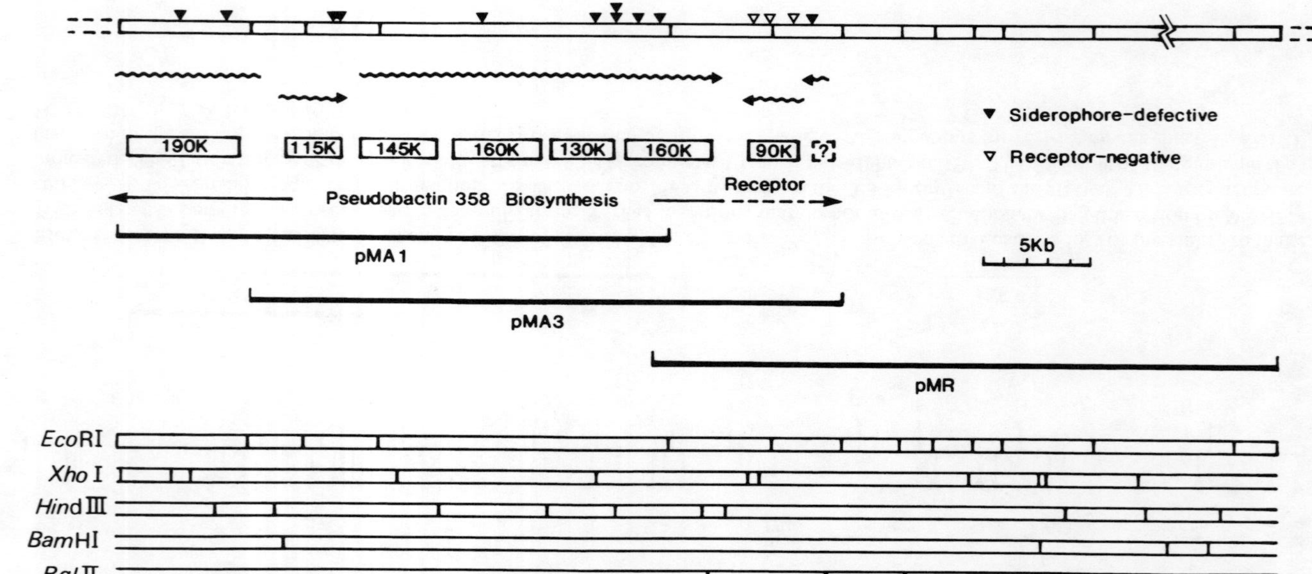

FIGURE 5. Genetic organization of gene cluster A, involved in siderophore biosynthesis and transport, present on the genome of *P. putida* WCS358. The orientations and directions of transcriptional units (wavy lines) and polypeptide products (boxes) are shown. Open and closed triangles refer to the Tn5 insertions of siderophore-defective and receptor-negative mutants, respectively. The restriction map at the bottom was combined from the data of the overlapping cosmid clones pMA1, pMA3, and pMR.

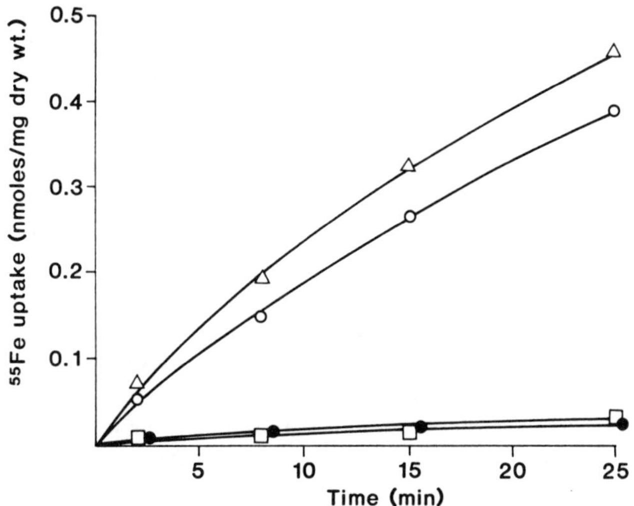

FIGURE 6. Pseudobactin 358-mediated iron uptake by cells of WCS374 (○), WCS374(pMR) (●), WCS374(pAK22) (△), and WCS374(pMR-36) (□) grown under iron limitation.

FepA (Lundrigan and Kadner, 1986), FhuA (Coulton et al., 1986), and IutA (Krone et al., 1985). This homology suggests the presence of a TonB-like protein in strain WCS358 that is required for Fe(III) transport and interaction of the receptor protein with this protein.

Strain WCS358 is able to utilize siderophores produced by many *Pseudomonas* soil isolates (P. A. H. M. Bakker, personal communication). Some of these siderophores were partially characterized and shown to be different from pseudobactin 358. Transposon Tn*5* mutants of strain WCS358, defective in synthesis of the 90-kilodalton outer membrane receptor protein, are still able to transport Fe(III) delivered by pseudobactin 358, although with a largely decreased efficiency (L. A. de Weger, personal communication). In contrast, no transport of Fe(III) via pseudobactin was observed in *Pseudomonas* sp. strain B10 Tn*5* mutants lacking the 85-kilodalton outer membrane receptor protein for ferric pseudobactin (Magazin et al., 1986).

FIGURE 7. Immunoblot analysis of cell envelope preparations run on a 9% sodium dodecyl sulfate-polyacrylamide gel, using an antiserum raised against a mixture of 90- and 92-kilodalton proteins of strain WCS358. Cell envelopes were isolated from cells that were grown under iron limitation. Lanes: 1, WCS374; 2 and 9, WCS358; 3, WCS374(pMR); 4, WCS374 (pMR-36); 5, WCS374(pMR-47); 6, WCS374 (pAK21); 7, WCS374(pAK22); 8, WCS374 (pMA3). Recombinant plasmid pMA3 also contains the receptor gene.

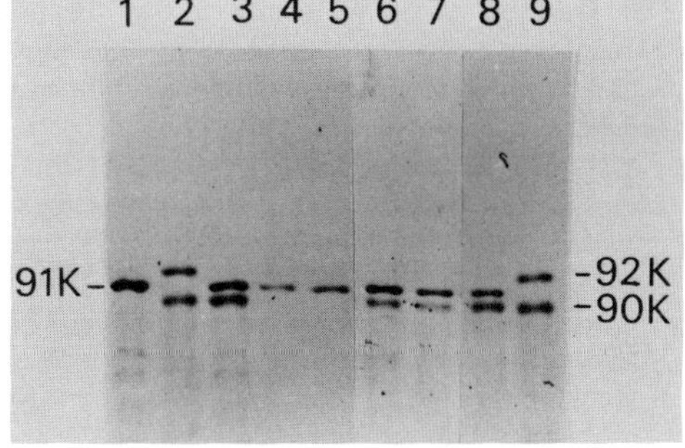

The Tn*5* mutants of strain WCS358 are also still able to utilize heterologous siderophores, including pseudobactins 374, BN2, BN7, and BN8, just like the wild-type strain. These results suggest that the 90-kilodalton protein is responsible for specific iron uptake via pseudobactin 358 only and that an alternative iron uptake system recognizes ferric pseudobactin 358 and heterologous ferric siderophores. An intriguing question is whether low-affinity iron transport via these other siderophores by strain WCS358 occurs by a single outer membrane receptor protein with low specificity or by several more specific receptors. The iron-regulated 92-kilodalton outer membrane protein may play a prominent role in this broad-specificity uptake system. We are now identifying the gene(s) responsible for this second uptake system. Recent research identified a second receptor that is responsible for iron uptake via a limited set of pseudobactins only. This finding indicates that in strain WCS358, at least three different uptake mechanisms operate to fulfill the iron requirements of the cell. A major difference with the situation in *E. coli* is that out of a large group of chemically very similar but distinct siderophores, selections are made via different receptors. A prediction here is that the receptors are probably highly related, as is already indicated by the immunological cross-reactivity of outer membrane proteins (receptors) of different strains.

ACKNOWLEDGMENTS. We thank P. A. H. M. Bakker, G. A. J. M. van der Hofstad, and L. A. de Weger for communicating results prior to publication.

These investigations were supported in part by the Netherlands Technology Foundation and by European Economic Community grant GBI-4-108 NL from the Bimolecular Engineering Programme.

LITERATURE CITED

Burr, T. J., and A. J. Caesor. 1984. Beneficial plant bacteria. *Crit. Rev. Plant Sci.* **2**:1–20.

Coulton, J. W., P. Mason, D. R. Cameron, G. Carmel, R. Jean, and H. N. Rode. 1986. Protein fusions of β-galactosidase to the ferrichrome-iron receptor of *Escherichia coli* K-12. *J. Bacteriol.* **165**:181–192.

de Weger, L. A., R. van Boxtel, B. van der Burg, R. A. Gruters, F. P. Geels, B. Schippers, and B. Lugtenberg. 1986. Siderophores and outer membrane proteins of antagonistic, plant growth-stimulating, root-colonizing *Pseudomonas* spp. *J. Bacteriol.* **165**:585–594.

Gross, D. C., and Y. S. Cody. 1985. Mechanisms of plant pathogenesis by *Pseudomonas* species. *Can. J. Microbiol.* **31**:403–410.

Heller, K., and R. J. Kadner. 1985. Nucleotide sequence of the gene for the vitamin B12 receptor protein in the outer membrane of *Escherichia coli. J. Bacteriol.* **161**:904–908.

Krone, W. J. A., F. Stegehuis, G. Koningstein, C. van Doorn, B. Roosendaal, F. K. de Graaf, and B. Oudega. 1985. Characterization of the pColV-K30 encoded cloacin DF13/aerobactin outer membrane receptor protein of *Escherichia coli*; isolation and purification of the protein and analysis of its nucleotide sequence and primary structure. *FEMS Microbiol. Lett.* **26**:153–161.

Leisinger, T., and R. Margraff. 1979. Secondary metabolites of the fluorescent pseudomonads. *Microbiol. Rev.* **43**:422–442.

Leong, J. 1986. Siderophores: their biochemistry and possible role in the biocontrol of plant pathogens. *Annu. Rev. Phytopathol.* **24**:187–209.

Lundrigan, M. D., and R. J. Kadner. 1986. Nucleotide sequence of the gene for the ferrienterochelin receptor FepA in *Escherichia coli. J. Biol. Chem.* **261**:10797–10801.

Magazin, M., J. C. Moores, and J. Leong. 1986. Cloning of the gene coding for the outer membrane receptor protein for ferric pseudobactin, a siderophore from a plant growth-promoting *Pseudomonas* strain. *J. Biol. Chem.* **261**:795–799.

Marugg, J. D., H. B. Nielander, A. J. G. Horrevoets, I. van Megen, I. van Genderen, and P. J. Weisbeek. 1988. Genetic organization and transcriptional analysis of a major gene cluster involved in siderophore biosynthesis in *Pseudomonas putida* WCS358. *J. Bacteriol.* **170:**1812–1819.

Marugg, J. D., M. van Spanje, W. P. M. Hoekstra, B. Schippers, and P. J. Weisbeek. 1985. Isolation and analysis of genes involved in siderophore biosynthesis in plant growth-stimulating *Pseudomonas putida* WCS358. *J. Bacteriol.* **164:**563–570.

Moores, J. C., M. Magazin, G. S. Ditta, and J. Leong. 1984. Cloning of genes involved in the biosynthesis of pseudobactin, a high-affinity iron transport agent of a plant growth-promoting *Pseudomonas* strain. *J. Bacteriol.* **157:**53–58.

Neilands, J. B. 1984. Methodology of siderophores. *Struct. Bonding* **58:**1–24.

Pressler, U., H. Staudenmaier, L. Zimmermann, and V. Braun. 1988. Genetics of the iron dicitrate transport system of *Escherichia coli*. *J. Bacteriol.* **170:**2716–2724.

Schippers, B., A. W. Bakker, and P. A. H. M. Bakker. 1987. Interactions of deleterious and beneficial rhizosphere microorganisms and the effect of cropping practices. *Annu. Rev. Phytopathol.* **25:**339–358.

Chapter 8

Structure, Function, Regulation, and Evolution of Genes Involved in Pathogenicity, the Hypersensitive Response, and Phaseolotoxin Immunity in the Bean Halo Blight Pathogen

M. N. Mindrinos, L. G. Rahme, R. D. Frederick, E. Hatziloukas, C. Grimm, and N. J. Panopoulos

The bean halo blight pathogen, *Pseudomonas syringae* pv. *phaseolicola*, provides a model for analysis of the genetic basis of the production of primary and secondary symptoms as well as the hypersensitive reaction (HR). This chapter presents a brief summary of previous work and some recent findings in our laboratories.

PRIMARY AND SECONDARY SYMPTOMS OF BEAN HALO BLIGHT AND THE HR

Pathogenic strains of *P. syringae* pv. *phaseolicola*, when inoculated on leaves or pods of susceptible cultivars of bean (compatible interaction), multiply in the intercellular spaces over a period of 4 to 7 days to attain high population levels (typically 10^5- to 10^7-fold above the initial inoculum). Symptoms usually appear several days postinoculation in the form of lesions that have a water-soaked appearance and may become progressively necrotic. We refer to this aspect of the disease phenotype as primary symptoms. The term secondary symptoms, as used here, refers to the systemic chlorosis that develops on beans after inoculation with strains that produce a low-molecular-weight phytotoxin, phaseolotoxin.

M. N. Mindrinos, L. G. Rahme, C. Frederick, C. Grimm, and N. J. Panopoulos • Department of Plant Pathology, University of California, Berkeley, California 94720.   *E. Hatziloukas* • Institute of Molecular Biology and Biotechnology, Foundation for Research and Technology-Hellas, Heraklion, Crete, Greece.

When the pathogen is inoculated on resistant bean cultivars or on nonhost plants (incompatible interactions), it multiplies only to a limited extent and usually elicits a localized necrotic response in the host within hours after inoculation (the HR). The HR is usually observed as a confluent necrosis of the inoculated tissue at high inoculum concentrations (5×10^6 CFU/ml or greater) or, with more dilute inoculum, as a necrosis of individual plant cells that are in direct contact with the pathogen or of a small number of cells in their immediate vicinity.

GENETIC CONTROL OF PRIMARY DISEASE SYMPTOMS AND THE HR

In earlier studies (Lindgren et al., 1986), we identified and cloned a group of genes that are required for the production of primary symptoms, as defined above, as well as for elicitation of the HR by *P. syringae* pv. *phaseolicola*. We designated these genes *hrp* (phonetic "harp"), for hypersensitive reaction and pathogenicity, to emphasize the fact that the phenotypic outcomes of compatible and incompatible interactions in which this bacterium engages have coincident genetic requirements on the part of the pathogen. Subsequent studies (Lindgren et al., 1988; C. Grimm and N. Panopoulos, unpublished data) showed that *hrp* DNA sequences are conserved among several pathovars of *P. syringae* and that functional homologs of several *hrp* genes exist in closely related members of this group. Phenotypically similar mutants and *hrp* genes were independently described in and have been cloned from other phytopathogenic *Pseudomonas* spp., both within and outside the *P. syringae* taxon (Boucher et al., 1987; Huang et al., 1988; Lindgren et al., 1988; T. Huyhn, B. J. Staskawicz, and D. Dahlbeck, submitted for publication).

Expression of the Hrp phenotype by *P. syringae* pv. *phaseolicola* requires the collective functions of genes encoded by a ca. 20-kilobase-pair (kb) region, which we have designated the *hrp* cluster, and by a separate locus, which, by agreement with others (Mukhopadhyay and Mills, 1988), is designated *hrpM*. We also infer from other studies (references in Keen and Staskawicz [1988]) that avirulence genes (*avr*) are also necessary for phenotypic expression of the HR, although not for the production of primary symptoms. A summary of our findings on the structure, organization, and function of the *hrp* genes in *P. syringae* pv. *phaseolicola* is presented below.

Genetic Organization of the *hrp* Cluster

The 20-kb *hrp* region has been extensively analyzed by insertional mutagenesis with a newly constructed reporter transposon, Tn*3*-Spice, by marker exchange and complementation analysis, and to some extent by DNA sequencing (Grimm and Panopoulos, 1989; Grimm et al., 1989; Lindgren et al., 1989; Rahme et al., 1989; L. Rahme, M. N. Mindrinos, and N. J. Panopoulos, manuscript in preparation). The region encodes *hrp* functions over its entire length, with only a short (0.5 to 1.0 kb) segment near its center apparently not encoding *hrp*-related functions. The direction of transcription in a ca. 9-kb segment and the genetic and physiological requirements for its expression have been determined by measuring the ice nucleation activity of genetic fusions between *hrp* sequences and a promoterless ice nucleation gene (*inaZ*). The fusions were constructed by insertional mutagenesis with Tn*3*-Spice or by cloning *hrp* DNA segments in plasmid vectors upstream of the *inaZ* gene and were examined for activity both in *hrp*[+]/*hrp*::*inaZ* merodiploids and in marker exchange *hrp*::*inaZ* haploids.

Three complementation groups have been defined in the 9-kb segment of the *hrp* cluster. One of these, designated *hrpAB*, comprises two functional units (*A* and *B*) that are apparently expressed from a single promoter, whereas the two others, designated *hrpC* and *hrpD*, are controlled by separate promoters. All of these units are transcribed in the same direction and, as discussed below, have the same physiological and genetic requirements for expression. The remainder of the *hrp* cluster is organized into at least four complementation groups (Rahme et al., in preparation) and includes the regulatory gene *hrpS* (see below).

Physiological Requirements for *hrpAB*, *hrpC*, and *hrpD* Expression

The *hrpD* locus was described by Lindgren et al. (1989) as inducible because it was actively expressed in the infected plant but not during growth in a nutritionally complex medium. This also holds true for *hrpAB* and *hrpC*. Conditions for in vitro expression of *hrpAB*, *hrpC*, and *hrpD* have now been established. Specifically, nutritional downshift of cultures that have been pregrown on complex medium leads to rapid induction of all the named genes, although the level of expression is modulated by the type of carbon source present in the medium (Rahme et al., in preparation). For convenience, the 9-kb segment encoding *hrpAB*, *hrpC*, and *hrpD* is referred to as the inducible segment of the *hrp* cluster, although (an)other *hrp* genes located elsewhere in the cluster show the same physiological requirements for expression (Rahme et al., in preparation).

In contrast with the *vir* genes of *Agrobacterium tumefaciens* and the common *nod* genes of *Rhizobium meliloti*, specific chemical signals of plant origin apparently are not required for *hrpAB*, *hrpC*, and *hrpD* expression in *P. syringae* pv. *phaseolicola*.

Genetic Requirements for *hrpAB*, *hrpC*, and *hrpD* Expression

Grimm and Panopoulos (1989) determined the nucleotide sequence of a gene (*hrpS*) located near the right end of the *hrp* cluster that encodes a protein with amino acid sequence similarity to several members of the NtrC family of procaryotic regulatory proteins (Ronson et al., 1987). This finding suggested that *hrpS* may be a regulatory locus, a prediction that subsequently was confirmed by comparing the ice nucleation activities of a *hrpD*::*inaZ* fusion in wild-type and *hrpS* backgrounds. DNA sequence analysis of the region upstream of *hrpS* revealed another open reading frame (ORF) that is also capable of encoding an NtrC-like protein (R. Grimm, N. J. Panopoulos, B. J. Staskawicz and D. Dahlbeck, manuscript in preparation). This gene has been designated *hrpR*. The deduced amino acid sequences of the HrpS and HrpR proteins share 62% identity

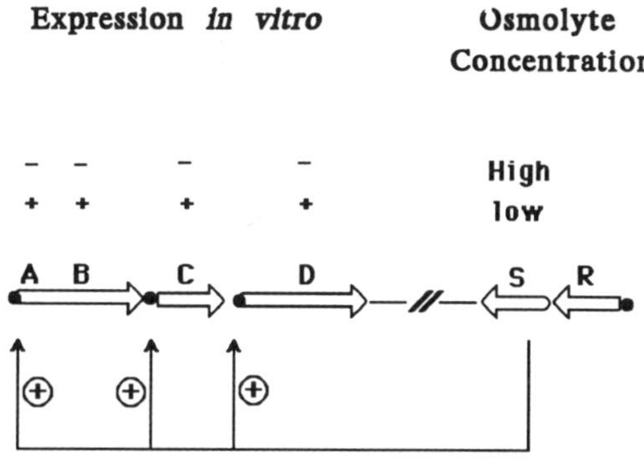

FIGURE 1. Tentative model of the genetic and physiological regulation of *hrp* genes in *P. syringae* pv. *phaseolicola*. A, B, C, D, S, and R represent the synonymous *hrp* genes discussed in the text. Symbols: ⊕, active promoters inferred from various studies; + and −, positive and negative effects, respectively. Direct interaction between the *hrpS* gene product and the promoters it regulates has not been experimentally tested. Gene regions are not drawn to scale.

with each other and about 40 to 46% identity with the highly conserved central domain of NtrC, NifA, and DctD (Grimm et al., in preparation).

In view of the sequence similarity between the putative HrpS and HrpR proteins, we sought to resolve their respective roles in activation of the *hrpAB*, -*C*, and -*D* genes. The experiments involved the construction of plasmids carrying either the *hrpS* or *hrpR* coding region under the control of the native or other promoters. These plasmids were introduced into three different genetic backgrounds: *hrpS4006*::Tn*5*, *hrpR4008*::Tn*5*, and Δ(*hrpS-hrpR*)*4010* (N. J. Mindrinos, L. Rahme, and N. J. Panopoulos, manuscript in preparation). Each mutant also carried either reporter insertions in the *hrp* loci or *inaZ* reporter plasmids with defined segments of the inducible region driving the expression of *inaZ*. In the absence of a functional *hrpS* gene, no expression of the *hrpAB*, -*C*, or -*D* promoter was obtained, either after nutritional downshift or after inoculation of bean leaves with the bacteria (the latter was tested only with *hrpD* reporter constructs). Absence of a functional *hrpR* region had only minor or no effect on the expression of reporter constructs (Fig. 1).

The *hrpS* and *hrpR* genes are transcribed in the same direction and appear to be transcriptionally linked. Since plasmids carrying the *hrpS* coding region expressed from different promoters permit activation of the inducible *hrpAB*, -*C*, and -*D* promoters in the Δ(*hrpS-hrpR*)*4010* background, the noninducible phenotype of *hrpR*::Tn*5* mutants is provisionally attributed to a polar effect on *hrpS* expression. Interestingly, expression of *hrpS* under the *lac*, *trp*, or *hrpR* promoter restores the Hrp[+] phenotype in the *hrpR*::Tn*5* mutant (Mindrinos et al., in preparation; Grimm et al., in preparation).

A novel feature of the regulation of these *hrp* genes is osmotic repression. Specifically, L. Rahme, M. N. Mindrinos, and N. J. Panopoulos (unpublished data) recently showed that expression of these genes in defined minimal medium is significantly reduced or effectively prevented by raising the osmolyte concentration. This effect is not relieved by addition of an osmoprotectant such as proline or betaine. Given the extensive knowledge of the molecular mechanisms of osmoregulation in other bacteria, this finding provides interesting leads for further study.

At present, we can only speculate about the possible significance of osmotic repression of *hrp* genes in the bacterium-plant interaction. Electrolyte leakage is normally associated with the early stages of the HR and may raise the concentration of osmolytes in the intercellular space to levels that prevent *hrp* gene expression. Similar electrolyte linkage occurs also in compatible interactions but at late stages of infection, when the primary lesions no longer expand. Since *hrp* genes are essential for multiplication of the pathogen in planta, osmotic repression of these genes may represent a front-line defense of plants against heterologous bacterial pathogens and may also be involved in the restriction of lesion size.

hrpM Locus of *P. syringae* pv. *phaseolicola*

The *hrpM* locus was independently characterized and recently sequenced in a related pathogen, *P. syringae* pv. *syringae* (Mukhopadhyay and Mills, 1988), which causes the brown spot disease on bean, as well as in *P. syringae* pv. *phaseolicola* (R. D. Frederick and N. J. Panopoulos, manuscript in preparation). It spans a ca. 4.5-kb region that is organized into an operon consisting of two ORFs (ORF1 and ORF2) capable of encoding polypeptides of 40 and 82 kilodaltons, respectively. An unusual feature of *hrpM* is the presence of two very long antiparallel ORFs (ORF3 and ORF4) roughly equal in size and in a codon-to-codon register arrangement with ORF1 and ORF2. Promoter fusion studies (Mukhopadhyay and Mills, 1988) indicated that only the later two ORFs were functional. The nucleotide sequence of *hrpM* from *P. syringae* pv. *phaseolicola* predicts a product of similar size for ORF1 but a slightly larger (by 52 amino acids) product for ORF2 compared with the corresponding regions in *P. syringae* pv. *syringae*. Alignment of the two sequences suggests a possible sequencing error in the published *P. syringae* pv. *syringae* sequence, probably between nucleotides 3456 and 3460, as being responsible for the apparent difference between the two pathovars in the size of the ORF2 product. Codon position divergence analysis of the two *hrpM* alleles is consistent with ORF1 and ORF2 being functional (Frederick and Panopoulos, in preparation). Thus, when ORF1 and ORF2 are aligned, the majority of variant nucleotides occur in the third position of the codons, as is the case with most gene families. By contrast, alignment of ORF3 and ORF4 produces variant nucleotides, mostly in the first codon positions. We have constructed *hrpM::inaZ* fusions in three of the four ORFs to test whether any transcription occurs in the orientation of ORF3 and ORF4.

GENETIC BASIS AND EVOLUTIONARY ORIGIN OF PHASEOLOTOXIN IMMUNITY

The chlorotic symptoms of bean halo blight are attributed to phaseolotoxin [($N\delta$-phosphosulfinyl)-ornithylalanylhomoarginine]. Peet et al. (1986) identified and cloned a separate cluster of genes that function in the synthesis of phaseolotoxin. The same cluster also carries a gene for ornithine carbamoyltransferase (OCTase), the target enzyme for phaseolotoxin in plant cells (Peet and Panopoulos, 1987). Unlike other OCTases, the enzyme encoded by this gene is

P. s. phaseolicola

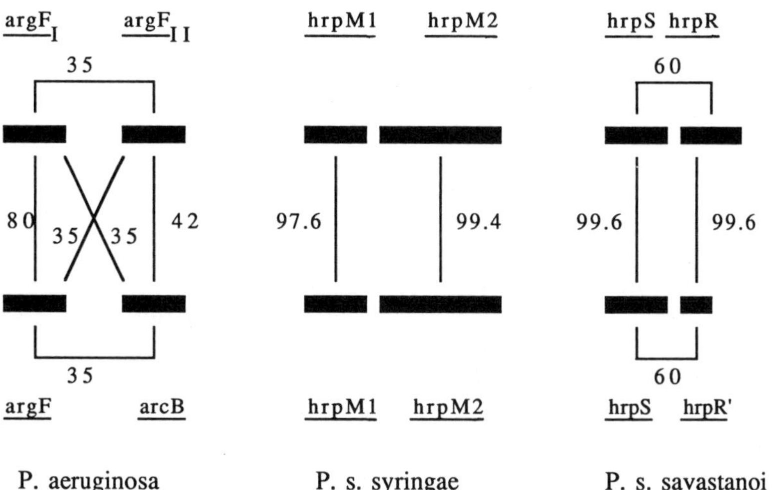

FIGURE 2. Amino acid sequence similarities between some gene products of *Pseudomonas* spp. discussed in the text. The *argF*$_I$ and *argF*$_{II}$ genes of *P. syringae* pv. *phaseolicola* encode the phaseolotoxin-sensitive and -resistant OCTases, respectively; *argF* and *arcB* of *P. aeruginosa* encode the anabolic and catabolic OCTases, respectively, found in this bacterium. The *hrpR* gene of *P. syringae* pv. *savastanoi* is only partially sequenced. Low similarity values have been rounded to the nearest integer.

insensitive to phaseolotoxin. The nucleotide sequence of this gene has recently been determined in our laboratory (E. Hatziloukas and N. J. Panopoulos, in preparation). The predicted amino acid sequence of the enzyme (327 residues) resembles more closely (about 42% similarity) the catabolic OCTase of *Pseudomonas aeruginosa* and slightly less other procaryotic and eucaryotic OCTases (Itoh et al., 1988). Transfer and expression of this gene in plants are in progress, with the aim of producing phaseolotoxin-resistant beans.

Comparisons of the deduced amino acid sequence of the phaseolotoxin-insensitive OCTase with those of nine other OCTases suggest that certain amino acid residues are critical in determining the insensitivity of this enzyme to the toxin. Among them is a glycine residue present in place of the first threonine of the highly conserved pentapeptide STRTR, which presumably constitutes part of the carbamoylphosphate-binding site.

P. syringae pv. *phaseolicola* also possesses a second OCTase gene that encodes a toxin-sensitive enzyme (Peet and Panopoulos, 1987). The nucleotide sequence of this gene has also been determined (Hatziloukas and Panopoulos, in preparation). Unlike the toxin-insensitive enzyme, this OCTase resembles the *P. aeruginosa* anabolic OCTase (Itoh et al., 1988) much more closely (80% amino acid sequence similarity) than it resembles either the toxin-insensitive enzyme (35% identity) or other bacterial OCTases. Our analysis suggests that the two OCTase genes did not originate from the same progenitor sequence in *P. syringae* pv. *phaseolicola*. Most likely, the gene encoding the toxin-insensitive enzyme originated from another, presently unknown source.

MOLECULAR EVOLUTION OF *hrp* GENES

Sequence divergence analysis of shared and unique genes connected with pathogenesis should provide some clues as to the evolutionary history of various members of the *P. syringae* taxon and the relationship between their radiation from a common ancestor(s) and the emergence of their hosts. The limited sequence data compiled thus far are shown in Fig. 2. The most similar sequences are those of the *hrpS* genes of the bean halo blight and olive knot pathogens. These genes appear to have diverged about 1 million years ago or less. The *hrpM* gene may have arisen from a common ancestor about 27 to 40 million years ago (Frederick and Panopoulos, in preparation). The *hrpS* and *hrpR* genes within a given genome predate both estimates by a considerable margin, which is difficult to approximate with the same precision because the differences in the third codon positions may have saturated (our unpublished data). If the *hrpS* and *hrpR* genes are products of gene duplication in a *P. syringae* "protopathogen," this event must have occurred considerably earlier than the time since the *hrpS*, *hrpR*, and *hrpM* genes found in the various pathovars separated from each other.

ACKNOWLEDGMENTS. This work was supported by grants from the National Science Foundation (DMB-8706129), the U.S. Department of Agriculture Science and Education Administration, the NATO Science for Stability Program, the European Economic Community, the Deutsche Forschungsgemeinschaft, and the General Secretariat of Research and Technology of Greece.

The assistance of Georgia Houlaki in typing the manuscript and preparing the figures is acknowledged.

LITERATURE CITED

Boucher, C. A., F. Van Gijsegem, P. A. Barberis, M. Arlat, and C. Zischek. 1987. *Pseudomonas solanacearum* genes controlling both pathogenicity on tomato and hypersensitivity on tobacco are clustered. *J. Bacteriol.* **169**:5626–5632.

Grimm, C., and N. J. Panopoulos. 1989. The predicted protein product of a pathogenicity locus from *Pseudomonas syringae* pv. *phaseolicola* is homologous to a highly conserved domain of several procaryotic regulatory proteins. *J. Bacteriol.* **171**:5031–5038.

Grimm, C., L. Rahme, R. Frederick, M. Mindrinos, P. Lindgren, and N. Panopoulos. 1989. The common pathogenicity genes of *Pseudomonas syringae* pathovars. *UCLA Symp. Mol. Cell. Biol.* **101**:49–55.

Huang, H.-C., R. Schuurink, T. P. Denny, M. M. Atkinson, J. C. Baker, I. Yucel, S. W. Hutcheson, and A. Collmer. 1988. Molecular cloning of a *Pseudomonas syringae* gene cluster that enables *Pseudomonas fluorescens* to elicit a hypersensitive response in tobacco. *J. Bacteriol.* **170**:4748–4756.

Itoh, Y., L. Soldati, V. Stalon, P. Flamagne, Y. Terawaki, T. Leisinger, and D. Haas. 1988. Anabolic ornithine carbamoyltransferase of *Pseudomonas aeruginosa*: nucleotide sequence and transcriptional control of the *argF* structural gene. *J. Bacteriol.* **170**:2725–2734.

Keen, N. T., and B. J. Staskawicz. 1988. Host range determinants of plant pathogens and symbionts. *Annu. Rev. Microbiol.* **42**:421–440.

Lindgren, P. B., R. Frederick, N. J. Panopoulos, D. Dahlbeck, B. J. Staskawicz, and S. E. Lindow. 1989. An ice nucleation reporter gene system: identification of an inducible pathogenicity gene in *Pseudomonas syringae* pv. *phaseolicola*. *EMBO J.* **8**:2490–3001.

Lindgren, P. B., N. J. Panopoulos, B. J. Staskawicz, and D. Dahlbeck. 1988. Genes required for pathogenicity and hypersensitivity are conserved and interchangeable among pathovars of *Pseudomonas syringae*. *Mol. Gen. Genet.* **211**:499–506.

Lindgren, P. B., R. C. Peet, and N. J. Panopoulos. 1986. Gene cluster of *Pseudomonas syringae* pv. *phaseolicola* controls pathogenicity on bean and hypersensitivity on non-host plants. *J. Bacteriol.* **168**:512–522.

Mukhopadhyay, P., and D. Mills. 1988. Molecular analysis of a pathogenicity locus in *Pseudomonas syringae* pv. *syringae*. *J. Bacteriol.* **170**:5479–5488.

Peet, R. C., P. B. Lindgren, D.K. Willis, and N. J. Panopoulos. 1986. Genetic analysis of phaseolotoxin production by *Pseudomonas syringae* pv. *phaseolicola*. *J. Bacteriol.* **166**:1096–1105.

Peet, R. C., and N. J. Panopoulos. 1987. Ornithine carbamoyltransferase genes and phaseolotoxin immunity in *Pseudomonas syringae* pv. *phaseolicola*. *EMBO J.* **6**:3585–3591.

Rahme, L., M. Mindrinos, C. Grimm, R. Frederick, P. Lindgren, and N. J. Panopoulos. 1989. Organization and expression of the *hrp* gene cluster of *Pseudomonas syringae* pv. *phaseolicola*, p. 303–314. *In* E. Tjamos and C. Beckman (ed.), *Vascular Wilt Diseases of Plants: Basic Studies and Control*. Springer-Verlag KG, Berlin.

Ronson, C. W., B. T. Nixon, and F. M. Ausubel. 1987. Conserved domains on bacterial regulatory proteins that respond to environmental stimuli. *Cell* **49**:579–581.

Chapter 9

Pseudomonas syringae Infection of *Arabidopsis thaliana* as a Model System for Studying Plant-Bacterial Interactions

Eric J. Schott, Keith R. Davis, Xinnian Dong, Michael Mindrinos, Pablo Guevara, and Frederick M. Ausubel

Over the past 3 years, we have developed a model plant pathogenesis system that uses *Arabidopsis thaliana* as the plant host and *Pseudomonas syringae* pv. *maculicola* as a model bacterial pathogen. In this chapter, we discuss the advantages of using this system to study plant pathogenesis and outline experimental strategies for identifying both plant and bacterial genes specifically involved in the pathogenic interaction.

ADVANTAGES OF *A. THALIANA* AS A PLANT HOST

A. thaliana has several advantages as a model system (Meyerowitz and Pruitt, 1985; Meyerowitz, 1987; Pang and Meyerowitz, 1987). First, *A. thaliana* is a true diploid, has a rapid generation time (6 to 8 weeks), is self-fertile, and produces copious numbers of small seeds that remain viable for many years. Second, among plant species in which the genome size has been determined, *A. thaliana* has the least amount of DNA (70 megabase pairs) per haploid nucleus (Leutwiler et al., 1984). Third, because *A. thaliana* can be transformed with *Agrobacterium tumefaciens* Ti plasmid vectors (Lloyd et al., 1986; Valvekens et al., 1988), it is possible to introduce and stably maintain genes of interest. Finally, several groups are developing restriction fragment length polymorphism and physical maps of the *A. thaliana* genome and correlating these maps with the genetic map already available (Koornneef et al., 1983; Chang et al., 1988; Nam et al., 1989). As the genetic and physical maps become more detailed, it will be possible to clone specific genes that have been identified only by mutation.

Eric J. Schott, Keith R. Davis, Xinnian Dong, Michael Mindrinos, Pablo Guevara, and Frederick M. Ausubel • Department of Genetics, Harvard Medical School, and Department of Molecular Biology, Massachusetts General Hospital, Boston, Massachusetts 02114.

PLANT DEFENSE RESPONSES

Although plants are continuously exposed to a variety of potentially pathogenic microorganisms, successful infections are rare. Plants utilize a diverse array of defense mechanisms to prevent microbial infections. Some of these defense strategies involve constitutively expressed physical and chemical barriers that provide a first line of defense against potential pathogens (Mansfield, 1983). Other defense mechanisms are specifically induced upon attempted infection. These induced defense responses include synthesis of polyphenolic lignins and hydroxy-proline-rich glycoproteins that are incorporated into plant cell walls, causing the walls to be more resistant to microbial invasion; synthesis of the hydrolases β-1,3-glucanase and chitinase (Metraux and Boller, 1986), which may inhibit fungi by degrading their cell walls; and synthesis and accumulation of antimicrobial compounds called phytoalexins (Bell, 1981; Collinge and Slusarenko, 1987; Darvill and Albersheim, 1984; Hahlbrock and Scheel, 1987; Corbin et al., 1987).

Some of the most detailed studies on the regulation of defense-related genes have involved characterization of the induction of genes encoding enzymes involved in phytoalexin biosynthesis in French bean (Lamb et al., 1986) and parsley (Hahlbrock and Scheel, 1987; Kombrink et al., 1986). The results of these studies indicate that there are groups of coordinately regulated genes that differ in the timing of their induction. Moreover, several of these genes, i.e., those encoding phenylalanine ammonia lyase (PAL), 4-coumarate coenzyme A ligase (4CL), and chalcone synthase, have been shown to be transcriptionally activated (Lamb et al., 1986; Kombrink et al., 1986). Other defense-related products have also been shown to be associated with increased steady-state levels of their mRNAs (Collinge and Slusarenko, 1987), suggesting that transcriptional activation may play a major role in defense gene expression.

GENETICS OF PLANT-PATHOGEN INTERACTIONS

Although it is thought that all plants possess a battery of defense genes, they do not always deploy these defenses effectively. A requisite for the effective expression of defense genes is the detection of the invading pathogen. Flor (1947) demonstrated in the flax rust system that resistance to a particular race of rust was frequently determined by a single dominant resistance gene in the host plant. Conversely, the different races of flax rust differed by single dominant avirulence genes. Flor (1947) postulated that the possession of a given avirulence gene by a pathogen triggers the expression of a hypersensitive response (HR) by the plant host, which carries the corresponding resistance gene. The HR is a complex process that includes rapid necrosis and desiccation of host tissue and interruption of the infection process. In practice, *avr* genes of pathogenic bacteria and fungi are defined as genes that elicit an HR from the plant host.

The existence of bacterial *avr* genes was first demonstrated by Staskawicz et al. (1984) for the soybean (*Glycine max*) pathogen *P. syringae* pv. *glycinae*. Race 4 of the pathogen normally causes disease on the soybean cultivars Harosoy and

Norchief, whereas race 6 causes disease only on Norchief. On Harosoy, race 6 elicits an HR and fails to cause disease. A single cloned gene from race 6 was found that when transferred to race 4 caused it to elicit an HR on Harosoy but not Norchief. One interpretation of these results is that *P. syringae* pv. *glycinae* race 6 contains a gene, *avrA*, that is specifically recognized by the soybean cultivar Harosoy. The simplest model is that the *avrA* gene product is recognized by the product of a Harosoy resistance gene.

During the past 5 years, a number of bacterial *avr* genes from *P. syringae* pv. *glycinae* have been cloned and sequenced (Tamaki et al., 1988; Napoli and Staskawicz, 1987). Avirulence genes have also been cloned from two other bacterial pathogens, *P. syringae* pv. *tomato* (Kobayashi et al., 1989) and *Xanthomonas campestris* pv. *malvacearum* (Gabriel et al., 1986). The biochemical functions of these *avr* genes are unknown.

In contrast to *avr* genes, bacterial pathogens have a variety of genes that contribute to their pathogenicity. Many pseudomonad pathogens produce toxins that enhance disease symptoms. Two of the best-characterized toxins are tabtoxin from *P. syringae* pv. *tabaci* and phaseolotoxin from *P. syringae* pv. *phaseolicola*. Tabtoxin inhibits glutamine synthetase, leading to toxic levels of ammonia in the leaf (Knight et al., 1986). Phaseolotoxin is an inhibitor of ornithine carbamoyl-transferase, leading to ornithine accumulation in affected tissues (Ferguson and Johnston, 1980). Other toxins include syringomycin from *P. syringae* pv. *syringae* (Xu and Gross, 1988) and coronatine from *P. syringae* pv. *tomato*. Coronatine is typical of pseudomonad toxins in that it is not specifically required for colonization and invasion of the host, but its production is important for the spread of lesions and the attainment of large bacterial populations in the leaf (Bender et al., 1987).

Hydrolytic enzymes have been implicated as pathogenicity factors of bacterial soft rot and wilt pathogens. These include pectate lyases from *Erwinia chrysanthemi* and *X. campestris* pv. *campestris* (Collmer et al., 1982; Daniels et al., 1984; Dow et al., 1987) and polygalacturanase and β-1,4-endoglucanase from *Pseudomonas solanacearum* (Schell et al., 1988; Roberts et al., 1988). Finally, extracellular polysaccharides have been shown to play an important role in pathogenesis, such as for the wilt pathogen *P. solanacearum* (Kelman, 1954; Whatley et al., 1980).

Recently, regulatory genes that are required for the activation of a variety of virulence factors as well as the *avr* genes have been identified in several *Pseudomonas* species (Lindgren et al., 1986; Boucher et al., 1986). Specifically, mutations in the *hrp* region of *P. syringae* pv. *phaseolicola* result not only in the loss of virulence on a susceptible host but also in the failure to activate transcription of the *avrB* gene (Lindgren et al., 1986). Interestingly, the *P. syringae* pv. *phaseolicola hrpS* gene product shares considerable homology with a highly conserved domain of a class of bacterial regulatory proteins that include *ntrC*, *nifA*, and *dctD* (Albright et al., 1989; Grimm and Panopoulos, 1989; Huynh et al., 1989). Because each of these regulators activates transcription in conjunction with the alternate sigma factor, NtrA (σ^{54}), it is likely that a *P. syringae* homolog of *ntrA* plays an essential role in pathogenesis. We are currently testing this hypothesis (see below).

RATIONALE FOR DEVELOPING THE *ARABIDOPSIS-PSEUDOMONAS* SYSTEM

Although progress has been made in identifying bacterial genes involved in pathogenesis and the elicitation of plant defenses, the mechanisms by which bacterial pathogens activate plant defenses are still unknown. Conversely, although advances have been made in identifying specific plant genes that are activated during attempted infection or treatment with compounds derived from microorganisms (elicitors; see Darvill and Albersheim [1984]), very little is known about the mechanisms involved in the activation of these defense-related genes. Because the plant-pathogen interaction necessarily involves two organisms, it would be desirable to be able to genetically manipulate both a bacterial pathogen and its host plant. Our major incentive in developing *A. thaliana* as a model host for *P. syringae* pv. *maculicola* is the potential of using a combination of genetic and biochemical-molecular biological approaches in *A. thaliana* as well as in *P. syringae* pv. *maculicola* to elucidate the mechanisms whereby the plant and pathogen recognize each other and how the recognition signals are transduced, causing the transcriptional activation of virulence genes in the pathogen and defense-related genes in the host.

PRELIMINARY RESULTS

P. syringae pv. *maculicola* Is an *A. thaliana* Pathogen

Because *A. thaliana* itself has no agronomic importance, there is virtually no published work on pathogens that infect it. However, since *A. thaliana* is a taxonomic relative of rapeseed, cabbage, and mustard, we reasoned that it might be susceptible to pathogens of these crop plants. After testing a number of potential pathogens, we focused our attention on *P. syringae* pv. *maculicola* because several strains that were virulent on *A. thaliana* were identified and because the *P. syringae* group contains some of the best-studied bacterial plant pathogens. Testing of these *P. syringae* pv. *maculicola* strains has been carried out in collaboration with Brian Staskawicz's laboratory at the University of California at Berkeley.

The initial goal with the *P. syringae* strains was to identify race-specific interactions that might be used to identify *A. thaliana* pathogen resistance genes. However, among 20 wild ecotypes of *A. thaliana* that were infiltrated with a variety of *P. syringae* strains, it was found that any particular *P. syringae* pv. *maculicola* strain elicited essentially the same response on all of the *A. thaliana* ecotypes tested. The *P. syringae* pv. *maculicola* strains could be divided into three categories, depending on the response of the *A. thaliana* plants to infiltration: the strains elicited either a susceptible (pathogenic) response, a hypersensitive response, or a null response. The susceptible and hypersensitive responses were typical of what is observed in other plant-pathogen systems. The null response was characterized by the lack of either a susceptible or a hypersensitive response when a larger number of bacteria were infiltrated into the host. Although a null interaction frequently indicates that a bacterium is a nonpathogen, in several cases null strains were able to elicit an HR in tobacco (nonhost resistance), something that a nonpathogen typically does not do.

Induction of *A. thaliana* Defense Genes by *P. syringae* pv. *maculicola*

We have examined the induction of several enzymatic activities and genes in *A. thaliana* that have been shown in other systems to be activated in response to pathogens (Davis and Hahlbrock, 1987; Edwards et al., 1985). Initially, we focused on the induction of genes coding for the following enzymes involved in phenylpropanoid metabolism: PAL, 4CL, caffeic acid *O*-methyltransferase, and peroxidase. We found that all of these enzymes were induced in *A. thaliana* tissue culture cells treated with the elicitor polygalacturonate lyase and that the induction of PAL and 4CL activities correlated with accumulation of mRNAs for these enzymes (Davis and Ausubel, 1989). More significantly, accumulation of PAL and 4CL mRNAs was also induced in planta in response to infiltration with *P. syringae* pv. *maculicola*. As expected, the levels of mRNA induction were different for the pathogenic and avirulent strains of the bacteria, similar to findings in other systems (Bell et al., 1986).

We have also been studying the *A. thaliana* β-1,3-glucanase gene family, which is likely to play an important defensive role in pathogen attack (Boller et al., 1983). The *A. thaliana* genome contains three β-1,3-glucanase genes, which are all adjacent to each other. The mRNAs corresponding to two of these genes accumulate in tissue culture cells treated with elicitor and in leaves infiltrated by *P. syringae* pv. *maculicola*.

Strategy for Identifying *A. thaliana* Pathogenesis Mutants

Two basic strategies are being used to identify *A. thaliana* mutants that display altered phenotypic responses to pathogens or elicitors. The first approach uses the three classes of *P. syringae* pv. *maculicola* strains described above to infiltrate mutagenized populations of *A. thaliana* and to screen for mutant plants that fail to display the typical phenotypic response. Using this first approach, we expect to identify mutants that fail to develop an HR (i.e., are susceptible) in response to an avirulent strain (type 1), are more resistant to a pathogenic strain (type 2), or are responsive to a null strain (type 3). On the basis of the model of plant-pathogen interaction described above, type 1 mutants should have defects in the detection of the product(s) of *avr* genes, possibly as a result of the lack of a receptor or signal transducer. Type 2 mutants should have gained the ability to recognize and respond to a normally pathogenic strain. Type 3 mutants should have either gained the ability to recognize a null strain or lost tolerance for its presence. Given these options, mutations that block the HR should be the easiest to identify, since they represent a loss of function.

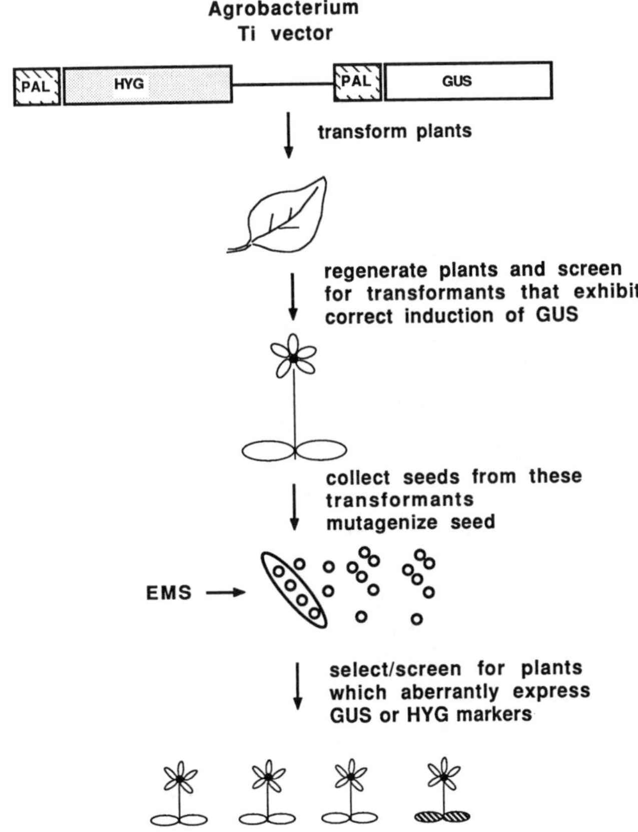

FIGURE 1. Experimental strategy for identifying *A. thaliana* mutants that contain altered *trans*-acting transcriptional factors that regulate the expression of pathogen-responsive genes. Abbreviations not given in text: HYG, hygromycin; GUS, β-glucuronidase; EMS, ethyl methanesulfonate.

The second approach for isolating *A. thaliana* mutations that result in a defective pathogenic response is to screen for mutants that fail to activate a specific pathogen-responsive gene. Transgenic *A. thaliana* plants that carry fusions of the PAL and β-1,3-glucanase gene promoters with readily assayed reporter genes such as that encoding β-glucuronidase (Jefferson et al., 1987) or chloramphenicol transacetylase are being constructed. Mutagenized plants carrying these fusions will be infiltrated with an appropriate *P. syringae* pv. *maculicola* strain. Subsequently, infected leaf ''punches'' will be assayed in microdilution plates for induction of the fusion (Fig. 1).

Genetics of *P. syringae* pv. *maculicola* Pathogenesis

In the past decade, genetic investigation of *P. syringae* pathovars has proceeded in two general directions. Genes whose presence in the bacterium causes it to be avirulent (that is, elicits an HR) have been identified. The other approach has been to identify genes that, when mutated, render the bacterium nonpathogenic. Our research on *P. syringae* pv. *maculicola* has proceeded in the same directions.

A library of an avirulent strain of *P. syringae* pv. *maculicola* was constructed in a wide-host-range cosmid vector that allows conjugation of library members to a virulent strain. Approximately 1,000 transconjugants were screened with the objective of finding clones that confer avirulence on the pathogenic recipient. Identifying specific *avr* genes in *P. syringae* pv. *maculicola* will allow us to set up genotype-specific screens for *A. thaliana* mutants that fail to respond to a particular *avr* gene. Maureen Whalen and Brian Staskawicz (personal communication) at the University of California at Berkeley have adopted a similar strategy.

We are also using gene libraries of both pathogenic and avirulent strains of *P. syringae* pv. *maculicola* to clone homologs to known bacterial signal transduction genes. For example, using a cloned *ntrA* (σ^{54}) gene from *P. aeruginosa* provided by Stephen Lory at the University of Washington, we have cloned a *P. syringae* pv. *maculicola ntrA* homolog that is able to complement phenotypically *ntrA* mutations in *Klebsiella pneumoniae* and *Escherichia coli*. We are now using these clones to construct *P. syringae* pv. *maculicola ntrA* deletion-insertion mutations. As described above, because of the homology between the *P. syringae* pv. *phaseolicola hrpS* gene and other positive regulators that require the NtrA sigma factor, we have hypothesized that *ntrA* will play an essential role in pathogenesis.

CONCLUSIONS

Our results to date show that *A. thaliana* plants and tissue cultures respond to bacterial pathogens and to elicitors in a manner similar to other plants and plant tissue cultures that have been studied. This finding suggests that the regulation of putative defense responses of *A. thaliana* is similar to the regulation of defense genes in other plants and that work in *A. thaliana* should provide insights into the regulation of defense responses in economically important plants. Finally, because we are now in a position to screen for the ability of a pathogen to activate a single pathogen-responsive gene in the host, it should be possible to identify specific bacterial signals that activate only a subset of plant defense genes as well as to elucidate the role that specific defense genes play in resistance to a given pathogen.

ACKNOWLEDGMENT. Unpublished work from our laboratory is supported by a grant from Hoechst AG to the Massachusetts General Hospital.

LITERATURE CITED

Albright, L. M., E. Huala, and F. M. Ausubel. 1989. Prokaryotic signal transduction mediated by sensor and regulator protein pairs. *Annu. Rev. Genet.* **23**:311–336.

Bell, A. A. 1981. Biochemical mechanisms of disease resistance. *Annu. Rev. Plant Physiol.* **23**:21–81.

Bell, J. N., T. B. Ryder, V. P. M. Wingate, J. A. Bailey, and C. J. Lamb. 1986. Differential accumulation of plant defense gene transcripts in a compatible and an incompatible plant-pathogen interaction. *Mol. Cell. Biol.* **6**:1615–1623.

Bender, C. L., H. E. Stone, J. J. Sims, and D. A. Cooksey. 1987. Reduced pathogen fitness of *Pseudomonas syringae* pv. *tomato* mutants defective in coronatine production. *Physiol. Mol. Plant Pathol.* **30:**273–283.

Boller, T., A. Gehri, F. Mauch, and U. Vogeli. 1983. Chitinase in bean leaves: induction by ethylene, purification, properties, and possible function. *Planta* **157:**22–31.

Boucher, C. A., A. Martinel, P. Barberis, G. Alloing, and C. Zischek. 1986. Virulence genes are carried on a megaplasmid of the pathogen *Pseudomonas solanacearum*. *Mol. Gen. Genet.* **205:**270–275.

Chang, C., J. L. Bowman, A. W. DeJohn, E. S. Lander, and E. M. Meyerowitz. 1988. Restriction fragment length polymorphism map for *Arabidopsis thaliana*. *Proc. Natl. Acad. Sci. USA* **85:**6856–6860.

Collinge, D. B., and A. J. Slusarenko. 1987. Plant gene expression in response to pathogens. *Plant Mol. Biol.* **9:**389–410.

Collmer, A., P. Bergman, and M. S. Mount. 1982. Pectate lyase regulation and bacterial soft rot pathogenesis, p. 395–422. *In* M. S. Mount and G. H. Lacy (ed.), *Phytopathogenic Prokaryotes*. Academic Press, Inc., New York.

Corbin, D. R., H. Sauer, and C. J. Lamb. 1987. Differential regulation of a hydroxyproline-rich glycoprotein gene family in wounded and infected plants. *Mol. Cell. Biol.* **7:**4337–4344.

Daniels, M. J., C. E. Barber, P. C. Turner, M. K. Sawczyc, R. J. W. Byrde, and A. H. Fielding. 1984. Cloning of genes involved in pathogenicity of *Xanthomonas campestris* pv. *campestris* using the broad host range plasmid pLAFR1. *EMBO J.* **3:**3323–3328.

Darvill, A. G., and P. Albersheim. 1984. Phytoalexins and their elicitors—a defense against microbial infection in plants. *Annu. Rev. Plant Physiol.* **35:**243–275.

Davis, K. R., and F. M. Ausubel. 1989. Characterization of elicitor-induced defense responses in suspension-cultured cells of *Arabidopsis*. *Mol. Plant Microbe Interact.* **2,** in press.

Davis, K. R., and K. Hahlbrock. 1987. Induction of defense responses in cultured parsley cells by plant cell wall fragments. *Plant Physiol.* **85:**1286–1290.

Dow, J. M., G. Scofield, K. Trafford, P. C. Turner, and M. J. Daniels. 1987. A gene cluster in *Xanthomonas campestris* pv. *campestris* required for pathogenicity controls the excretion of polygalacturonase and other enzymes. *Physiol. Mol. Plant Pathol.* **31:**261–271.

Edwards, K., C. L. Cramer, G. P. Bolwell, R. A. Dixon, W. Schuch, and C. J. Lamb. 1985. Rapid transient induction of phenylalanine ammonia-lyase mRNA in elicitor-treated bean cells. *Proc. Natl. Acad. Sci. USA* **82:**6731–6735.

Ferguson, A. R., and J. S. Johnston. 1980. Phaseolotoxin chlorosis, ornithine accumulation, and inhibition of ornithine transcarbamoyltransferase in different plants. *Physiol. Plant Pathol.* **16:**269–275.

Flor, A. H. 1947. Host-parasite interactions in flax rust—its genetics and other implications. *Phytopathology* **45:**680–685.

Gabriel, D. W., A. Burgess, and G. R. Lazo. 1986. Gene-for-gene interactions of five cloned avirulence genes from *Xanthomonas campestris* pv. *malvacearum* with specific resistance genes in cotton. *Proc. Natl. Acad. Sci. USA* **83:**6415–6419.

Grimm, C., and N. J. Panopoulos. 1989. The predicted protein product of a pathogenicity locus from *Pseudomonas syringae* pv. *phaseolicola* is homologous to a highly conserved domain of several procaryotic regulatory proteins. *J. Bacteriol.* **171:**5031–5038.

Hahlbrock, K., and D. Scheel. 1987. Biochemical responses of plants to pathogens, p. 229–254. *In* I. Chet (ed.), *Innovative Approaches to Plant Disease Control*. John Wiley & Sons, Inc., New York.

Huynh, T. V., D. Dahlbeck, and B. J. Staskawicz. 1989. Bacterial blight of soybean: regulation of a pathogen gene determining host cultivar specificity. *Science* **245:**1374–1377.

Jefferson, R. A., T. A. Kavanagh, and M. W. Bevan. 1987. GUS fusions: beta-glucuronidase as a sensitive and versatile gene fusion marker in higher plants. *EMBO J.* **6:**3901–3907.

Kelman, A. 1954. The relationship of pathogenicity of *Pseudomonas solanacearum* to colony appearance on tetrazolium medium. *Phytopathology* **44:**693–695.

Knight, T. J., R. D. Durbin, and P. J. Langston-Unkefer. 1986. Effects of tabtoxinine-β-lactam on nitrogen metabolism in *Avena sativa* L. roots. *Plant Physiol.* **82:**1045–1050.

Kobayashi, D. Y., S. J. Tamaki, and N. T. Keen. 1989. Cloned avirulence genes from the tomato pathogen *Pseudomonas syringae* pv. tomato confer cultivar specificity on soybean. *Proc. Natl. Acad. Sci. USA* **86:**157–161.

Kombrink, E., J. Bollmann, K. D. Hauffe, W. Knogge, D. Scheel, E. Schmelzer, I. Somssich, and K. Hahlbrock. 1986. Biochemical responses of non-host plant cells to fungi and fungal elicitors, p. 253–262. *In* J. A. Bailey (ed.), *Biology and Molecular Biology of Plant-Pathogen Interactions.* NATO ASI Ser., vol. H1. Springer-Verlag KG, Berlin.

Koornneef, M., J. van Eden, C. J. Hanhart, P. Stam, F. J. Braaksma, and W. J. Feenstra. 1983. Linkage map of *Arabidopsis thaliana. J. Hered.* **74:**265–272.

Lamb, C. J., D. R. Corbin, M. A. Lawton, N. Sauer, and V. P. M. Wingate. 1986. Recognition and response in plant:pathogen interactions, p. 333–344. *In* B. Lugtenberg (ed.), *Recognition in Microbe-Plant Symbiotic Interactions.* Springer-Verlag KG, Berlin.

Leutwiler, L. S., R. B. Hough-Evans, and E. M. Meyerowitz. 1984. The DNA of *Arabidopsis thaliana. Mol. Gen. Genet.* **194:**15–23.

Lindgren, P. B., R. C. Peet, and N. J. Panopoulos. 1986. A gene cluster of *Pseudomonas syringae* pv. *phaseolicola* controls pathogenicity on bean and hypersensitivity on non-host plants. *J. Bacteriol.* **169:**512–522.

Lloyd, A. M., A. R. Barnason, S. G. Rogers, M. C. Byrne, R. T. Fraley, and R. B. Horsch. 1986. Transformation of *Arabidopsis* with *Agrobacterium tumefaciens. Science* **234:**464–466.

Mansfield, J. 1983. Antimicrobial compounds, p. 237–265. *In* J. A. Callow (ed.), *Biochemical Plant Pathology.* John Wiley & Sons, Inc., New York.

Metraux, J. P., and T. Boller. 1986. Local and systemic induction of chitinase in cucumber plants in response to viral, bacterial, and fungal infections. *Physiol. Mol. Plant Pathol.* **28:**161–169.

Meyerowitz, E. M. 1987. *Arabidopsis thaliana. Annu. Rev. Genet.* **21:**93–111.

Meyerowitz, E. M., and R. E. Pruitt. 1985. *Arabidopsis thaliana* and plant molecular genetics. *Science* **229:**1214–1218.

Nam, H.-G., J. Giraudat, B. den Boer, F. Moonan, W. D. B. Loos, B. M. Hauge, and H. M. Goodman. 1989. Restriction fragment length polymorphism linkage map of *Arabidopsis thaliana. Plant Cell* **1:**699–705.

Napoli, C., and B. J. Staskawicz. 1987. Molecular characterization and nucleic acid sequence of an avirulence gene from race 6 of *Pseudomonas syringae* pv. *glycinae. J. Bacteriol.* **169:**572–578.

Pang, P. P., and E. M. Meyerowitz. 1987. *Arabidopsis thaliana*: a model system for plant molecular biology. *Bio/Technology* **5:**1177–1181.

Roberts, D. P., T. P. Denny, and M. A. Schell. 1988. Cloning of the *egl* gene of *Pseudomonas solanacearum* and analysis of its role in phytopathogenicity. *J. Bacteriol.* **170:**1445–1451.

Schell, M. A., D. P. Roberts, and T. P. Denny. 1988. Analysis of the *Pseudomonas solanacearum* polygalacturonase encoded by *pglA* and its involvement in phytopathogenicity. *J. Bacteriol.* **170:**4501–4508.

Staskawicz, B. J., D. Dahlbeck, and N. Keen. 1984. Cloned avirulence gene of *Pseudomonas syringae* pv. *glycinae* determines race-specific incompatibility on *Glycine max. Proc. Natl. Acad. Sci. USA* **81:**6024–6028.

Staskawicz, B. J., D. Dahlbeck, N. Keen, and C. Napoli. 1987. Molecular characterization of cloned avirulence genes from race 0 and race 1 of *Pseudomonas syringae* pv. *glycinae. J. Bacteriol.* **169:**5789–5792.

Tamaki, S., D. Dahlbeck, B. J. Staskawicz, and N. Keen. 1988. Characterization and expression of two avirulence genes cloned from *Pseudomonas syringae* pv. *glycinae. J. Bacteriol.* **170:**4846–4854.

Valvekens, D., M. van Montagu, and M. van Lijsebettens. 1988. *Agrobacterium tumefaciens* mediated transformation of *Arabidopsis thaliana* root explants by using kanamycin selection. *Proc. Natl. Acad. Sci. USA* **85:**5536–5540.

Whatley, M. H., N. Hunter, M. A. Cantrell, C. A. Hendrick, L. Sequiera, and K. Keegstra. 1980. Lipopolysaccharide composition of the wilt pathogen *Pseudomonas solanacearum*: correlation to the hypersensitivity response in tobacco. *Plant Physiol.* **65:**557–559.

Xu, G.-W., and D. C. Gross. 1988. Evaluation of the role of syringomycin in plant pathogenesis by using Tn*5* mutants of *Pseudomonas syringae* pv. *syringae* defective in syringomycin production. *Appl. Environ. Microbiol.* **54:**1345–1353.

Chapter 10

Rhizobium meliloti Genes Involved in Exopolysaccharide Production and Infection of Alfalfa Nodules

M. Keller, W. Arnold, D. Kapp, P. Müller, K. Niehaus, M. Schmidt, J. Quandt, W. M. Weng, and A. Pühler

The gram-negative soil bacterium *Rhizobium meliloti* is able to fix atmospheric nitrogen in symbiosis with alfalfa (*Medicago sativa*). This process takes place in root nodules that are colonized by the microsymbiont. One important step in nodule formation is the synthesis of the infection thread. It has been found that acidic exopolysaccharides (EPS) play an essential role in infection thread formation. Mutants lacking the ability to synthesize acidic EPS fail to invade root nodules (Leigh et al., 1985; Finan et al., 1985; Müller et al., 1988b). In this chapter, we describe *R. meliloti* genes that are involved in EPS production and nodule infection.

ISOLATION AND ANALYSIS OF *R. MELILOTI* INFECTION MUTANTS ALTERED IN EPS PRODUCTION

After Tn5 mutagenesis of *R. meliloti* 2011, several symbiotic mutants could be isolated (Pühler et al., 1986). A specific group of mutants could be characterized by their defects in nodule infection (Inf⁻). Inf⁻ mutants induce ineffective alfalfa nodules that lack infection threads and are therefore devoid of bacteroids (Müller et al., 1988b). Such empty nodules were described by several other researchers (Leigh et al., 1985; Finan et al., 1985; Finan et al., 1986). The Inf⁻ mutants isolated in our laboratory could be subdivided into two classes (Müller et al., 1988b). One class of mutants produces acidic EPS lacking the terminal

M. Keller, W. Arnold, D. Kapp, K. Niehaus, M. Schmidt, J. Quandt, W. M. Weng, and A. Pühler ● Faculty of Biology, Department of Genetics, University of Bielefeld, Postbox 8640, D-4800 Bielefeld 1, Federal Republic of Germany. *P. Müller* ● Department of Biology/Botany, Philipps University Marburg, Karl-von-Frisch Strasse, D-3550 Marburg, Federal Republic of Germany.

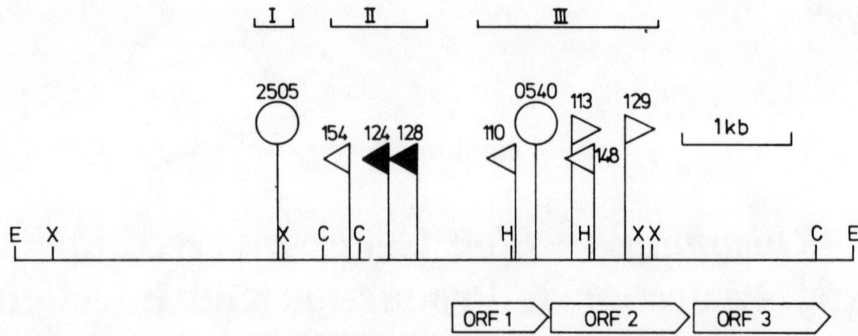

FIGURE 1. Genetic analysis of the 7.8-kb *Eco*RI fragment located on megaplasmid 2 of *R. meliloti*. Tn5 (○) and Tn5-*lacZ* (◀, ◁) insertions are numbered. The flags indicate the transcription direction of the promoterless *lacZ* gene of transposon Tn5-*lacZ*. ◁, EPS⁻ Inf⁻ phenotype; ◀, EPS⁺ Inf⁺ phenotype of the corresponding mutant. The transposon mutations are grouped in three regions (I, II, and III). The open bars below the map represent the sequenced ORFs. Abbreviations for restriction enzyme sites: E, *Eco*RI; X, *Xho*I; C, *Cla*I; H, *Hin*dIII.

pyruvyl residue (EPS*). Mutations leading to EPS* were located on the chromosome in a region recently described to be responsible for nodule development (Dylan et al., 1986; Geremia et al., 1987).

Mutations of the other class completely abolished the production of acidic EPS. These mutants can easily be distinguished from the wild type because they do not fluoresce on Cellufluor-white agar when viewed under UV light (Hynes et al., 1986; Müller et al., 1988b; Keller et al., 1988). Tn5 insertions responsible for the EPS⁻ Inf⁻ phenotype could be located on the second megaplasmid of *R. meliloti* (Hynes et al., 1986). Several complementing cosmids were isolated and physically mapped (Müller et al., 1988a). Tn5 insertions were localized on a 7.8-kilobase-pair (kb) *Eco*RI fragment, which was further analyzed.

THREE DEFINED DNA REGIONS ON A 7.8-KB FRAGMENT OF MEGAPLASMID 2 ARE INVOLVED IN EPS SYNTHESIS AND NODULE INFECTION

To obtain more information about the 7.8-kb *Eco*RI fragment of megaplasmid 2, we carried out a fragment-specific Tn5-*lacZ* mutagenesis. With this approach, it was possible to identify gene regions involved in EPS synthesis and nodule infection and to analyze the transcriptional activity at the insertion site of Tn5-*lacZ* (Keller et al., 1988). According to the location of the different Tn5 or Tn5-*lacZ* insertions, we defined at least three regions (I, II, and III) on the 7.8-kb fragment that are responsible for nodule invasion, EPS synthesis, or both (Fig. 1; Keller et al., 1988).

Mutations in regions I and III showed a clear Inf⁻ EPS⁻ phenotype, emphasizing the correlation between EPS production and nodule invasion. Insertions in region II exhibited a somewhat more complicated phenotype.

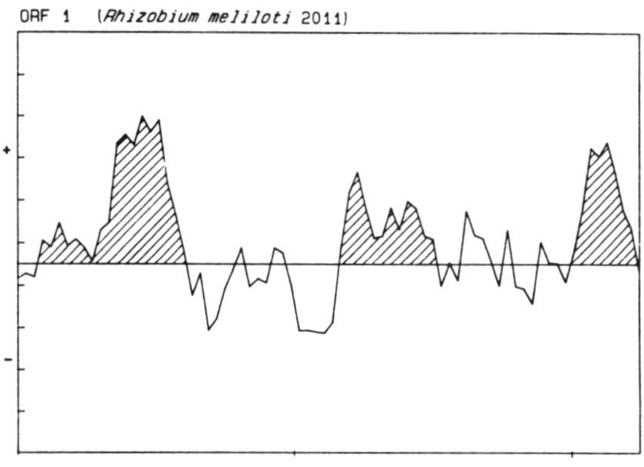

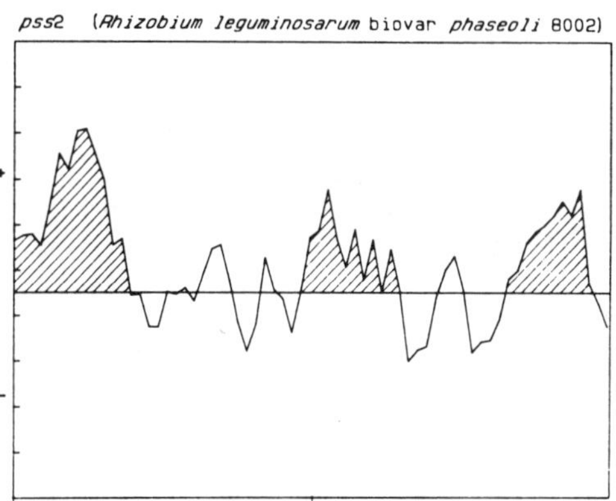

FIGURE 2. Analysis of the polypeptides encoded by the *R. meliloti* ORF1 and the *R. leguminosarum* bv. *phaseoli pss2* gene. The hydropathic plot (Kyte and Doolittle, 1982) is divided into hydrophobic (+) and hydrophilic (−) regions. The hatched areas mark clusters of amino acids in hydrophobic domains present in both polypeptides at equivalent regions.

Insertion 154 also caused an Inf⁻ EPS⁻ phenotype, but the corresponding mutant exhibited weak UV fluorescence on Cellufluor-containing agar. In contrast to the wild type and other EPS⁻ mutants, the *R. meliloti* mutant Rm154 could also be stained with Congo red and aniline blue, probably indicating the production of an unusual polysaccharide. Insertions 124 and 128 had no negative effect on the symbiotic properties of *R. meliloti*, but mutants harboring these insertions produced different amounts of EPS. Mutant Rm124 produced 300% and mutant Rm128 produced only 30% of the wild-type level of EPS. For regions II and III, we could also demonstrate by transcriptional *lacZ* fusions that some EPS genes are translated not only in the free-living but also in the symbiotic state.

SEQUENCE ANALYSIS OF THE DNA REGION III LOCATED ON MEGAPLASMID 2 REVEALED THREE ORFS

For a more detailed analysis, we started to sequence the 7.8-kb *Eco*RI fragment. In DNA region III, we identified three open reading frames (ORFs)

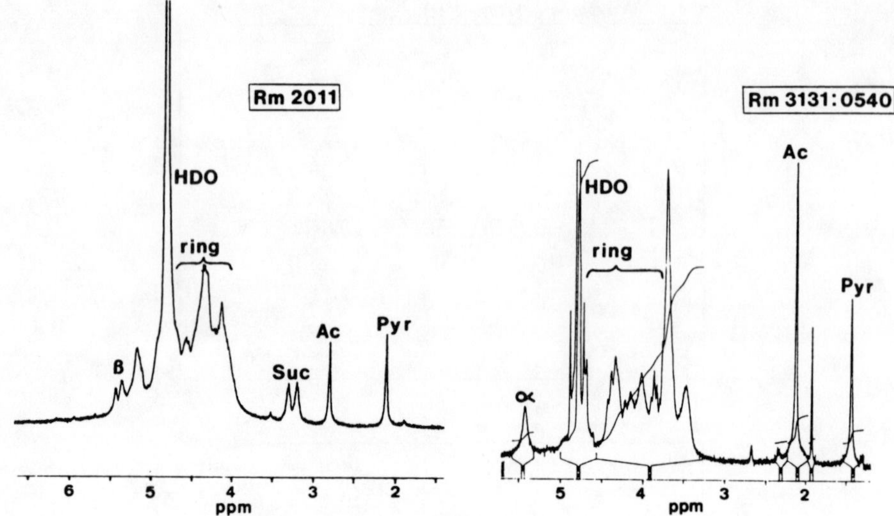

FIGURE 3. Proton NMR spectra of EPS produced by *R. meliloti* wild-type strain 2011 and the *R. meliloti* double mutant RmJQ46 (Rm3131:0540). The spectrum of EPS produced by *R. meliloti* 2011 was recorded at 20°C, and the spectrum of EPS produced by RmJQ46 was recorded at 80°C. The proton NMR spectrum of EPS from RmJQ46 differed significantly from the spectrum obtained from the wild-type EPS. A strong signal at 5.4 ppm indicates a high amount of α-anomeric glycosidic linkages in the EPS of RmJQ46, whereas in the wild-type EPS only β-anomeric linkages are observed. The signals from the ring protons of the sugars (4.5 to 3.4 ppm) indicate the main differences between the two EPS species. The signals at 3.3 and 3.2 ppm in the spectrum of wild-type EPS are missing in the spectrum of the EPS of RmJQ46, indicating that no succinyl group is present. The signals from methyl protons of acetate and pyruvate are present in both spectra. Abbreviations: α, α-anomeric protons; β, β-anomeric protons; HDO, hemideuterated water; ring, ring protons of the sugars; Suc, methyl protons of the succinyl groups; Ac, methyl protons of the acetyl groups; Pyr, methyl protons of the pyruvyl groups.

running from left to right (Fig. 1). The direction of transcription is in accordance with data obtained by operon fusions with *lacZ* monitor genes (Keller et al., 1988). Two of the identified ORFs (ORF1 and ORF2) have already been described (Müller et al., 1988a). ORF1 codes for a polypeptide of 226 amino acids that showed 37% homology with a polypeptide involved in EPS synthesis of *Rhizobium leguminosarum* bv. *phaseoli* encoded by a gene named *pss2* (Borthakur et al., 1988). When the hydrophobicities of these two polypeptides were compared (Fig. 2), the structural homology of the two polypeptides could clearly be seen. The hydropathic plot revealed hydrophobic domains at the N terminus, the center, and the C terminus of each protein (Fig. 2).

ORF2, separated from ORF1 by 52 base pairs, codes for a polypeptide of 407 amino acids. This ORF reveals homology to a sequence motif of 15 amino acids of the mouse testicular lactate dehydrogenase. This motif is responsible for binding the coenzyme NADH/H$^+$ (Pan et al., 1980). A comparison of the amino acid sequence of ORF3 with sequences in a protein data bank (R.16.0) did not reveal any clear relationship to known protein sequences.

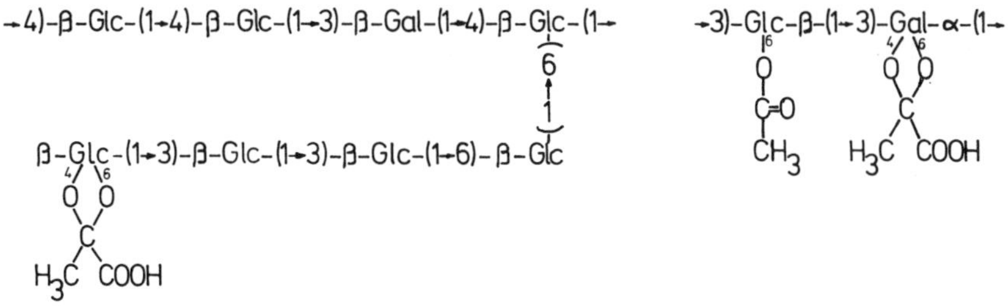

FIGURE 4. Chemical structure of repeating units of the two EPS of *R. meliloti*. The structure of the succinoglucan (EPSI; left) was published by Jansson et al. (1977); the structure of EPSII (right) was recently published by Glazebrook and Walker (1989). Abbreviations: Glc, glucose; Gal, galactose.

ORF1, ORF2, and ORF3 seem to be cotranscribed, since we could not identify any transcriptional signals in the noncoding regions between them. When we compared our genetic map of the 7.8-kb *Eco*RI fragment with the map recently published by Long et al. (1988), it became evident that at least ORF1 and ORF2 are part of the *exoF* complementation group.

R. MELILOTI MUTANTS PRODUCING A NOVEL EPS CAN INFECT ALFALFA NODULES

To identify new gene regions involved in EPS synthesis, we carried out an additional Tn*5* mutagenesis, using the Tn*5* delivering plasmid 2011 (Simon et al., 1983). We isolated several mutants with alterations in surface polysaccharides. Among these, one mutant (Rm3131) turned out to be of special interest. It showed a mucoid colony morphology, but only weak UV fluorescence could be observed when it was grown on Cellufluor-containing agar (data not shown). Further investigations of this mutant revealed that the Tn*5* insertion was located on the chromosome and that this mutant did not produce the acidic EPS (succinoglucan) of the *R. meliloti* 2011 wild-type strain. Nevertheless, this mutant was able to infect alfalfa nodules. We were able to isolate small amounts of EPS from cultures of this mutant. Larger amounts of EPS were isolated from a double mutant (RmJQ46) constructed by transduction of the Tn*5* insertion 0540 (region III in Fig. 1) into mutant Rm3131. ^{13}C and ^{1}H nuclear magnetic resonance (NMR) analyses of the EPS isolated from Rm3131 and RmJQ46 showed that the two mutants synthesized the same EPS. We were able to demonstrate that this EPS is different in structure from the succinoglucan produced by the wild-type strain. Our ^{1}H NMR data (Fig. 3) correlate well with the structure of EPSII (EPSb) previously published by Glazebrook and Walker (1989) and Zhan et al. (1989) (Fig. 4).

CONCLUSIONS

The results presented in this chapter demonstrate that EPS of *R. meliloti* are molecules important for the infection process of alfalfa root nodules. However, it remains to be determined which structural part of the EPS is responsible for efficient infection thread formation, since there are large differences between the succinoglucan and the novel EPS of *R. meliloti*.

ACKNOWLEDGMENTS. We thank Victor Wray, GBF Braunschweig, for discussion and measurement of the proton NMR spectra. We are indebted to A. Kleickmann for excellent technical assistance.

This work was supported by grant Pu 28/13-2 from Deutsche Forschungsgemeinschaft. K.N. was financed by Studienstiftung des Deutschen Volkes.

LITERATURE CITED

Borthakur, D., R. F. Barker, J. W. Latchford, L. Rossen, and A. W. B. Johnston. 1988. Analysis of *pss* genes of *Rhizobium leguminosarum* required for exopolysaccharide synthesis and nodulation of peas: their primary structure and their interaction with *psi* and other nodulation genes. *Mol. Gen. Genet.* **213**:155–162.

Dylan, T., L. Ielpi, S. Stanfield, L. Kashyap, C. Douglas, M. Yanofsky, E. Nester, D. R. Helinski, and G. Ditta. 1986. *Rhizobium meliloti* genes required for nodule development are related to chromosomal virulence genes in *Agrobacterium tumefaciens*. *Proc. Natl. Acad. Sci. USA* **83**:4403–4407.

Finan, T. M., A. M. Hirsch, J. A. Leigh, E. Johansen, G. A. Kuldau, S. Deegan, G. C. Walker, and E. R. Signer. 1985. Symbiotic mutants of *Rhizobium meliloti* that uncouple plant from bacterial differentiation. *Cell* **40**:869–877.

Finan, T. M., B. Kunkel, G. F. De Vos, and E. R. Signer. 1986. A second symbiotic megaplasmid in *Rhizobium meliloti* encodes exopolysaccharide and thiamine genes. *J. Bacteriol.* **167**:66–72.

Geremia, R. A., S. Cavaignac, A. Zorreguieta, N. Toro, J. Olivares, and R. A. Ugalde. 1987. A *Rhizobium meliloti* mutant that forms ineffective pseudonodules in alfalfa produces normal exopolysaccharide but fails to form β-(1→2) glucan. *J. Bacteriol.* **169**:880–884.

Glazebrook, J., and G. C. Walker. 1989. A novel exopolysaccharide can function in place of the Calcofluor-binding exopolysaccharide in nodulation of alfalfa by *Rhizobium meliloti*. *Cell* **56**:661–672.

Hynes, M. F., R. Simon, P. Müller, K. Niehaus, M. Labes, and A. Pühler. 1986. The two megaplasmids of *Rhizobium meliloti* are involved in the effective nodulation of alfalfa. *Mol. Gen. Genet.* **202**:356–362.

Jansson, P.-E., L. Kenne, B. Lindberg, H. Ljunggren, J. Lönngren, U. Ruden, and S. Svensson. 1977. Demonstration of an octasaccharide repeating unit in the extracellular polysaccharide of *Rhizobium meliloti* by sequential degradation. *J. Am. Chem. Soc.* **99**:3812–3815.

Keller, M., P. Müller, R. Simon, and A. Pühler. 1988. *Rhizobium meliloti* genes for exopolysaccharide synthesis and nodule infection located on megaplasmid 2 are actively transcribed during symbiosis. *Mol. Plant Microbe Interact.* **1**:267–274.

Kyte, J., and R. F. Doolittle. 1982. A simple method for displaying the hydropathic character of proteins. *J. Mol. Biol.* **157**:105–132.

Leigh, J. A., E. R. Signer, and G. C. Walker. 1985. Exopolysaccharide deficient mutants of *Rhizobium meliloti* that form ineffective nodules. *Proc. Natl. Acad. Sci. USA* **82**:6231–6235.

Long, S., J. W. Reed, J. Himawan, and G. C. Walker. 1988. Genetic analysis of a cluster of genes required for synthesis of the Calcofluor-binding exopolysaccharide of *Rhizobium meliloti*. *J. Bacteriol.* **170**:4239–4248.

Müller, P., B. Enenkel, A. Hillemann, D. Kapp, M. Keller, J. Quandt, and A. Pühler. 1988a. Genetic analysis of two DNA regions of the *Rhizobium meliloti* genome involved in the infection process of alfalfa nodules, p. 26–32. *In* R. Palacios and D. P. S. Verma (ed.), *Molecular Genetics of Plant-Microbe Interactions*. APS Press, St. Paul, Minn.

Müller, P., M. Hynes, D. Kapp, K. Niehaus, and A. Pühler. 1988b. The two classes of *Rhizobium meliloti* infection mutants differ in exopolysaccharide production and in coinoculation properties with nodulation mutants. *Mol. Gen. Genet.* **211**:17–26.

Pan, Y. E., S. Huang, J. P. Marciniszyn, Jr., C. Lee, and S. Li. 1980. The preliminary amino acid sequence of mouse testicular lactate dehydrogenase. *Hoppe-Seyler's Z. Physiol. Chem.* **361:** 795–799.

Pühler, A., M. F. Hynes, D. Kapp, P. Müller, and K. Niehaus. 1986. Infection mutants of *Rhizobium meliloti* are altered in acidic exopolysaccharide production, p. 29–37. *In* B. Lugtenberg (ed.), *Recognition in Microbe-Plant Symbiotic and Pathogenic Interactions*. Springer-Verlag KG, Berlin.

Simon, R., U. Priefer, and A. Pühler. 1983. A broad host range mobilization system for *in vivo* genetic engineering: transposon mutagenesis in Gram negative bacteria. *Bio/Technology* **1:**784–791.

Simon, R., J. Quandt, and W. Klipp. 1989. New derivatives of transposon Tn*5* suitable for mobilization of replicons, generation of operon fusions and induction of genes in Gram-negative bacteria. *Gene* **80:**161–169.

Zhan, H., S. B. Levery, C. C. Lee, and J. A. Leigh. 1989. A second exopolysaccharide of *Rhizobium meliloti* strain SU47 that can function in root nodule invasion. *Proc. Natl. Acad. Sci. USA* **86:**3055–3059.

Part III

BIOTRANSFORMATIONS

Chapter 11

Site-Directed Mutagenesis of the *Pseudomonas cam* Operon

Matthew D. Davies, Hideo Koga, Tadao Horiuchi, and Stephen G. Sligar

Beginning over 20 years ago, pioneering work in the Gunsalus laboratory showed that camphor could be used as the sole source of carbon and energy by a soil pseudomonad (Hedegaard and Gunsalus, 1965). This example provided the scientific community with a host of prototypic systems for the elucidation of molecular mechanisms of secondary metabolism. Experimental work on the ability of pseudomonads to use a wide variety of foodstuffs brought to light the concept of "metabolic plasmids" (Rheinwald et al., 1973). In camphor degradation, a 140-megadalton plasmid (Chakrabarty, 1976) has genes clustered in an operon which encode proteins that initiate monoterpene ring fission through alkaline hydroxylation, dehydrogenation, and then lactone formation through Bayer-Villiger chemistry (Fig. 1).

Although the 11 steps leading to acetate and isobutyrate represent interesting chemical biotransformations, the first step was the most exciting. The functionalization of an unactivated alkane is difficult chemistry, even without the degree of stereo- and regiospecificity seen in the 5-exo-hydroxylation of camphor. This oxygenation event is catalyzed by a soluble three-protein system linking pyridine nucleotide dehydrogenation by a flavin adenine dinucleotide flavoprotein (putidaredoxin reductase) to iron-sulfur protein (putidaredoxin)-mediated electron transport to the cytochrome. In the early 1970s, P-450$_{cam}$, obtained in absolute purity and high yield, served as the best model for the ubiquitous P-450s found in mammalian microsomal and mitochondrial fractions. Enzymatically active eucaryotic counterparts were isolated and purified to homogeneity through the diligence of the Coon laboratory several years later (Lu and Coon, 1968). Along with other members of the P-450 family, the bacterial enzymes continue to serve

Matthew D. Davies and Stephen G. Sligar ● Department of Biochemistry, University of Illinois, Urbana, Illinois 61801. *Hideo Koga and Tadao Horiuchi* ● Faculty of Pharmaceutical Sciences, Kyushu University, Fukuoka 812, Japan.

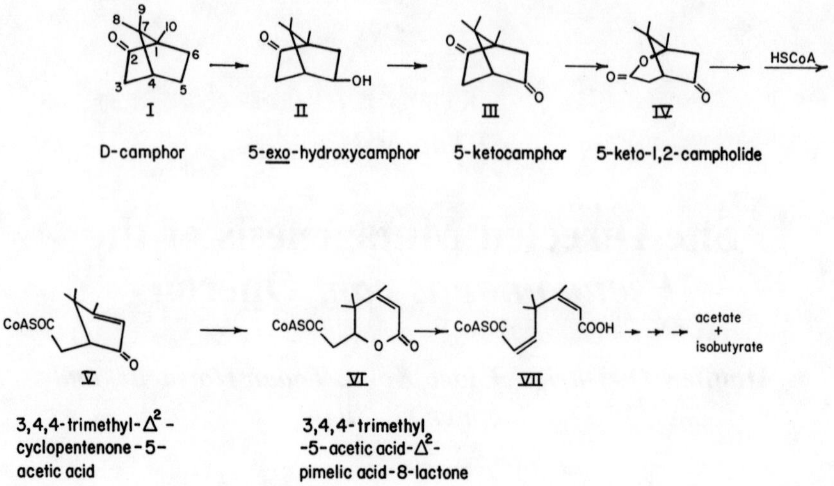

FIGURE 1. Pathway of camphor conversion to acetate and isobutyrate in *Pseudomonas putida* (ATCC 17453). Cytochrome P-450$_{cam}$ in the presence of NADH and its electron transport chain hydroxylates D-camphor at the 5-exo position. HSCoA, Coenzyme A; CoASOC, thioester-linked coenzyme A.

as an experimental system for understanding general problems of protein recognition, electron transport, and oxygen activation (for a review, see Sligar and Murray, 1986).

Our focus in this chapter will be on the utilization of recombinant DNA techniques, building on the breadth of biophysical and chemical data accumulated on the native components, to probe structure-function relationships necessary for camphor hydroxylation. To utilize site-directed mutagenesis, one needs a gene to mutate. Again, our work has benefited from the efforts and generosity of the Gunsalus laboratory. Hideo Koga, a visiting scientist from Kyushu University working with Dr. Gunsalus, cloned the operon containing the genes for P-450$_{cam}$, putidaredoxin, putidaredoxin reductase, 5-alcohol dehydrogenase, and a camphor operon regulatory protein (Koga et al., 1986). The operon structure is given in Fig. 2. The genetic manipulations of the *camA*, *camB*, and *camC* genes will be discussed separately.

PUTIDAREDOXIN REDUCTASE

The flavoprotein component of the camphor hydroxylase is a 48,000-dalton protein containing flavin adenine dinucleotide as a prosthetic group (Roome et al., 1983). Figure 3 shows the translated sequence (Koga et al., 1989). One of the interesting questions regarding the regulation of the *cam* operon concerns the mechanism by which the flavoprotein is expressed at some 10-fold lower levels than either putidaredoxin or P-450$_{cam}$, even though all three are on the same operon with the reductase between the two highly expressed proteins. The reductase gene translation is initiated by an unusual GTG codon. We expect that

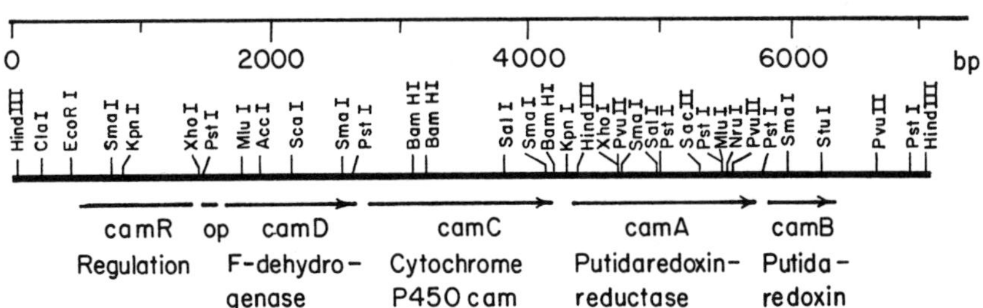

FIGURE 2. Physical and functional map of the camphor hydroxylase (*camDCAB*) operon. The protein product of CamR is a negative regulator which responds to camphor as an inducer of coordinate expression of the *camDCAB* genes (Koga et al., 1986). bp, Base pairs; op, operator.

this codon is responsible for the poor expression level. To increase the level of flavoprotein production for a myriad of biophysical characterizations, we mutated the wild-type codon to ATG. The synthetic oligonucleotide is shown in Fig. 4. The ATG-initiated gene was transferred to a pUC vector and transformed into *Escherichia coli* TB-1. The reductase expressed to roughly 10% of the total soluble cell protein, which is comparable to the expression of putidaredoxin and P-450$_{cam}$ in the same expression system.

PUTIDAREDOXIN

Hideo Koga, a visiting scientist from Kyushu University working with I. C. Gunsalus, cloned the P-450 *cam* gene during his stay (April 1980 through March 1982). After his return to Japan, he and his colleagues succeeded in cloning genes for NADH-putidaredoxin reductase, putidaredoxin, 5-alcohol dehydrogenase, and a camphor operon regulatory protein (Koga et al., 1986, 1989). The translated nucleotide sequence is given in Fig. 5 (Koga et al., 1989). Putidaredoxin is expressed to roughly 8% of the soluble cell protein. Our mutational analysis of putidaredoxin centers on refining chemical and enzymatic modification studies to further clarify the role played by particular residues in binding and electron transfer. In a system similar to that of camphor hydroxylase, chemical modification of bovine adrenal cortex ferredoxin implicated its surface carboxylates in binding to its reductase and P-450$_{scc}$ (Lambeth et al., 1984). Similarly, chemical modification of analogous carboxylates numbering 58, 65, and 67 in putidaredoxin decreased its association with putidaredoxin reductase (Geren et al., 1986). T. Nagamune in our laboratory has replaced the suspect carboxylates with the corresponding amines and lysine. Unfortunately, it appears that the proteins with replacements at positions 65 and 67 are expressed at less than 10% of the wild-type expression. Analysis of binding reactions for the position 58 mutant protein is under way.

Most interestingly, however, are a series of mutants which alter the single tryptophan at putidaredoxin's carboxyl terminus. Studies begun in the Gunsalus laboratory over 15 years ago (Sligar et al., 1974) suggested a role for this residue

```
               10             20             30             40             50             60
A C A C A T G G G A G T G C G T G C T A A G T G A A C G C A A A C G A C A A C G T G G T C A T C G T C G G T A C C G G A
                          Met Asn Ala Asn Asp Asn Val Val Ile Val Gly Thr Gly

               70             80             90            100            110            120
C T G G C T G G C G T T G A G G T C G C C T T C G G C C T G C G C G C C A G C G G C T G G G A A G G C A A T A T C C G G
Leu Ala Gly Val Glu Val Ala Phe Gly Leu Arg Ala Ser Gly Trp Glu Gly Asn Ile Arg

              130            140            150            160            170            180
T T G G T G G G G G A T G C G A C G G T A A T T C C C C A T C A C C T A C C A C C G C T A T C C A A A G C T T A C T T G
Leu Val Gly Asp Ala Thr Val Ile Pro His His Leu Pro Pro Leu Ser Lys Ala Tyr Leu

              190            200            210            220            230            240
G C C G G C A A A G C C A C A G C G G A A A G C C T G T A C C T G A G A A C C C C A G A T G C C T A T G C A G C G C A G
Ala Gly Lys Ala Thr Ala Glu Ser Leu Tyr Leu Arg Thr Pro Asp Ala Tyr Ala Ala Gln

              250            260            270            280            290            300
A A C A T C C A A C T A C T C G G A G G C A C A C A G G T A A C G G C T A T C A A C C G C G A C C G A C A G C A A G T A
Asn Ile Gln Leu Leu Gly Gly Thr Gln Val Thr Ala Ile Asn Arg Asp Arg Gln Gln Val

              310            320            330            340            350            360
A T C C T A T C G G A T G G C C G G G C A C T G G A T T A C G A C C G G C T G G T A T T G G C T A C C G G A G G G C G T
Ile Leu Ser Asp Gly Arg Ala Leu Asp Tyr Asp Arg Leu Val Leu Ala Thr Gly Gly Arg

              370            380            390            400            410            420
C C A A G A C C C C T A C C G G T G G C C A G T G G C G C A G T T G G A A A G G C G A A C A A C T T T C G A T A C C T G
Pro Arg Pro Leu Pro Val Ala Ser Gly Ala Val Gly Lys Ala Asn Asn Phe Arg Tyr Leu

              430            440            450            460            470            480
C G C A C A C T C G A G G A C G C C G A G T G C A T T C G C C G G C A G C T G A T T G C G G A T A A C C G T C T G G T G
Arg Thr Leu Glu Asp Ala Glu Cys Ile Arg Arg Gln Leu Ile Ala Asp Asn Arg Leu Val

              490            500            510            520            530            540
G T G A T T G G T G G C G G C T A C A T T G G C C T T G A A G T G G C T G C C A C C G C C A T C A A G G C G A A C A T G
Val Ile Gly Gly Gly Tyr Ile Gly Leu Glu Val Ala Ala Thr Ala Ile Lys Ala Asn Met

              550            560            570            580            590            600
C A C G T C A C C C T G C T T G A T A C G G C A G C C C G G G T T C T G G A G C G G G T T A C C G C C C C G C C G G T A
His Val Thr Leu Leu Asp Thr Ala Ala Arg Val Leu Glu Arg Val Thr Ala Pro Pro Val

              610            620            630            640            650            660
T C G G C C T T T T A C G A G C A C C T A C A C C G C G A A G C C G G C G T T G A C A T A C G A A C C G G C A C G C A G
Ser Ala Phe Tyr Glu His Leu His Arg Glu Ala Gly Val Asp Ile Arg Thr Gly Thr Gln

              670            680            690            700            710            720
G T G T G C G G G T T C G A G A T G T C G A C C G A C C A A C A G A A G G T T A C C G C C G T C C T C T G C G A G G A C
Val Cys Gly Phe Glu Met Ser Thr Asp Gln Gln Lys Val Thr Ala Val Leu Cys Glu Asp

              730            740            750            760            770            780
G G C A C A A G G C T G C C A G C G G A T C T G G T A A T C G C C G G G A T T G G C C T G A T A C C A A A C T G C G A G
Gly Thr Arg Leu Pro Ala Asp Leu Val Ile Ala Gly Ile Gly Leu Ile Pro Asn Cys Glu

              790            800            810            820            830            840
T T G G C C A G T G C G G C C G G C C T G C A G G T T G A T A A C G G C A T C G T G A T C A A C G A A C A C A T G C A G
Leu Ala Ser Ala Ala Gly Leu Gln Val Asp Asn Gly Ile Val Ile Asn Glu His Met Gln

              850            860            870            880            890            900
A C C T C T G A T C C C T T G A T C A T G G C C G T C G G C G A C T G T G C C C G A T T T C A C A G T C A G C T C T A T
Thr Ser Asp Pro Leu Ile Met Ala Val Gly Asp Cys Ala Arg Phe His Ser Gln Leu Tyr

              910            920            930            940            950            960
```

```
G A C C G C T G G G T G C G T A T C G A A T C G G T G C C C A A T G C C T T G G A G C A G G C A C G A A A G A T C G C C
Asp  Arg  Trp  Val  Arg  Ile  Glu  Ser  Val  Pro  Asn  Ala  Leu  Glu  Gln  Ala  Arg  Lys  Ile  Ala

        970              980              990             1000             1010             1020
G C C A T C C T C T G T G G C A A G G T G C C A C G C G A T G A G G C G G C G C C C T G G T T C T G G T C C G A T C A G
Ala  Ile  Leu  Cys  Gly  Lys  Val  Pro  Arg  Asp  Glu  Ala  Ala  Pro  Trp  Phe  Trp  Ser  Asp  Gln

       1030             1040             1050             1060             1070             1080
T A T G A G A T C G G A T T G A A G A T G G T C G G A C T G T C C G A A G G G T A C G A C C G G A T C A T T G T C C G C
Tyr  Glu  Ile  Gly  Leu  Lys  Met  Val  Gly  Leu  Ser  Glu  Gly  Tyr  Asp  Arg  Ile  Ile  Val  Arg

       1090             1100             1110             1120             1130             1140
G G C T C T T T G G C G C A A C C C G A C T T C A G C G T T T T C T A C C T G C A G G G A G A C C G G G T A T T G G C G
Gly  Ser  Leu  Ala  Gln  Pro  Asp  Phe  Ser  Val  Phe  Tyr  Leu  Gln  Gly  Asp  Arg  Val  Leu  Ala

       1150             1160             1170             1180             1190             1200
G T C G A T A C A G T G A A C C G T C C A G T G G A G T T C A A C C A G T C A A A A C A A A T A A T C A C G G A T C G T
Val  Asp  Thr  Val  Asn  Arg  Pro  Val  Glu  Phe  Asn  Gln  Ser  Lys  Gln  Ile  Ile  Thr  Asp  Arg

       1210             1220             1230             1240             1250             1260
T T G C C G G T T G A A C C A A A C C T A C T C G G T G A C G A A A G C G T G C C G T T A A A G G A A A T C A T C G C C
Leu  Pro  Val  Glu  Pro  Asn  Leu  Leu  Gly  Asp  Glu  Ser  Val  Pro  Leu  Lys  Glu  Ile  Ile  Ala

       1270             1280             1290
G C C G C C A A A G C T G A A C T G A G T A G T G C C T G A
Ala  Ala  Lys  Ala  Glu  Leu  Ser  Ser  Ala  ***
```

FIGURE 3. Translated genetic sequence and upstream region of putidaredoxin reductase (*camA*) from *P. putida*. Note the GTG translation initiation codon.

```
                10               20               30               40               50
A A T T C G G G A G T G C G T G C T A A A T G A A C G C A A A C G A C A A C G T G G T C A T C G T C G G T A C
                               Met  Asn  Ala  Asn  Asp  Asn  Val  Val  Ile  Val  Gly  Thr
```

FIGURE 4. Synthetic oligonucleotide for conversion of the wild-type GTG initiation codon to ATG. The oligonucleotide and its complement were cloned between the vector's *Eco*RI site and a *Kpn*I site beginning at nucleotide 52 of the putidaredoxin reductase sequence.

```
          10            20            30            40            50            60
ATAGCGTGTGAGGATAAACAGATGTCTAAAGTAGTGTATGTGTCACATGATGGAACGCGT
                    Met Ser Lys Val Val Tyr Val Ser His Asp Gly Thr. Arg

          70            80            90           100           110           120
CGCGAACTGGATGTGGCGGATGGCGTCAGCCTGATGCAGGCTGCAGTCTCCAATGGTATC
Arg Glu Leu Asp Val Ala Asp Gly Val Ser Leu Met Gln Ala Ala Val Ser Asn Gly Ile

         130           140           150           160           170           180
TACGATATTGTCGGTGATTGTGGCGGCAGCGCCAGCTGCCACCTGCCATGTCTATGTG
Tyr Asp Ile Val Gly Asp Cys Gly Gly Ser Ala Ser Cys Ala Thr Cys His Val Tyr Val

         190           200           210           220           230           240
AACGAAGCGTTCACGGACAAGGTGCCCGCCGCCAACGAGCGGGAAATCGGCATGCTGGAG
Asn Glu Ala Phe Thr Asp Lys Val Pro Ala Ala Asn Glu Arg Glu Ile Gly Met Leu Glu

         250           260           270           280           290           300
TGCGTCACGGCCGAACTGAAGCCGAACAGCAGGCTCTGCTGCCAGATCATCATGACGCCC
Cys Val Thr Ala Glu Leu Lys Pro Asn Ser Arg Leu Cys Cys Gln Ile Ile Met Thr Pro

         310           320           330           340
GAGCTGGATGGCATCGTGGTCGATGTTCCCGATAGGCAATGGTAA
Glu Leu Asp Gly Ile Val Val Asp Val Pro Asp Arg Gln Trp ***
```

FIGURE 5. Translated genetic sequence and upstream region of putidaredoxin (*camB*) from *P. putida*.

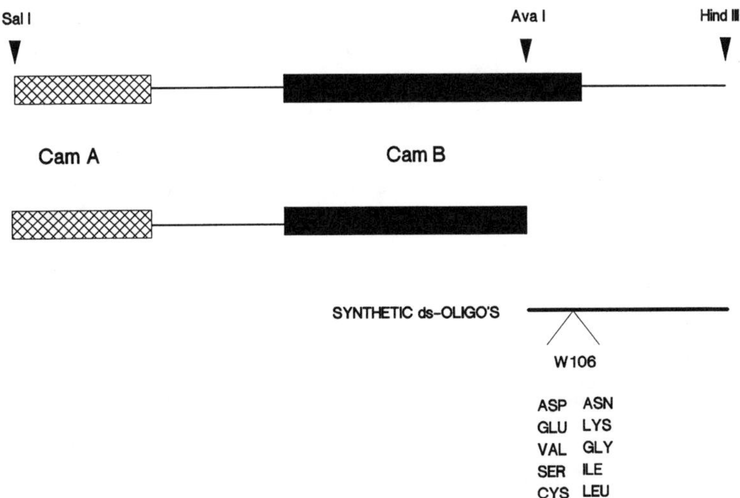

FIGURE 6. Genetic construction of C-terminal mutant putidaredoxins. The mutant oligonucleotide and the *Sal*I-to-*Ava*I fragment were cloned into a pUC vector and expressed in *E. coli*.

in the formation of a complex with P-450 and/or in the electron transfer event between iron-sulfur and heme center. We have replaced the C-terminal tryptophan with a variety of aromatic, nonpolar, and charged residues, as shown schematically in Fig. 6.

Ling Qin in our laboratory has measured the first electron transfer from putidaredoxin to P-450$_{cam}$ by laser photolysis. At concentrations of protein that saturate the protein-protein association, the rate of ferric-ferrous reduction of the heme iron should be concentration independent, aside from the second-order direct reduction of P-450$_{cam}$ without putidaredoxin involvement. Figure 7 shows the observed rate constants for approach to equilibrium between the two proteins as a function of P-450$_{cam}$ concentrations. Clearly there is much more efficient electron transfer when the residue at position 106 is aromatic. Is this the first defined ''pi-electron'' pathway in a native electron transfer event? Preliminary results suggest that mutants at position 106 still form a tight complex with P-450$_{cam}$. Clearly either tryptophan 106 provides a unique orientation for the donor-acceptor pair, or it is involved in a super-exchange mechanism for the shuttle of electrons into the P-450$_{cam}$ heme.

CYTOCHROME P-450$_{cam}$

The cytochrome P-450$_{cam}$ peptide forms an active site at the molecule's center. The amino acid side chains contact substrate and oxygen next to the thiolate-ligated heme. The active site as a whole directs the binding and activation of dioxygen, with subsequent use of one atom for regiospecific hydroxylation of substrate and the reduction of the remaining atom to water. The involvement of

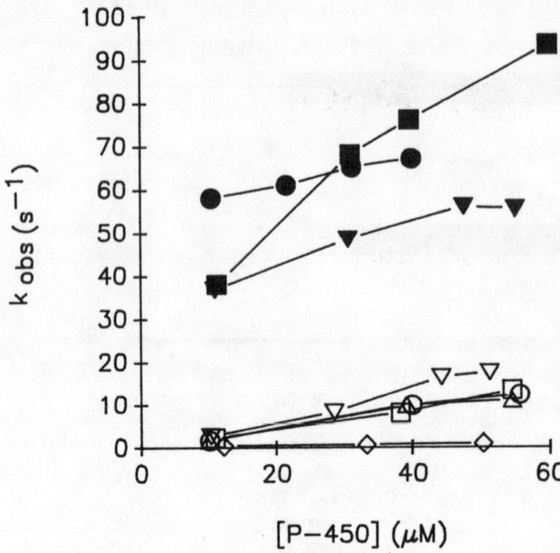

FIGURE 7. Observed rate constants for the reduction of P-450$_{cam}$ by mutant and wild-type putidaredoxins. Putidaredoxin reduction was initiated by a laser flash in the presence of methyl viologen. The formation of ferrous P-450$_{cam}$ was followed by 432 nm. Symbols: ●, wild-type protein; putidaredoxin in which the residue at position 106 has been replaced with tyrosine (■), phenylalanine (▼), valine (○), leucine (△), aspartic acid (□), lysine (◇), or a termination codon (▽).

particular peptide residues in this rich catalytic process is currently under investigation using mutational analysis. One of the first experimental targets was the role of specific active site residues in the positioning of the substrate at the active site. These experiments are published (Atkins and Sligar, 1988, 1989) and will only be summarized here. Crystallographic data show that camphor is held at the active site by aliphatic contacts and a hydrogen bond from tyrosine 96 to camphor's carbonyl (Poulos et al., 1987). Mutational events directed at disrupting these contacts lead to the predictable observation that loosening the contacts causes deterioration of the strict regiospecificity of camphor hydroxylation and that tightening the contacts increases, although only slightly, the regiospecific hydroxylation of smaller camphor analogs. Two other measures of substrate binding disruption, the ability of camphor to exclude water from the wild-type active site and the stoichiometric coupling of NADH oxidation to hydroxylated product formation, were measured using the mutant proteins. Neither of these properties of the wild-type enzyme was completely preserved when the active site was enlarged or when the substrate was a smaller monoterpene. Further mutational work aimed at creating hydroxylation specificity for a variety of substrates continues in our laboratory.

The unique spectral features of the P-450 class of heme proteins result from the presence of a thiolate ligand, as initially suggested by Mason et al. (1965) (for a recent review, see Dawson, 1988). When the primary sequences of P-450$_{cam}$ (Haniu et al., 1982) and P-450LM2 were determined by classical protein sequencing, two regions of homology containing cysteine residues were observed. These two regions, called HR1 and HR2 (homologous region), are seen in the sequences of nearly 100 P-450 genes to date (Nebert and Gonzales, 1987), with HR1 being somewhat more conserved than HR2. Although there are a couple of cases where HR1 does not contain a cysteine residue, there was earlier heated discussion regarding which was the heme ligand. Several authors proposed that cysteine 136 (in the P-450$_{cam}$ numbering) contained in HR1 was the heme ligand (Haniu et al.,

1983; Tarr et al., 1983), and indeed the first presentations of the X-ray crystal structure had this cysteine as the axial ligand. Mutagenesis was used to determine the role of C-136 in the bacterial P-450$_{cam}$ system by replacing it with serine. When the X-ray structure was refined with the primary sequence determined from the cloned P-450$_{cam}$ gene (Unger et al., 1986), it was clear that C-357 was the axial ligand and C-136 was on the surface some 20 Å (2 nm) from the heme iron. The C136S mutant of P-450$_{cam}$ appears identical to the wild type in substrate binding, spin state conversion, and the ability to hydroxylate camphor with absolute stereo- and regiospecificity. The role of the HR1 region in the P-450 systems remains elusive.

The camphor hydroxylase operon has provided a beautiful system for the application of state-of-the-art techniques of chemistry, biophysics, and most recently, recombinant DNA technology. Clearly, the "nose" of I. C. Gunsalus goes beyond wine. In discovering camphor catabolism in *Pseudomonas*, Dr. Gunsalus provided an example of metabolic diversity the crux of which is cytochrome P-450$_{cam}$. His work in purifying the enzymes and cloning the genes for the cytochrome and its electron transport chain set the stage for continued discovery of nature's secrets regarding oxygen and carbon chain utilization.

ACKNOWLEDGMENTS. The work in our laboratory is supported by Public Health Service grants from the National Institutes of Health (GM33775 and GM31756).

LITERATURE CITED

Atkins, W. M., and S. G. Sligar. 1988. The roles of active site hydrogen bonding in cytochrome P-450$_{cam}$ as revealed by site-directed mutagenesis. *J. Biol. Chem.* **263:**18842–18849.

Atkins, W. M., and S. G. Sligar. 1989. Molecular recognition in cytochrome P-450: alteration of regioselective alkane hydroxylation via protein engineering. *J. Am. Chem. Soc.* **111:**2715–2717.

Chakrabarty, A. M. 1976. Plasmids in Pseudomonas. *Annu. Rev. Genet.* **10:**7–30.

Dawson, J. H. 1988. Probing structure-function relations in heme-containing oxygenases and peroxidases. *Science* **240:**433–439.

Geren, L., J. Tuls, P. O'Brien, F. Millet, and J. A. Peterson. 1986. The involvement of carboxylate groups of putidaredoxin in the reaction with putidaredoxin reductase. *J. Biol. Chem.* **261:**15491–15495.

Haniu, M., L. G. Armes, K. T. Yasunobu, B. A. Shastry, and I. C. Gunsalus. 1982. Amino acid sequence of the *Pseudomonas putida* cytochrome P-450. II. Cyanogen bromide peptides, acid cleavage peptides, and the complete sequence. *J. Biol. Chem.* **257:**12664–12671.

Haniu, M., K. T. Yasunobu, and I. C. Gunsalus. 1983. Heme binding and substrate-protected cysteine residues in P-450$_{cam}$. *Biochem. Biophys. Res. Commun.* **116:**30–36.

Hedegaard, J., and I. C. Gunsalus. 1965. Mixed function oxidation. IV. An induced methylene hydroxylase in camphor oxidation. *J. Biol. Chem.* **240:**4038–4043.

Koga, H., H. Aramaki, E. Yamaguchi, K. Takeuchi, T. Horiuchi, and I. C. Gunsalus. 1986. *camR*, a negative regulator locus of the cytochrome P-450$_{cam}$ hydroxylase operon. *J. Bacteriol.* **166:**1089–1095.

Koga, H., E. Yamaguchi, K. Matsunaga, H. Aramaki, and T. Horiuchi. 1989. Cloning and nucleotide sequences of NADH putidaredoxin reductase gene *camA* and putidaredoxin gene *camB* involved in cytochrome P-450$_{cam}$ hydroxylase of *Pseudomonas putida*. *J. Biochem.* **106:**831–836.

Lambeth, J. D., L. M. Green, and F. Millet. 1984. Adrenodoxin interaction with adrenodoxin reductase and cytochrome P-450$_{scc}$. *J. Biol. Chem.* **259:**10025–10029.

Lu, A. Y. H., and M. J. Coon. 1968. Role of hemoprotein P-450 in fatty acid-hydroxylation in a soluble enzyme system from liver microsomes. *J. Biol. Chem.* **243:**1331–1332.

Mason, H. S., J. C. North, and M. Vanneste. 1965. Microsomal mixed-function oxidations: the metabolism of xenobiotics. *Fed. Proc.* **24:**1172–1180.

Nebert, D. W., and F. J. Gonzales. 1987. P-450 genes: structure, evolution, and regulation. *Annu. Rev. Biochem.* **56:**945–993.

Poulos, T. L., B. C. Finzel, and A. J. Howard. 1987. High-resolution crystal structure of cytochrome P-450$_{cam}$. *J. Mol. Biol.* **195:**687–700.

Rheinwald, J. G., A. M. Chakrabarty, and I. C. Gunsalus. 1973. A transmissible plasmid controlling camphor oxidation in *Pseudomonas putida*. Proc. Natl. Acad. Sci. USA **70:**885–889.

Roome, P. W., Jr., J. C. Philley, and J. A. Peterson. 1983. Purification and properties of putidaredoxin reductase. *J. Biol. Chem.* **258:**2593–2598.

Sligar, S. G., and R. I. Murray. 1986. Cytochrome P-450$_{cam}$ and other bacterial P-450 enzymes, p. 429–443. *In* P. Ortiz de Montellano (ed.), *Cytochrome P-450: Structure, Mechanism, and Biochemistry*. Plenum Publishing Corp., New York.

Sligar, S. G., P. G. DeBrunner, J. D. Lipscomb, M. J. Namtvedt, and I. C. Gunsalus. 1974. A role of the putidaredoxin COOH-terminus in P-450cam (cytochrome m) hydroxylations. *Proc. Natl. Acad. Sci. USA* **71:**3906–3910.

Tarr, G. E., S. D. Black, V. S. Fujita, and M. J. Coon. 1983. Complete amino acid sequence and predicted membrane topology of phenobarbital-induced cytochrome P-450 (isozyme 2) from rabbit liver microsome. *Proc. Natl. Acad. Sci. USA* **80:**6552–6556.

Unger, B. P., I. C. Gunsalus, and S. G. Sligar. 1986. Nucleotide sequence of the *Pseudomonas putida* cytochrome P-450$_{cam}$ gene and its expression in *Escherichia coli*. *J. Biol. Chem.* **261:**1158–1163.

Chapter 12

Biphenyl/Polychlorinated Biphenyl Catabolic Gene (*bph* Operon): Organization, Function, and Molecular Relationship in Various Pseudomonads

Kensuke Furukawa, Nobuki Hayase, and Kazunari Taira

Since identification of polychlorinated biphenyl (PCB) residues in the environment in 1966, these widespread and persistent pollutants have become of greater global concern. They are recognized to be present in great abundance in the ecosystem, similar to 2,2-bis(*p*-chlorophenyl)1,1,1-trichloroethane (DDT) and its metabolites. It has been shown that biphenyl-utilizing bacteria are ubiquitously distributed in the environment and can cometabolize many PCB congeners to chlorobenzoic acids (Ahmed and Focht, 1973; Furukawa and Matsumura, 1976; Ruisinger et al., 1976; Yagi and Sudo, 1980; Furukawa, 1982; Bedard et al., 1986; Bedard et al., 1987) through the oxidative routes as illustrated in Fig. 1 (Catelani et al., 1971; Furukawa et al., 1978; Furukawa et al., 1979). Molecular oxygen is introduced at the 2,3 position of the nonchlorinated or less chlorinated ring to produce a dihydrodiol compound (2,3-dihydroxy-4-phenylhexa-4,6-diene) (Fig. 1, compound II) by the action of a biphenyl dioxygenase (product of the *bphA* gene). The dihydrodiol is then dehydrogenated to a 2,3-dihydroxybiphenyl (Fig. 1, compound III) by a dihydrodiol dehydrogenase (product of *bphB*). The 2,3-dihydroxybiphenyl is cleaved at the 1,2 position by a 2,3-dihydroxybiphenyl dioxygenase (23OHBPO; product of *bphC*) to produce the *meta*-cleavage compound 2-hydroxy-6-oxo-6-phenylhexa-2,4-dienoic acid (Fig. 1, compound IV). The *meta*-cleavage compound is hydrolyzed to the corresponding benzoic acid (Fig. 1, compound V) by a hydrolase (product of *bphD*). Thus, at least four enzymes are involved in the oxidative degradation of PCBs to chlorobenzoic

---

Kensuke Furukawa ● Department of Agricultural Chemistry, Kyushu University, Fukuoka 812, Japan.   ***Nobuki Hayase*** ● Biotechnology Laboratory, Kobe Steel Ltd., Tsukuba, Ibaraki 305, Japan.   ***Kazunari Taira*** ● Fermentation Research Institute, Agency of Industrial Science and Technology, Tsukuba Science City, Ibaraki 305, Japan.

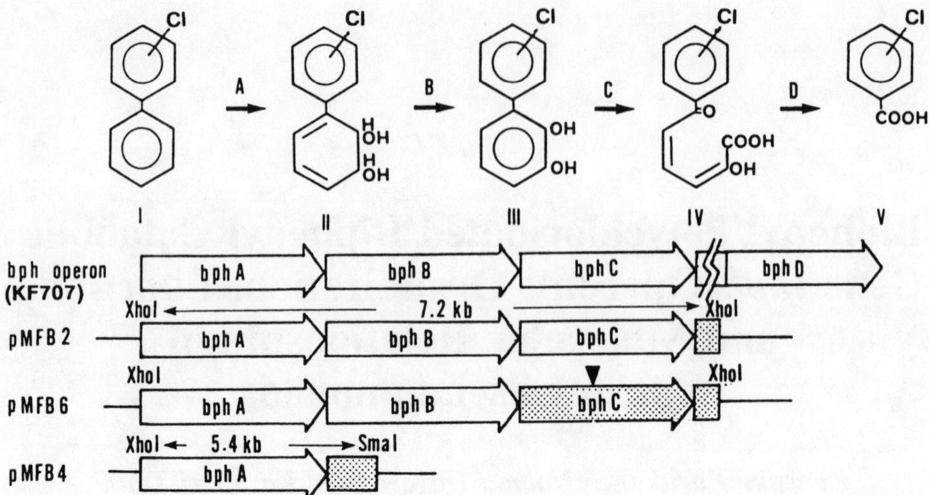

FIGURE 1. Degradative pathway of biphenyl/PCB by soil bacteria and *bph* genes from *P. pseudoalcaligenes*. (Top) Compounds: I, biphenyl/PCB; II, 2,3-dihydroxy-4-phenylhexa-4,6-diene (dihydrodiol compound); III, 2,3-dihydroxybiphenyl; IV, 2-hydroxy-6-oxo-6-phenylhexa-2,4-dienoic acid (ring *meta*-cleavage compound); V, benzoic acid. Enzymes: A, biphenyl dioxygenase; B, dihydrodiol dehydrogenase; C, 2,3-dihydroxybiphenyl dioxygenase; D, *meta*-cleavage compound hydrolase. (Bottom) Organization of the *bph* operon of *P. pseudoalcaligenes* KF707 and the structures of plasmids pMFB2, pMFB6, and pMFB4. In vitro mutation at the *Cla*I site within the *bphC* gene of pMFB6 is shown by an arrowhead.

acids. Most of the biphenyl-utilizing strains cannot degrade chlorobenzoic acids any further, and therefore the corresponding chlorobenzoates accumulate during PCB catabolism. Biphenyl/PCB-degrading bacteria have been isolated from various soils of different places. They are usually gram-negative soil bacteria that include species of *Pseudomonas*, *Achromobacter*, *Alcaligenes*, *Acinetobacter*, and *Moraxella*. Gram-positive bacteria such as *Arthrobacter* spp. have also been isolated (Ruisinger et al., 1976; Furukawa and Chakrabarty, 1982). This chapter describes the organization, function, and molecular relationships of biphenyl/PCB catabolic genes in various soil bacteria.

bphABCXD OPERON IN *P. PSEUDOALCALIGENES* KF707

A gene cluster encoding biphenyl/PCB-degrading enzymes was cloned from the chromosomal DNA of *Pseudomonas pseudoalcaligenes* KF707 (Furukawa and Miyazaki, 1986). The cloned *Xho*I 7.2-kilobase-pair (kb) DNA fragment contained the genes *bphA* (encoding biphenyl dioxygenase), *bphB* (encoding dihydrodiol dehydrogenase), and *bphC* (encoding 23OHBPO). *Pseudomonas aeruginosa* PAO1161 carrying recombinant plasmid pMFB2 (pKT230 containing the 7.2-kb *bphABC* operon at the unique *Xho*I site) converts biphenyl/PCBs into *meta*-cleavage yellow compounds (Furukawa and Miyazaki, 1986). The *bphD*

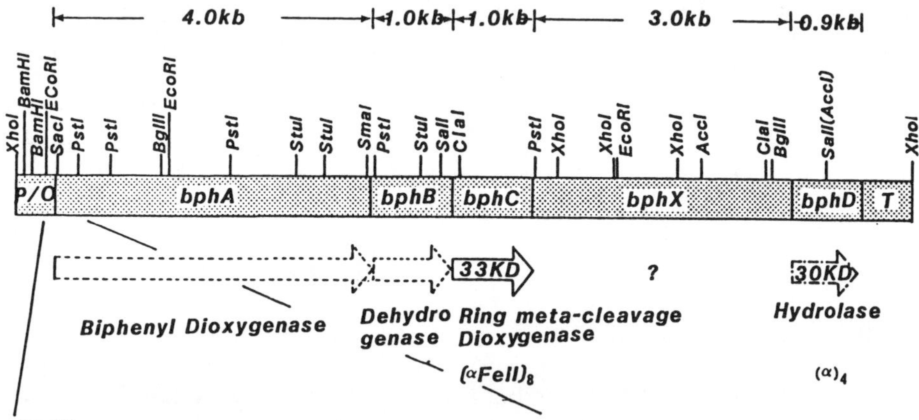

FIGURE 2. Organization of the *bph* operon in *P. pseudoalcaligenes* KF707 and partial nucleotide sequences of the upstream region of the gene. +1, Transcriptional start site; RBS, putative ribosome-binding site; KD, kilodaltons.

(encoding the ring *meta*-cleavage compound hydrolase) has also been cloned (K. Furukawa and S. Yamashita, manuscript in preparation). *Escherichia coli* JM109 carrying recombinant plasmid pFYD177 (pHSG396 [Takara Shuzo Co. Ltd., Kyoto, Japan] containing *bphD* [*Xho*I 3.0-kb DNA] at the *Xho*I site [5.2 kb]) readily converted the ring *meta*-cleavage yellow compound to benzoic acid. Subcloning, deletion analysis, and transposon (Tn*5-21* Tc^r; kindly provided by R. Simon, Bielefeld Universität, Bielefeld, Federal Republic of Germany) mutagenesis of the cloned *bph* genes revealed that the biphenyl/PCB catabolic *bph* operon of *P. pseudoalcaligenes* KF707 is organized as presented in Fig. 2. *bphA* starts just downstream of the *Eco*RI site and extends ca. 4 kb in length. Biphenyl dioxygenase encoded by *bphA* would most likely be a multicomponent enzyme that usually consists of several nonidentical subunits, as in the case of other aromatic dioxygenases such as benzene dioxygenase (Axcell and Geary, 1975; Crutcher and Geary, 1979; Geary et al., 1984; Irie et al., 1987), toluene dioxygenase (Subramanian et al., 1979; Subramanian et al., 1981; Subramanian et al., 1985), naphthalene dioxygenase (Ensley et al., 1982; Ensley and Gibson, 1983), benzoate dioxygenase (Yamaguchi et al., 1975; Yamaguchi and Fujisawa, 1978, 1982), and toluate dioxygenase (Harayama et al., 1986). The *bphB* gene is located downstream of *bphA* and extends ca. 1 kb, and the *bphC* gene (ca. 1 kb) immediately follows *bphB*. The *bphD* gene is not located just downstream of *bphC*. There is an extra ca. 3-kb DNA segment (*bphX*) between *bphC* and *bphD*.

The function of the putative *bphX* gene has not yet been elucidated. The *bph* operon in *P. pseudoalcaligenes* KF707 is thus organized as *bphABCXD* (Fig. 2). The transcriptional start site (+1 in Fig. 2) of the *bph* operon (KF707) has been determined by reverse transcriptase mapping. This transcriptional initiation site is located 104 base pairs upstream from the start codon of the *bphA* cistron. We could not find any consensus promoter sequence upstream of the +1 site.

bphABCD OPERON IN *P. PUTIDA* KF715

By using *bph* genes of *P. pseudoalcaligenes* KF707 as DNA probes, *bph* genes of another PCB-degrading strain, *Pseudomonas putida* KF715, have been cloned. Both *bphABC* (KF707) and *bphD* (KF707) probes were hybridized to a 9.4-kb fragment of the *Xho*I-digested chromosomal DNA of strain KF715. The DNA fragments of around 9 to 10 kb in size were electroeluted and ligated into the unique *Xho*I site of pHSG396 and transformed into *E. coli* JM109. The transformants that converted 2,3-dihydroxybiphenyl to a ring *meta*-cleavage yellow compound were screened. One transformant thus obtained harbored a recombinant plasmid, pYH715 (11.6 kb), that contained the *Xho*I 9.4-kb DNA fragment from *P. putida* KF715 and was capable of converting 4-chlorobiphenyl to 4-chlorobenzoic acid, indicating that the cloned fragment carried the *bphABCD* genes. The 9.5-kb DNA fragment was successively deleted by exonuclease III in the direction *bphD* → *bphA*. The functions of deleted plasmids were analyzed from accumulation of metabolic intermediates from 4-chlorobiphenyl. The gene order was determined to be *bphA-bphB-bphC-bphD*. Sequence analysis revealed that there did not exist the extra DNA segment, *bphX*, that was observed in *P. pseudoalcaligenes* KF707. The upstream regions of the *bphA* genes of strains KF707 and KF715 are extremely similar in restriction profile (Fig. 2). Partial nucleotide sequence and reverse transcriptase mapping also revealed that the transcriptional initiation site of *bphABCD* (KF715) is identical with that of *bphABCXD* (KF707).

bphC GENES AND 23OHBPOs: COMPARATIVE STUDIES IN SOME PCB-DEGRADING STRAINS

The *bphC* gene product, 23OHBPO, catalyzes the oxidative ring cleavage of 2,3-dihydroxybiphenyl to 2-hydroxy-6-oxo-6-phenylhexa-2,4-dienoic acid (Fig. 1, compound IV). This is one of the key reactions in the degradation of PCBs. The 23OHBPOs were purified from *P. pseudoalcaligenes* KF707, which was isolated in Kitakyushu, Japan (Furukawa and Miyazaki, 1986), and *Pseudomonas paucimobilis* Q1, which was isolated in Chicago, Ill. (Furukawa et al., 1983). Table 1 shows some of the enzymatic properties of 23OHBPOs in strain KF707 and Q1 (Furukawa and Arimura, 1987; Taira et al., 1988). Both enzymes have molecular weights of ca. 260,000. They are composed of eight identical subunits of molecular weight ca. 33,000. Since ferrous ion [Fe(II)] as a cofactor is essential for

TABLE 1

Enzymatic properties of 23OHBPOs of *P. pseudoalcaligenes* KF707 and *P. paucimobilis* Q1

Strain	V_{max} (s^{-1}) of substrate:		
	23OHBP	34OHBP	Catechol
KF707	330	<1	~3
Q1	150	<1	33

enzymatic activity, the structure of each enzyme is thought to be $[\alpha Fe(II)]_8$. Both 23OHBPOs are specific for 2,3-dihydroxybiphenyl, and they do not oxidize a positional isomer such as 2,3-dihydroxybiphenyl. Despite the close similarities between these enzymes, there are some differences; although the 23OHBPO of Q1 can oxidize catechol with a catalytic efficiency of almost one-quarter (1/4 V_{max}) with respect to the natural substrate, 2,3-dihydroxybiphenyl, catechol is nearly inert with respect to the 23OHBPO of KF707.

The nucleotide sequences of the *bphC* genes of strains KF707 and Q1 were then determined (Furukawa et al., 1987; Taira et al., 1988), and the deduced amino acid sequences were compared with each other and with the sequence of catechol 2,3-dioxygenase encoded by *xylE* on the TOL plasmid pWW0 (Nakai et al., 1983a; Nakai et al., 1983b) (Fig. 3). The *bphC* (KF707) gene exhibits approximately 60% homology with the *bphC* (Q1) gene when the nucleotide sequences are optimally aligned. Reflecting their origin from *Pseudomonas* spp., all three genes possess high G+C contents of 60, 62, and 57 mol% for *bphC* (KF707), *bphC* (Q1), and *xylE*, respectively. The overall homology between 23OHBPO of KF707 (297

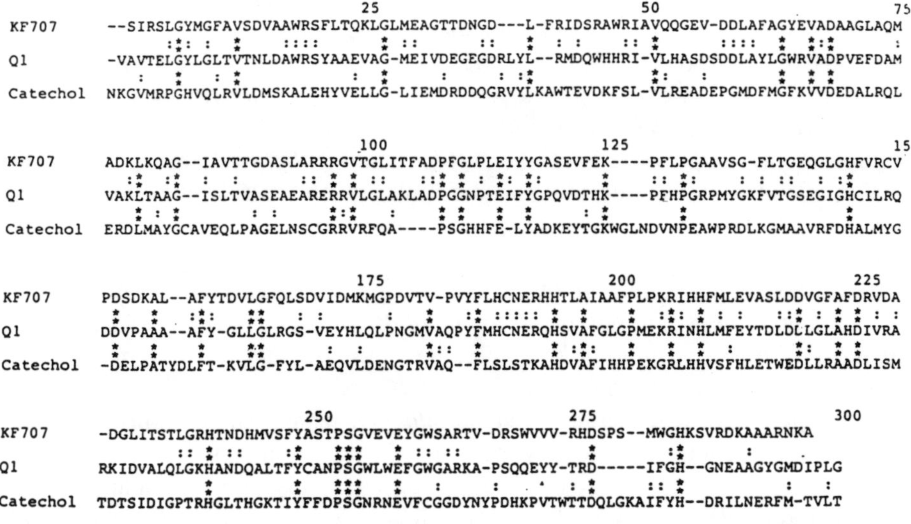

FIGURE 3. Comparison of amino acid sequences of 23OHBPOs from strains KF707 and Q1 and catechol 2,3-dioxygenase, represented by KF707, Q1, and catechol, respectively. Identical amino acids are indicated by colons; double asterisks represent conserved amino acid residues among the three dioxygenases.

amino acids) and 23OHBPO of Q1 (298 amino acids) at the amino acid level is 38%. Catechol 2,3-dioxygenase (307 amino acids) exhibits 26 and 24% homology with 23OHBPOs from KF707 and Q1, respectively. The homology of 38% between these 23OHBPOs is not considered high, considering that both of these enzymes are of *Pseudomonas* origin. Even though there are some short segments of identity between the two 23OHBPOs (Fig. 3), antibodies raised against the 23OHBPO from Q1 did not cross-react with the KF707 enzyme, and vice versa. Thus, a sequence of high homology such as residues 185 to 194 (KF707 numbering), Try-Phe-Leu-His-Cys-Asn-Glu-Arg-His-His, despite its relatively high hydrophilicity, may line the binding pocket and confer substrate specificity, or it may constitute the catalytic system. Otherwise, these regions of high homology could be exposed and targeted as antigenic recognition sites.

The *bphC* gene from *P. putida* KF715 has also been sequenced. The DNA-derived protein sequence indicates a primary structure of 292 amino acids, and the overall homology between 23OHBPOs from strains KF707 (297 amino acids) and KF715 is as high as 91.4% (N. Hayase, K. Taira, and K. Furukawa, *J. Bacteriol.*, in press).

DISTRIBUTION AND GENETIC HOMOLOGY OF *bph* GENES AMONG VARIOUS PCB DEGRADERS

The molecular relationship of chromosomal genes encoding biphenyl/PCB catabolism was investigated in various soil bacteria, including species of *Pseudomonas*, *Achromobacter*, *Alcaligenes*, *Moraxella*, and *Arthrobacter*. The *bphA* gene as well as a *bphC* gene containing part of the *bphB* gene of *P. pseudoalcaligenes* KF707 were used as DNA probes. Among 15 strains tested, five *Pseudomonas* strains and one *Alcaligenes* strain possessed the *bphABC* gene cluster on a *Xho*I 7.2-kb DNA fragment identical to that of strain KF707. The restriction profiles of these *Xho*I 7.2-kb fragments containing *bphABC* genes were very similar, if not identical, despite the dissimilarity of the flanking chromosomal regions. Among the other *Pseudomonas* strains, *P. putida* KF715 possessed homologous *bphABCD* genes on 9.4-kb *Xho*I DNA fragments. One *Achromobacter* strain possessed similar *bphABCD* genes on the 9.4-kb *Xho*I DNA fragment. One *Pseudomonas* strain possessed the *bphABC* genes on two *Xho*I fragments of 6.0 and 2.5 kb. Five other strains, including a gram-positive *Arthrobacter* strain, showed no significant homology with *bphABC* (KF707). The *bphC* gene cloned from another PCB degrader, *P. paucimobilis* Q1, which was the only American isolate, lacked genetic homology with any of 15 other biphenyl/PCB degraders, all of which were isolated in Japan. Thus, there are many chromosomal biphenyl/PCB-degrading genes; some of them are nearly identical and others are quite different, and they may be classified into three groups. The existence of nearly identical chromosomal genes among many strains may imply a common ancestry of the *bph* genes among such strains.

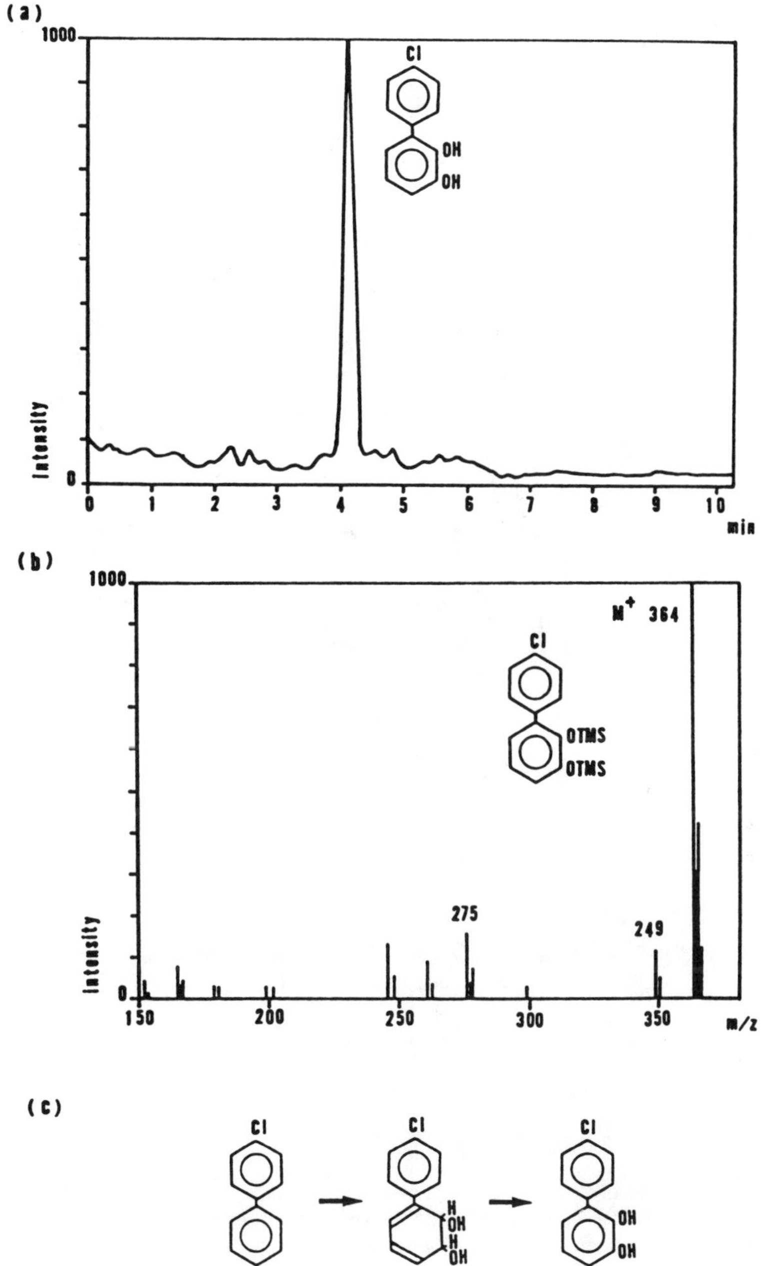

FIGURE 4. Production of dihydroxy compounds from 4-chlorobiphenyl by *P. aeruginosa* KF274 carrying pMFB6. (a) Gas chromatography-mass spectrometry total ion monitor of an ethyl acetate extract. (b) Mass spectrum of the trimethylsilyl derivative of the product. (c) Proposed conversion of 4-chlorobiphenyl to a dihydroxy compound by strain KF274.

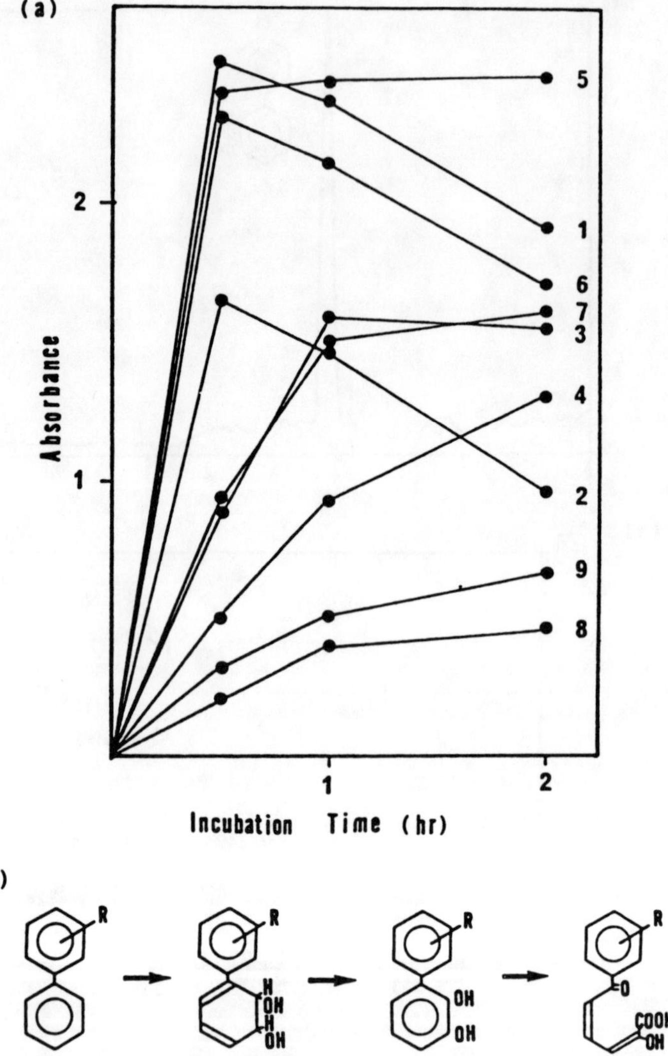

FIGURE 5. Production of ring *meta*-cleavage compounds from various biphenyls and diphenylmethane by *P. aeruginosa* KF258 carrying pMFB2. (a) Time course of production of ring *meta*-cleavage compounds. The absorption maximum of each *meta*-cleavage compound was monitored: biphenyl (1), 434 nm; 4-chlorobiphenyl (2), 430 nm; 3,4-dichlorobiphenyl (3), 436 nm; 2,4,5-trichlorobiphenyl (4), 390 nm; 2-bromobiphenyl (5), 400 nm; 4-methylbiphenyl (6), 436 nm; 2-nitrobiphenyl (7), 385 nm; 4-biphenylmethanol (8), 400 nm; diphenylmethane (9), 390 nm. (b) Proposed conversion of various biphenyl and diphenylmethane compounds by strain KF258.

PRODUCTION OF CATABOLIC INTERMEDIATES OF VARIOUS BIPHENYL-RELATED COMPOUNDS BY THE RECOMBINANT STRAINS CARRYING VARIOUS SETS OF *bph* GENES

Catabolic intermediates of various biphenyl compounds could be efficiently produced by *P. aeruginosa* carrying recombinant plasmids containing a set of the cloned *bph* genes (Furukawa and Suzuki, 1988). A dihydrodiol compound was produced by the strain carrying pMFB4 (Fig. 1), containing the *bphA* gene (encoding biphenyl dioxygenase). A dihydroxy compound was produced from 4-chlorobiphenyl by the strain carrying plasmid PMFB6, containing *bphA* and *bphB* (encoding dihydrodiol dehydrogenase) (Fig. 4). The same strain converted biphenyl to tetrahydroxybiphenyl via dihydroxybiphenyl. Ring *meta*-cleavage yellow compounds were produced from biphenyl and its derivatives substituted with a methyl, chloro, bromo, or nitro group on one of the biphenyl rings by strains carrying pMFB2, containing *bphA*, *bphB*, and *bphC* (encoding dihydroxybiphenyl dioxygenase) (Fig. 5). Diphenylmethane, dibenzyl, and diphenyl ether could be converted to the corresponding intermediates by these strains. Finally, a biphenyl-assimilating strain could be constructed by introducing the broad-host-range plasmid pNHF715 (pKT230 containing the *bphABCD* genes of *P. putida* KF715) into benzoate-utilizing *P. putida* AC30, *P. aeruginosa* PAO1161, and *Achromobacter xerosis* IFO 12668. It might be also possible to construct strains that can utilize certain PCB congeners as a sole source of carbon and energy if plasmid pNHF715 could be introduced and expressed in the chlorobenzoate degraders.

LITERATURE CITED

Ahmed, M., and D. D. Focht. 1973. Degradation of polychlorinated biphenyls by two species of *Achromobacter*. *Can. J. Microbiol.* **19:**47–52.

Axcell, B. C., and P. J. Geary. 1975. Purification of soluble benzoate-oxidizing system from a strain of *Pseudomonas*. *Biochem. J.* **146:**173–183.

Bedard, D. L., R. Unterman, L. H. Bopp, M. J. Brennan, M. L. Haberl, and C. Johnson. 1986. Rapid assay for screening and characterizing microorganisms for the ability to degrade polychlorinated biphenyls. *Appl. Environ. Microbiol.* **51:**761–768.

Bedard, D. L., R. E. Wagner, M. J. Brennan, M. L. Haberl, and J. F. Brown, Jr. 1987. Extensive degradation of Aroclors and environmentally transformed polychlorinated biphenyls by *Alcaligenes eutrophus* H850. *Appl. Environ. Microbiol.* **53:**1094–1102.

Catelani, D., C. Sorlini, and V. Treccani. 1971. The metabolism of biphenyl by *Pseudomonas putida*. *Experientia* **27:**1173–1174.

Crutcher, S. E., and P. J. Geary. 1979. Properties of the iron-sulphur proteins of the benzene dioxygenase system from *Pseudomonas putida*. *Biochem. J.* **177:**393–400.

Ensley, B. D., and D. T. Gibson. 1983. Naphthalene dioxygenase: purification and properties of a terminal oxygenase component. *J. Bacteriol.* **155:**505–511.

Ensley, B. D., D. T. Gibson, and A. L. Laborde. 1982. Oxidation of naphthalene by a multicomponent enzyme system from *Pseudomonas* sp. strain NCIB 9816. *J. Bacteriol.* **149:**948–954.

Furukawa, K. 1982. Microbial degradation of polychlorinated biphenyls, p. 33–57. *In* A. M. Chakrabarty (ed.), *Biodegradation and Detoxification of Environmental Pollutants*. CRC Press, Inc., Boca Raton, Fla.

Furukawa, K., and N. Arimura. 1987. Purification and properties of 2,3-dihydroxybiphenyl dioxygenase from polychlorinated biphenyl-degrading *Pseudomonas pseudoalcaligenes* and *Pseudomonas aeruginosa* carrying the cloned *bphABC* gene. *J. Bacteriol.* **169:**924–927.

120   Furukawa et al.

Furukawa, K., N. Arimura, and T. Miyazaki. 1987. Nucleotide sequence of the 2,3-dihydroxybiphenyl dioxygenase gene of *Pseudomonas pseudoalcaligenes*. *J. Bacteriol.* **169**:427–429.

Furukawa, K., and A. M. Chakrabarty. 1982. Involvement of plasmids in total degradation of chlorinated biphenyls. *Appl. Environ. Microbiol.* **44**:619–626.

Furukawa, K., and F. Matsumura. 1976. Microbial metabolism of polychlorinated biphenyls. Studies on the relative degradability of polychlorinated biphenyl components by *Alcaligenes* sp. *J. Agric. Food Chem.* **42**:543–548.

Furukawa, K., and T. Miyazaki. 1986. Cloning of a gene cluster encoding biphenyl and chlorobiphenyl degradation in *Pseudomonas pseudoalcaligenes*. *J. Bacteriol.* **166**:392–398.

Furukawa, K., J. R. Simon, and A. M. Chakrabarty. 1983. Common induction and regulation of biphenyl, xylene/toluene, and salicylate catabolism in *Pseudomonas paucimobilis*. *J. Bacteriol.* **154**:1356–1362.

Furukawa, K., and H. Suzuki. 1988. Gene manipulation of catabolic activities for production of intermediates of various biphenyl compounds. *Appl. Microbiol. Biotechnol.* **29**:363–369.

Furukawa, K., N. Tomizuka, and A. Kamibayashi. 1979. Effect of chlorine substitution on the bacterial metabolism of various polychlorinated biphenyls. *Appl. Environ. Microbiol.* **38**:301–310.

Furukawa, K., K. Tonomura, and A. Kamibayashi. 1978. Effect of chlorine substitution on the biodegradability of polychlorinated biphenyls. *Appl. Environ. Microbiol.* **35**:223–227.

Geary, P. J., F. Saboowalla, D. Patil, and R. Cammack. 1984. An investigation of the iron-sulphur proteins of benzene dioxygenase from *Pseudomonas putida* by electron-spin-resonance spectroscopy. *Biochem. J.* **217**:667–673.

Harayama, S., M. Rekik, and K. N. Timmis. 1986. Genetic analysis of a relaxed substrate specificity aromatic ring dioxygenase, toluene 1,2-dioxygenase, encoded by TOL plasmid pWW0 of *Pseudomonas putida*. *Mol. Gen. Genet.* **202**:226–234.

Irie, S., S. Doi, T. Yorifuji, M. Takagi, and K. Yano. 1987. Nucleotide sequencing and characterization of soluble benzene-oxidizing system from a strain of *Pseudomonas putida*. *J. Bacteriol.* **169**:5174–5179.

Nakai, C., K. Hori, H. Kagamiyama, T. Nakazawa, and M. Nozaki. 1983a. Purification, subunit structure, and partial amino acid sequence of metapyrocatechase. *J. Biol. Chem.* **258**:2916–2922.

Nakai, C., H. Kagamiyama, M. Nozaki, T. Nakazawa, S. Inouye, Y. Ebina, and A. Nakazawa. 1983b. Complete nucleotide sequence of the metapyrocatechase gene on the TOL plasmid of *Pseudomonas putida* mt-2. *J. Biol. Chem.* **258**:2923–2928.

Ruisinger, S., U. Klages, and F. Lingrens. 1976. Abbau der 4-Chlorobenzoesaure durch eine *Arthrobacter* Species. *Arch. Microbiol.* **110**:253–256.

Subramanian, V., T.-N. Liu, W. K. Teh, and D. T. Gibson. 1979. Toluene dioxygenase: purification of an iron-sulfur protein by affinity chromatography. *Biochem. Biophys. Res. Commun.* **91**:1131–1139.

Subramanian, V., T.-N. Liu, W.-K. Yeh, M. Narro, and D. T. Gibson. 1981. Purification and properties of NADH feredosin$_{\text{TOL}}$ reductase. *J. Biol. Chem.* **256**:2723–2730.

Subramanian, V., T.-N. Liu, W.-K. Yeh, C. H. Serdar, L. P. Wackett, and D. T. Gibson. 1985. Purification and properties of ferredoxin$_{\text{TOL}}$, a component of toluene dioxygenase from *Pseudomonas putida* F1. *J. Biol. Chem.* **260**:2355–2363.

Taira, K., N. Hayase, N. Arimura, S. Yamashita, T. Miyazaki, and K. Furukawa. 1988. Cloning and nucletoide sequence of the 2,3-dihydroxybiphenyl dioxygenase gene from the PCB-degrading strain of *Pseudomonas paucimobilis* Q1. *Biochemistry* **27**:3990–3996.

Yagi, O., and R. Sudo. 1980. Degradation of polychlorinated biphenyls by microorganisms. *J. Water Pollut. Control Fed.* **52**:1035–1043.

Yamaguchi, M., and H. Fujisawa. 1978. Characterization of NADH-cytochrome c reductase, a component of benzoate 1,2-dioxygenase system from *Pseudomonas arvilla* c-1. *J. Biol. Chem.* **253**:8848–8853.

Yamaguchi, M., and H. Fujisawa. 1982. Subunit structure of oxygenase component in benzoate-1,2-dioxygenase system from *Pseudomonas arvilla* c-1. *J. Biol. Chem.* **257**:12497–12502.

Yamaguchi, M., T. Yamauchi, and H. Fujisawa. 1975. Studies on mechanism of double hydroxylation. I. Evidence for participation of NADH-cytochrome c reductase in the reaction of benzoate 1,2-dioxygenase (benzoate hydroxylase). *Biochem. Biophys. Res. Commun.* **67**:264–271.

Chapter 13

Biotransformations Catalyzed by Toluene Dioxygenase from *Pseudomonas putida* F1

D. T. Gibson, G. J. Zylstra, and S. Chauhan

In 1926, den Dooren de Jong published his dissertation listing 80 organic compounds that could support the growth of *Pseudomonas putida* (L. E. den Dooren de Jong, Ph.D. thesis, University of Rotterdam, Rotterdam, The Netherlands, 1926). Since that time, pseudomonads have played an important role in our current understanding of the pathways and mechanisms used by bacteria for the degradation of a wide range of biosynthetic and man-made compounds.

It is a characteristic of aerobic organisms that the vast majority of enzymatic oxidations are mediated by the removal of hydrogen and electrons rather than the insertion of molecular oxygen into organic substrates (Dagley, 1972). However, in 1955 Hayaishi and his colleagues showed that pyrocatechase (catechol:oxygen 1,2-oxidoreductase; EC 1.13.1.1) from a *Pseudomonas* species incorporated both atoms of molecular oxygen into catechol to form *cis,cis*-muconate (Hayaishi et al., 1955). Subsequent studies revealed that at least two hydroxyl substituents are required for oxygenative fission of the benzenoid nucleus. Metabolic pathways are now known for the degradation of catechol, protocatechuate, homoprotocatechuate, 5-methoxyprotocatechuate, hydroxyquinol, gentisate, and homogentisate (Dagley, 1986). Precursors of many of these substrates are found in the environment in the form of natural products. For example, lignin depolymerization by fungi leads to the formation of aromatic acids, aldehydes, alcohols, and alkyl ethers that can serve as carbon and energy sources for a variety of microorganisms (Kirk, 1984).

Aromatic hydrocarbons, ranging in size from benzene to benzo[a]pyrene, are also known to be metabolized by microorganisms (Gibson and Subramanian, 1984). These compounds are not synthesized by living organisms. They are formed by the pyrolysis of organic material. The structures formed are dependent on the pyrolysis temperature. For example, at high temperatures (2,000°C),

---

D. T. Gibson, G. J. Zylstra, and S. Chauhan • Department of Microbiology and Biocatalysis Research Group, The University of Iowa, Iowa City, Iowa 52242.

unsubstituted polycyclic hydrocarbons are the major products, whereas the aromatic hydrocarbons formed by diagenesis (~150°C) usually contain alkyl substituents. The latter are the types of molecules found in crude petroleum (Blumer, 1976). Some sources of aromatic hydrocarbons in the environment include crude oil, forest and prairie fires, combustion of fossil fuels, coal liquefaction and gasification processes, motor vehicle emissions, and industrial contamination. It is clear that living organisms have been in contact with aromatic hydrocarbons throughout evolutionary periods of time, and therefore one would predict that microorganisms would have evolved the enzymes necessary to convert them to carbon dioxide and water. This supposition is supported by the fact that it is relatively easy to isolate bacteria that can utilize simple aromatic hydrocarbons as the sole sources of carbon and energy for growth. Since at least two hydroxyl groups are required for fission of the aromatic nucleus, we originally focused our attention on the initial reactions utilized by a strain of *P. putida* to incorporate oxygen into benzene and toluene. These studies led to the discovery of a novel hydroxylation reaction and, more recently, to the use of chiral aromatic hydrocarbon metabolites in the synthesis of new polymers and pharmaceutical products.

HISTORICAL PERSPECTIVE

In 1965, one of us (D.T.G.) joined the laboratory of the late Reino E. Kallio in the Department of Microbiology at the University of Illinois. Those were exciting times. Two blocks away, I. C. Gunsalus and his students were dissecting the (+)-camphor methylene hydroxylase system from camphor-grown cells of *P. putida* (Cushman et al., 1967). In the previous year, a unique cytochrome of unknown function was detected in liver microsomes. This cytochrome, when reduced with dithionite in the presence of carbon monoxide, gave a characteristic absorption maximum at 450 nm (Omura and Sato, 1964). At the National Institutes of Health, studies were being conducted on the mechanism of action of phenylalanine hydroxylase in an attempt to explain the retention of deuterium in the tyrosine formed from *p*-deuterophenylalanine by a *Pseudomonas* species (Guroff et al., 1966). In those early days, we had no idea that in these three different laboratories we were witnessing the birth of the cytochrome P-450 field and its relationship to drug metabolism, chemical carcinogenesis, and oxygen fixation.

At that time, our own studies were directed toward elucidating the mechanisms used by bacteria to degrade aromatic hydrocarbons. Previous work had shown that bacteria oxidize benzene through catechol to tricarboxylic acid cycle intermediates (Marr and Stone, 1961). In their studies at the National Institutes of Health, Jerina and his colleagues demonstrated that liver microsomes oxidize benzene to benzene 1,2-oxide as the first oxygenated product. The oxide was extremely unstable and could undergo isomerization to phenol, enzymatic hydration to form *trans*-1,2-dihydroxy-1,2-dihydrobenzene (*trans*-benzene dihydrodiol), or conjugation with glutathione to yield premercapturic acids (Jerina et al., 1968). Figure 1 shows the reactions involving *trans*-benzene dihydrodiol.

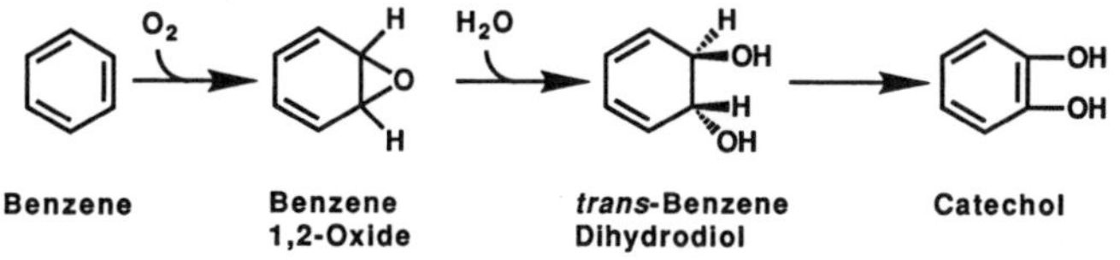

FIGURE 1. Oxidation of benzene through *trans*-benzene dihydrodiol by mammalian microsomes.

Analogous reactions had been suggested previously for the bacterial oxidation of benzene to catechol (Marr and Stone, 1961).

We isolated a fluorescent pseudomonad that could utilize ethylbenzene as the sole source of carbon and energy for growth. This organism, identified as *P. putida* biotype B, was obtained from soil at the edge of Boneyard Creek near the University of Illinois campus. Cells grown with ethylbenzene or toluene rapidly oxidized benzene, toluene, ethylbenzene, catechol, 3-methylcatechol, 4-methylcatechol, and, to a lesser extent, phenol, *o*-cresol, and *m*-cresol. The most surprising result was that both whole cells and cell extracts rapidly oxidized *cis*-1,2-dihydroxy-1,2-dihydrobenzene (*cis*-benzene dihydrodiol). In contrast, little activity was observed with *trans*-benzene dihydrodiol. Radioisotope-trapping experiments indicated that *cis*-benzene dihydrodiol is an intermediate in benzene degradation, and this was confirmed by the isolation of a mutant, *P. putida* 39/D, that accumulated *cis*-benzene dihydrodiol in the culture medium after growth on glucose in the presence of benzene. Experiments with ^{18}O showed that both oxygen atoms in the dihydrodiol were derived from atmospheric oxygen. Cell extracts prepared from toluene-grown cells catalyzed the NAD^+-dependent oxidation of *cis*-benzene dihydrodiol to catechol. The latter compound was oxidized to a yellow ring-fission product whose absorption spectra in acid, neutral, and alkaline solutions were identical to those given by 2-hydroxymuconic semialdehyde. The initial reactions in the oxidation of benzene by *P. putida* are shown in Fig. 2.

P. putida 39/D also oxidized toluene to a dihydrodiol that was isolated in crystalline form. This product was unstable and, at pH values below 7.0, spontaneously eliminated water to yield *o*-cresol. The position and relative stereochemistry of the hydroxyl groups in the dihydrodiol were determined by proton magnetic resonance spectrometry of a Diels-Alder adduct. The latter was formed by reacting the diacetate of toluene dihydrodiol with maleic anhydride. The absolute stereochemistry of the metabolite was determined by X-ray crystallography of a Diels-Alder adduct formed from the diacetate by reaction with 4-(*p*-bromophenyl)-1,2,4-triazoline dione. The absolute stereochemistry of the

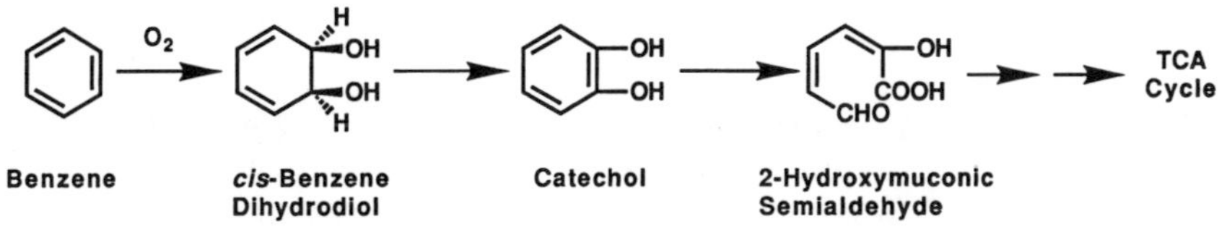

FIGURE 2. Oxidation of benzene to 2-hydroxymuconic semialdehyde by *P. putida*.

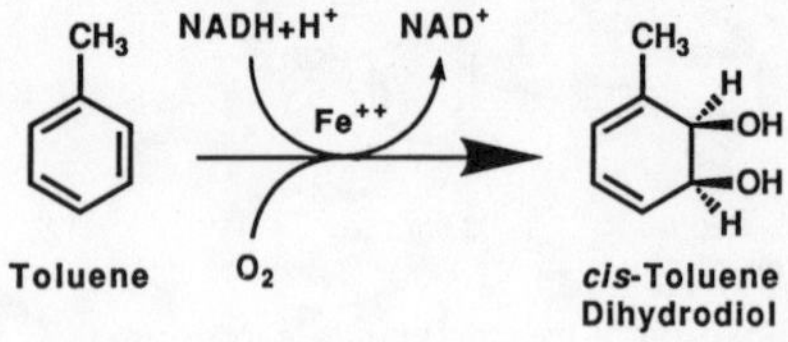

FIGURE 3. Oxidation of toluene to *cis*-toluene dihydrodiol by *P. putida*.

toluene dihydrodiol was also determined by converting it to methyladipic acid of known absolute stereochemistry and by application of the dibenzoate chirality rule of Nakanishi and Harada. These experiments confirmed that the product formed from toluene is $(+)$-*cis*-(1*S*,2*R*)-dihydroxy-3-methylcyclohexa-3,5-diene (*cis*-toluene dihydrodiol). References pertaining to the studies mentioned above may be found in Gibson and Subramanian (1984).

TOLUENE DIOXYGENASE

Crude cell extracts prepared from toluene-grown cells of *P. putida* oxidize toluene to *cis*-toluene dihydrodiol (Fig. 3). The enzyme was designated toluene dioxygenase; enzyme activity is dependent on the presence of NADH and oxygen. In addition, the rate of toluene oxidation is stimulated by ferrous iron (Yeh et al., 1977). Subsequent studies led to the isolation of three protein components that are essential for toluene dioxygenase activity. These have been characterized as a flavoprotein (ferredoxin$_{TOL}$ reductase), a [2Fe · 2S] ferredoxin (ferredoxin$_{TOL}$), and an iron sulfur protein (ISP$_{TOL}$). All of these proteins have been purified to homogeneity, and their properties are summarized in Table 1. Spectrophotometric studies showed that electrons are transferred from NADH to the terminal oxygenase by the sequence shown in Fig. 4.

Figure 4 also shows the gene designations for the individual components of toluene dioxygenase. Mutants defective in each of the three proteins were obtained by mutagenesis with nitrosoguanidine, followed by a selection procedure that involved the use of the redox dye nitroblue tetrazolium. Mutants defective in the structural genes for 3-methylcatechol 2,3-dioxygenase and 2-hydroxy-6-oxo-2,4-heptadienoate hydrolase were also isolated during these experiments (Finette et al., 1984). It was at this point in our studies that we gave *P. putida* the strain designation F1.

CLONING, NUCLEOTIDE SEQUENCE, AND EXPRESSION OF TOLUENE DIOXYGENASE GENES IN *E. coli*

The genes encoding the first four enzymes in toluene degradation (Fig. 5) are coordinately induced and form part of the *tod* operon (Finette and Gibson, 1988). DNA from *P. putida* F1 was cleaved with *Eco*RI, and the resulting fragments were cloned into *Escherichia coli* HB101 by using the cosmid cloning vector pLAFR1

TABLE 1
Properties of the components of toluene dioxygenase

Component	Physical property					
	Mol wt	Subunit mol wt	Redox group	λ_{max} ($\in$ mM^{-1} cm^{-1})	Iron content (g-atom/mol)	Acid-labile sulfur content (g-atom/mol)
Ferredoxin$_{TOL}$ reductase[a]	46,000	46,000	FAD (1:1)	274 372 448 (10.4)		
Ferredoxin$_{TOL}$[b]	15,400	15,400		278 327 (13.95) 460 (7.75)	2	2
ISP$_{TOL}$[c]	151,000	52,500 and 20,800		278 326 (12.46) 450 (7.58)	4	4

[a] From Subramanian et al. (1981).
[b] From Subramanian et al. (1985).
[c] From Subramanian et al. (1979) and Gibson et al. (1982).

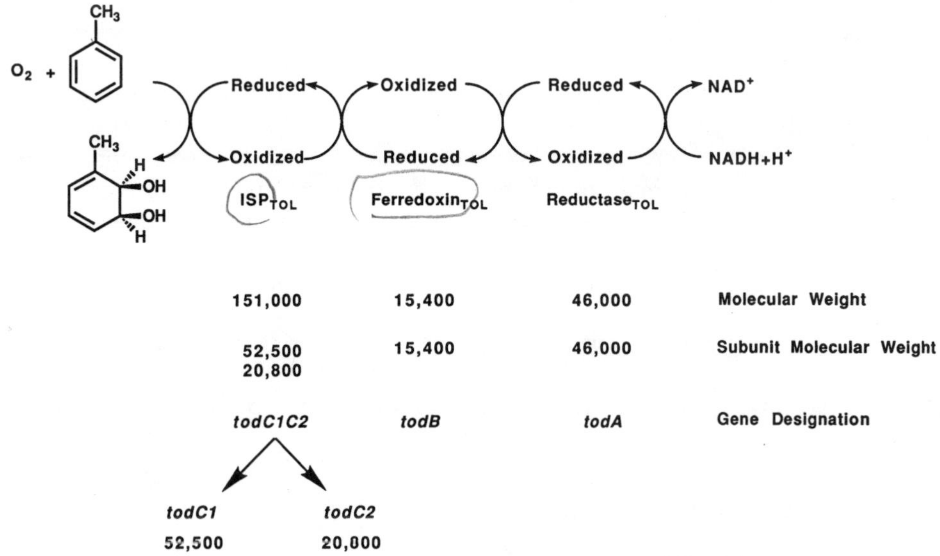

FIGURE 4. Organization and gene designation of the components of toluene dioxygenase from *P. putida* F1.

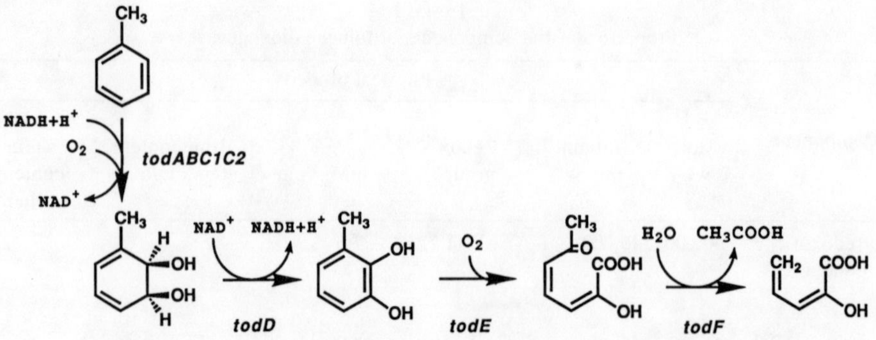

FIGURE 5. Initial reactions in the oxidation of toluene by *P. putida* F1.

(W. R. McCombie, *Abstr. Annu. Meet. Am. Soc. Microbiol. 1985*, K53, p. 155). One tetracycline-resistant recombinant was shown to contain a plasmid (pDTG301) that complemented mutations in all of the structural genes for the enzymes shown in Fig. 5. Digestion of pDTG301 with *Eco*RI gave two fragments that were 14 and 11 kilobases in size. Each fragment was cloned separately into pKT230 and transformed into *E. coli* BHB2600. The 11-kilobase fragment (pDTG351) complemented mutations in the *todABC1C2DE* genes shown in Fig. 5, whereas the 14-kilobase fragment did not complement any of the *tod* mutants. Subsequent subcloning experiments and complementation analyses showed that the genes in the *tod* operon are transcribed in the order *todC1C2BADE* (Zylstra et al., 1988).

The nucleotide sequence of the *todC1C2BADE* genes has been determined. Six open reading frames were detected in the region sequenced. Each gene was identified by comparison of the deduced amino acid sequence with the N-terminal amino acid sequence determined for the purified proteins isolated from toluene-grown cells of *P. putida* F1 (Zylstra and Gibson, 1989). In this study, a clone of *E. coli* JM109 that contains the four structural genes of toluene dioxygenase under the control of the *tac* promoter was constructed by using the expression vector pKK223-3. The recombinant organism *E. coli* JM109(pDTG601), after induction with isopropyl-β-D-thiogalactopyranoside, oxidized toluene to *cis*-toluene dihydrodiol.

SUBSTRATE SPECIFICITY OF TOLUENE DIOXYGENASE

Toluene dioxygenase is a remarkable enzyme that has the ability to oxidize a wide range of substrates. In many instances, the enzyme produces optically pure hydroxylated products. For example, toluene is oxidized to (+)-(1*S*,2*R*)-dihydroxy-3-methylcyclohexa-3,5-diene. The same absolute stereochemistry is found in the dihydrodiols formed from ethylbenzene, chlorobenzene, *p*-fluorotoluene, and biphenyl (Ziffer et al., 1977). In addition, toluene dioxygenase oxidizes (±)-3-methylcyclohexene to *cis*-diols that have the same absolute stereochemistry

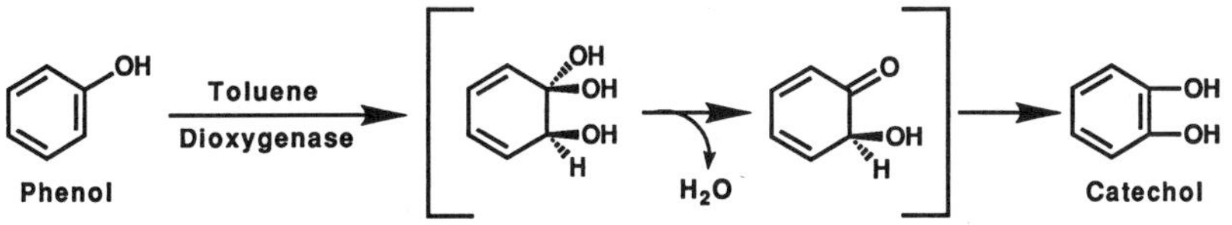

FIGURE 6. Proposed mechanism of phenol oxidation by toluene dioxygenase from *P. putida* F1.

about the carbon atoms bearing the hydroxyl groups (Ziffer and Gibson, 1975). The relative importance of steric and electronic factors can be seen in *p*-halogenated toluene derivatives, in which the size of the halogen increases as its electronegativity decreases in the series of F, Cl, and Br. All three *p*-halogenated substrates are oxidized to *cis*-dihydrodiols. However, only *p*-fluorotoluene dihydrodiol is optically active. Apparently, the enzyme cannot distinguish between the volumes of a methyl, chloro, or bromo substituent, and the electronegativity of the substituents does not influence the course of the oxidation (Ziffer et al., 1977).

Toluene dioxygenase can also function as a monooxygenase and oxidizes the benzylic carbon atom of indan to yield (−)-1(*R*)-indanol. The enzyme also oxidizes indene to (−)-*cis*-(1*S*,2*R*)-dihydroxyindan and (+)-(1*S*)-indenol. Both of these metabolites were of low optical purity (Wackett et al., 1988).

Phenol and certain substituted phenols are oxidized to the corresponding catechols by toluene dioxygenase (Spain and Gibson, 1988). Catechol formation was observed with *P. putida* F39/D, which contains a defect in the structural gene for *cis*-toluene dihydrodiol dehydrogenase (Gibson et al., 1970). These observations suggest that toluene dioxygenase catalyzes dioxygenation of phenol to form the first intermediate shown in Fig. 6. This intermediate is a hydrated ketone that would readily rearomatize to give catechol (Spain et al., 1989).

Toluene dioxygenase has also been implicated in the degradation of trichloroethylene (Nelson et al., 1988). This has been confirmed by demonstrating that toluene-induced cells of *P. putida* F1 degrade trichloroethylene, whereas a mutant defective in *todC*, the gene encoding the terminal component of toluene dioxygenase, and a mutant lacking the *todC1C2BADEF* genes of the *tod* operon do not (Wackett and Gibson, 1988). These observations have also been confirmed (Zylstra et al., 1989) with the cloned toluene dioxygenase synthesized by *E. coli* JM109(pDTG601).

Substrates oxidized by *P. putida* F39/D and *E. coli* JM109(pDTG601) are listed in Table 2.

SIGNIFICANCE OF TOLUENE DIOXYGENASE IN ORGANIC SYNTHESIS

The oxidation of benzene to *cis*-benzene dihydrodiol by toluene dioxygenase is a facile reaction that cannot be accomplished in significant yield by conventional chemical processes. Imperial Chemical Industries, U.K., have used a mutant strain of *P. putida* to produce kilogram amounts of *cis*-benzene dihydrodiol. Acetylation of the dihydrodiol, followed by free-radical polymerization,

TABLE 2

Substrates oxidized by toluene dioxygenase

Substrate	Major product(s)[a]	Organism	
		P. putida F39/D	*E. coli* JM109(pDTG601)
Benzene	*cis*-1,2-Dihydrodiol	+	+
Toluene	*cis*-2,3-Dihydrodiol	+	+
Ethylbenzene	*cis*-2,3-Dihydrodiol	+	+
Propylbenzene	*cis*-2,3-Dihydrodiol	+	+
Cyanobenzene	*cis*-2,3-Dihydrodiol	+	NT[b]
Fluorobenzene	*cis*-2,3-Dihydrodiol	+	NT
Chlorobenzene	*cis*-2,3-Dihydrodiol	+	+
Bromobenzene	*cis*-2,3-Dihydrodiol	+	NT
Trifluorotoluene	*cis*-2,3-Dihydrodiol	+	+
Anisole	*cis*-2,3-Dihydrodiol	+	+
Styrene	*cis*-2,3-Dihydrodiol	+	NT
4-Fluorotoluene	*cis*-2,3-Dihydrodiol	+	+
4-Chlorotoluene	*cis*-2,3-Dihydrodiol	+	+
4-Bromotoluene	*cis*-2,3-Dihydrodiol	+	NT
1,2-Dimethylbenzene	2,3-Dimethylphenol	NT	+
1,3-Dimethylbenzene	2,4-Dimethylphenol	+	+
1,4-Dimethylbenzene	*cis*-2,3-Dihydrodiol	+	+
1,2-Dichlorobenzene	*cis*-3,4-Dihydrodiol	+	+
1,3-Dichlorobenzene	*cis*-4,5-Dihydrodiol	+	+
1,4-Dichlorobenzene	*cis*-2,3-Dihydrodiol	+	+
Biphenyl	*cis*-2,3-Dihydrodiol	+	+
2-Chlorobiphenyl	*cis*-2,3-Dihydrodiol[c]	NT	+
3-Chlorobiphenyl	*cis*-2,3-Dihydrodiol[c]	NT	+
4-Chlorobiphenyl	*cis*-2,3-Dihydrodiol[c]	NT	+
Naphthalene	*cis*-1,2-Dihydrodiol	+	+
2-Chlorophenol	3-Chlorocatechol	NT	+
3-Chlorophenol	3-Chlorocatechol	NT	+
4-Chlorophenol	4-Chlorocatechol	NT	+
2-Methylphenol	3-Methylcatechol	NT	+
3-Methylphenol	3-Methylcatechol	NT	+
4-Methylphenol	4-Methylcatechol	NT	+
Indan	1-Indanol	+	+
Indene	*cis*-1,2-Dihydroxyindan	+	+
	1-Indanone	+	+
	1-Indenol	+	+
Indole	Indigo	+	+
Trichloroethylene	Unidentified	+	+

[a] Monosubstituents arbitrarily assigned position 1.
[b] NT, Not tested.
[c] Hydroxylation occurs on the unsubstituted ring.

gave a soluble high-molecular-weight polymer that was converted by heat to polyphenylene. The latter is a polymer of commercial interest with properties that may find application in the organic semiconductor field (Ballard et al., 1983). *cis*-Benzene dihydrodiol has also been used as a precursor in the synthesis of ($\pm$)-pinitol. Interest in polyhydroxylated cyclohexanes is related to their potential

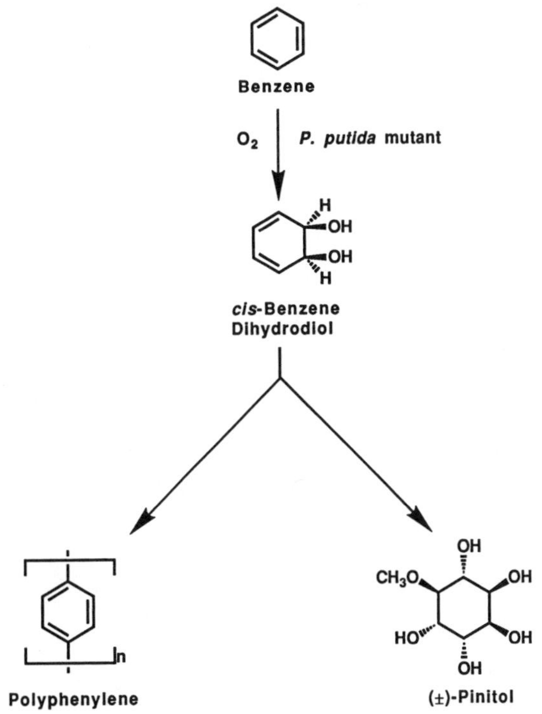

FIGURE 7. *cis*-Benzene dihydrodiol as a precursor in the synthesis of polyphenylene and (±)-pinitol.

use in the synthesis of inositol-1,4,5-triphosphate derivatives (Ley et al., 1987). The products formed from *cis*-benzene dihydrodiol are shown in Fig. 7.

Toluene dioxygenase oxidizes toluene to a single enantiomer of *cis*-toluene dihydrodiol. In an elegant series of experiments, Hudlicky and his colleagues have shown that the dihydrodiol can serve as a versatile chiral intermediate in the synthesis of prostaglandin, terpene, and cyclohexene oxide synthons (Hudlicky et al., 1988). Two examples of these synthons (Fig. 8) are intermediates of pharmaceutical interest. The prostaglandin synthon utilizes the chiral features of *cis*-toluene dihydrodiol, whereas the reactions leading to the terpene synthons transfer chirality to the methyl group. The diol can also be converted to cyclohexene oxides, a class of compounds known to have antitumor properties.

CONCLUSION

The mechanism of dioxygen fixation by toluene dioxygenase forms a major objective of our research program. The cloning and expression of the individual genes encoding the four structural proteins of the dioxygenase complex will permit detailed studies on the mechanism of electron transport from NADH to the terminal dioxygenase, the molecular interactions between the four proteins, and

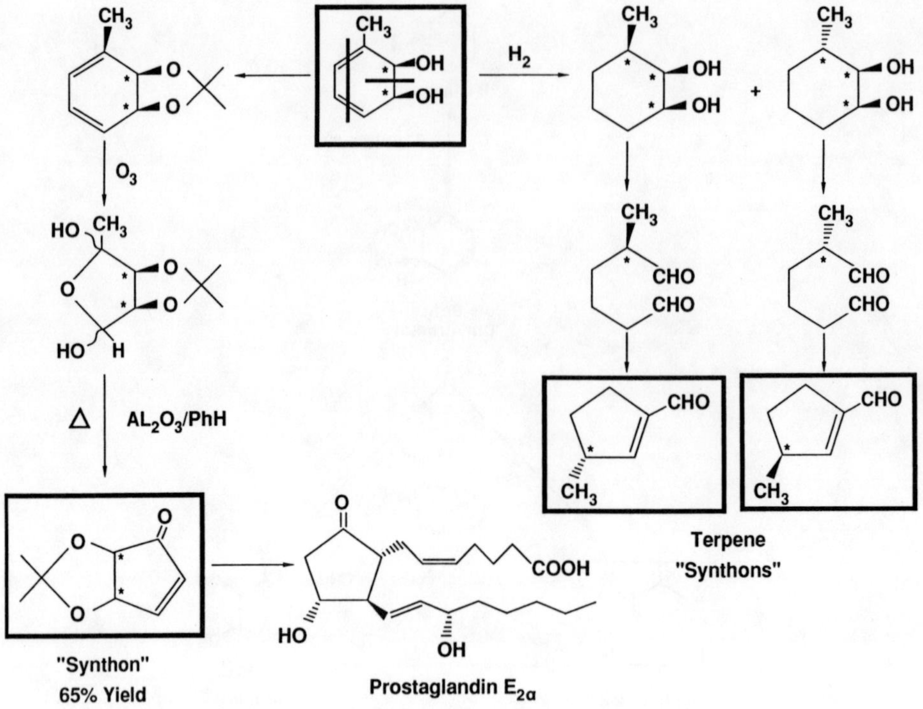

FIGURE 8. Reactions involved in the conversion of enantiomerically pure *cis*-toluene dihydrodiol to prostaglandin and terpene synthons. (Adapted from Hudlicky et al. [1988].)

the role of iron in the activation of molecular oxygen. In addition, the relaxed substrate specificity of the enzyme can be exploited to provide further information on the mechanism of oxygen fixation.

An unexpected benefit of the enantiomeric specificity of toluene dioxygenase can be seen in the use of the chiral properties of *cis*-toluene dihydrodiol to synthesize products of pharmaceutical interest. The broad range of substrates oxidized by toluene dioxygenase suggests that several other chiral synthons may be useful precursors in the synthesis of a variety of specialty chemicals.

ACKNOWLEDGMENTS. This work was supported in part by Public Health Service grant GM29909 from the National Institute of General Medical Sciences and grant AFOSR-88-6225 from the U.S. Air Force Office of Scientific Research. G.J.Z. is a recipient of Public Health Service National Research Service award 1 F32 GM13091 from the National Institute of General Medical Sciences.

We thank Sharon Gaffney for assistance in preparing the manuscript.

LITERATURE CITED

Ballard, D. G. H., A. Courtis, A. Shirley, and S. C. Taylor. 1983. A biotech route to polyphenylene. *J. Chem. Soc. Chem. Commun.* **1983**:954–955.

Blumer, M. 1976. Polycyclic aromatic hydrocarbons in the environment. *Sci. Am.* **234**:34–41.

Cushman, D. W., R. L. Tsai, and I. C. Gunsalus. 1967. The ferroprotein component of a methylene hydroxylase. *Biochem. Biophys. Res. Commun.* **26**:577–583.

Dagley, S. 1972. Microbial degradation of stable chemical structures: general features of metabolic pathways, p. 1–16. *In Degradation of Synthetic Organic Molecules in the Biosphere.* National Academy of Sciences, Washington, D.C.

Dagley, S. 1986. Biochemistry of aromatic hydrocarbon degradation in pseudomonads, p. 527–555. *In* J. R. Sokatch and L. N. Ornston (ed.), *The Bacteria,* vol. 10. *The Biology of Pseudomonas.* Academic Press, Inc., Orlando, Fla.

Finette, B. A., and D. T. Gibson. 1988. Initial studies on the regulation of toluene degradation by *Pseudomonas putida* F1. *Biocatalysis* 2:29–37.

Finette, B. A., V. Subramanian, and D. T. Gibson. 1984. Isolation and characterization of *Pseudomonas putida* PpF1 mutants defective in the toluene dioxygenase enzyme system. *J. Bacteriol.* 160:1003–1009.

Gibson, D. T., M. Hensley, H. Yoshioka, and T. J. Mabry. 1970. Formation of (+)-*cis*-2,3-dihydroxy-1-methylcyclohexa-4,6-diene from toluene by *Pseudomonas putida. Biochemistry* 7:3795–3802.

Gibson, D. T., and V. Subramanian. 1984. Microbial degradation of aromatic hydrocarbons, p. 181–252. *In* D. T. Gibson (ed.), *Microbial Degradation of Organic Compounds.* Marcel Dekker, Inc., New York.

Gibson, D. T., W.-K. Yeh, T.-N. Liu, and V. Subramanian. 1982. Toluene dioxygenase: a multicomponent enzyme system from *Pseudomonas putida,* p. 51–62. *In* M. Nozaki, S. Yamamoto, Y. Ishimura, M. J. Coon, L. Ernster, and R. W. Estabrook (ed.), *Oxygenases and Oxygen Metabolism.* Academic Press, Inc., New York.

Guroff, G., C. A. Reifsnyder, and J. Daly. 1966. Retention of deuterium in *p*-tyrosine formed enzymatically from *p*-deuterophenylalanine. *Biochem. Biophys. Res. Commun.* 24:720–724.

Hayaishi, O., M. Katagiri, and S. Rothberg. 1955. Mechanism of the pyrocatechase reaction. *J. Am. Chem. Soc.* 77:5440–5441.

Hudlicky, T., H. Luna, G. Barbieri, and L. D. Kwart. 1988. Enantioselective synthesis through microbial oxidation of arenes. I. Efficient preparation of terpene and prostanoid synthons. *J. Am. Chem. Soc.* 110:4735–4741.

Jerina, D. M., J. Daly, B. Witkop, P. Zaltzman-Nirenberg, and S. Udenfriend. 1968. Role of the arene oxide-oxepin system in the metabolism of aromatic substrates. *Arch. Biochem.* 28:176–182.

Kirk, T. K. 1984. Degradation of lignin, p. 399–438. *In* D. T. Gibson (ed.), *Microbial Degradation of Organic Compounds.* Marcel Dekker, Inc., New York.

Ley, S. V., F. Sternfeld, and S. Taylor. 1987. Microbial oxidation in synthesis: a six step preparation of (±)-pinitol from benzene. *Tetrahedron Lett.* 28:225–226.

Marr, E. K., and R. W. Stone. 1961. Bacterial oxidation of benzene. *J. Bacteriol.* 81:425–430.

Nelson, M. J., S. O. Montgomery, and P. H. Pritchard. 1988. Trichloroethylene metabolism by microorganisms that degrade aromatic compounds. *Appl. Environ. Microbiol.* 54:604–606.

Omura, T., and R. Sato. 1964. The carbon monoxide-binding pigment of liver microsomes I. Evidence for its hemoprotein nature. *J. Biol. Chem.* 239:2370–2378.

Spain, J. C., and D. T. Gibson. 1988. Oxidation of substituted phenols by *Pseudomonas putida* F1 and *Pseudomonas* sp. strain JS6. *Appl. Environ. Microbiol.* 54:1399–1404.

Spain, J. C., G. J. Zylstra, C. K. Blake, and D. T. Gibson. 1989. Monohydroxylation of phenol and 2,5-dichlorophenol by toluene dioxygenase in *Pseudomonas putida* F1. *Appl. Environ. Microbiol.* 55:2648–2652.

Subramanian, V., T.-N. Liu, W.-K. Yeh, and D. T. Gibson. 1979. Toluene dioxygenase: purification of an iron sulfur protein by affinity chromatography. *Biochem. Biophys. Res. Commun.* 91:1131–1139.

Subramanian, V., T.-N. Liu, W.-K. Yeh, M. Narro, and D. T. Gibson. 1981. Purification and properties of NADH-ferredoxin$_{TOL}$ reductase. *J. Biol. Chem.* 256:2723–2730.

Subramanian, V., T.-N. Liu, W.-K. Yeh, C. M. Serdar, L. P. Wackett, and D. T. Gibson. 1985. Purification and properties of ferredoxin$_{TOL}$: a component of toluene dioxygenase from *Pseudomonas putida* F1. *J. Biol. Chem.* 260:2355–2363.

Wackett, L. P., and D. T. Gibson. 1988. Degradation of trichloroethylene by toluene dioxygenase in whole-cell studies with *Pseudomonas putida* F1. *Appl. Environ. Microbiol.* 54:1703–1708.

Wackett, L. P., L. D. Kwart, and D. T. Gibson. 1988. Benzylic monooxygenation catalyzed by toluene dioxygenase from *Pseudomonas putida. Biochemistry* 27:1360–1367.

Yeh, W.-K., D. T. Gibson, and T.-N. Liu. 1977. Toluene dioxygenase: a multicomponent enzyme system. *Biochem. Biophys. Res. Commun.* **78:**401–410.

Ziffer, H., and D. T. Gibson. 1975. Relative and absolute stereochemistry of diols obtained from microbial oxidation of 3-methylcyclohexene. *Tetrahedron Lett.* **25:**2137–2138.

Ziffer, H., K. Kabuto, D. T. Gibson, and V. M. Kobal. 1977. The absolute stereochemistry of several *cis*-dihydrodiols microbially produced from substituted benzenes. *Tetrahedron* **33:**2491–2496.

Zylstra, G. J., and D. T. Gibson. 1989. Toluene degradation by *Pseudomonas putida* F1: nucleotide sequence of the *todC1C2BADE* genes and their expression in *Escherichia coli*. *J. Biol. Chem.* **264:**14940–14946.

Zylstra, G. J., W. R. McCombie, D. T. Gibson, and B. A. Finette. 1988. Toluene degradation by *Pseudomonas putida* F1: genetic organization of the *tod* operon. *Appl. Environ. Microbiol.* **54:**1498–1503.

Zylstra, G. J., L. P. Wackett, and D. T. Gibson. 1989. Trichloroethylene degradation by *Escherichia coli* containing the cloned *Pseudomonas putida* F1 toluene dioxygenase genes. *Appl. Environ. Microbiol.* **55:**3162–3166.

Chapter 14

Regulatory Systems for Expression of *xyl* Genes on the TOL Plasmid

Teruko Nakazawa, Sachiye Inouye, and Atsushi Nakazawa

Pseudomonas spp., natural habitants in soil and water, have abilities to dissimilate a wide range of organic compounds of both biological and nonbiological origins. Their metabolic versatility is often directed by plasmid-borne genes and gene clusters encoding catabolic enzymes (Frantz and Chakrabarty, 1986). Expression of such genes in *Pseudomonas* spp. is expected to be finely controlled, because survival and propagation of the bacteria depend on the utilization of a variety of compounds existing in low concentrations in the environment. In addition, *Pseudomonas* spp. may have more chance to be exposed to toxic substances in the environment than do other microorganisms, such as enteric bacteria. To adapt themselves to such unfavorable conditions, *Pseudomonas* spp. may have developed regulatory systems of gene expression that are distinct from the well-characterized systems in *Escherichia coli*.

In this chapter, we summarize the molecular mechanism of the regulation of gene expression on the TOL plasmid (Worsey and Williams, 1975) in response to aromatic hydrocarbons, alcohols, and carboxylic acids (summarized in Fig. 1; Inouye et al., 1987a; Ramos et al., 1987).

OPERON ORGANIZATION

The genes for the catabolic enzymes on the TOL plasmid are localized in a 56-kilobase-pair transposon (Tsuda and Iino, 1987) and are organized in two operons (Nakazawa et al., 1980; Franklin et al., 1981); one is the *xylCAB* operon, which is responsible for the upper catabolic pathway from xylenes and toluene to aromatic carboxylic acids (*m*-toluate and benzoate), and the other is the *xylDLEGF* operon, which directs the lower catabolic pathway from the aromatic

---

Teruko Nakazawa ● Department of Microbiology, Yamaguchi University School of Medicine, Ube, Yamaguchi 755, Japan. *Sachiye Inouye and Atsushi Nakazawa* ● Department of Biochemistry, Yamaguchi University School of Medicine, Ube, Yamaguchi 755, Japan.

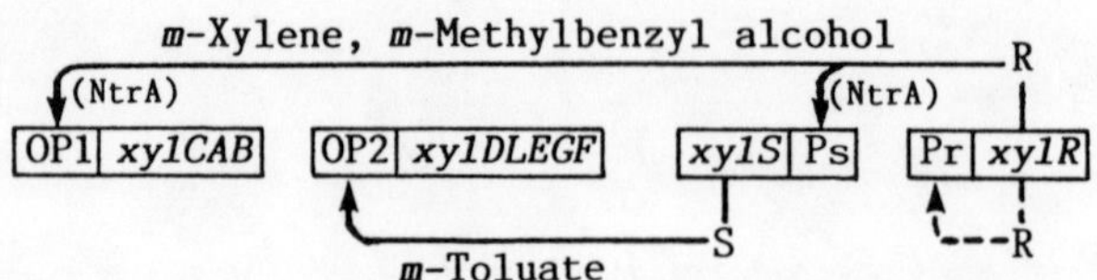

FIGURE 1. Regulation of *xyl* genes on the TOL plasmid. Arrows with solid and broken lines indicate positive and negative control, respectively.

carboxylic acids to compounds that enter the tricarboxylic acid cycle (Harayama et al., 1986a; Harayama et al., 1986b). Two regulatory genes, *xylR* and *xylS*, positively control these operons (Inouye et al., 1981, 1983; Franklin et al., 1981, 1983). In the presence of *m*-xylene or *m*-methylbenzyl alcohol, the *xylR* product (XylR) activates expression of both *xylCAB* and *xylS*. The activation of these genes occurs at the transcriptional level and depends on NtrA (RpoN) RNA polymerase. The *xylS* product (XylS) thus amplified in turn activates the *xylDLEGF* operon (Inouye et al., 1987b; Mermod et al., 1987). In the presence of *m*-toluate, XylS at a noninduced level activates the *xylDLEGF* operon. In contrast to other *xyl* genes, the *xylR* gene is constitutively expressed and repressed by its own product (Inouye et al., 1987a).

THE *xylR* AND *xylS* PRODUCTS ARE TRANSCRIPTIONAL ACTIVATORS

The role of the regulatory genes was analyzed in a system consisting of a pair of compatible plasmids (Inouye et al., 1983). One plasmid contained either the promoter of the *xylCAB* operon (OP1) fused to *xylE* or the *xylDLEGF* operon with its own promoter (OP2), and the other plasmid contained *xylR*, *xylS*, or both. Synthesis of the *xylE* product, catechol 2,3-dioxygenase, was monitored to determine expression from OP1 or OP2. The results indicated that XylR and XylS are *trans*-acting factors which activate expression. For inducible expression of the *xylCAB* operon by *m*-xylene, only XylR is required, whereas both XylR and XylS are required for the expression of *xylDLEGF*. On the other hand, large amounts of XylS alone are sufficient for the induction of *xylDLEGF*. Activation at the transcriptional level of the *xyl* operons was verified, and the transcription start sites were determined by S1 nuclease and reverse transcriptase mapping analysis (Inouye et al., 1984a, 1984b).

XylR ACTIVATES *xylS* EXPRESSION

The expression of gene *xylS* in *Pseudomonas putida* was determined with an RSF1010-derived plasmid containing a fusion of the *xylS* promoter (Ps) to *xylE* and the regulatory genes (Inouye et al., 1987a). Inducible expression of *xylS* by *m*-xylene was dependent on XylR, and XylS had neither a stimulatory nor an inhibitory effect on its own expression. Analysis of *xylS* transcripts by primer extension (Inouye et al., 1987a) or by S1 nuclease protection (Ramos et al., 1987) led to the same conclusion, indicating that XylR activates *xylS* expression at the transcriptional level.

OVERPRODUCED XylS CAN ACTIVATE THE *xylDLEGF* OPERON

The activation of OP2 is remarkably stimulated by XylS, which is overproduced in *E. coli* with the aid of the *tac* promoter (Inouye et al., 1987b), suggesting that large amounts of XylS can compensate for its poor ability to activate OP2 transcription in the absence of *m*-toluate. A direct and specific binding of *m*-toluate to XylS should lead to the formation of active XylS, as evidenced by the isolation of *xylS* mutants having altered inducer specificity (Ramos et al., 1986). Higher production of XylS appears to have a deleterious effect on the host cell; this may be due to the DNA-binding nature of the protein, as predicted by a helix-turn-helix motif (Pabo and Sauer, 1984) in the 321-amino-acid sequence (Inouye et al., 1986).

EXPRESSION OF *xylR* IS AUTOGENOUSLY REGULATED

Expression of *xylR* has a key role in the regulatory system for *xyl* gene expression (Fig. 1). Transcription of *xylR* is constitutive and unaffected by the addition of aromatic inducers (Inouye et al., 1985). Transcription starts at two sites separated by 27 base pairs in both *P. putida* and *E. coli*. Each start site has a structure similar to that of the *E. coli* canonical promoters at   35 and 10 which is recognized by the major RNA polymerase containing σ^{70} (Reznikoff et al., 1985). This may account for the high expression of *xylR* in *E. coli* as well as in *P. putida* (Inouye et al., 1985). Further quantitative analysis indicated that *xylR* expression is repressed by its own product (Inouye et al., 1987a).

The *xylR* promoter shares the upstream regulatory region of *xylS*, which is divergently transcribed from *xylR* (Fig. 2). The putative sequence involved in the XylR-mediated activation of *xylS* may be used for the autogenous repression of *xylR*.

NtrA IS REQUIRED FOR XylR-MEDIATED EXPRESSION OF
xylCAB AND *xylS*

The nucleotide sequences of the promoter regions of *xylS* and *xylCAB* have homology to the consensus sequences of nitrogen-regulated (*ntr*) and nitrogen fixation (*nif*) promoters: TGGC at −24 and TTGC at −12 (Fig. 2). Activation of *xylCAB* and *xylS* by XylR in *E. coli* is dependent on the *ntrA* gene (Dixon, 1986; Inouye et al., 1987a), whose product is a specific sigma factor (σ^{60}) for the *ntr*/*nif* promoters (Hunt and Magasanik, 1985; Hirschman et al., 1985). Furthermore, the basal-level (XylR-independent) expression of *xylCAB* and *xylS* is also dependent on NtrA (Ramos et al., 1987; Inouye et al., unpublished observation).

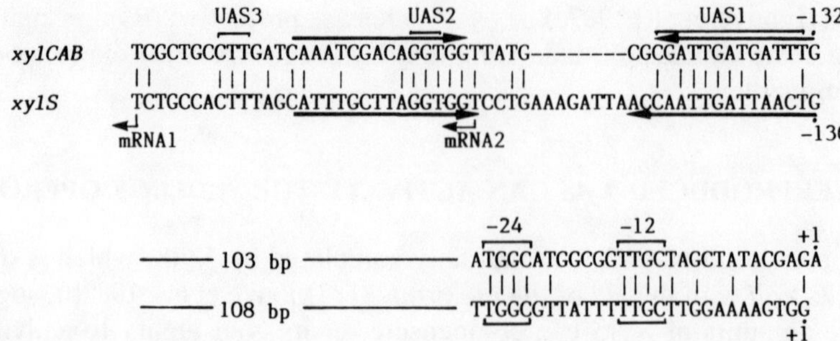

FIGURE 2. UASs (UAS1, UAS2, and UAS3) and the promoters (−24 and −12) of *xylCAB* and *xylS*. Nucleotides are numbered from the transcription start sites. Inverted repeats are indicated by horizontal arrows, and homologous bases are joined by lines. mRNA1 and mRNA2 represent transcriptional start sites of *xylR*. bp, Base pairs.

The consensus sequence for *ntr/nif* promoters is also found in some other *Pseudomonas* promoters such as the *P. aeruginosa* pilin promoter (Johnson et al., 1986) and the carboxypeptidase G2 promoter (Minton and Clark, 1985). Pilin gene expression might be controlled by environmental stimuli such that pilin adheres to the surface of animal cells for colonization. The *ntrA* (*rpoN*) gene of *P. aeruginosa* was cloned in *E. coli* (Ishimoto and Lory, 1989). The isolated clone was able to complement the *rpoN*-negative phenotype of *E. coli* and was used to produce an *ntrA* mutant of *P. aeruginosa* that was defective in pilin formation.

P. PUTIDA NtrA IS HIGHLY HOMOLOGOUS TO *AZOTOBACTER* NtrA

P. putida ntrA has been cloned and sequenced (Inouye et al., 1989). The isolated clone complemented an *ntrA*-negative phenotype of *E. coli* with respect to the XylR-mediated expression of OP1-*xylE* in response to *m*-xylene. The nucleotide sequence of the coding region of the *ntrA* gene as well as the 5′- and the 3′-flanking regions resemble those of *Azotobacter vinelandii* (Merrick et al., 1987). Comparison of the amino acid sequence of the *P. putida* NtrA with those of NtrAs from other bacteria is schematically illustrated in Fig. 3. *P. putida* NtrA is strikingly homologous to *Azotobacter* NtrA (81.7%) but less so to *Klebsiella* NtrA (52.6% [Merrick and Gibbins, 1985]) or *Rhizobium* NtrA (36.1% [Ronson et al., 1987a]). The conserved regions similar to procaryotic sigma factors and the β′ subunit of *E. coli* RNA polymerase may play a role in the protein-protein interaction between NtrA and core RNA polymerase (Merrick et al., 1987). A helix-turn-helix motif is also found in *P. putida* NtrA, suggesting that this may be a DNA-binding protein.

NtrA requires an activator to initiate transcription. Thus, XylR, NtrC, and NifA are required for transcriptional activation of *xyl* genes, a wide range of nitrogen-regulated genes, and nitrogen fixation genes, respectively (Hirshman et al., 1985; Hunt and Magasanik, 1985; Gussin et al., 1986). The conserved

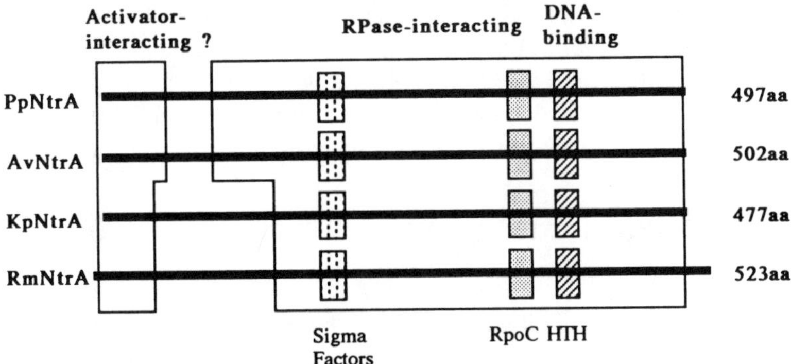

FIGURE 3. Amino acid sequence homology and functional domains of NtrAs. PpNtrA, *P. putida* NtrA; AvNtrA, *A. vinelandii* NtrA; KpNtrA, *Klebsiella pneumoniae* NtrA; RmNtrA, *R. meliloti* NtrA; HTH, helix-turn-helix motif; aa, amino acids.

sequence found in the N-terminal portion of NtrA might play a role in the interaction between NtrA and these activators.

XylR HAS A PUTATIVE NtrA-BINDING DOMAIN

The 566-amino-acid sequence of XylR (Inouye et al., 1988) has two characteristic regions that are homologous to the NtrC (Buikema et al., 1985) and NifA (Drummond et al., 1986) sequences. The C-terminal region contains a helix-turn-helix motif, suggesting that XylR is also a DNA-binding protein. The central region of XylR corresponds to the NtrA-interacting domain of NtrC or NifA.

No homology among XylR, NtrC, and NifA was found in the N-terminal regions. The N-terminal region of NtrC was suggested to act as a receptor for signals transmitted by a sensory protein, NtrB (Nixon et al., 1986). In the case of XylR, such a sensorlike protein may not be required. XylR and an inducer are sufficient for the activation of *xylCAB* and *xylS*.

xylCAB HAS A UAS

An upstream activator sequence (UAS) is required for efficient NifA-mediated activation of *nif* promoters. It is normally located 100 to 150 base pairs upstream from the transcription start site and is characterized by a DNA sequence with twofold rotational symmetry (Buck et al., 1986).

Deletion analysis of the upstream region of *xylCAB* has shown that there is a UAS between −133 and −174 which is required for efficient XylR-mediated transcription in response to *m*-xylene (Fig. 2; S. Inouye, A. Nakazawa, and T. Nakazawa, manuscript in preparation). Furthermore, results of phasing experiments that involved inserting half and whole turns of DNA between the UAS and the promoter suggested that the two sites are brought together via loop formation by the action of XylR (Inouye et al., in preparation).

The upstream region of *xylS* shares significant sequence homology with that of *xylCAB* (Fig. 2). In addition to the *ntr/nif* consensus sequence around −12 and −24, the sequence between −137 and −185 is highly homologous to the UAS of *xylCAB*. A twofold rotational symmetry of the UASs of *xylCAB* and *xylS* suggests that an oligomeric form of XylR binds to the sequences.

NtrA CONTROLS EXPRESSION OF DIVERSE PHYSIOLOGICAL FUNCTIONS

The *ntrA* gene was initially identified on the basis of its role in the activation of nitrogen-regulated operons. It seems likely, however, that *ntrA* has a broader physiological role than originally thought. Consistent with this idea, the *ntrA* gene is required for the XylR-mediated activation of *xyl* genes in *P. putida*, the DctD-mediated activation of the C4-dicarboxylate transport gene *dctA* in *Rhizobium meliloti* (Ronson et al., 1987a), and the formation of pilin in *P. aeruginosa* (Ishimoto and Lory, 1989). The *ntrA* gene is also responsible for the diverse metabolic activity of *Alcaligenes eutrophus* and *Pseudomonas facilis* (Römmermann et al., 1989) and possibly for expression of a set of *fla* genes of *Caulobacter crescentus* (Nifa et al., 1989). Among these functions, xylene and toluene catabolism by *P. putida* and hydrogen-oxidizing and -denitrifying activities of *A. eutrophus* are known to be controlled by plasmids (Kortlüke et al., 1987). These plasmids contain an activator gene in addition to structural genes.

CONCLUSIONS

Although it is not clear why *xylR* as well as *ntrC*, *nifA*, and *dctD* have evolved to use NtrA rather than the *rpoD* product σ^{70} for transcription, these genes seem to play a role in response to rather poor nutritional conditions in the environment. The *ntr/nif* system is active when the nitrogen source is limited, whereas the XylR and DctD systems are used by bacteria when the carbon source is restricted to xylene and dicarboxylic acids, respectively.

The *ntrA*-regulated genes usually share a common mechanism of transcriptional activation that responds to environmental stimuli by two-component signal-transducing systems (Ronson et al., 1987b). The system involving XylR appears to be exceptional because it does not require sensory elements. For this catabolic system, substrates are aromatic hydrocarbons and alcohols that are toxic for cellular activity, although they exist in low concentrations in the environment. Therefore, rapid and efficient degradation of these aromatic compounds would be beneficial to the cell in terms of both detoxification of deleterious substances and acquisition of metabolic energy. The substrates for the XylR-mediated catabolic system can be regarded as an alarm signal to the cell as well.

LITERATURE CITED

Buck, M., S. Miller, M. Drummond, and R. Dixon. 1986. Upstream activator sequences are present in the promoters of nitrogen fixation genes. *Nature* (London) **320**:374–378.

Buikema, W. J., W. W. Szeto, P. V. Lemley, W. H. Orme-Johnson, and F. M. Ausubel. 1985. Nitrogen fixation specific regulatory genes of *Klebsiella pneumoniae* and *Rhizobium meliloti* share homology with the general regulatory gene *ntrC* of *K. pneumoniae*. *Nucleic Acids Res.* **13**:4539–4555.

Dixon, R. 1986. The *xylABC* promoter from the *Pseudomonas putida* TOL plasmid is activated by nitrogen regulatory genes in *Escherichia coli*. *Mol. Gen. Genet.* **203**:129–136.

Drummond, M., P. Whitty, and J. Wootton. 1986. Sequences and domain relationships of *ntrC* and *nifA* from *Klebsiella pneumoniae*: homology to other regulatory proteins. *EMBO J.* **5**:441–447.

Franklin, F. C. H., M. Bagdasarian, M. M. Bagdasarian, and K. N. Timmis. 1981. Molecular and functional analysis of the TOL plasmid from *Pseudomonas putida* and cloning of genes for regulated aromatic ring *meta*-cleavage pathway. *Proc. Natl. Acad. Sci. USA* **78**:7458–7462.

Franklin, F. C. H., P. R. Lehrbach, R. Lurz, B. Rückert, M. Bagdasarian, and K. N. Timmis. 1983. Localization and functional analysis of transcription mutations in regulatory genes of the TOL catabolic pathway. *J. Bacteriol.* **154**:676–685.

Frantz, B., and A. M. Chakrabarty. 1986. Degradative plasmids in *Pseudomonas*, p. 295–323. *In* I. Gunsalus, J. R. Sokatch, and L. N. Ornston (ed.), *The Bacteria*, vol. 10. *The Biology of Pseudomonas*. Academic Press, Inc., Orlando, Fla.

Gussin, G. N., C. W. Ronson, and F. M. Ausubel. 1986. Regulation of nitrogen fixation genes. *Annu. Rev. Genet.* **20**:567–591.

Harayama, S., R. A. Leppik, M. Rekik, N. Mermod, P. R. Lehrbach, W. Reineke, and K. N. Timmis. 1986a. Gene order of the TOL catabolic plasmid upper pathway operon and oxidation of both toluene and benzylalcohol by the *xylA* product. *J. Bacteriol.* **167**:455–460.

Harayama, S., M. Rekik, and K. N. Timmis. 1986b. Genetic analysis of a relaxed substrate specificity aromatic ring dioxygenase, toluene 1,2-dioxygenase, encoded by TOL plasmid pWWO of *Pseudomonas putida*. *Mol. Gen. Genet.* **202**:226–234.

Hirschman, J., P.-K. Wong, K. Sei, J. Keener, and S. Kustu. 1985. Products of nitrogen regulatory genes *ntrA* and *ntrC* of enteric bacteria activate *glnA* transcription in vitro: evidence that the *ntrA* product is a σ factor. *Proc. Natl. Acad. Sci. USA* **82**:7525–7529.

Hunt, T. P., and B. Magasanik. 1985. Transcription of *glnA* by purified *Escherichia coli* components: core RNA polymerase and the products of *glnF*, *glnG* and *glnL*. *Proc. Natl. Acad. Sci. USA* **82**:8453–8457.

Inouye, S., A. Nakazawa, and T. Nakazawa. 1981. Molecular cloning of gene *xylS* on the TOL plasmid: evidence for positive regulation of the *xylDEGF* operon by *xylS*. *J. Bacteriol.* **148**:413–418.

Inouye, S., A. Nakazawa, and T. Nakazawa. 1983. Molecular cloning of regulatory gene *xylR* and operator-promoter regions of the *xylABC* and *xylDEGF* operons of the TOL plasmid. *J. Bacteriol.* **155**:1192–1199.

Inouye, S., A. Nakazawa, and T. Nakazawa. 1984a. Nucleotide sequence surrounding the transcription initiation site of *xylABC* operon on TOL plasmid of *Pseudomonas putida*. *Proc. Natl. Acad. Sci. USA* **81**:1688–1691.

Inouye, S., A. Nakazawa, and T. Nakazawa. 1984b. Nucleotide sequence of the operator-promoter region of the *xylDEGF* operon on TOL plasmid in *Pseudomonas putida*. *Gene* **29**:323–330.

Inouye, S., A. Nakazawa, and T. Nakazawa. 1985. Determination of the transcription initiation site and identification of the protein product of the regulatory gene *xylR* for *xyl* operons on the TOL plasmid. *J. Bacteriol.* **163**:863–869.

Inouye, S., A. Nakazawa, and T. Nakazawa. 1986. Nucleotide sequence of the regulatory gene *xylS* on the *Pseudomonas putida* TOL plasmid and identification of the protein product. *Gene* **44**:235–242.

Inouye, S., A. Nakazawa, and T. Nakazawa. 1987a. Expression of the regulatory gene *xylS* on the TOL plasmid is positively controlled by the *xylR* gene product. *Proc. Natl. Acad. Sci. USA* **84**:5182–5186.

Inouye, S., A. Nakazawa, and T. Nakazawa. 1987b. Overproduction of the *xylS* gene product and activation of the *xylDLEGF* operon on the TOL plasmid. *J. Bacteriol.* **169**:3587–3592.

Inouye, S., A. Nakazawa, and T. Nakazawa. 1988. Nucleotide sequence of the regulatory gene *xylR* of the TOL plasmid from *Pseudomonas putida*. *Gene* **66**:301–306.

Inouye, S., A. Nakazawa, and T. Nakazawa. 1989. Cloning and sequence analysis of the *ntrA* (*rpoN*) gene of *Pseudomonas putida*. *Gene* **85**:145–151.

Ishimoto, K. S., and S. Lory. 1989. Formation of pilin in *Pseudomonas aeruginosa* requires the alternative σ factor (RpoN) of RNA polymerase. *Proc. Natl. Acad. Sci. USA* **86**:1954–1957.

Johnson, K., M. L. Parker, and S. Lory. 1986. Nucleotide sequence and transcriptional initiation site of two *Pseudomonas aeruginosa* pilin genes. *J. Biol. Chem.* **261**:15703–15708.

Kortlüke, C., G. Hogrefe, G. Eberz, A. Pühler, and B. Friedrich. 1987. Genes of lithoautotrophic metabolism are clustered on the megaplasmid pHGl in *Alcaligenes eutrophus*. *Mol. Gen. Genet.* **210**:122–128.

Mermod, N., J. L. Ramos, A. Bairoch, and K. N. Timmis. 1987. The *xylS* gene positive regulator of TOL plasmid pWWO: identification, sequence analysis and overproduction leading to constitutive expression of *meta*-cleavage pathway operon. *Mol. Gen. Genet.* **207**:349–354.

Merrick, M. J., and J. R. Gibbins. 1985. The nucleotide sequence of the nitrogen-regulation gene *ntrA* of *Klebsiella pneumoniae* and comparison with conserved features in bacterial RNA polymerase sigma factors. *Nucleic Acids Res.* **13**:7607–7620.

Merrick, M., J. Gibbins, and A. Toukdarian. 1987. The nucleotide sequence of the sigma factor gene *ntrA* (*rpoN*) of *Azotobacter vinelandii*: analysis of conserved sequences in NtrA proteins. *Mol. Gen. Genet.* **210**:323–330.

Minton, N. P., and P. Clark. 1985. Identification of the promoter of the *Pseudomonas* gene coding for carboxypeptidase G2. *J. Mol. Appl. Genet.* **3**:26–35.

Nakazawa, T., S. Inouye, and A. Nakazawa. 1980. Physical and functional mapping of RP4-TOL plasmid recombinants: analysis of insertion and deletion mutants. *J. Bacteriol.* **144**:222–231.

Nifa, A. J., D. A. Mullin, G. Ramakrishnan, and A. Newton. 1989. *Escherichia coli* σ^{54} RNA polymerase recognizes *Caulobacter crescentus flbG* and *flaN* flagellar gene promoters in vitro. *J. Bacteriol.* **171**:383–391.

Nixon, B. T., C. W. Ronson, and F. M. Ausubel. 1986. Two-component regulatory systems responsive to environmental stimuli share strongly conserved domains with the nitrogen assimilation regulatory genes *ntrB* and *ntrC*. *Proc. Natl. Acad. Sci. USA* **83**:7850–7854.

Pabo, C. O., and R. T. Sauer. 1984. Protein-DNA recognition. *Annu. Rev. Genet.* **53**:293–321.

Ramos, J. L., N. Mermod, and K. N. Timmis. 1987. Regulatory circuit controlling transcription of TOL plasmid operon encoding *meta*-cleavage pathway for degradation of alkylbenzoates by *Pseudomonas*. *Mol. Microbiol.* **1**:293–300.

Ramos, J. L., A. Stolz, W. Reineke, and K. N. Timmis. 1986. Altered effector specificities in regulators of gene expression: TOL plasmid *xylS* mutants and their use to engineer expansion of the range of aromatics degraded by bacteria. *Proc. Natl. Acad. Sci. USA* **83**:8467–8471.

Reznikoff, W. S., D. A. Siegele, D. W. Cowing, and C. A. Gross. 1985. The regulation of transcription initiation in bacteria. *Annu. Rev. Genet.* **19**:355–387.

Römmermann, D., J. Warrelmann, R. A. Bender, and B. Friedrich. 1989. An *rpoN*-like gene of *Alcaligenes eutrophus* and *Pseudomonas facilis* controls expression of diverse metabolic pathways, including hydrogen oxidation. *J. Bacteriol.* **171**:1089–1099.

Ronson, C. W., B. T. Nixon, L. M. Albright, and F. M. Ausubel. 1987a. *Rhizobium meliloti ntrA* (*rpoN*) gene is required for diverse metabolic functions. *J. Bacteriol.* **169**:2424–2431.

Ronson, C. W., B. T. Nixon, and F. M. Ausubel. 1987b. Conserved domains in bacterial regulatory genes that respond to environmental stimuli. *Cell* **49**:571–581.

Tsuda, M., and T. Iino. 1987. Genetic analysis of a transposon carrying toluene degrading genes on a TOL plasmid pWWO. *Mol. Gen. Genet.* **210**:270–276.

Worsey, M. J., and P. A. Williams. 1975. Metabolism of toluene and xylenes by *Pseudomonas putida* (*arvilla*) mt-2: evidence for a new function of the TOL plasmid. *J. Bacteriol.* **124**:7–13.

Chapter 15

Oxidation of Alkanes by *Pseudomonas oleovorans*

Bernard Witholt, Joke Sijtsema, Menno Kok, and Gerrit Eggink

One of the potential applications of biotechnology is in the production of fine and medium-priced chemicals such as amino acids, vitamins, steroids, oxidized aromatic compounds, long-chain epoxides, dialcohols, dialdehydes, and dicarboxylic acids. The latter can in principle be prepared enzymatically by oxidizing aromatic and aliphatic compounds with oxygenases, which incorporate molecular oxygen directly into organic substrates with high selectivity.

Oxygenases are widespread among *Pseudomonas* species. The oxygenases of *Pseudomonas* species are usually encoded by genes located on large catabolic plasmids (Frantz and Chakrabarty, 1986), such as the CAM, NAH, SAL, XYL, TOL, and OCT plasmids, which determine the first step in the oxidation of camphor, naphthalene, salicylate, *p*- and *m*-xylene, and *n*-alkanes, respectively. These oxygenases are complexes of enzymes that need cofactors (NADH or NADPH) for activity, and whole cells are therefore preferred to isolated enzymes for biotechnological applications. Given these considerations, *Pseudomonas* strains are interesting candidates for the bioconversion of aromatic and aliphatic compounds (Sokatch and Ornston, 1986).

Pseudomonas oleovorans is a well-studied example of such a strain. It can grow on alkanes as well as on water-soluble substrates such as citrate, pyruvate, and malate (Stanier et al., 1966). Growth on alkanes depends on the presence in the cell of the OCT plasmid, which contains about 15% of the total genetic information of the bacterium (Chakrabarty et al., 1973; Fennewald et al., 1978). The enzymology of alkane oxidation was worked out in the late 1960s and early 1970s by Coon and co-workers, who showed that three proteins are involved in the first oxidation step by alkane hydroxylase (McKenna and Coon, 1970; Ueda et al., 1972; Peterson and Coon, 1968). Shapiro and co-workers studied the genetics of the system in the late 1970s and showed that these proteins are encoded and

---

Bernard Witholt, Joke Sijtsema, Menno Kok, and Gerrit Eggink • Laboratory of Biochemistry, Groningen Biotechnology Center, Nijenborgh 16, 9747 AG Groningen, The Netherlands.

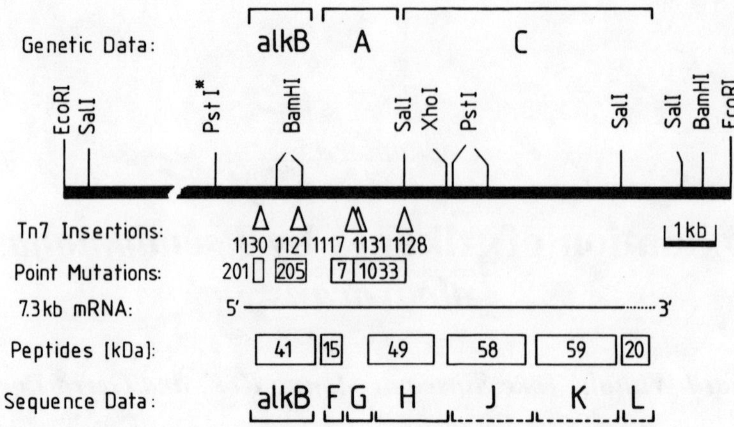

FIGURE 1. Genetic structure and nomenclature of the *alkBAC* operon. The *alkBAC* operon is transcribed as a single 7.3-kb mRNA and encodes seven polypeptides (Eggink et al., 1987b). Previous genetic experiments have shown that *alkB* encodes the 41-kDa cytoplasmic membrane component, *alkA* encodes at least one of the two soluble components of alkane hydroxylase, and *alkC* encodes several functions that have not been well defined. On the basis of peptide and sequencing data, we have introduced the nomenclature shown for the seven cistrons encoded by the *alkBAC* operon. The sizes of the polypeptide products of *alkB* (46 kDa), *alkF* (15 kDa), *alkH* (53 kDa), *alkJ* (61 kDa), *alkK* (59 kDa), and *alkL* (25 kDa) as determined by DNA sequencing are in good agreement with the apparent molecular weights of the *alk* translation products determined by minicell-labeling experiments (Eggink et al., 1987b). Mutations affecting alkane oxidation activity are indicated by boxes (*N*-methyl-*N'*-nitro-*N*-nitrosoguanidine mutations) and arrows (Tn7 insertions).

regulated by the *alk* system, which is located on the OCT plasmid. A number of mutants were obtained, which allowed the identification of several structural and regulatory genes (Benson et al., 1979; Fennewald and Shapiro, 1977; Fennewald et al., 1979; Owen et al., 1984).

STRUCTURE OF THE *alk* REGULON

We have cloned sequences encoding *alk* genes which complement various structural and regulatory mutants from the collection of Shapiro and co-workers. Two sequences have been characterized in detail.

alkB-L Sequence

One sequence complemented *alkB*, *alkA*, and *alkC* mutations (Fig. 1) and was taken to encode two enzymatic activities: alkane hydroxylation and alcohol dehydrogenation. Analysis of the peptides encoded in *Escherichia coli* minicells by subclones of the DNA fragment of Fig. 1 showed that six peptides were formed. Table 1 lists these peptides (AlkB to AlkL); positions of the respective genes are shown in Fig. 1 (Eggink et al., 1987b). Using R-loop electron microscopy, we identified a single 7.3-kilobase-pair (kb) mRNA species that was formed

TABLE 1
Characteristics of the gene products of the *alk* regulon

| Gene | Molecular size (kDa) of gene product on SDS-PAGE[a] | Sequence-derived information | | Function | Reference |
		Molecular size (kDa)	No. of amino acids		
alkB	41	45.7	401	Alkane hydroxylase	Kok et al., 1989b Benson et al., 1979
alkF	15	14.6	132	Rubredoxin 1	Kok et al., 1989a
alkG	20	18.7	172	Rubredoxin 2	Peterson and Coon, 1968 Kok et al., 1989a
alkH	49	52.7	483	Aldehyde dehydrogenase	Kok et al., 1989a
alkJ	58	60.9	558	Alkanol dehydrogenase	Owen et al., 1984 Eggink, unpublished data
alkK	59	59.3	546	Unknown	Eggink, unpublished data
alkL	20	25.0	230	Unknown	Eggink, unpublished data
alkS	99			*alk* regulatory protein	Eggink et al., 1988
alkT	48	41.1	385	Rubredoxin reductase	Eggink et al., in press Ueda et al., 1972

[a] SDS-PAGE, Sodium dodecyl sulfate-polyacrylamide gel electrophoresis.

on induction of the *alk* system and hybridized with the cloned *alk* operon at the position shown in Fig. 1 (Eggink et al., 1987b).

We have sequenced the *alkB-L* operon. Table 1 lists several characteristics derived from the sequence data. The gene positions are shown in Fig. 1.

The positional overlap in Fig. 1 between the sequenced gene positions, the 7.3-kb mRNA transcript, and the gene products as expressed from subclones in *E. coli* minicells is satisfying. A gap that we originally observed between the 15- and 49-kilodalton (kDa) peptides (Eggink et al., 1987b) has now been accounted for. It contains the *alkG* gene, which encodes rubredoxin 2 (Kok et al., 1989a).

The fact that we could identify a single 7.3-kb mRNA transcript implies that the entire *alkB-L* operon is transcribed as one large message. The expression of the different genes of this message differs considerably.

alkST Sequence

The second *alk* sequence complemented regulatory mutations and was found to encode AlkS and AlkT by expression experiments in *E. coli* minicells (Eggink et al., 1988). We initially assumed both AlkS and AlkT to be regulatory proteins, but sequence analysis of the *alkT* gene showed it to be rubredoxin reductase (Table 1). Figure 2 summarizes the information available on the *alkST* sequence.

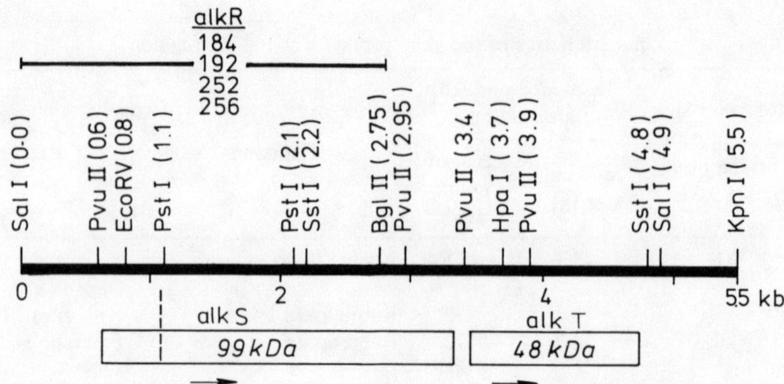

FIGURE 2. Genetic organization of the *alkR* locus. Symbols: □, proteins encoded by the *alkR* locus; →, proposed direction of transcription of the corresponding cistrons. The region in which the *alkR* mutations (256, 252, 192, and 184) were mapped is given above the restriction map.

Components of the Alkane Oxidation System

A model for the localization of the various gene products is shown in Fig. 3, which also shows the enzymatic reactions and cofactors associated with each of the alkane oxidation enzymes. The localization of AlkS, the positive regulator of the *alk* system, is speculative (Benson, 1979), and the functions of AlkK and AlkL are not yet known.

The alkane hydroxylase complex is encoded by *alkB* (the membrane-bound

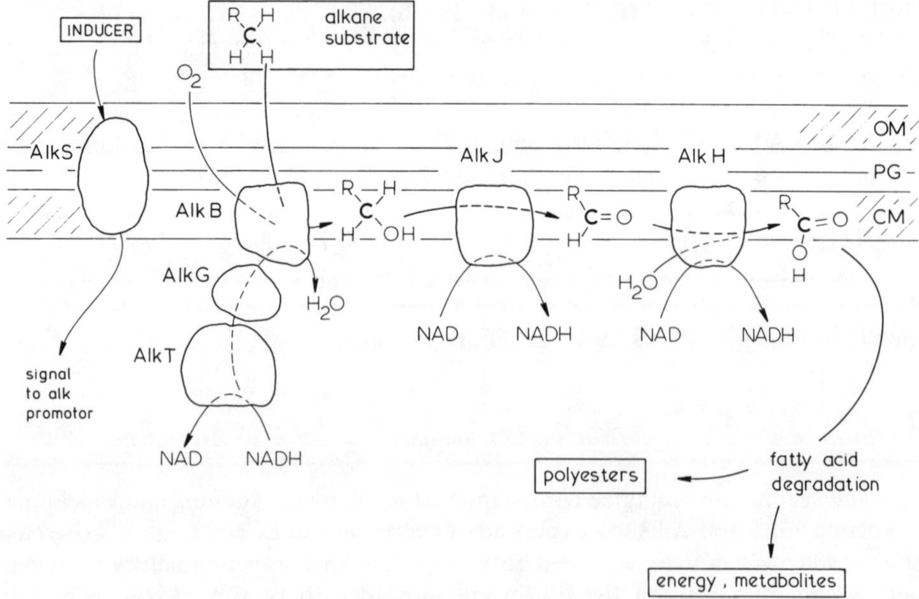

FIGURE 3. Model for the cellular localization of the alkane oxidation system.

monooxygenase), *alkG* (rubredoxin), and *alkT* (rubredoxin reductase). Alcohol and aldehyde dehydrogenases are encoded by *alkJ* and *alkH*, respectively.

STRUCTURE OF THE ALKANE HYDROXYLASE COMPLEX

Coon and co-workers have purified the three components of the alkane hydroxylase system (McKenna and Coon, 1970; Peterson and Coon, 1968; Ueda et al., 1972) and have reconstituted the active complex from these purified components and added phospholipids (Ruettinger et al., 1974).

We purified alkane monooxygenase (AlkB) and sequenced the N-terminal amino acids to establish its relationship to the *alkB* gene (Kok et al., 1989b). The *alkB* nucleotide sequence predicts an amino acid sequence with eight potential membrane-spanning segments and several hydrophilic loops and shows limited stretches of homology only to *p*-hydroxybenzoic acid hydroxylase and tyrosinase (Kok et al., 1989b). There is no homology to sequenced P-450 cytochromes.

The amino acid sequence of *P. oleovorans* rubredoxin has been determined (Benson et al., 1971). Except for minor deviations, this sequence is identical to that predicted from the nucleotide sequence of *alkG*. We do not yet understand the role of *alkF*, which is closely related to *alkG*, but it is not essential for alkane oxidation by *Pseudomonas* strains (Kok et al., 1989a).

Rubredoxin reductase has been purified, and its amino acid composition has been determined (Ueda et al., 1972). The amino acid composition predicted from the *alkT* nucleotide sequence is in full agreement with the experimentally determined amino acid composition; genetic data also identify *alkT* as the gene encoding rubredoxin reductase (G. Eggink et al., *J. Mol. Biol.*, in press). Analysis of the *alkT* sequence has identified fingerprints for NAD and FAD binding. These have allowed us to construct a model for rubredoxin reductase based on glutathione reductase, another NAD-binding flavoprotein for which the three-dimensional structure is known.

We hope to be able to use some of this information to develop a model for the interactions between the components of the alkane hydroxylase system. We do not, however, expect to be able to describe a stable three-component complex because AlkB, AlkG, and AlkT are not present in equimolar amounts in fully induced cells.

TRANSCRIPTION AND TRANSLATION OF THE *alk* SEQUENCES

The *alkB-L* operon is transcribed as a single 7.3-kb mRNA species (Eggink et al., 1987b). Induction by alkanes requires the *alkS* gene product, which acts as a positive regulator on the *alk* promoter. The *alkB-L* promoter lies within a 182-base-pair region immediately preceding the *alk* mRNA transcription initiation site (Kok et al., 1989b).

The *alk* transcript begins with a 96-nucleotide leader that can fold in two stem-loop structures. The A+T content of this leader is 62%, very high compared with those of the *Pseudomonas putida* chromosome and the OCT plasmid (Fennewald et al., 1978).

TABLE 2

Ribosome-binding sites of the *alkBFGH* and *alkT* genes

Site	Organism	Sequence
16S rRNA	*E. coli*	3'–auuCCUCCacuag
	P. aeruginosa	3'–auuCCUCUc...g
Consensus	*E. coli*	5'- GGAGG........AUG..A/U
	Pseudomonas spp.	5'- AGGAGA (..) AUG
	alkB	5'–auuGGAGAacaccaa AUGcuU
	alkF	5'–auaGGAGAguggaga AUGucA
	alkG	5'–cauGGUGAugagu AUGgcU
	alkH	5'–ucaGGACAaaauaaaa AUGacc
	alkT	5'–accGGAGAgagaauu AUGgcA

The *alkST* operon also appears to be transcribed as a single message, as determined by R-loop electron microscopy experiments (G. Eggink, unpublished data). However, we have not yet examined the structure of this message in detail.

As to translation efficiencies, AlkB accounts for 1.5% of the total cell protein under full induction (about 35,000 copies of AlkB per cell), whereas AlkG accounts for 0.2% of the total cell protein, or 10,000 copies per cell.

On the basis of the results of Coon and co-workers, fully induced cells contain at most 1,000 copies of AlkT per cell. Only a few dozen copies per cell of the regulatory protein AlkS should be enough for a well-functioning *alk* regulon. Thus, the transcription of the *alkB-L* and the *alkST* operons and the translation efficiencies of the *alkB-L* messages are quite heterogeneous.

RIBOSOME-BINDING SITES AND CODON USAGE OF THE *alk* GENES

The *alk* ribosome-binding sites generally agree reasonably well with the *Pseudomonas* and *E. coli* consensus sequences, although their spacing is more suggestive of the *E. coli* sequence (Table 2).

Codon usage in the *alk* sequences differs from that of both *Pseudomonas* and *E. coli* chromosomal genes. Table 3 shows the leucine codon usage as a rather striking example of these differences.

The G+C content of the *alk* genes (47%) is very low compared with that of the *P. putida* (62.5%) and *P. aeruginosa* (67.2%) chromosomes. Both the G+C content and the codon usage of the *alk* genes suggest that these genes may have originated from an unrelated organism.

EXPRESSION OF *alk* GENES IN *E. COLI* AND *P. PUTIDA*

The *alk* genes have been cloned in various combinations in suitable vectors (Eggink et al., 1987a). One vector (pGEc47) contains all *alkB-L* and *alkST* sequences and encodes the entire alkane-to-alkanoic acid oxidation pathway. Another vector (pGEc41) contains only *alkBFG(H)* and *alkST* sequences and

TABLE 3
Comparison of codon usage for *alk* genes with usage of *Pseudomonas* and *E. coli* genes[a]

Codon	Codon usage for leucine (%)			
	alkBFGH	*P. putida*[b]	*P. aeruginosa*[c]	*E. coli*[d]
UUA	9	3	1	3
UUG	22	15	3	4
CUU	28	4	3	6
CUC	10	17	32	6
CUA	9	5	1	1
CUG	22	56	60	80

[a] From Kok et al. (1989a).
[b] *catB clcD xylE xylS camC bphC*.
[c] *cpg-2 pmi* hemolysin.
[d] *lpp lamB tufB* EF-G IF-3 *recA*.

therefore encodes only alkane hydroxylase activity. Such fusion plasmids have been introduced into *P. putida* strains that contain no plasmids. They show the expected growth behavior (Table 4).

The fusion plasmids have also been introduced into *E. coli*. Interestingly, *E. coli* cells not only produced the *alk* gene products (Fig. 4) but also functioned as expected. If there is fatty acid degradation (the *fadR* mutation causes constitutive expression of the *E. coli fad* genes), *E. coli* containing the *alk* genes can grow on alkanes (Table 4).

The reason why it is useful to have these fusion plasmids is that they allow the construction of partial oxidation pathways in *Pseudomonas* or *E. coli* strains. These permit a selected number of enzymatic degradation steps to be carried out while blocking subsequent steps. By using such partial oxidation pathways, it is possible to produce alcohols or aldehydes.

GROWTH OF *P. OLEOVORANS* IN TWO-PHASE BIOREACTORS

P. oleovorans grows well in simple salt media if a carbon source is present. This can be a water-soluble substrate such as citrate, glucose, or pyruvate. When

TABLE 4
Growth on octane of *Pseudomonas* spp. and *E. coli* transformed with OCT-related plasmids

Strain	Host	Plasmid	*alk* genes	Growth on octane
GPo1	*P. oleovorans*	OCT	*alkB-L, alkST*	+++
GPp7	*P. putida*	pGEc47	*alkB-L, alkST*	+++
GPp9	*P. putida*	pGEc41	*alkBFG, alkST*	++
GPp10	*P. putida (alcA)*[a]	pGEc47	*alkB-L, alkST*	++
GPp11	*P. putida (alcA)*	pGEc41	*alkBFG, alkST*	−
DH1	*E. coli*			−
GEc92	DH1	pGEc47	*alkB-L, alkST*	−
GEc93	DH1 *(fadR)*[b]	pGEc47	*alkB-L, alkST*	++
GEc136	DIl1 *(fadR)*	pGEc41	*alkBFG, alkST*	+

[a] *alcA* is a chromosomal alcohol dehydrogenase mutant.
[b] *fadR* is a chromosomal fatty acid degradation regulatory mutant.

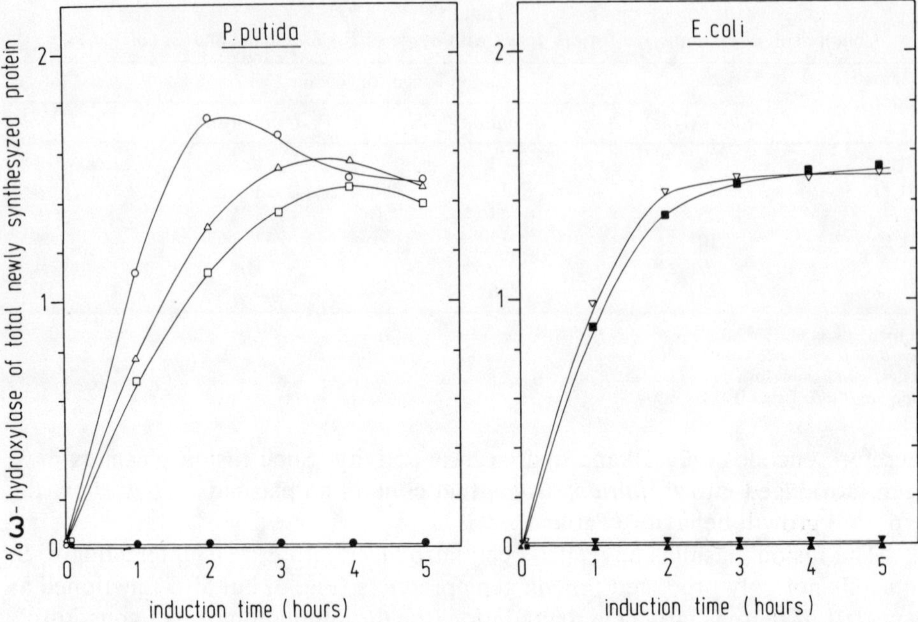

FIGURE 4. Induction kinetics of alkane hydroxylase (*alkB*) in *P. putida* and *E. coli*. Cells were pulse-chase labeled with [^{35}S]methionine, and AlkB was immunoprecipitated. The percentage of alkane hydroxylase relative to newly synthesized total protein was calculated for the different time points. (Left) *P. oleovorans* noninduced (●); *P. oleovorans* induced (○); PpS124 (PpG1, CAM-OCT) induced (△); GPp7 (PpG1, pGEc47) induced (□). (Right) *E. coli* DH1 induced (▼); GEc93 (DH1, *fadR*, pGEc47) noninduced (▲); GEc93 induced (▽); GEc92 (DH1, pGEc47) induced (■).

alkanes are added, usually 20% (vol/vol), the *alk* system (either on the OCT plasmid or on one of the fusion plasmids) is induced via the *alkS* gene product. A water-soluble carbon source is necessary for growth of strains that produce some of the alkane-oxidizing enzymes but not the entire set, as a result of which they cannot grow on alkanes. Since pyruvate shows absolutely no repression effect, it is the substrate of choice in experiments with recombinant strains.

After initiation of transcription of *alk* genes, the corresponding gene products are synthesized and accumulate in the cell membrane and cell cytoplasm. Maximum enzyme levels are reached within 2 h (Fig. 4). As they accumulate, these enzymes begin oxidizing alkanes. If all of the enzymes are present, the alkanes are oxidized completely and are used for cell metabolism. In that case, there is little or no accumulation of intermediates.

If only alkane hydroxylase is present (pGEc41), alkanol accumulates a little and is oxidized only by the chromosomally encoded alcohol dehydrogenase. When *P. putida* PpS81, which has an *alcA* mutation in the chromosome, is used as the host organism, there is neither plasmid nor chromosomal alcohol dehydrogenase. As a result, alkanol is not oxidized to alkanal. Therefore, alkanol accumulates, and the cells grow on the alternate carbon source, the water-soluble pyruvate.

Aside from the specific carbon source being used, the cells must in all cases survive in the two-phase system. This is a not trivial consideration, since apolar solvents tend to damage cell membranes. Moreover, in a two-phase system there is a potentially enormous interfacial surface (as alkane droplets in the aqueous phase become smaller), and cell damage at the interface may be considerable.

Progress in our laboratory with two-phase systems in shaker cultures was slow because it is very difficult to regulate phase mixing, O_2 levels, and bacterial dispersion in Erlenmeyer flasks. For these reasons, we have developed computer-controlled bioreactors in which temperature, pH, stirrer speed, O_2 concentration, and O_2 flux can be measured and regulated continuously. By using suitable materials, damage to reactor parts due to apolar solvents can be avoided or minimized. The fact that these reactors can be operated reproducibly is especially important.

With use of the computer-controlled bioreactors, all of these parameters can be regulated reproducibly, and we are now able to run multiple small-scale (500- to 1,000-ml) two-phase fermentations simultaneously. Optimal fermentation conditions are as follows: temperature, 30°C; pH, 6.9 to 7.0; agitation, 500 to 1,000 rpm; dissolved oxygen tension, above 50% air saturation; air flow, 120 ml/min; percent (vol/vol) octane or octene, 20 to 95; medium, minimal salts medium containing N, P, S, Mg, and microelements.

Two points are especially interesting. First, the maximum growth rate of *Pseudomonas* spp. is totally independent of the volume ratio of octane or octene relative to the total medium volume. Second, very high stirring speeds can be used. These have no effect on the maximum growth rate, but they do affect maximum cell densities.

Both of these observations were unexpected because earlier experiments with flask cultures had pointed toward considerable cell damage at high apolar phase contents and high shaking speeds. Clearly, however, these early results were due to other factors. With the much more reproducible two-phase reactors, it has become clear that stirring speeds (at least up to 1,500 rpm) affect aeration rates but not cell survival, whereas the relative size of the apolar phase is essentially irrelevant to the cells, all of which occupy the aqueous phase.

CONCLUSIONS AND PERSPECTIVES

The alkane oxidation system of *P. oleovorans* can be manipulated and expressed in various other bacteria. With the use of two-liquid-phase bioreactors, improved bioconversion rates can be obtained.

Further work in our laboratory is directed at modifications of the *alk* system to increase enzyme activity and longevity and to alter the substrate range of this system. The supply and regeneration of intracellular cofactor is of interest. An exploration of the potential of gram-negative organisms in the presence of bulk apolar phases has been initiated.

ACKNOWLEDGMENT. We thank Jim Shapiro for many stimulating discussions and unlimited hospitality.

LITERATURE CITED

Benson, A., K. Tomoda, J. Chang, G. Matsueda, E. T. Lode, M. J. Coon, and K. T. Yasunobu. 1971. Evolutionary and phylogenetic relationships of rubredoxin-containing microbes. *Biochem. Biophys. Res. Commun.* **42:**640–646.

Benson, S. 1979. Local anesthetics block induction of the *Pseudomonas alk* regulon. *J. Bacteriol.* **140:**1123–1125.

Benson, S., M. Oppici, J. Shapiro, and M. Fennewald. 1979. Regulation of membrane peptides by the *Pseudomonas* plasmid *alk* regulon. *J. Bacteriol.* **140:**754–762.

Chakrabarty, A. M., G. Chou, and I. C. Gunsalus. 1973. Genetic regulations of octane dissimilation plasmid in *Pseudomonas. Proc. Natl. Acad. Sci. USA* **70:**1137–1140.

Eggink, G., H. Engel, W. G. Meijer, J. Otten, J. Kingma, and B. Witholt. 1988. Alkane utilization in *Pseudomonas oleovorans*: structure and function of the regulatory locus *alkR. J. Biol. Chem.* **263:**13400–13405.

Eggink, G., R. G. Lageveen, B. Altenburg, and B. Witholt. 1987a. Controlled and functional expression of the *Pseudomonas oleovorans* alkane utilizing system in *Pseudomonas putida* and *Escherichia coli. J. Biol. Chem.* **262:**17712–17718.

Eggink, G., P. H. van Lelyveld, A. Arnberg, N. Arfman, C. Witteveen, and B. Witholt. 1987b. Structure of the *Pseudomonas putida alkBAC* operon. *J. Biol. Chem.* **262:**6400–6406.

Fennewald, M., S. Benson, M. Oppici, and J. Shapiro. 1979. Insertion element analysis and mapping of the *Pseudomonas* plasmid *alk* regulon. *J. Bacteriol.* **139:**940–952.

Fennewald, M., W. Prevatt, R. Meijer, and J. A. Shapiro. 1978. Isolation of Inc. P-2 plasmid DNA from *Pseudomonas aeruginosa. Plasmid* **1:**164–173.

Fennewald, M., and J. Shapiro. 1977. Regulatory mutations of the *Pseudomonas* plasmid *alk* regulon. *J. Bacteriol.* **132:**622–627.

Frantz, B., and A. M. Chakrabarty. 1986. Degradative plasmids in *Pseudomonas*, p. 295–317. *In* J. R. Sokatch and L. N. Ornston (ed.), *The Bacteria*, vol. 10. *The Biology of Pseudomonas.* Academic Press, Inc., Orlando, Fla.

Kok, M., R. Oldenhuis, M. P. G. van der Linden, C. H. Meulenberg, J. Kingma, and B. Witholt. 1989a. The *Pseudomonas oleovorans alkBAC* operon encodes two structurally related rubredoxins and an aldehyde dehydrogenase. *J. Biol. Chem.* **264:**5442–5451.

Kok, M., R. Oldenhuis, M. P. G. van der Linden, P. Raatjes, J. Kingma, P. H. van Lelyveld, and B. Witholt. 1989b. The *Pseudomonas oleovorans* alkane hydroxylase gene: sequence and expression. *J. Biol. Chem.* **264:**5435–5441.

McKenna, E. J., and M. J. Coon. 1970. Enzymatic ω-oxidation. IV. Purification and properties of the ω-hydroxylase of *Pseudomonas oleovorans. J. Biol. Chem.* **245:**3882–3889.

Owen, D. J., G. Eggink, B. Hauer, M. Kok, D. L. McBeth, Y. L. Yang, and J. A. Shapiro. 1984. Physical structure, genetic content and expression of the *alkBAC* operon. *Mol. Gen. Genet.* **197:**373–383.

Peterson, J. A., and M. J. Coon. 1968. Enzymatic ω-oxidation. III. Purification and properties of rubredoxin, a component of the ω-hydroxylation system of *Pseudomonas oleovorans. J. Biol. Chem.* **243:**320–334.

Ruettinger, R. T., S. T. Olson, R. F. Boyer, and M. J. Coon. 1974. Identification of the alkane hydroxylase of *Pseudomonas oleovorans* as a nonheme iron protein requiring phospholipids for catalytic activity. *Biochem. Biophys. Res. Commun.* **57:**1011–1017.

Sokatch, J. R., and L. N. Ornston (ed.). 1986. *The Bacteria*, vol. 10. *The Biology of Pseudomonas.* Academic Press, Inc., Orlando, Fla.

Stanier, R. Y., N. J. Palleroni, and M. Doudoroff. 1966. The aerobic *Pseudomonads*: a taxonomic study. *J. Gen. Microbiol.* **43:**159–271.

Ueda, T., E. T. Lode, and M. J. Coon. 1972. Enzymatic ω-hydroxylation. VI. Isolation of homogeneous reduced diphosphopyridine nucleotide rubredoxin reductase. *J. Biol. Chem.* **247:**2109–2116.

Chapter 16

Organization and Regulation of the *mva* Operon of *Pseudomonas mevalonii*[†]

Victor W. Rodwell, Douglas H. Anderson, Michael J. Beach, John F. Gill, Jr., Tuajuanda C. Jordan-Starck, David S. Scher, and Yuli Wang

INTERMEDIARY METABOLISM

P. mevalonii Can Utilize Mevalonate as Its Sole Source of Carbon

R-Mevalonate was initially discovered as a factor that stimulated growth of *Lactobacillus acidophilus* (Skeggs et al., 1956). While considerable research over the past 35 years has addressed the central role of mevalonate in isoprenoid biosynthesis in *Saccharomyces cerevisiae* and animal tissues, less is known of its metabolism in bacteria.

We have investigated the catabolism of mevalonate in *Pseudomonas mevalonii* [initially termed *Pseudomonas* sp. M (Gill et al., 1984, 1985)], an organism we isolated from soil by aerobic elective culture on ammonium *R,S*-mevalonate (pH 8.0) as the sole source of carbon (Gill et al., 1984). Only the *R* isomer is utilized for growth, which ceases after approximately 50% of racemic mevalonate has been removed from the medium.

Catabolism of Mevalonate Leads to a Two-Carbon Economy

Figure 1 depicts the intermediates in mevalonate catabolism by *P. mevalonii*. After internalization, *R*-mevalonate is oxidatively acylated to 3-hydroxy-3-meth-

[†] Journal paper no. 12,134 from the Purdue University Agricultural Experiment Station.

Victor W. Rodwell and Yuli Wang ● Department of Biochemistry, Purdue University, West Lafayette, Indiana 47907.   *Douglas H. Anderson* ● Department of Clinical Biochemistry, Banting Institute, University of Toronto, 100 College Street, Toronto, Ontario, Canada M5G 1L5.   *Michael J. Beach* ● Hepatitis Branch, Centers for Disease Control, Atlanta, Georgia 30333.   *John F. Gill, Jr.* ● Protein Chemistry Division, Boehringer Mannheim Diagnostics, 9115 Hague Road, Indianapolis, Indiana 46250.   *Tuajuanda C. Jordan-Starck* ● Department of Pharmacology and Cell Biophysics, University of Cincinnati College of Medicine, Cincinnati, Ohio 45267.   *David S. Scher* ● Boehringer Ingelheim Pharmaceuticals, Ridgefield, Connecticut 06877.

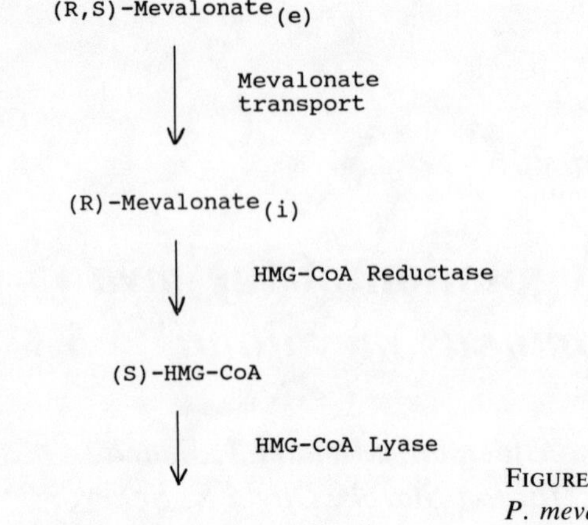

FIGURE 1. Intermediates in catabolism of mevalonate by *P. mevalonii*. (e), External mevalonate; (i), internal mevalonate.

ylglutaryl coenzyme A (HMG-CoA) in a reaction catalyzed by HMG-CoA reductase (EC 1.1.1.88) (Gill et al., 1985). HMG-CoA is then cleaved to acetoacetate and acetyl-CoA by HMG-CoA lyase (EC 4.1.3.4). Further catabolism of acetyl-CoA involves known reactions of two-carbon metabolism. Acetoacetate, which can also serve as a sole source of carbon for growth, presumably is catabolized to acetyl-CoA by reactions as yet unidentified in *P. mevalonii*.

ENZYMOLOGY

R-Mevalonate Enters via a High-Affinity Active Transport System

Growth of cells on *R*,*S*-mevalonate induces transport activity 40- to 65-fold. Transport is maximal at pH 7.0 and at 30°C. The inferred K_m for *R*-mevalonate is 44 μM, and the V_{max} is 26 nmol of *R*-mevalonate transported per min per mg (dry weight) of cells. Transport, which is energy dependent, is blocked by azide, cyanide, or *m*-chlorophenylhydrazone.

Structural features of mevalonate that might be involved in substrate recognition for transport include the primary hydroxyl group, the carboxylate group, and the chiral center at carbon 3, which bears both a methyl and a secondary hydroxyl group. The system is not, however, a general acid or general alcohol transport system. Of 16 structural analogs of mevalonate tested, only mevaldehyde and the mevalonate catabolite acetoacetate (Fig. 1) competed with mevalonate for transport.

The First Intracellular Reaction of Mevalonate Catabolism Is Catalyzed by HMG-CoA Reductase

P. mevalonii grown on mevalonate has up to 800-fold-induced levels of HMG-CoA reductase. This enzyme, which can be purified to electrophoretic

Mevalonate + 2 NAD$^+$ + CoASH ---> HMG-CoA + 2 NADH + 2 H$^+$

HMG-CoA + 2 NADH + 2 H$^+$ ---> Mevalonate + 2 NAD$^+$ + CoASH

Mevaldehyde + NADH + H$^+$ ---> Mevalonate + NAD$^+$

Mevaldehyde + NAD$^+$ + CoASH ---> HMG-CoA + NADH + H$^+$

FIGURE 2. Reactions catalyzed by *P. mevalonii* HMG-CoA reductase. CoASH, Reduced coenzyme A.

homogeneity in over 50% yield (final specific activity, 60 μmol of NAD$^+$ reduced per min per mg of protein [Gill et al., 1985]), interconverts reduced coenzyme A (K_m = 0.05 mM) plus *R*-mevalonate (K_m = 0.11 mM) and *S*-HMG-CoA (K_m = 0.15 mM). The K_m values for NAD$^+$ and NADH are 0.37 and 0.17 mM, respectively. In addition to both overall reactions, the enzyme also catalyzes two half-reactions (Fig. 2) (Jordan-Starck and Rodwell, 1989a, 1989b). A homotetramer (M_r, 45,538) of identical subunits (one subunit contains 428 amino acids), HMG-CoA reductase is a slightly acidic protein (53% of the charged residues are negative) with a hydropathy profile typical for a soluble, hydrophilic protein (Beach and Rodwell, 1989). It lacks the N-terminal multiple hydrophobic segments thought to function as membrane anchor domains for eucaryotic HMG-CoA reductases (Chin et al., 1984) and exhibits only a limited structural similarity to the C-terminal domain of the eucaryotic enzymes (Chin et al., 1984; Basson et al., 1986).

Cysteine Residues Play No Essential Role in Catalysis or Substrate Recognition by *P. mevalonii* HMG-CoA Reductase

Each subunit of HMG-CoA reductase contains only two cysteine residues, Cys-156 and Cys-296 (Beach and Rodwell, 1989). Evidence suggestive of a catalytic role of these residues includes (i) the susceptibility of HMG-CoA reductase to reagents such as *N*-ethylmaleimide (NEM) that derivatize sulfhydryl groups, (ii) the ability of the substrate HMG-CoA to protect against inactivation by NEM (Jordan-Starck and Rodwell, 1989a) and (iii) the postulated role of a thiohemiacetal intermediate during interconversion of mevalonate and HMG-CoA via the putative enzyme-bound intermediate, mevaldehyde.

The availability of cloned, sequenced HMG-CoA reductase (see below) permitted us to use site-directed mutagenesis to inquire whether either cysteine played a key role in the enzymatic mechanism. We replaced either or both cysteine (C) residues by alanine (A) residues, generating HMG-CoA reductase mutants C156A and C296A and the cysteine-free mutant C156/296A (Jordan-Starck and Rodwell, 1989b). Alanine was selected to minimize changes in shape or net charge at neutral pH and because it cannot function as a nucleophile. We expressed these mutants in *Escherichia coli* and assayed cell extracts for HMG-CoA reductase activity. Both crude and purified mutant forms of the enzyme were as active as the native enzyme, and their abilities to bind all substrates of all four catalyzed reactions (Fig. 2) were indistinguishable from that of the wild-type enzyme. Thus, neither cysteine residue plays any essential role in catalysis, substrate recognition, or substrate binding by HMG-CoA reductase.

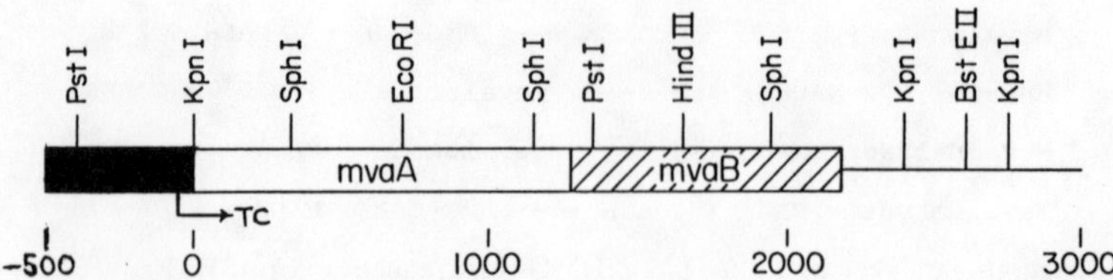

FIGURE 3. Organization of the *mva* operon. Shown are *mvaA* (▢), which encodes HMG-CoA reductase, *mvaB* (▨), which encodes HMG-CoA lyase, the region upstream of *mvaA* that contains the *mva* promoter (▮), and selected restriction endonuclease cleavage sites. The first nucleotide of the initiator methionine codon of *mvaA* is assigned coordinate 1. Transcription (TC) initiates at coordinate −56. *mvaA* maps from coordinates 1 to 1287, and *mvaB* maps from coordinates 1299 to 2202. The nucleotide sequence has been determined for the region from −500 to 2800.

Mutant C296A, but not mutant C156A or the cysteine-free mutant C156/296A, was sensitive to inhibition by NEM. The NEM-reactive residue thus is Cys-156. The ability of NEM to inactivate forms of the enzyme that retain Cys-156 thus probably reflects either an adverse conformational change brought about by addition of a bulky group or inhibition of an essential conformational change (Jordan-Starck and Rodwell, 1989a, 1989b).

HMG-CoA Lyase Cleaves HMG-CoA to Acetyl-CoA and Acetoacetate

Although HMG-CoA lyase activity is induced severalfold by growth of *P. mevalonii* on mevalonate, succinate-grown cells provide a less expensive source of the enzyme. HMG-CoA lyase from succinate-grown cells, purified 650-fold by ammonium sulfate, DEAE-Sepharose, and dye ligand chromatography, has a specific activity of 22 μmol of HMG-CoA cleaved per min per mg of protein but is electrophoretically heterogeneous. The substrate is *S*-HMG-CoA, for which the inferred K_m is about 100 μM. The lyase probably is monomeric. Activity is over 10-fold higher at the pH optimum, pH 8.8, than at pH 7 and is virtually undetectable below pH 6.5. A divalent cation is essential for activity, and Mn^{2+} is preferred. After treatment with EDTA, concentrations that produce half-maximal activation are 20, 120, and 30,000 μM for Mn^{2+}, Mg^{2+}, and Ca^{2+}, respectively. However, at or above 1 mM, Mg^{2+} and Mn^{2+} are equally effective. A reduced thiol is also required for activity (Scher and Rodwell, 1989).

MOLECULAR BIOLOGY OF THE *mva* OPERON

Organization of the *mva* Operon

Figure 3 summarizes the organization of the *mva* operon. The nucleotide sequence from −500 to 2,800 base pairs (bp) relative to the first nucleotide of the initiator methionine codon of *mvaA* as coordinate +1 has been determined (Beach and Rodwell, 1989; Anderson and Rodwell, 1989; Wang et al., 1989).

Codon Usage Resembles That for Other *Pseudomonas* Genes

The high G+C content (65% for *mvaA* [Beach and Rodwell, 1989]; 67% for *mvaB* [Anderson and Rodwell, 1989]) reflects a strong preference (80%) for G or

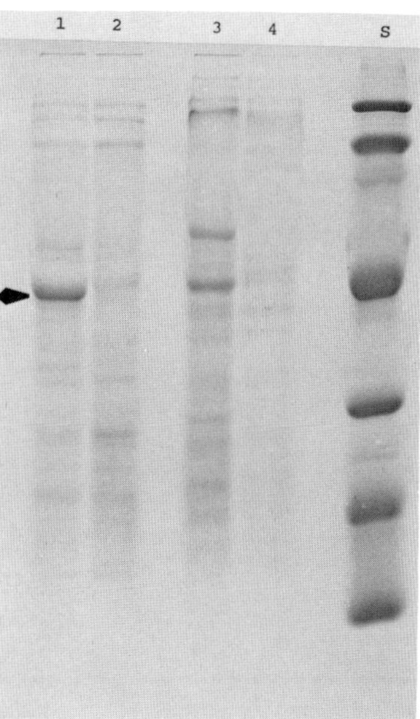

FIGURE 4. Overexpression of HMG-CoA reductase protein in transformed *E. coli*. *E. coli* transformed with pHMGR-1 (contains *mvaA* cloned behind the *tac* promoter) was grown in the presence (lane 1) or absence (lane 2) of isopropylthiogalactoside. *P. mevalonii* was grown on mevalonate (lane 3) or glucose (lane 4). Lanes 1 through 4 contained 15 μg of protein. After sodium dodecyl sulfate-polyacrylamide gel electrophoresis, the gel was stained with Coomassie blue. The arrow indicates the band corresponding to HMG-CoA reductase. Lane S contained protein standards with the indicated M_r values: phosphorylase *b* (94,000), bovine serum albumin (67,000), ovalbumin (43,000), carbonic anhydrase (30,000), soybean trypsin inhibitor (20,100), and alpha-lactalbumin (14,000) (Beach and Rodwell, 1989).

C in the degenerate base position. An exception is the use of GAA rather than GAG for glutamate 60% of the time in *mvaB* and 70% of the time in *mvaA*.

mvaA Encodes HMG-CoA Reductase

We have cloned, sequenced, and overexpressed in *E. coli* the 1,287-bp gene *mvaA*, the structural gene for HMG-CoA reductase. The amino acid composition of HMG-CoA reductase agrees with that predicted from the nucleotide sequence, and DNA-derived sequences are identical to all experimentally determined peptide sequences (Beach and Rodwell, 1989).

Overexpression of *mvaA* in *E. coli* yields large quantities of HMG-CoA reductase (Fig. 4). The overexpressed enzyme, which may be purified to homogeneity in high yield (over 80 mg of electrophoretically homogeneous protein per liter of cells), catalyzes all four HMG-CoA reductase reactions (Fig. 2).

mvaB Encodes HMG-CoA Lyase

We have cloned, sequenced, and overexpressed in *E. coli* the gene *mvaB*, which encodes HMG-CoA lyase, a cytosolic protein of 301 aminoacyl residues with a predicted molecular weight of 31,600. A proposed ribosome-binding site having 75% identity with the 3′ end of the 16S rRNA of *P. aeruginosa* is present 9 bp upstream of the initiator methionine codon of *mvaB*. No characteristics associated with Rho-independent terminators were apparent.

No strongly hydrophobic domains are evident in the inferred protein sequence, and computer searches of data banks revealed no proteins with a strong

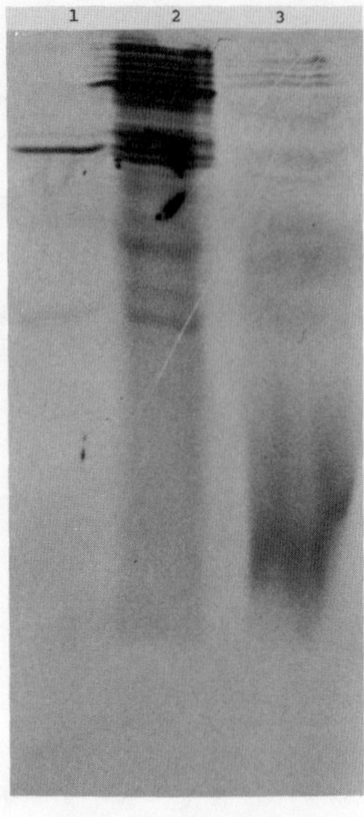

FIGURE 5. Autoradiograph after sodium dodecyl sulfate-polyacryla-mide gel electrophoresis of ^{35}S-labeled proteins encoded by *mvaB*. Log-phase, cysteine-starved *E. coli* JM103 cells containing plasmids pGP1-2 (encodes phage T7 RNA polymerase) and pT7-2600 (contains *mvaB* cloned behind the φ10 promoter of phage T7) in the presence (lane 1) or absence (lane 2) of rifampin or pGP1-2 plus pT7-7 (lacks the *mvaB* insert) in the presence of rifampin (lane 3) were incubated in the presence of L-[^{35}S]cysteine (Anderson and Rodwell, 1989).

similarity to the *mvaB* gene product. When placed under the control of the φ10 promoter of phage T7 and expressed in *E. coli* in the presence of rifampin, the *mvaB* gene product is visualized as a polypeptide of molecular weight 32,000, the approximate size predicted from the DNA sequence (Fig. 5).

Induced cell extracts of *E. coli* have HMG-CoA lyase levels over 40-fold above basal levels and a specific activity (165 ± 15 nmol/min per mg) of a magnitude comparable to that of fully induced *P. mevalonii* (230 ± 20 nmol/min per mg).

The Region from −60 to −140 bp Upstream of *mvaA* May Be Significant for Regulation of the *mva* Operon

While the G+C content of the upstream region (62%) is only slightly less than that of *mvaA* (65%) or *mvaB* (67%), the region from −60 to −140 bp immediately upstream of the transcription initiation site has a G+C content (50%) significantly below that of the coding region, of the upstream region as a whole, or of *Pseudomonas* spp. in general. Relatively A+T-rich regions, reported for several highly expressed genes, may facilitate binding of RNA polymerase (Cole et al., 1982) and/or facilitate formation of the open complex (Lin and Wilson, 1988). The upstream region from −60 to −140 bp thus may have significance for regulation of the *mva* operon.

Transcription Initiates 56 bp Upstream of the Translation Start Site

Transcription is initiated at −56 bp relative to the first base of the initiator methionine codon of *mvaA* (Fig. 3). The promoter exhibits a strong sequence

FIGURE 6. Comparison of the region from −12 to −24 of the *mva* promoter (numbered relative to the transcription start site as coordinate +1) with the recognition sequence for the σ^{54} factor encoded by *ntrA*.

```
                       -24                              -12
                        C      C                                A
Consensus      T | G  G |   A     (5 bp)  T  T     | G  C |
                        T      T                                T
mva              G | G  G | C  A  C(5 bp)  C  T     | G  C | A
```

homology with the recognition sequence for the core of the σ^{54} factor encoded by *ntrA* (Harschman et al., 1985; Merrick and Gibbins, 1985) (Fig. 6).

REGULATION OF THE *mva* OPERON

The Rise in HMG-CoA Reductase Activity That Follows Induction Reflects Increased Levels of HMG-CoA Reductase Protein and *mvaA* mRNA

While increases in activity that follow induction in procaryotes generally reflect increased levels of a given protein and its mRNA, the activity of mammalian HMG-CoA reductase (Kennelly and Rodwell, 1985) and of certain bacterial enzymes (Cozzone, 1988) may also be regulated by posttranslational phosphorylation. We therefore used specific antibody to measure HMG-CoA reductase protein levels in induced and noninduced cells. We calculate that 2 to 4% of the protein of mevalonate-grown cells is HMG-CoA reductase, a value which agrees with the quantity calculated from data for the catalytic activity of crude extracts and the specific activity of homogeneous enzyme.

Mevalonate-grown cells also contain high levels of *mvaA*-specific RNA. Densitometric scanning after S1 nuclease mapping revealed at least 200-fold-higher levels of *mvaA*-specific RNA than in glucose-grown cells. Elevations in HMG-CoA reductase activity that follow induction thus appear to reflect primarily, and probably exclusively, increased levels of *mvaA* mRNA and of reductase protein.

Deletion Analysis and Band Shift Data Suggest the Importance of a Region Upstream of the *mva* Promoter for the Response to Mevalonate

The region upstream of the *mva* promoter contains elements that respond to mevalonate induction. This was shown in two ways. Deletions from the 5' end were prepared, fused to *lacZ*, transformed into *E. coli*, conjugated into *P. mevalonii*, and tested for their ability to respond to mevalonate by production of β-galactosidase. In addition, preliminary band shift experiments confirmed the importance of the same region to the response to mevalonate (Y. Wang and V. W. Rodwell, unpublished observations).

ACKNOWLEDGMENTS. This work was funded by Public Health Service grant GM 33457 from the National Institutes of Health. M.J.B. was supported in part by Public Health Service training grant GM 07211 from the National Institutes of Health. T.C.J.-S. was supported in part by a National Institutes of Health Minority Access to Research Careers Predoctoral Fellowship (GM 09886).

LITERATURE CITED

Anderson, D. H., and V. W. Rodwell. 1989. Nucleotide sequence and expression in *Escherichia coli* of the 3-hydroxy-3-methylglutaryl coenzyme A lyase gene of *Pseudomonas mevalonii*. *J. Bacteriol.* **171:**6468–6472.

Basson, M. E., M. Thorness, and J. Rine. 1986. *Saccharomyces cerevisiae* contains two functional genes encoding 3-hydroxy-3-methylglutaryl coenzyme A reductase. *Proc. Natl. Acad. Sci. USA* **83:**5563–5567.

Beach, M. J., and V. W. Rodwell. 1989. Cloning, sequencing, and overexpression of *mvaA*, which encodes *Pseudomonas mevalonii* 3-hydroxy-3-methylglutaryl coenzyme A reductase. *J. Bacteriol.* **171:**2994–3001.

Chin, D. J., G. Gil, D. W. Russell, L. Liscum, K. L. Luskey, S. K. Basu, H. Okayama, P. Berg, J. L. Goldstein, and M. S. Brown. 1984. Nucleotide sequence of 3-hydroxy-3-methylglutaryl coenzyme A reductase, a glycoprotein of endoplasmic reticulum. *Nature* (London) **308:**613–617.

Cole, S. T., E. Bremer, I. Hindennach, and U. Henning. 1982. Characterization of the promoters for the *ompA* gene which encodes a major outer membrane protein of *Escherichia coli*. *Mol. Gen. Genet.* **188:**472–479.

Cozzone, A. J. 1988. Protein phosphorylation in prokaryotes. *Annu. Rev. Microbiol.* **42:**97–125.

Gill, J. F., Jr., M. J. Beach, and V. W. Rodwell. 1984. Transport of mevalonate by *Pseudomonas* sp. strain M. *J. Bacteriol.* **160:**294–298.

Gill, J. F., Jr., M. J. Beach, and V. W. Rodwell. 1985. Mevalonate utilization in *Pseudomonas* sp. M. Purification and characterization of an inducible 3-hydroxy-3-methylglutaryl coenzyme A reductase. *J. Biol. Chem.* **260:**9393–9398.

Harschman, J. P., K. Wong, K. Sei, J. Keener, and S. Kustu. 1985. Products of nitrogen regulatory genes *ntrA* and *ntrC* of enteric bacteria activate *glnA* transcription *in vitro*: evidence that the *ntrA* product is a sigma factor. *Proc. Natl. Acad. Sci. USA* **82:**7525–7529.

Jordan-Starck, T. C., and V. W. Rodwell. 1989a. *Pseudomonas mevalonii* HMG-CoA reductase. Characterization and chemical modification. *J. Biol. Chem.* **264:**17913–17918.

Jordan-Starck, T. C., and V. W. Rodwell. 1989b. Role of cysteine residues in *Pseudomonas mevalonii* HMG-CoA reductase. Site-directed mutagenesis and characterization of the mutant enzymes. *J. Biol. Chem.* **264:**17919–17923.

Kennelly, P. J., and V. W. Rodwell. 1985. Regulation of HMG-CoA reductase by phosphorylation-dephosphorylation. *J. Lipid Res.* **26:**903–914.

Lin, E., and D. B. Wilson. 1988. Transcription of the *celE* gene in *Thermomonospora fusca*. *J. Bacteriol.* **170:**3838–3842.

Merrick, M. J., and J. R. Gibbins. 1985. The nucleotide sequence of the nitrogen-regulation gene *ntrA* of *Klebsiella pneumoniae* and comparison with conserved features in bacterial RNA polymerase sigma factors. *Nucleic Acids Res.* **13:**7607–7620.

Scher, D. S., and V. W. Rodwell. 1989. 3-Hydroxy-3-methylglutaryl coenzyme A lyase from *Pseudomonas mevalonii*. *Biochim. Biophys. Acta* **1003:**321–326.

Skeggs, H. R., L. D. Wright, E. L. Cresson, G. D. E. McRae, C. H. Hoffman, D. E. Wolf, and K. Folkers. 1956. Discovery of a new acetate-replacing factor. *J. Bacteriol.* **72:**519–524.

Wang, Y., M. J. Beach, and V. W. Rodwell. 1989. *S*-3-Hydroxy-3-methylglutaryl coenzyme A reductase, a product of the *mva* operon of *Pseudomonas mevalonii*, is regulated at the transcriptional level. *J. Bacteriol.* **171:**5567–5571.

Chapter 17

Genetics of Vanillate and Sodium Dodecyl Sulfate Degradation in *Pseudomonas*

John Davison, Françoise Brunel, and Angelika Phanopoulos

Pseudomonads are remarkable in their catabolic ability, being able to degrade a wide variety of aromatic and aliphatic compounds and to utilize them as carbon sources (Frantz and Chakrabarty, 1986; Dagley, 1986). The bacterium used in this study, *Pseudomonas* sp. strain ATCC 19151, was isolated from the Baltimore Back River sewage plant by Hsu (1965) on the basis of its ability to utilize sodium dodecyl sulfate (SDS) as a sole carbon and sulfur source. SDS is produced in enormous amounts and is a common pollutant. However, it does not seem to pose environmental or health problems, probably because it is rapidly degraded in the environment by bacteria. This same *Pseudomonas* isolate is also able to degrade vanillate (3-methoxy-4-hydroxybenzoate). Vanillate is a product of the degradation of lignin by white rot fungi, a reaction necessary for the carbon cycle of the planet. In its chlorinated form, vanillate is a major pollutant, being liberated in vast quantities by the wood pulp bleaching process. Vanillate is also found in the root exudates of plants.

Although the biochemistry of SDS and vanillate degradation has been studied in pseudomonads (Hsu, 1965; Dodgson et al., 1982; Ribbons, 1971), nothing is known about the genetics. In this brief review, the cloning, characterization, and nucleotide sequencing of the genes responsible for vanillate and SDS degradation are summarized.

VANILLATE DEMETHYLASE GENES

The vanillate degradation genes (*van*) from *Pseudomonas* sp. ATCC 19151 were isolated from a cosmid gene bank constructed in a wide-host-range vector

John Davison ● Transgene s.a., Rue de Molsheim 11, 67000 Strasbourg, France.   *Angelika Phanopoulos* ● Unit of Molecular Biology, International Institute of Cellular and Molecular Pathology, 75 Avenue Hippocrate, 1200 Brussels, Belgium.   *Françoise Brunel* ● European Patent Office, Erhardtstrasse 27, D-8000 Munich, Federal Republic of Germany.

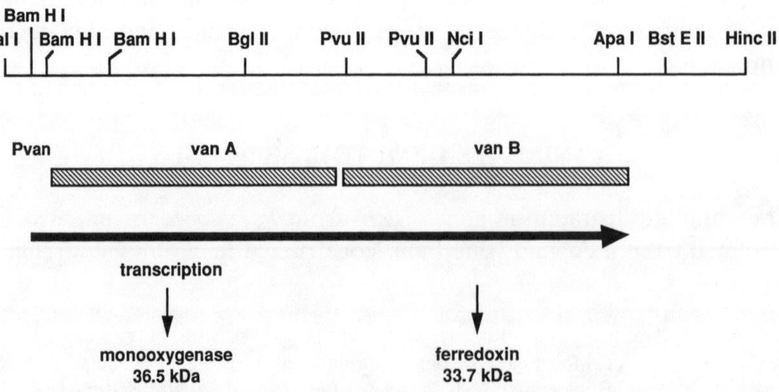

FIGURE 1. Vanillate demethylase reaction.

(Davison et al., 1987; J. Davison, F. Brunel, K. Kaniga, and N. Chevalier, this volume). The *van* clones were identified by their ability to complement *van* mutants of *Pseudomonas* sp. strain ATCC 19151 that were able to grow on protocatechuate as a carbon source but had lost the ability to grow on vanillate (Brunel and Davison, 1988; Fig. 1). All available *van* mutants were complemented by a 2,598-base-pair fragment that contained two open reading frames, *vanA* and *vanB*, able to code for polypeptides of 36 and 33 kilodaltons, respectively. The biological significance of these open reading frames was verified by deletion analysis and by complementation of the *van* mutants, which could thus be divided into two complementation groups, *vanA* and *vanB* (Fig. 2). The *vanA* and *vanB* gene products were radiolabeled in *Escherichia coli*, using the bacteriophage T7 RNA polymerase system, and two polypeptides, corresponding in size and location to those predicted by nucleotide sequence analysis, were detected.

The predicted amino acid sequences of the *vanA* and *vanB* polypeptides were compared with those in the NBRF Protein Identification Resource. The *vanB* polypeptide exhibits similarity to the ferredoxin family and probably serves for electron transport in the monooxygenase reaction (Ribbons, 1971; Bernhardt and Kuthan, 1983; Dagley, 1986). The *vanA* polypeptide failed to show convincing sequence similarity to other known polypeptides but is likely to be the monooxygenase. Transfer of the *vanAB* clone to other species of *Pseudomonas* gave interesting results (Brunel and Davison, 1988). *Pseudomonas oleovorans* GP01

FIGURE 2. Genetic and physical map of the *van* operon.

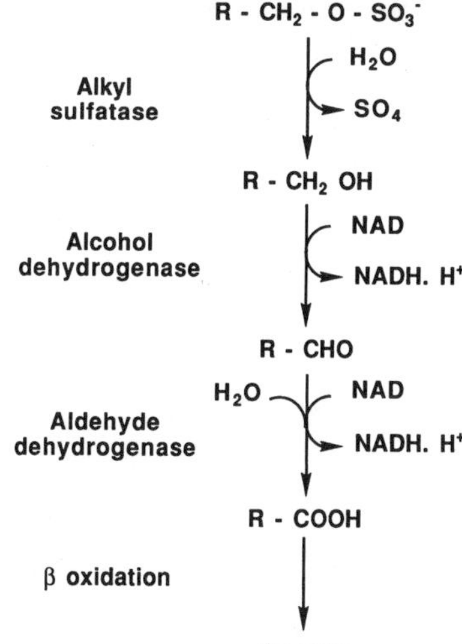

FIGURE 3. Degradation of SDS by *Pseudomonas* sp. strain ATCC 19151.

can utilize protocatechuate but not vanillate as a carbon source, and transfer of the *vanAB* clone to *P. oleovorans* conferred the ability to use vanillate. *Pseudomonas aeruginosa* PAO2175 can naturally use vanillate as a carbon source, but mutants (*vtu*; vanillate utilization) unable to do so were kindly made available by H. Matsumoto. All *vtu* mutants could be complemented by the *vanAB* clone. However, deletions containing only *vanA* or *vanB* failed to complement any *vtu* mutant. A probable explanation for this may lie in the specificity of interaction between the monooxygenase component and its electron transport ferredoxin component, such that a functional vanillate demethylase cannot be formed by mixed polypeptides from different species.

Fusion of the *van* promoter region to the *E. coli* galactokinase gene shows that transcription of the *van* genes is induced sixfold by growth on vanillate (F. Brunel, unpublished results). Nothing is yet known about the mechanism of this induction. It is possible that a third unidentified *van* gene codes for a repressor or activator protein.

SDS DEGRADATION GENES

Mutants of *Pseudomonas* sp. strain ATCC 19151 that were unable to utilize SDS as a carbon source but retained the ability to use dodecanol were isolated and shown to lack alkyl sulfatase activity (Fig. 3). The mutants permitted identification of complementing clones from the same cosmid gene bank that yielded the *van* clones. Complementation analysis using subclones and deletions permitted the *sds* mutants to be divided into two groups, *sdsA* and *sdsB*. Nucleotide sequence analysis confirmed the existence of two open reading frames that were transcribed in opposite directions (Fig. 4; A. Phanopoulos et al., manuscript in preparation). Expression studies in both *E. coli* and *Pseudomonas* spp., using the

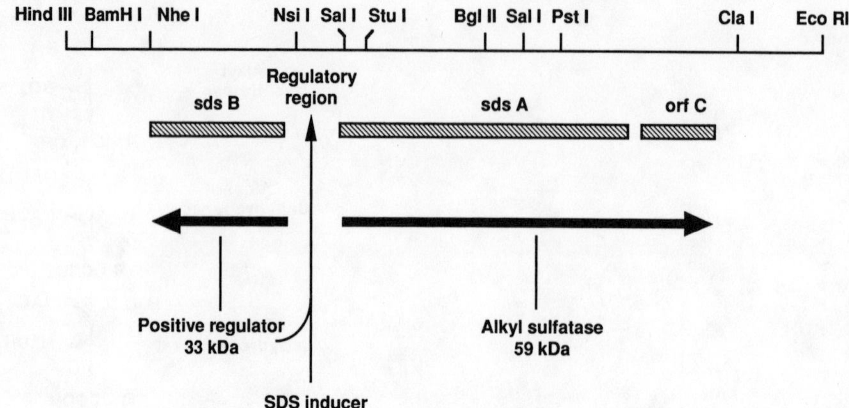

FIGURE 4. Genetic and physical map of the *sds* genes.

phage T7 RNA polymerase system, were used to verify the utilization and location of the *sdsA* and *sdsB* open reading frames.

The predicted amino acid sequences of the *sdsA* and *sdsB* polypeptides were compared with those of all known proteins in the NBRF Protein Identification Resource. For the *sdsA* protein, no significant similarities were found. This result may not be surprising, since this enzyme seems to be the first alkyl sulfatase for which the sequence has been determined. For the *sdsB* protein, homologies were found with the newly discovered LysR family of positive regulators of transcription (Table 1; Henikoff et al., 1988; Chang et al., 1989; M. Chang, D. W. Essar, and I. P. Crawford, this volume). All of these activator proteins are (i) positive activators of transcription, (ii) DNA-binding proteins (helix-turn-helix domain), (iii) homologous to each other at the N terminus, (iv) often autogenously

TABLE 1

Members of the LysR family of activator proteins

Organism	Gene	Function
Escherichia coli	*lysR*	Activator
	ilvY	Activator
	cysB	Activator
	oxyR	Activator
Enterobacter cloacae	*ampR*	Activator
Rhizobium meliloti	*nodD*	Activator
Rhizobium leguminosarum	*nodD*	Activator
Rhizobium trifolii	*nodD*	Activator
Rhizobium sp.	*nodD1*	Activator
Bradyrhizobium sp.	*nodD*	Activator
Salmonella typhimurium	*cysB*	Activator
Pseudomonas aeruginosa	*trpI*	Activator
Pseudomonas putida	*trpI*	Activator
	catM	Repressor
	nahR	Activator
Lactococcus lactis	*mleR*	Activator

```
SDS   ATCCA    CAACAACAACGAGCCGACC

VAN   ATCCAATACAACAACAACGAG  GACC


n1    ATCCAA  ACAA  T    CAA         TTTTACCAATC
n6    TCCCAA  ACAA  T    CGA         TTTTCACACTC
n2    ATCCAA  ACAA  T    CGA         TTTTACCAATC
n3    ATAAAA  ACAA  T    CGA         TTTTACCAATC
n4    ATCCTC  ATAA  T    CGA         TTTTACCAATC
n5    GTCCAA  ACAA  T    CGA         TTTTACTAATC
```

FIGURE 5. Comparison of the 5'-flanking region of *sdsA* with those of *vanAB* and *nodD*.

regulated, and (v) often divergently transcribed from the genes they control. When *sdsA* is cloned under control of another promoter, it is able to complement an *sdsB* mutation for growth on SDS. This finding confirms the interpretation that the role of *sdsB* is only to facilitate transcription of the *sdsA* gene and that it takes no part in SDS biodegradation. Our present hypothesis of the regulation of *sdsA* is shown in Fig. 4.

Experiments are in progress to determine whether the *sdsB* gene product is a DNA-binding protein and whether, like certain other members of the LysR family, it has a negative effect on its own transcription. Recently, Rostas et al. (1986) identified a regulatory region (the *nod* box) upstream of several genes regulated by the *nodD* activator (Table 1). The intergenic region between *sdsA* and *sdsB* has strong similarity to the 5' end of the *nod* box (Fig. 5). Curiously, there is also considerable homology between the upstream region of the *vanAB* operon and both the *sds* and *nod* regulatory regions.

Finally, it is worthwhile mentioning that whereas many degradative genes are plasmid borne (Frantz and Chakrabarty, 1986), the *van* and *sds* genes are chromosomally located. The G+C content of the *sds* and *van* genes is high (69%), and in accordance with the predictions of Bibb et al. (1984), GC utilization in the third base pair of the codon is extremely high (>90%), giving a very biased codon utilization (Brunel and Davison, 1988; Phanopoulos et al., in preparation). Since open reading frames are frequent in G+C-rich DNA, this property is most useful for the identification of probable translated reading frames.

ACKNOWLEDGMENTS. This research was carried out under research contract BAP-0048-B of the Commission of the European Communities. A.P. is grateful for a CEC-BAP training fellowship. J.D. acknowledges support from the Cystic Fibrosis Foundation.

We are grateful for extensive discussions with A. M. Chakrabarty (during the tenure of North Atlantic Treaty Organization grant 0177/87), P. Terpstra, I. P. Crawford, I. C. Gunsalus, V. Venturi, and A. Menendez-Alarcon. We also thank N. Chevalier for expert technical assistance and P. Mulder for nucleotide sequence analysis and typing of the manuscript.

LITERATURE CITED

Bernhardt, F. H., and H. Kuthan. 1983. Kinetics of reduction of putidamonooxin by NADH-putidamonooxin oxidoreductase, sodium dithionite and superoxide radicals. *Eur. J. Biochem.* **130:**99–103.

Bibb, M. J., P. R. Findlay, and M. W. Johnson. 1984. The relationship between base composition and codon usage in bacterial genes and its use for the simple and reliable identification of protein-coding sequences. *Gene* **30:**157–166.

Brunel, F., and J. Davison. 1988. Cloning and sequencing of *Pseudomonas* genes encoding vanillate demethylase. *J. Bacteriol.* **170:**4924–4930.

Chang, M., A. Hadero, and I. P. Crawford. 1989. Sequence of the *Pseudomonas aeruginosa trpI* activator gene and relatedness of *trpI* to other procaryotic regulatory genes. *J. Bacteriol.* **171:**172–183.

Dagley, S. 1986. Biochemistry of aromatic hydrocarbons degradation in *Pseudomonads*, p. 527–555. *In* I. C. Gunsalus, J. R. Sokatch, and L. N. Ornston (ed.), *The Bacteria*, vol. 10. *The Biology of Pseudomonas*. Academic Press, Inc., Orlando, Fla.

Davison, J., M. Heusterspreute, and F. Brunel. 1987. Restriction site bank vectors for cloning in Gram-negative bacteria and yeast. *Methods Enzymol.* **153:**34–54.

Dodgson, K. S., G. F. White, and J. W. Fitzgerald. 1982. The alkylsulfatases, p. 9–48. *In Sulfatases of Microbial Origin*, vol. 1. CRC Press, Inc., Boca Raton, Fla.

Frantz, B., and A. M. Chakrabarty. 1986. Degradative plasmids in *Pseudomonas*, p. 295–325. *In* I. C. Gunsalus, J. R. Sokatch, and L. N. Ornston (ed.), *The Bacteria*, vol. 10. *The Biology of Pseudomonas*. Academic Press, Inc., Orlando, Fla.

Henikoff, S., G. W. Haughn, J. M. Calvo, and J. C. Wallace. 1988. A large family of bacterial activator proteins. *Proc. Natl. Acad. Sci. USA* **85:**6602–6606.

Hsu, Y. C. 1965. Detergent-splitting enzyme from Pseudomonas. *Nature* (London) **207:**385–388.

Ribbons, D. W. 1971. Requirement of two protein fractions for O-demethylase activity in *Pseudomonas testosteroni*. *FEBS Lett.* **12:**161–165.

Rostas, K., E. Kondorosi, B. Horvath, A. Simoncsits, and A. Kondorosi. 1986. Conservation of extended promoter regions of nodulation genes in *Rhizobium*. *Proc. Natl. Acad. Sci. USA* **83:**1757–1761.

Chapter 18

Regulation of the Naphthalene Degradation Genes of Plasmid NAH7: Example of a Generalized Positive Control System in *Pseudomonas* and Related Bacteria

Mark A. Schell

Members of the genus *Pseudomonas* have long been recognized for their ability to metabolize a wide variety of both natural and synthetic organic compounds as sole carbon and energy sources (Stanier et al., 1966). Subsequent work in many laboratories established that in certain cases the genetic information encoding some catabolic abilities is located on degradative plasmids (reviewed by Frantz and Chakrabarty [1986]). Whereas the enzymology of many plasmid encoded pathways has been elucidated, only recently, with the advent of molecular genetic and recombinant DNA techniques, have the many similarities in enzymology, organization, regulation, and evolution of degradative genes become evident. Application of rapid DNA sequence determination methods and computerized DNA sequence data base homology searches has further shown that some plasmids contain very similar genes although they are involved in degradation of apparently dissimilar substrates. For example, plasmid NAH7, encoding metabolism of naphthalene, and plasmid TOL pWWO, encoding toluene degradation, contain two different genes, *nahH* and *xylE*, both encoding catechol 2,3-dioxygenase, that are greater than 80% similar in DNA and protein sequence (Harayama et al., 1987; Ghosal et al., 1988). It was further suggested that the isofunctional genes *xylEFG* (on TOL) and *nahHIN* (on NAH7) may have evolved from a common ancestor (Harayama et al., 1987). Furthermore, evidence that plasmid genes encoding chlorocatechol degradation are related to chromosomal genes for catechol degradation has been presented (Aldrich et al., 1987; Frantz and Chakrabarty, 1987). All of these data suggest that many degradative genes are related by common ancestry and that substantial genetic exchange and interaction has occurred among various plasmids and the host chromosomes.

Mark A. Schell ● Department of Microbiology, University of Georgia, Athens, Georgia 30602.

Recent evidence suggests that the regulatory genes for certain aromatic hydrocarbon degradation genes are also very similar to one another. Regulatory genes for degradation of naphthalene, chlorobenzoate, 2,4-dichlorophenoxyacetic acid, and catechol appear to be related, since they are members of the LysR family of positive transcriptional activators (Henikoff et al., 1988; Schell and Sukordhaman, 1989; R. K. Rothmel, W. Coco, T. Aldrich, and A. M. Chakrabarty, *Abstr. Annu. Meet. Am. Soc. Microbiol. 1989*, K-60, p. 255). In this chapter, recent developments in genetic and biochemical analysis of the organization and regulation of naphthalene degradation genes will be discussed. The focus will be on plasmid NAH7 and the *nahR* gene that it uses to regulate its naphthalene degradation genes, because it is one of the most extensively studied plasmid-borne degradative gene systems in *Pseudomonas* spp. However, knowledge about the NAH7 regulatory system has implications for the many other systems with LysR-type activators, which probably use a very similar control mechanism.

MOLECULAR RELATIONSHIPS AMONG NAPHTHALENE DEGRADATION PLASMIDS

The majority of reports indicate that the genes for utilization of naphthalene as a sole carbon and energy source are plasmid encoded. Only indirect evidence for partial chromosomal location has ever been reported (Zuniga et al., 1981). Many naphthalene degradation plasmids have been reported, but only a few have been molecularly characterized to any great extent (reviewed by Yen and Serdar [1989]). The best characterized at the molecular level is NAH7 (Dunn and Gunsalus, 1973), followed by pWW60-1 (Cane and Williams, 1986), NAH2/NAH3 (Connors and Barnsley, 1982), pDTG1 (Yen and Serdar, 1989), and pNAH484 from *Pseudomonas putida* ATCC 17484 (S. Chung, M.S. thesis, University of Georgia, Athens, 1989). It should be noted that all of these plasmids except NAH7 and pNAH484 were derived from variants of one strain, *P. putida* NCIB 9816. Nevertheless, most Southern hybridization studies indicate that many of the naphthalene degradation genes on all of these plasmids are homologous in DNA sequence to those on NAH7. Although significant restriction fragment length polymorphisms and metabolic differences exist among these plasmids, most can be explained by relatively minor genetic variations. For example, restriction endonuclease digest patterns of pWW60-1, pNAH484, and NAH7 are very different, yet the *nahABC* regions on all three plasmids are highly homologous (Chung, M.S. thesis). Furthermore, it has been observed that the DNA sequences of the *nahA* cistrons encoding the ferredoxin component of naphthalene dioxygenase on these three plasmids are greater than 90% homologous (M. A. Schell, unpublished observation). Metabolic and regulatory differences among some naphthalene degradation plasmids are easily explained by the presence of inserted DNA sequences near *nahH* on pWW60-1 (Cane and Williams, 1986) and in *nahA* on SAL1 (Yen et al., 1983).

Most evidence indicates that the enzymes and genes for metabolism of naphthalene at least as far as catechol (i.e., *nahA* to *-G*) are conserved on NAH7, SAL1, pWW60-1, and pNAH484. Moreover, positive regulation of naphthalene degradation genes by salicylate (Barnsley, 1975, 1976) and the regulatory gene *nahR* appears to occur on NAH7 (Schell, 1985), pWW60-1 (Cane and Williams, 1986), SAL1, and pNAH484 (Chung, M.S. thesis). It is likely that many of the described naphthalene degradation plasmids are closely related and may share a common ancestor. Furthermore, knowledge concerning regulation and organization of naphthalene degradation genes on NAH7 has direct implications for these other plasmids.

ORGANIZATION OF NAH7 NAPHTHALENE DEGRADATION GENES

The NAH7-encoded pathway for metabolism of naphthalene via salicylate involves 14 enzymatic steps (Davies and Evans, 1964) (Fig. 1). The polar effects of Tn*5* insertions in NAH7 (Yen and Gunsalus, 1982) localized many naphthalene degradation genes and indicated that the *nah* genes are organized in two coordinately controlled operons: *nah* (or *nah-1*) and *sal* (or *nah-2*). Gene sizes and locations were further refined by subcloning and deletion experiments (Schell, 1983, 1985; Harayama et al., 1987). *nahF* is probably located between *nahC* and *nahD*, since the apparent polar effects of Tn*5* insertions in *nahC* dramatically lowered the levels of the *nahD*, *nahE*, and *nahF* gene products, whereas Tn*5* insertions in *nahD* did not affect levels of *nahF* gene product (Yen and Gunsalus, 1982). These results are summarized in Fig. 2, which shows the probable locations and sizes of the *nah* and *sal* genes on a partial restriction endonuclease cleavage map of NAH7. Although it is likely that *nahE* follows *nahD*, its exact location and size are not known. The location of *nahM* is totally unknown. The complete nucleotide sequences of *nahA* (Kurkela et al., 1988; B. Ensley et al., unpublished data), *nahH* (Ghosal et al., 1988), and *nahG* (I.-S. You, D. Ghosal, and I. C. Gunsalus, *Abstr. Annu. Meet. Am. Soc. Microbiol. 1989*, H-206, p. 204) have been determined.

Transcription of both *nah* and *sal* is increased over 20-fold by the inducer salicylate (Schell, 1985), consistent with the magnitude of salicylate-induced increases in *nah* enzyme levels reported by Barnsley (1975, 1976). The *nah* operon probably produces a large salicylate-induced polycistronic transcript containing the *nahABCFDE* sequences, whereas induction of *sal* operon transcription results in synthesis of a polycistronic mRNA containing *nahGHINLK* (Fig. 2). *nah* encodes metabolism of naphthalene to salicylate; *sal* encodes metabolism of salicylate to pyruvate and acetaldehyde (Fig. 1). *nahM* expression is not induced by salicylate and shows no polar effects from Tn*5* insertions in *nah* or *sal* (Yen and Gunsalus, 1982) and thus probably is not part of either the *nah* or *sal* operon.

In at least two other cases, plasmid-borne degradative genes encoding the metabolism of aromatic hydrocarbons are organized in two operons. In both cases, as with NAH7, pWW60-1, and pNAH484, the first operon encodes oxidation of an aromatic hydrocarbon to a direct precursor of a catechol; the second operon encodes a hydroxylase enzyme (which converts this precursor to

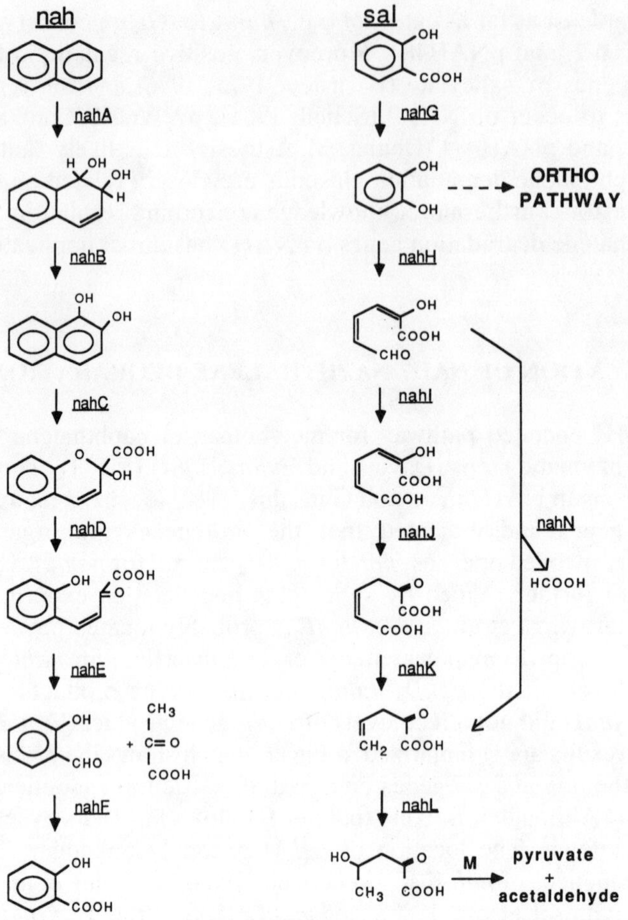

FIGURE 1. Metabolism of naphthalene encoded by plasmid NAH7. Naphthalene is degraded by a series of 14 enzymatic reactions. The 13 catalyzed by specific *nah* gene products from NAH7 are naphthalene dioxygenase (*nahA*), *cis*-dihydrodiol naphthalene dehydrogenase (*nahB*), 1,2-dihydroxynaphthalene dioxygenase (*nahC*), 2-hydroxychromene-2-carboxylate isomerase (*nahD*), 2-hydroxybenzalpyruvate aldolase (*nahE*), salicylaldehyde dehydrogenase (*nahF*), salicylate hydroxylase (*nahG*), catechol 2,3-dioxygenase (*nahH*), 2-hydroxymuconate semialdehyde dehydrogenase (*nahI*), 4-oxalocrotonate tautomerase (*nahJ*), 4-oxalocrotonate decarboxylase (*nahK*), 2-oxopent-4-enoate hydratase (*nahL*), and 2-hydroxymuconic semialdehyde hydrolase (*nahN*). The final step producing pyruvate and acetaldehyde is catalyzed by 2-oxo-4-hydroxypentanoate aldolase (M), which is not encoded by *nah* or *sal*. Catechol may also be metabolized by the chromosomally encoded *ortho* pathway.

a catechol) and the enzymes for its further metabolism via the *ortho*- or *meta*-cleavage pathway. For example, in the TOL plasmid pWWO, two coordinately regulated operons (*xyl* OP1 and OP2) are found, one encoding metabolism of toluene to benzoate and the other encoding metabolism of benzoate to pyruvate and acetylaldehyde (Inouye et al., 1986, 1987). Whereas the enzymatic activities encoded by one of the *xyl* operons are very similar to those of the *sal* operon, the regulatory system for *xyl* genes appears to be very different from that used by

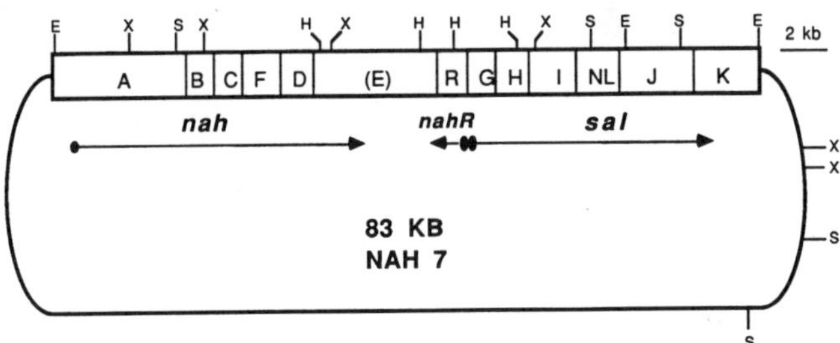

FIGURE 2. Physical and genetic map of naphthalene degradation genes and plasmid NAH7. Map shows approximate location and extent of each *nah* gene encoding enzyme activities shown in Fig. 1. Sizes and directions of transcription units, *nah*, *nahR*, and *sal*, are indicated by arrows. Abbreviations for restriction sites: S, *Sma*I; X, *Xho*I; H, *Hin*dIII; E, *Eco*RI. The *Hin*dIII and *Eco*RI cleavage sites in the NAH7 vector portion are not shown. kb, Kilobase pairs.

NAH7 (Nakazawa et al., 1985; Inouye et al., 1987). Plasmid pJP4 from *Alcaligenes eutrophus* encodes the metabolism of 2,4-dichlorophenoxyacetic acid and also has its degradative genes organized in two coordinately regulated operons (Streber et al., 1987). The similar dual-operon organization of degradative genes on metabolic plasmids appears to be common and probably results from a similar mode of evolution.

CHARACTERIZATION OF THE *nahR* LOCUS

Yen and Gunsalus (1982) initially described the *nahR* locus as a region located upstream of *nahG* in which Tn5 insertions simultaneously inactivated salicylate-induced expression of all *nah* and *sal* genes. It was subsequently reported that salicylate-induced high-level expression of *nah* and *sal* in *Escherichia coli* (Schell, 1983) and in *P. putida* (Grund and Gunsalus, 1983) required the presence of a region containing the *nahR* locus. A detailed localization of the *nahR* locus by Tn5 mutagenesis was reported later (Yen and Gunsalus, 1985).

A 1.6-kilobase-pair DNA fragment from the *nahR* region was cloned and shown in *trans* to fully complement a *nahR*::Tn5 mutant and to confer salicylate-inducible transcription activation of the *nah* operon promoter (P_{nah}) in both *P. putida* and *E. coli* (Schell, 1985). Maxicell experiments showed that the same fragment encodes a 36-kilodalton (kDa) polypeptide; a 400-base-pair (bp) deletion introduced into the fragment abolished both production of the 36-kDa polypeptide and *trans* activation of transcription from the *sal* operon promoter (P_{sal}) (Schell and Wender, 1986). The presence of the *nahR* gene and the 36-kDa polypeptide was also correlated with a DNA-binding activity that was specific for DNA fragments containing either P_{nah} or P_{sal} (Schell and Faris, 1987; Schell and Poser, 1989; You et al., 1988).

You and Gunsalus (1986) reported two complementation groups at the *nahR* locus; however, biochemical evidence for the production of two polypeptides from the *nahR* locus is lacking (Schell and Wender, 1986). Production of a 23-kDa polypeptide in *E. coli* maxicells from a fragment containing only part of *nahR* (i.e.,

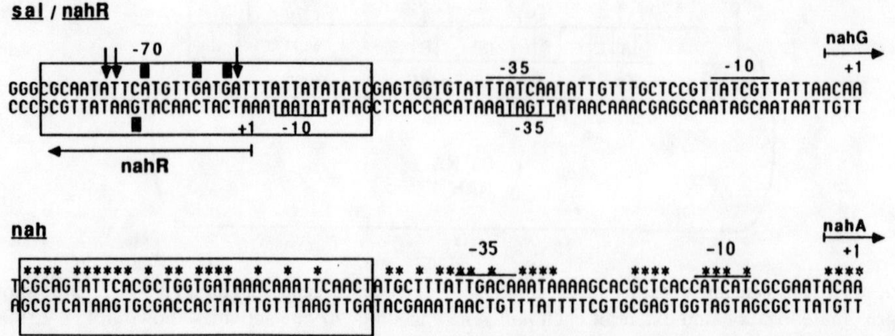

FIGURE 3. Regulatory sequences of the *nah* and *sal* promoters. The nucleotide sequences (−83 to +1) of the *nah* (lower line) and the divergent *sal* and *nahR* (upper line) promoters are shown; the putative −35 and −10 RNA polymerase recognition sites are underlined. Transcription start sites (+1) are indicated. Homologous nucleotides found in both promoters are marked with asterisks. Boxed regions designate sequences protected from DNase I by NahR protein. Other symbols: ↓, nucleotide position where mutation inactivated NahR binding and/or transcription activation; ■, nucleotide position that showed altered reactivity with dimethyl sulfate in vivo only in the presence of *nahR* and salicylate.

lacking the first 300 bp) has been reported (You and Gunsalus, 1988). However, this polypeptide was not produced from intact *nahR* or fragments lacking only the first 100 bp of *nahR*.

Experiments with *sal* promoter fusion plasmids and the cloned *nahR* gene in *E. coli* and *P. putida* strongly suggest that *nahR* is the only gene involved in positive regulation of *nah* and *sal* (Schell, 1985; Schell and Wender, 1986). Experiments with fusion plasmids also indicate that salicylate is probably the natural inducer, since only salicylate (not naphthalene or salicylaldehyde) can induce expression from P_{sal} in *E. coli* or *P. putida* cells that cannot metabolize naphthalene or salicylate. *nah* and *sal* are not catabolite repressed, since full salicylate induction of *nah* and *sal* enzymes occurs in cells grown in minimal succinate, minimal glucose, or complex rich media (Schell, unpublished data). Most evidence suggests that in vivo *nahR* produces only one polypeptide, the 36-kDa positive regulatory protein NahR, which binds to the promoters of *nah* and *sal* and activates their transcription after interaction with salicylate.

INTERACTIONS OF NahR WITH THE *nah* AND *sal* PROMOTERS

The transcription start sites and DNA sequences of the coordinately regulated *nah* and *sal* promoters were located by S1 nuclease mapping experiments and DNA sequencing (Schell, 1986). Comparison of sequences of P_{nah} and P_{sal} showed extensive homology between the two promoters in the −80 to −60 region (81%) and in the −40 to −28 region (75%) (Fig. 3). Analysis of transcriptional fusions of P_{sal} sequences between −83 and +27 to the *galK* gene in *E. coli* showed that only *nahR* and salicylate are required to activate transcription initiation from the −83 to +27 P_{sal} fragment (Schell and Wender, 1986). Deletion of P_{sal}

sequences between −83 and −45 resulted in a loss of only its ability to be transcriptionally activated by *nahR* and salicylate, not its uninduced expression. Similar results were obtained with analogous P_{nah} fusion plasmids (Schell and Faris, 1987).

Binding of NahR to the −82 to −47 sequences of P_{sal} and P_{nah} was suggested by gel retardation assays with crude extracts of *P. putida* and *E. coli* cells containing *nahR* (Schell and Faris, 1987; Schell and Poser, 1989) and was confirmed by DNase I protection experiments with partially purified NahR protein (Schell and Poser, 1989) (Fig. 3). Salicylate did not dramatically affect the location or extent of NahR binding. Saturation mutagenesis experiments with the NahR-binding site of P_{sal} suggests that nucleotides −74, −73, and −61 are involved in binding and activation by NahR protein (Schell and Poser, 1989). Surprisingly, mutations at seven other positions within the NahR-binding site had only minor effects on the ability of the promoter to be activated by NahR, suggesting that relatively few nucleotides in the DNase I-protected region are involved in actual protein-DNA contact. Preliminary in vivo footprinting experiments suggest major contacts between NahR and P_{sal} at positions −71, −70, −65, and −62 in salicylate-induced cells (Fig. 3) (S. Smith and M. Schell, manuscript in preparation). The IlvY protein, a LysR-type transcription activator, makes very similar contacts at analogous positions of its target site at the *ilvC* promoter (Wek and Hatfield, 1988). Preliminary evidence indicates that three other LysR-type activators, TrpI, NodD, and AmpR, also bind to an analogous region of their target promoters (ca. −80 to −50).

The available evidence suggests that the NahR protein (in the presence or absence of salicylate) binds to the −82 to −47 region of both P_{sal} and P_{nah} via direct interactions with several nucleotides in the recognition sequence TATT CAnGnTGnTGA, located between −75 and −61. The inducer salicylate probably alters the interaction of the bound NahR protein with the promoter or RNA polymerase, resulting in increased transcription from P_{sal} (S. Smith and M. Schell, unpublished data). It is likely that other LysR-type activators (e.g., IlvY and NodD) interact with their target promoters in a similar manner. NahR apparently can activate both *P. putida* and *E. coli* RNA polymerase to increase the transcription rate from P_{sal}. This is not unexpected, since many *Pseudomonas* genes are expressed from their own promoters in *E. coli*, albeit at low levels. Furthermore, *E. coli* and *P. putida* RNA polymerases have been reported to be antigenically related and to recognize promoters in a similar manner (Gregerov et al., 1984).

TRANSCRIPTION REGULATION OF *nahR*

The transcription start site and promoter of *nahR* were located by S1 nuclease mapping and DNA sequence analysis (Schell, 1986). Transcription of *nahR* is constitutive and starts approximately 65 bp upstream of the *sal* operon transcription start site but proceeds in the opposite direction (Fig. 3). The divergent *sal* and *nahR* promoters overlap at −35. This places the transcription start site of *nahR* within the NahR-binding site of the *sal* promoter, indicating a potential for autoregulation of *nahR* transcription by its own product. A 2.5-fold decrease in transcription from the *nahR* promoter was apparently caused by the presence of the *nahR* gene in *trans* (Schell and Faris, 1987). Mutations resulting in *sal* and *nahR* promoters that cannot bind NahR do not dramatically increase the synthesis of NahR protein (Schell, unpublished data). If *nahR* was strongly autoregulated, larger increases would be expected. At present, it appears that autoregulation of *nahR* transcription by its own product occurs only to a limited extent. Low-level autoregulation of other LysR-type transcription activators (e.g., AmpR, IlvY, and NodD) has also been reported (Rossen et al., 1985; Wek and Hatfield, 1988). The purpose and operation of the overlapping, divergent *sal* and *nahR* promoters remain to be clarified.

UBIQUITY OF NahR-LIKE PROTEINS AND REGULATORY SYSTEMS

The DNA and deduced amino acid sequences of *nahR* were recently reported; a computer search revealed that NahR is very similar in DNA (45%) and amino acid sequence (47%) to NodD (Egelhoff et al., 1985), a transcriptional activator of the *nod* genes of *Rhizobium meliloti* (Schell and Sukordhaman, 1989). This observation and other similarities in promoter sequences, target sites, and inducer recognition led to the suggestion that *nahR* and *nodD* evolved from a common ancestor.

Further analysis indicated that NahR is a member of the LysR family of transcription activators described by Henikoff et al. (1988). Distinguishing characteristics of family members are as follows: (i) all are nearly identical size (300 ± 20 amino acids) positive activators of transcription, (ii) all share major amino acid sequence similarities in their N-terminal halves, and (iii) all are transcribed from promoters that are very close to (usually overlapping) and divergent from the promoters of one set of structural genes they control. Since the initial discovery of the LysR family, several new members in addition to NahR have been proposed: TrpI, MleR, CatM, and ClcR (Table 1). LysR-type activators are found in diverse genera, in both gram-positive and gram-negative bacteria, and on both chromosomes and plasmids. The types of genes regulated by LysR-type activators include genes for amino acid biosynthesis, degradation of various aromatic compounds, antibiotic resistance, and malolactic fermentation. Initially, it appeared that LysR family members evolved from a common ancestral transcriptional activator gene. Alternatively, the diversity of LysR-like regulatory systems may suggest convergent evolution of a widespread and fundamental control system or mechanism. It is difficult to suggest common ancestry when the G+C content of LysR-type genes varies from 70 to 40% unless these genes diverged a long time ago. Moreover, certain pairs of family members appear to be more similar to one another (Renault et al., 1989; Chang et al., 1989; Schell and Sukordhaman, 1989). For example, NahR and NodD are similar in both amino acid and DNA sequence but similar to many other family members mostly at the amino acid level; in the first 250 bp, TfdO is very similar to ClcR in DNA (65%)

TABLE 1
LysR family of transcriptional activators

Activator	Source	Gene and enzyme regulated	Reference
LysR	*Escherichia coli*	*lysA*, diaminopimelate decarboxylase	Stragier et al., 1983
AmpR	*Enterobacter cloacae*	*ampC*, cephalosporinase	Honore et al., 1986
IlvY	*Escherichia coli*	*ilvC*, acetohydroxy acid isomeroreductase	Wek and Hatfield, 1986
NodD	*Rhizobium* (plasmid pSym)	*nod*, nodulation for N_2 fixation symbiosis	Applebaum et al., 1988
TfdO[a]	*Alcaligenes eutrophus* (plasmid pJP4)	Unknown, dichlorophenoxyacetate degradation?	Streber et al., 1987
LeuO	*Escherichia coli*	Unknown	Henikoff et al., 1988
CysB	*Escherichia coli*	*cys*, cysteine biosynthesis	Ostrowski et al., 1987
ClcR	*Pseudomonas putida* (plasmid pAC27)	*clcABD*, chlorocatechol degradation	Frantz and Chakrabarty, 1987
MetR	*Salmonella typhimurium*	*met*, methionine biosynthesis	Plaman and Stauffer, 1987
NahR	*Pseudomonas putida* (plasmid NAH7)	*nah*, *sal*, naphthalene degradation	Schell and Sukhordhaman, 1989
CatR	*Pseudomonas putida*	*catBC*, catechol degradation	R. K. Rothmel and A. M. Chakrabarty, personal communication
CatM[b]	*Acinetobacter calcoaceticus*	*catBC*, catechol degradation	Neidle et al., 1989
TrpI	*Pseudomonas aeruginosa*	*trpBA*, tryptophan synthetase	Chang et al., 1989
MleR	*Lactococcus lactis*	Unknown, malolactic fermentation	Renault et al., 1989

[a] Also called TfdS.
[b] Behaves as repressor, not activator.

and protein (80%) sequence but simlar to CatM (60%) only at the amino acid level (Fig. 4). Moreover, ClcR, CatM, and possibly TfdO are involved in controlling genes encoding very similar enzymes, albeit in three different bacteria. These results suggest the existence of possible subfamilies of LysR-type activators. However, the relationships between different LysR-family members remain to be clarified.

Nearly all of the highly conserved amino acid similarities in LysR-type activators are found in the first 170 residues, residues 1 to 75 in particular. Within this region (ca. residues 20 to 50), a possible helix-turn-helix motif (HTH) was identified (Henikoff et al., 1988). The HTH is a structural motif found in many DNA-binding proteins (Pabo and Sauer, 1984; Dodd and Egan, 1987; Brennan and Matthews, 1989) and in certain cases has been shown to contain amino acids that directly interact with DNA to mediate DNA binding (Jordan and Pabo, 1988; Wohlberger et al., 1988). Five different amino acid substitutions within this HTH region of NahR result in a loss of DNA binding, transcriptional activation, or both (M. Schell, P. Brown, and S. Raju, *J. Biol. Chem.*, in press) (Fig. 4), further supporting the involvement of this region of LysR-type activators in DNA

```
                     HELIX -TURN- HELIX

                   ::          :          : :            :
LDLNLLV----LL-DRRVS--A±-L-LTQPAhS-AL-RLRT-----LF-R-      NahR/NodD    consensus
**   *     *  *   *   ** *'**** **  *  *+         ** *
MEFR-LRYFhAVAEEGNhGAAA±RLHhSQPPhTRQIQALEQELGh-LFERT  ClcR/TfdO/CatM consensus

     L                                           V          ClcR
     Q      A                        H    H    L            TfdO
  L  H    T V  QS SK       C A       K    E    Q     G       CatM
```

FIGURE 4. Probable DNA-binding domains of NahR and related regulatory proteins. The top line gives the consensus sequence of the NH_2-terminal amino acid sequences of NahR/NodD (residues 5 to 56) in single-letter code. :, Position of a substitution mutation that decreased NahR binding, transcription activation, or both. The second line shows the consensus sequence for the analogous region of ClcR, TfdO, and CatM (residues 1 to 52). *, Position of similar residues in both consensus sequences. Residues at variance with the consensus sequence of ClcR, TfdO, CatM are given below. Amino acid similarities used in addition to identities were T = S, K = R, D = E, and h = V, I or L; ± = R or E. Region of predicted HTH is indicated at the top.

binding. Conservation of the HTH motif and flanking sequences involved in DNA binding may be the predominant basis for relatedness of the LysR family members, since conserved similarities in the C-terminal half are sparse. Comparison of several LysR-type activators that regulate aromatic compound degradation genes shows a highly conserved amino acid sequence in the center of the HTH region between the two putative helices (Fig. 4). It is possible that the N-terminal domain of LysR-type activators is an expanded HTH motif that is commonly utilized in many transcription activators and that the mechanism of binding and transcription activation it mediates is a conserved, fundamental mechanism used in many procaryotic systems. Differences in DNA target site specificity and inducer specificity, however, remain to be explored, as does the anomaly of the CatM protein (Neidle et al., 1989). Although CatM has been suggested to be a member of the LysR family, it behaves like a repressor in regulating *catBC*. It is also significantly shorter than other LysR proteins (50 residues) and possibly lacks the transcription activation domain.

ACKNOWLEDGMENTS. I thank E. Neidle and N. Ornston for CatM sequence data, S. Smith for preparation of figures, and P. Bates for typing the manuscript.

Some of the research reported here was supported by Public Health Service grant GM 32255-07 from the National Institutes of Health.

LITERATURE CITED

Aldrich, T. L., B. Frantz, J. Gill, J. J. Kilbane, and A. M. Chakrabarty. 1987. Cloning and complete nucleotide sequence determination of the *catB* gene encoding *cis,cis* muconate lactonizing enzyme. *Gene* **52**:185–195.

Applebaum, E. R., D. V. Thompson, K. Idler, and N. Chartrain. 1988. *Rhizobium japonicum* USDA 191 has two *nodD* genes that differ in primary structure and function. *J. Bacteriol.* **170**:12–20.

Barnsley, E. A. 1975. Induction of the enzymes of naphthalene metabolism in *Pseudomonas* by salicylate and 2-aminobenzoate. *J. Gen. Microbiol.* **88**:193–196.

Barnsley, E. A. 1976. Role and regulation of the *ortho* and *meta* pathways of catechol metabolism in pseudomonads metabolizing naphthalene and salicylate. *J. Bacteriol.* **125**:404–408.

Brennan, R. G., and B. W. Matthews. 1989. The helix-turn-helix DNA binding motif. *J. Biol. Chem.* **264**:1903–1906.

Cane, P., and P. A. Williams. 1986. A restriction map of naphthalene catabolic plasmid pWW60-1 and the location of some of its catabolic genes. *J. Gen. Microbiol.* **132**:2919–2929.

Chang, M., A. Hadero, and I. P. Crawford. 1989. Sequence of the *Pseudomonas aeruginosa trpI* activator gene and relatedness of *trpI* to other procaryotic regulatory genes. *J. Bacteriol.* **171**:172–183.

Connors, M. A., and E. A. Barnsley. 1982. Naphthalene plasmids in pseudomonads. *J. Bacteriol.* **149**:1096–1101.

Davies, J. I., and W. C. Evans. 1964. Oxidative metabolism of naphthalene by soil pseudomonads. *Biochem. J.* **91**:251–261.

Dodd, I. B., and J. B. Egan. 1987. Systematic method for the detection of potential Cro-like DNA-binding regions in proteins. *J. Mol. Biol.* **194**:557–564.

Dunn, N. W., and I. C. Gunsalus. 1973. Transmissible plasmid encoding early enzymes of naphthalene oxidation in *Pseudomonas putida*. *J. Bacteriol.* **144**:974–979.

Egelhoff, T. T., R. F. Fisher, T. W. Jacobs, J. T. Mulligan, and S. R. Long. 1985. Nucleotide sequence of *Rhizobium meliloti* 1021 nodulation genes: *nodD* is read divergently from *nodABC*. *DNA* **4**:241–248.

Frantz, B., and A. M. Chakrabarty. 1986. Degradative plasmids in *Pseudomonas*, p. 295–323. *In* J. R. Sokatch and L. N. Ornston (ed.), *The Bacteria*, vol. 10. *The Biology of Pseudomonas*. Academic Press, Inc., Orlando, Fla.

Frantz, B., and A. M. Chakrabarty. 1987. Organization and nucleotide sequence determination of a gene cluster involved in 3-chlorocatechol degradation. *Proc. Natl. Acad. Sci. USA* **84**:4460–4464.

Ghosal, D., I.-S. You, and I. C. Gunsalus. 1988. Nucleotide sequence and expression of gene *nahH* of plasmid NAH7 and homology with gene *xylE* of TOL pWWO. *Gene* **55**:19–28.

Gregerov, A. I., A. Chencik, V. Aivasasashrilli, R. S. Beabealashvilli, and V. G. Nikiforov. 1984. *Escherichia coli* and *Pseudomonas putida* RNA polymerases display identical contacts with promoters. *Mol. Gen. Genet.* **195**:511–515.

Grund, A. D., and I. C. Gunsalus. 1983. Cloning of genes for naphthalene metabolism in *Pseudomonas putida*. *J. Bacteriol.* **156**:89–94.

Harayama, S., M. Rekik, A. Wasserfallen, and A. Bairoch. 1987. Evolutionary relationships between catabolic pathways for aromatics: conservation of gene order and nucleotide sequences of catechol oxidation genes of pWWO and NAH7 plasmids. *Mol. Gen. Genet.* **210**:241–247.

Henikoff, S., G. Haughn, J. Calvo, and J. C. Wallace. 1988. A large family of bacterial activator proteins. *Proc. Natl. Acad. Sci. USA* **85**:6602–6606.

Honore, N., M. H. Nicolas, and S. T. Cole. 1986. Inducible cephalosporinase production in clinical isolates of *Enterobacter cloacae* is controlled by a regulatory gene that has been deleted from *Escherichia coli*. *EMBO J.* **5**:3709–3714.

Inouye, S., A. Nakazawa, and T. Nakazawa. 1986. Determination of the transcription initiation site and identification of the protein product of regulatory gene *xylR* for *xyl* operons on the TOL plasmid. *J. Bacteriol.* **163**:863–869.

Inouye, S., A. Nakazawa, and T. Nakazawa. 1987. Expression of the regulatory gene *xylS* on TOL plasmid is positively controlled by the *xylR* gene product. *Proc. Natl. Acad. Sci. USA* **84**:5182–5186.

Jordan, S. R., and C. Pabo. 1988. Structure of the lambda complex at 2.5 Å resolution: details of repressor-operator interactions. *Science* **242**:893–899.

Kurkela, S., H. Lehväslaiho, E. T. Palva, and T. H. Teeri. 1988. Cloning and nucleotide sequence and characterization of genes encoding naphthalene dioxygenase of *Pseudomonas putida* strain NCIB 9816. *Gene* **73**:355–362.

Nakazawa, T., S. Inouye, and A. Nakazawa. 1985. Positive regulation of transcription initiation of *xyl* operons on TOL plasmid, p. 415–429 *In* D. Helinski, S. Cohen, D. Clewell, D. Jackson, and A. Hollaender (ed.), *Plasmids in Bacteria*. Plenum Publishing Corp., New York.

Neidle, E., C. Hartnett, and L. N. Ornston. 1989. Characterization of *Acinetobacter calcoaceticus catM*, a repressor gene homologous in sequence to transcriptional activator genes. *J. Bacteriol.* **171**:5410–5421.

Ostrowski, J. G., G. Jagura-Burdzy, and N. M. Kedrich. 1987. DNA sequences of the *cysB* regions of *Salmonella typhimurium* and *Escherichia coli*. *J. Biol. Chem.* **262**:5999–6005.

Pabo, C. O., and R. J. Sauer. 1984. Protein DNA recognition. *Annu. Rev. Biochem.* **53**:293–321.

Plaman, L. S., and G. V. Stauffer. 1987. Nucleotide sequence of the *Salmonella typhimurium metR* gene and the *metR-metE* control region. *J. Bacteriol.* **169:**3932–3937.

Renault, P., C. Gaillardin, and H. Heslot. 1989. Product of the *Lactococcus lactis* gene required for malolactic fermentation is homologous to a family of positive regulators. *J. Bacteriol.* **171:** 3108–3114.

Rossen, L., C. A. Shearman, A. W. B. Johnston, and J. A. Downie. 1985. The *nodD* regulatory gene of *Rhizobium leguminosarum* is autoregulatory and in the presence of plant exudate induces the *nodABC* genes. *EMBO J.* **4:**3369–3373.

Schell, M. A. 1983. Cloning and expression in *Escherichia coli* of the naphthalene degradation genes from plasmid NAH7. *J. Bacteriol.* **153:**822–828.

Schell, M. A. 1985. Transcriptional control of the *nah* and *sal* hydrocarbon-degradation operons by the *nahR* gene product. *Gene* **36:**301–309.

Schell, M. A. 1986. Homology between nucleotide sequences of promoter regions of *nah* and *sal* operons of NAH7 plasmid of *Pseudomonas putida. Proc. Natl. Acad. Sci. USA* **83:**369–373.

Schell, M. A., and E. Faris. 1987. Transcriptional regulation of the *nah* and *sal* naphthalene degradation operons of plasmid NAH7 of *Pseudomonas putida*, p. 455–458. *In* W. Reznikoff, R. Burgess, C. Gross, and M. Record (ed.), *RNA Polymerase and the Regulation of Transcription.* Elsevier Science Publishing, Inc., New York.

Schell, M. A., and E. Poser. 1989. Demonstration, characterization, and mutational analysis of NahR protein binding in *nah* and *sal* promoters. *J. Bacteriol.* **171:**837–846.

Schell, M. A., and M. Sukordhaman. 1989. Evidence that the transcription activator encoded by the *nahR* gene of *Pseudomonas putida* is evolutionarily related to the transcription activators encoded by the *nodD* gene of *Rhizobium. J. Bacteriol.* **171:**1952–1959.

Schell, M. A., and P. Wender. 1986. Identification of the *nahR* gene product and nucleotide sequences required for its activation of the *sal* operon. *J. Bacteriol.* **166:**9–14.

Stanier, R. Y., N. J. Palleroni, and M. Doudoroff. 1966. Aerobic Pseudomonads: a taxonomic study. *J. Gen. Microbiol.* **43:**159–271.

Stragier, P., O. Danas, and J.-C. Patte. 1983. Regulation and diaminopimelate decarboxylase synthesis in *Escherichia coli*. III. Nucleotide sequence and regulation of the *lysR* gene. *J. Mol. Biol.* **168:**333–350.

Streber, W. R., K. N. Timmis, and M. H. Zenk. 1987. Analysis, cloning, and high-level expression of 2,4-dichlorophenoxyacetate monooxygenase gene *tfdA* of *Alcaligenes eutrophus* JMP134. *J. Bacteriol.* **169:**2950–2955.

Wek, R. C., and W. Hatfield. 1986. Nucleotide sequence and *in vivo* expression of the *ilvY* and *ilvC* genes in *Escherichia coli* K12. *J. Biol. Chem.* **261:**2441–2450.

Wek, R. C., and W. Hatfield. 1988. Transcriptional activation at adjacent operators in the divergent-overlapping *ilvY* and *ilvC* promoters of *Escherichia coli. J. Mol. Biol.* **203:**643–663.

Wohlberger, C., Y. Dong, M. Ptashne, and S. C. Harrison. 1988. Structure of phage 434 Cro/DNA complex. *Nature* (London) **355:**789–795.

Yen, K.-M., and I. C. Gunsalus. 1982. Plasmid gene organization: naphthalene/salicylate oxidation. *Proc. Natl. Acad. Sci. USA* **79:**874–878.

Yen, K.-M., and I. C. Gunsalus. 1985. Regulation of naphthalene catabolic plasmid NAH7. *J. Bacteriol.* **162:**1008–1013.

Yen, K.-M., and C. Serdar. 1989. Genetics of naphthalene metabolism in Pseudomonads. *Crit. Rev. Microbiol.* **15:**247–268.

Yen, K.-M., M. Sullivan, and I. C. Gunsalus. 1983. Electron microscope heteroduplex mapping of naphthalene oxidation genes on the NAH7 and SAL1 plasmids. *Plasmid* **9:**105–111.

You, I.-S., D. Ghosal, and I. C. Gunsalus. 1988. Nucleotide sequence of plasmid NAH7 gene *nahR* and DNA binding of the *nahR* product. *J. Bacteriol.* **170:**5409–5415.

You, I.-S., and I. C. Gunsalus. 1986. Regulation of the *nah* and *sal* operons of plasmid NAH7: evidence for a new function of *nahR. Biochem. Biophys. Res. Commun.* **141:**986–992.

Zuniga, M. C., D. R. Durham, and R. A. Welch. 1981. Plasmid and chromosome-mediated dissimilation of naphthalene and salicylate in *Pseudomonas putida* PMD-1. *J. Bacteriol.* **147:** 836–843.

Chapter 19

Organization and Regulation of the Operon Encoding the Branched-Chain Keto Acid Dehydrogenase of *Pseudomonas putida*

Gayle Burns, K. T. Madhusudhan, K. Hatter, and J. R. Sokatch

Soil and water pseudomonads are metabolically omnivorous organisms whose role in nature is to dissimilate natural and man-made organic chemicals. Figure 1 shows the pathways for the conversion of branched-chain amino acids to intermediates that are then oxidized by the tricarboxylic acid cycle. Branched-chain keto acid dehydrogenase catalyzes reaction 3 in Fig. 1 and is common to the metabolism of all three branched-chain amino acids. The complex is induced by branched-chain keto acids (Martin et al., 1973) that are formed by transamination of L amino acids (Fig. 1, reaction 1) or by deamination of D amino acids (Fig. 1, reaction 2).

Branched-chain keto acid dehydrogenase has recently been the subject of considerable research. The first objective was to purify the enzyme to determine whether it was a multienzyme complex with the general architecture of pyruvate and 2-ketoglutarate dehydrogenases. In addition, branched-chain keto acid dehydrogenase is defective in the human genetic disease maple syrup urine disease, and autoantibodies are formed against the E2 component in primary biliary cirrhosis (Fussey et al., 1989). Therefore, there is considerable interest in the enzyme from a medical point of view.

Branched-chain keto acid dehydrogenase is indeed a multienzyme complex with surprisingly similar properties for the *Pseudomonas* and mammalian complexes. The reactions catalyzed by the components of the complex are shown in Fig. 2. The cofactor for the E1 component is thiamine pyrophosphate, and together these components catalyze the decarboxylation of all three branched-chain keto acids, with reduction of lipoic acid, the prosthetic group of the E2 component. E2 catalyzes transacylation between its lipoic acid residue and the

---

Gayle Burns, K. T. Madhusudhan, K. Hatter, and J. R. Sokatch ● Department of Biochemistry and Molecular Biology, The University of Oklahoma Health Sciences Center, P.O. Box 26901, Oklahoma City, Oklahoma 73190.

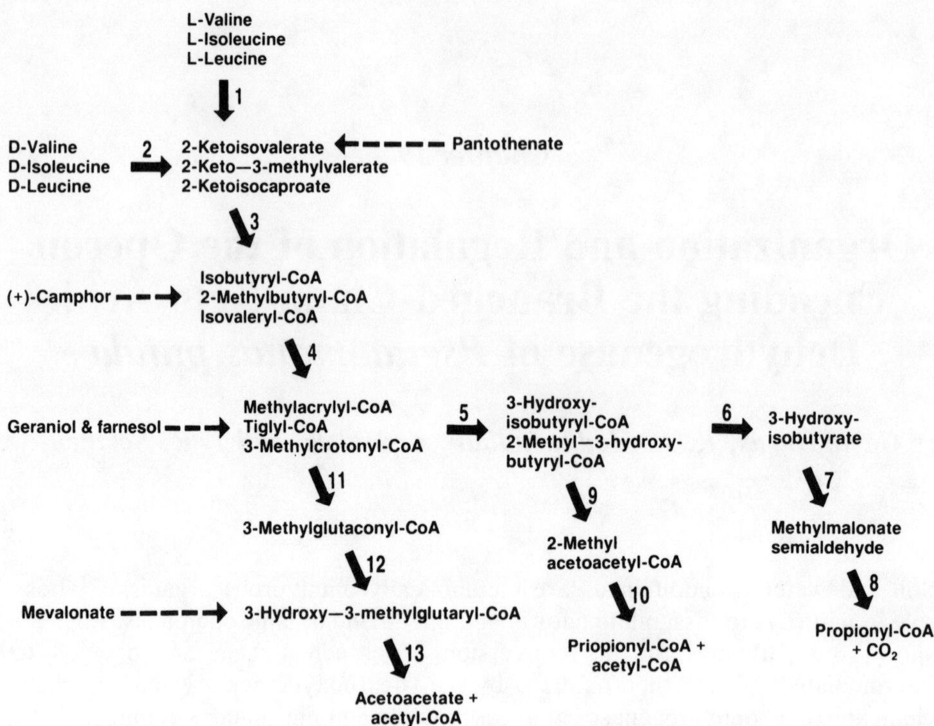

FIGURE 1. Pathways for metabolism of branched-chain amino acids by bacteria.

thiol group of coenzyme A. The E3 component is lipoic dehydrogenase and catalyzes the oxidation of dihydrolipoic acid to lipoic acid.

Branched-chain keto acid dehydrogenase has been purified from *Pseudomonas putida* (Sokatch et al., 1981b) and *Pseudomonas aeruginosa* (McCully et al., 1986) and consists of four polypeptides, as does the mammalian complex (Paxton and Harris, 1982; Pettit et al., 1978). In all cases, the E1 component is composed

FIGURE 2. Reactions catalyzed by components of branched-chain keto acid dehydrogenase.

of E1α and E1β subunits, whereas the E2 and E3 components are single polypeptides.

There are many similarities between the complexes from *Pseudomonas* spp. and from mammals. As noted above, all complexes consist of four polypeptides with similar molecular masses for the corresponding components. Mammalian pyruvate dehydrogenase also consists of four polypeptides (Reed, 1974); however, *Escherichia coli* (Reed, 1974) and *P. aeruginosa* (Jeyaseelan et al., 1980) pyruvate dehydrogenases are composed of three polypeptides with a single large E1 component. One question, then, is whether the large E1 component of *E. coli* divided into E1α and E1β subunits during evolution.

There are some significant differences between the *Pseudomonas* and mammalian branched-chain keto acid dehydrogenases. The mammalian complexes are regulated by phosphorylation of E1α (Paxton and Harris, 1982). In contrast, the *Pseudomonas* branched-chain keto acid dehydrogenase is regulated allosterically by L branched-chain amino acids, with L-valine being the best activator (Sokatch et al., 1981b). In addition, it is likely that all keto acid dehydrogenases from mammals have the same E3 component, whereas in *Pseudomonas* spp. there are separate lipoamide dehydrogenases, LPD-Val for branched-chain keto acid dehydrogenase (Sokatch et al., 1981a) and LPD-Glc for pyruvate and 2-ketoglutarate dehydrogenases (Burns et al., 1989b) and the glycine oxidation complex (Sokatch and Burns, 1984). There is also a third lipoamide dehydrogenase in *P. putida*, LPD-3, whose function is still undetermined (Burns et al., 1989b).

CLONING OF THE *bkd* OPERON

After the properties of the purified complex had been determined, we turned our attention to the structure of the components. The question of the evolutionary relationship of *Pseudomonas* branched-chain keto acid dehydrogenase to *E. coli* pyruvate dehydrogenase could be addressed by a comparison of the primary structures of the components of the two complexes, since the nucleotide sequence of the *E. coli* pyruvate dehydrogenase gene had been reported. In addition, it would be interesting to compare the regulation of both complexes.

The structural genes for the branched-chain keto acid dehydrogenase of the *P. putida* complex were cloned into pKT230, a broad-host-range vector for gram-negative bacteria (Bagdsarian et al., 1981). Positive clones were detected by complementation of several mutants affected in structural genes encoding the components of the branched-chain keto acid dehydrogenase operon (Sykes et al., 1987). These mutants regained the ability to grow on agar with branched-chain amino acids as sole carbon sources. The recombinant clone, pSS1-1, was expressed constitutively in *P. putida* mutants, indicating that the regulatory region had not been cloned. All of the dehydrogenase genes were subcloned into pUC and expressed in *E. coli* from the *lac* promoter (Sykes et al., 1987). These studies established the gene order of the *bkd* operon (Fig. 3) and the direction of transcription. Southern blots using a 1.45-kilobase-pair probe encoding E1α and part of E1β identified a transcript of about 6 kilobase pairs (Burns et al., 1989a)

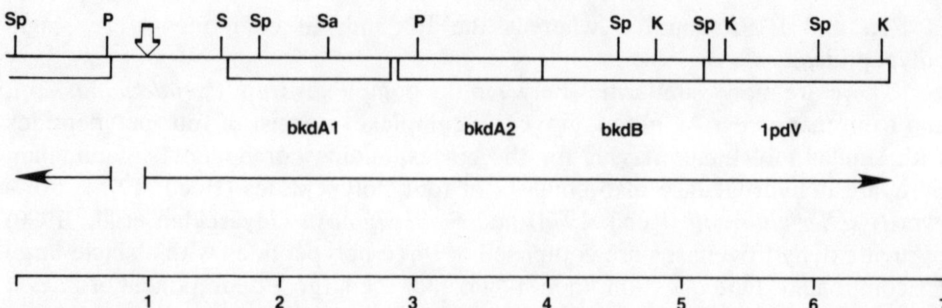

FIGURE 3. Organization of the *bkd* operon. *bkdA1*, *bkdA2*, *bkdB*, and *lpdV* are genes encoding E1α, E1β, E2, and LPD-Val, respectively. Abbreviations for restriction enzymes: K, *Kpn*I; P, *Pst*I; S, *Sst*I; Sa, *Sal*I; Sp, *Sph*I. Bottom scale gives distances in kilobases.

that was somewhat longer than the coding region of 4.9 kilobase pairs. Recent studies from our laboratory have located the start of transcription 592 base pairs upstream of the coding region for *bkdA1*. Therefore, the structural genes encoding the components of the branched-chain keto acid dehydrogenase of *P. putida* are transcribed from a single promoter.

ORGANIZATION OF THE OPERON

The gene order is *bkdA1-bkdA2-bkdB-lpdV*, encoding E1α, E1β, E2, and LPD-Val, the latter being the specific E3 component of *P. putida* branched-chain keto acid dehydrogenase. The coding region is tightly linked, with only 42 intergenic bases. Curiously, most of the intergenic space is between *bkdA1* and *bkdA2*. All of the mature proteins except LPD-Val lack an N-terminal methionine. There are good potential ribosome-binding sites preceding each structural gene. There is a strong Rho-independent terminator preceded by two in-frame stop codons immediately after the *lpdV* gene. The G+C content of the coding region is 65.2%; the G+C content of the leader region between the start of transcription and *bkdA1* is 56.9%. No open reading frame(s) could be detected in this region in any of the six possible frames.

NUCLEOTIDE SEQUENCES OF *bkdA1* AND *bkdA2*

Translation of *bkdA1* and *bkdA2* yielded proteins with molecular weights of 45,158 and 37,007, respectively, when the N-terminal methionine was omitted (Burns et al., 1988a). The protein with an M_r of 37,007 corresponded to the 37-kilodalton protein observed in sodium dodecyl sulfate-polyacrylamide gels (Sokatch et al., 1981b). The 45,158-M_r protein corresponded to the 39-kilodalton protein observed on sodium dodecyl sulfate-polyacrylamide gels (Sokatch et al., 1981b). There was no similarity to the E1 component of *E. coli* pyruvate (Stephens et al., 1983b) or 2-ketoglutarate dehydrogenase (Darlison et al., 1984). There was,

```
                        310        320        330
      P. putida      RAGPHSTSDDPSKYRPADDWSHF-P
                     : :.:::::::.: ::...:. ...
      Rat liver      RIGHHSTSDDSSAYRSVDEVNYWDK
                        290   *    300   *    310
```

FIGURE 4. Alignment of E1α subunits from *P. putida* (Burns et al., 1988a) and rat liver branched-chain keto acid dehydrogenases (Zhang et al., 1987). The amino acids of the rat liver subunit marked with an asterisk are phosphorylated. Numbers represent the amino acid residues of the respective proteins.

however, distinct similarity to the E1α subunit of rat liver branched-chain keto acid dehydrogenase (Zhang et al., 1987). In particular, the region of the rat liver E1α subunit that is phosphorylated was found to be highly conserved in *Pseudomonas* branched-chain keto acid dehydrogenase (Fig. 4). It seems very likely that E1α of rat liver and *Pseudomonas* branched-chain keto acid dehydrogenases are functionally equivalent even though the latter is not phosphorylated. Although it is not shown in Fig. 4, there was also considerable similarity to the human pyruvate dehydrogenase E1α subunit in the region that is phosphorylated (Dahl et al., 1987; Koike et al., 1988).

NUCLEOTIDE SEQUENCE OF *bkdB*

The nucleotide sequence of *bkdB* encoded a protein of M_r 45,003 minus the N-terminal methionine (Burns et al., 1988b). This corresponds to the 47-kilodalton protein observed on sodium dodecyl sulfate-polyacrylamide gels (Sokatch et al., 1981b). There was a single lipoyl domain, compared with the three lipoyl domains of the *E. coli* pyruvate dehydrogenase (Fig. 5). There was considerable similarity of the E2 component of *Pseudomonas* branched-chain keto acid dehydrogenase to the E2 component of *E. coli* pyruvate (Stephens et al., 1983a) and 2-ketoglutarate dehydrogenases (Spencer et al., 1984).

NUCLEOTIDE SEQUENCE OF *lpdV*

The final gene in the *bkd* operon is *lpdV*, which encodes LPD-Val (Burns et al., 1989a). The molecular weight of the encoded protein is 48,164 (48,949, including FAD). LPD-Val has considerable similarity to other lipoamide dehydrogenases, particularly in the highly conserved redox-active disulfide active site. LPD-Val is the specific E3 component of *P. putida*. Branched-chain keto acid dehydrogenase is the only known example of this specificity. There is no obvious reason for this specificity in the primary structure of the encoded protein. However, the region of LPD-Val that is thought to bind to the E2 component has the least similarity to the other lipoamide dehydrogenases whose structures have been reported (Pons et al., 1988; Stephens et al., 1983c; Westphal et al., 1988).

P. PUTIDA HAS THREE LIPOAMIDE DEHYDROGENASES

We have recently reported the existence of a third lipoamide dehydrogenase, LPD-3, in *P. putida*. The function of LPD-3 is still unknown; however, it was

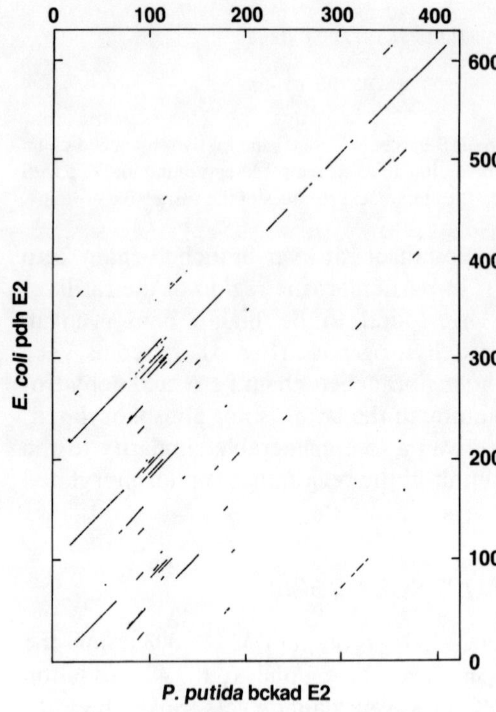

FIGURE 5. Comparison of amino acid sequences of E2 components from *E. coli* pyruvate dehydrogenase (Stephens et al., 1983a) and *P. putida* branched-chain keto acid dehydrogenases (Burns et al., 1988b). The similarity of the single lipoyl domain from E2 of *P. putida* to the three lipoyl domains of E2 from *E. coli* is evident.

discovered in a mutant of *P. putida* lacking LPD-Glc (Burns et al., 1989b). This mutant, *P. putida* JS348, was unusual in that it lacked 2-ketoglutarate dehydrogenase, but it apparently had a normal pyruvate dehydrogenase, unlike the *E. coli* *lpd* mutants (Guest, 1978). Other LPD-Glc-negative mutants of *P. putida* lacked both pyruvate and 2-ketoglutarate dehydrogenases. *P. putida* JS348 did, however, have some lipoamide dehydrogenase activity, and that protein was purified from cell extracts of strain JS348. The N-terminal amino acid sequences of purified LDP-Glc and LPD-3 were determined and found to be different from each other and from that of LPD-Val (Fig. 6). The function of LPD-3 is now being investigated.

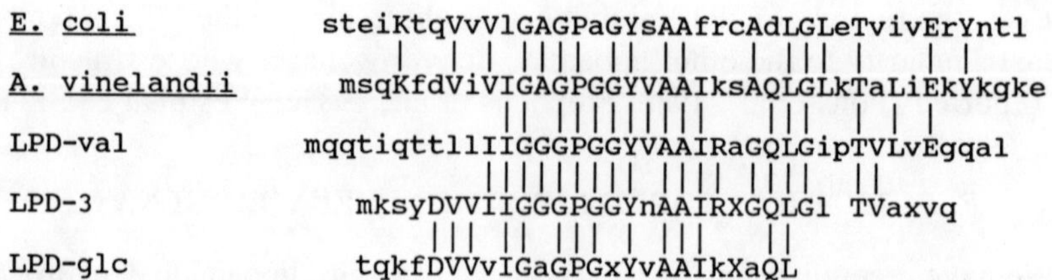

FIGURE 6. Comparison of N-terminal sequences of procaryotic lipoamide dehydrogenases.

CONCLUSIONS

One of the early hypotheses in this study was that branched-chain keto acid dehydrogenase evolved from the procaryotic pyruvate dehydrogenase, possibly by splitting the large E1 component into E1α and E1β subunits. This was quickly shown to be incorrect, since the E1α and E1β subunits of *P. putida* branched-chain keto acid dehydrogenase have no similarity to the large E1 components of pyruvate dehydrogenase. In fact, the relationship that was discovered is between the *P. putida* branched-chain keto acid dehydrogenase and mammalian pyruvate and branched-chain keto acid dehydrogenases. The finding that the region of the mammalian complexes which is phosphorylated is conserved in *Pseudomonas* spp. was both surprising and interesting. The conclusion is that the E1 component of procaryotic pyruvate dehydrogenase is an evolutionary dead end, since it does not have similarity to any other proteins whose structures have been reported.

The question of why *Pseudomonas* spp. have three lipoamide dehydrogenases when other species seem to have a single functional protein is also unanswered. It is possible that other species of bacteria have multiple lipoamide dehydrogenases that have not been discovered, and the same could be true of mammals. In *Pseudomonas* spp., LPD-Glc is absolutely specific for pyruvate and 2-ketoglutarate dehydrogenases and for the glycine oxidation complex. LPD-Val is specific for branched-chain keto acid dehydrogenase. It is not clear whether this arrangement confers any advantage to pseudomonads, since apparently mammals make do with a single lipoamide dehydrogenase for all three complexes. Since the pseudomonads are relatively ancient organisms, this may simply be an example of early evolution of lipoamide dehydrogenase that was not conserved.

ACKNOWLEDGMENTS. This research was supported by Public Health Service grants DK 21727 and GM 30428 from the National Institutes of Health.

LITERATURE CITED

Bagdasarian, M., R. Lurz, B. Rückert, F. C. H. Franklin, M. M. Bagdasarian, J. Frey, and K. N. Timmis. 1981. Specific purpose plasmid cloning vectors. II. Broad host range, copy number RSF1010-derived vectors, and a host-vector system for gene cloning in *Pseudomonas*. *Gene* **16**:237–247.

Burns, G., T. Brown, K. Hatter, J. M. Idriss, and J. R. Sokatch. 1988a. Similarity of the E1 subunits of branched-chain-oxoacid dehydrogenase from *Pseudomonas putida* to the corresponding subunits of mammalian branched-chain-oxoacid and pyruvate dehydrogenases. *Eur. J. Biochem.* **176:** 311–317.

Burns, G., T. Brown, K. Hatter, and J. R. Sokatch. 1988b. Comparison of the amino acid sequences of the transacylase components of branched chain oxoacid dehydrogenase of *Pseudomonas putida*, and the pyruvate and 2-oxoglutarate dehydrogenases of Escherichia coli. *Eur. J. Biochem.* **176:**165–169.

Burns, G., T. Brown, K. Hatter, and J. R. Sokatch. 1989a. Sequence analysis of the lpdV gene for lipoamide dehydrogenase of branched chain oxoacid dehydrogenase of *Pseudomonas putida*. *Eur. J. Biochem.* **179:**61–69.

Burns, G., P. J. Sykes, K. Hatter, and J. R. Sokatch. 1989b. Isolation of a third lipoamide dehydrogenase from *Pseudomonas putida*. *J. Bacteriol.* **171:**665–668.

Dahl, H.-H. M., S. M. Hunt, W. M. Hutchinson, and G. K. Brown. 1987. The human pyruvate dehydrogenase complex. Isolation of cDNA clones for the E1α subunit, sequence analysis and characterization of the mRNA. *J. Biol. Chem.* **262:**7398–7403.

184   Burns et al.

Darlison, M. G., M. E. Spencer, and J. R. Guest. 1984. Nucleotide sequence of the sucA gene encoding the 2-oxoglutarate dehydrogenase of *Escherichia coli. Eur. J. Biochem.* **141**:351–359.

Fussey, S. P. M., J. R. Guest, O. F. W. James, M. F. Bassendine, and S. J. Yeaman. 1989. Identification and analysis of the major M2 autoantigens in primary biliary cirrhosis. *Proc. Natl. Acad. Sci. USA* **85**:8654–8658.

Guest, J. R. 1978. Aspects of the molecular biology of lipoamide dehydrogenase. *Adv. Neurol.* **21**:219–244.

Jeyaseelan, K., J. R. Guest, and J. Visser. 1980. The pyruvate dehydrogenase complex of *Pseudomonas aeruginosa* PAO. Purification, properties and characterization of mutants. *J. Gen. Microbiol.* **120**:393–402.

Koike, K., S. Ohta, Y. Urata, Y. Kagawa, and M. Koike. 1988. Cloning and sequencing of cDNAs encoding α and β subunits of human pyruvate dehydrogenase. *Proc. Natl. Acad. Sci. USA* **85**:41–45.

Martin, R. R., V. D. Marshall, J. R. Sokatch, and L. Unger. 1973. Common enzymes of branched chain amino acid catabolism in *Pseudomonas aeruginosa* PAO. *J. Bacteriol.* **115**:198–204.

McCully, V., G. Burns, and J. R. Sokatch. 1986. Resolution of branched-chain oxo acid dehydrogenase complex of *Pseudomonas putida. Biochem. J.* **233**:737–742.

Paxton, R., and R. A. Harris. 1982. Isolation of rabbit liver branched chain alpha-ketoacid dehydrogenase and regulation by phosphorylation. *J. Biol. Chem.* **257**:14433–14439.

Pettit, F. H., S. J. Yeaman, and L. J. Reed. 1978. Purification and characterization of branched chain α-ketoacid dehydrogenase complex of bovine kidney. *Proc. Natl. Acad. Sci. USA* **75**:4881–4885.

Pons, G., C. Raefsky-Estrin, D. J. Carothers, R. A. Pepin, A. A. Javed, B. W. Jesse, M. K. Ganapathi, D. Samols, and M. S. Patel. 1988. Cloning and cDNA sequence of the dihydrolipoamide dehydrogenase component of human α-ketoacid dehydrogenase complexes. *Proc. Natl. Acad. Sci. USA* **85**:1422–1426.

Reed, L. J. 1974. Multienzyme complexes. *Acc. Chem. Res.* **7**:40–46.

Sokatch, J. R., and G. Burns. 1984. Oxidation of glycine by Pseudomonas putida requires a specific lipoamide dehydrogenase. *Arch. Biochem. Biophys.* **228**:660–666.

Sokatch, J. R., V. McCully, J. Gebrosky, and D. J. Sokatch. 1981a. Isolation of a specific lipoamide dehydrogenase for a branched-chain keto acid dehydrogenase from *Pseudomonas putida. J. Bacteriol.* **148**:639–646.

Sokatch, J. R., V. McCully, and C. M. Roberts. 1981b. Purification of a branched-chain keto acid dehydrogenase from *Pseudomonas putida. J. Bacteriol.* **148**:647–652.

Spencer, M. E., M. G. Darlison, P. E. Stephens, I. K. Duckenfield, and J. R. Guest. 1984. Nucleotide sequence of the sucB gene encoding the dihydrolipoamide succinyltransferase of *Escherichia coli* K12 and homology with the corresponding acetyltransferase. *Eur. J. Biochem.* **141**:361–374.

Stephens, P. E., M. G. Darlison, H. M. Lewis, and J. R. Guest. 1983a. Pyruvate dehydrogenase complex of *Escherichia coli* K12: nucleotide sequence encoding the dihydrolipoamide acetyltransferase component. *Eur. J. Biochem.* **133**:481–489.

Stephens, P. E., M. G. Darlison, H. M. Lewis, and J. R. Guest. 1983b. The pyruvate dehydrogenase complex of *Escherichia coli* K12: nucleotide sequence encoding the pyruvate dehydrogenase component. *Eur. J. Biochem.* **133**:155–162.

Stephens, P. E., H. M. Lewis, M. G. Darlison, and J. R. Guest. 1983c. Nucleotide sequence of the lipoamide dehydrogenase gene of *Escherichia coli* K12. *Eur. J. Biochem.* **135**:519–527.

Sykes, P. J., G. Burns, J. Menard, K. Hatter, and J. R. Sokatch. 1987. Molecular cloning of genes encoding branched-chain keto acid dehydrogenase of *Pseudomonas putida. J. Bacteriol.* **169**:1619–1625.

Westphal, A. H., and A. de Kok. 1988. Lipoamide dehydrogenase from *Azotobacter vinelandii*: molecular cloning, organization and sequence analysis of the gene. *Eur. J. Biochem.* **172**:299–305.

Zhang, B., M. J. Kuntz, G. W. Goodwin, R. A. Harris, and D. W. Crabb. 1987. Molecular cloning of a cDNA for the E1α subunit of rat liver branched chain α-ketoacid dehydrogenase. *J. Biol. Chem.* **262**:15220–15224.

Chapter 20

Enzymes of Haloaromatics Degradation: Variations of *Alcaligenes* on a Theme by *Pseudomonas*

Michael Schlömann, Dietmar H. Pieper, and Hans-Joachim Knackmuss

THE THEME: SEPARATE SETS OF ENZYMES EFFECTING THE DEGRADATION OF CATECHOL AND HALOCATECHOLS

For the aerobic bacterial degradation of mono- and dichlorinated aromatic compounds, several different pathways have been described. They include breakage of the carbon-halogen bond as the first step by hydrolytic, oxygenolytic, or reductive mechanisms, as well as modifications of the gentisate pathway, the *meta* cleavage of chloroprotocatechuate, and the degradation via *ortho* cleavage of halosubstituted catechols (for recent reviews, see Reineke [1984], Müller and Lingens [1986], Rochkind-Dubinsky et al. [1987], and Reineke and Knackmuss [1988]). The latter pathway has initially been found to be adopted for the breakdown of chlorosubstituted phenoxyacetates, benzoates, and phenols (Bollag et al., 1968; Tiedje et al., 1969; Evans et al., 1971a; Evans et al., 1971b; Dorn et al., 1974; Knackmuss and Hellwig, 1978). More recently, the degradation of mono- and dichlorinated benzenes and anilines via *ortho* cleavage has been described (Reineke and Knackmuss, 1984; Zeyer et al., 1985; Surovtseva et al., 1986; De Bont et al., 1986; Schraa et al., 1986; Haigler et al., 1988).

The enzymology of this degradative route was first investigated in the 3-chlorobenzoate (3CB)-utilizing strain *Pseudomonas* sp. strain B13. During grown with 3CB, this organism synthesizes four enzymes, which are not induced, when benzoate is supplied as the carbon source (Fig. 1; Dorn and Knackmuss,

---

Michael Schlömann ● Department of Biology, Yale University, New Haven, Connecticut 06511.   *Dietmar H. Pieper* ● Gesellschaft für Strahlen- und Umweltforschung, Ingolstädter Landstrasse 1, D-8042 Neuherberg, Federal Republic of Germany.   *Hans-Joachim Knackmuss* ● Institut für Mikrobiologie der Universität Stuttgart, Azenbergstrasse 18, D-7000 Stuttgart 1, Federal Republic of Germany.

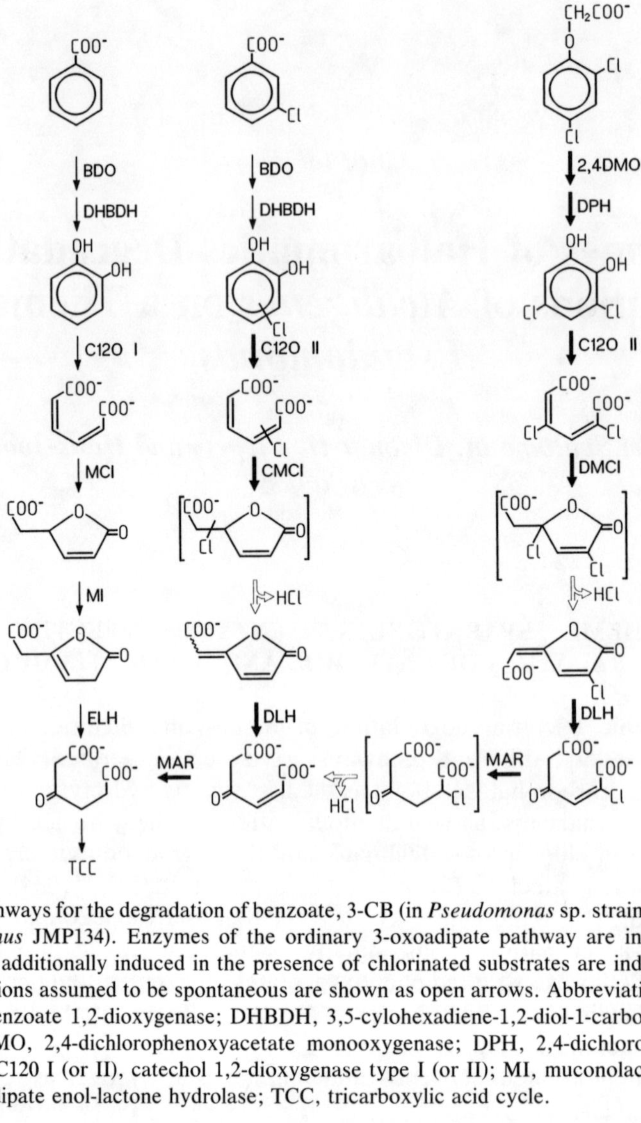

FIGURE 1. Pathways for the degradation of benzoate, 3-CB (in *Pseudomonas* sp. strain B13), and 2,4-D (in *A. eutrophus* JMP134). Enzymes of the ordinary 3-oxoadipate pathway are indicated by light arrows; those additionally induced in the presence of chlorinated substrates are indicated by heavy arrows. Reactions assumed to be spontaneous are shown as open arrows. Abbreviations not given in text: BDO, benzoate 1,2-dioxygenase; DHBDH, 3,5-cylohexadiene-1,2-diol-1-carboxylate dehydrogenase; 2,4DMO, 2,4-dichlorophenoxyacetate monooxygenase; DPH, 2,4-dichlorophenoxyacetate hydroxylase; C12O I (or II), catechol 1,2-dioxygenase type I (or II); MI, muconolactone isomerase; ELH, 3-oxoadipate enol-lactone hydrolase; TCC, tricarboxylic acid cycle.

1978; Schmidt and Knackmuss, 1980; Reineke, 1984). The first three of these enzymes, the catechol 1,2-dioxygenase type II (EC 1.13.11.1), the chloromuconate cycloisomerase (or muconate cycloisomerase type II; CMCI; EC 5.5.1.7), and the dienelactone hydrolase (DLH; EC 3.1.1.45), catalyze reactions analogous to those of the well-known 3-oxoadipate pathway. The fourth, however, the maleylacetate reductase (MAR; EC 1.3.1.32), has no equivalent among the enzymes of this pathway.

The molecular genetics of the chlorocatechol-degrading enzyme sequence in strain B13 has been investigated only to a limited extent (Weisshaar et al., 1987). The corresponding genes encoded by pAC27, on the other hand, have been cloned and sequenced. Hybridization studies between pAC25 (the evolutionary precursor of pAC27) and pWR1, isolated from strain B13 (Chatterjee and Chakrabarty, 1983), as well as partial amino acid sequences of the respective DLHs (Frantz et al., 1987) suggest that the chlorocatechol degradation genes of these plasmids are very similar or even identical.

The 2,4-dichlorophenoxyacetate (2,4-D)-utilizing strain *Alcaligenes eutrophus* JMP134, which harbors plasmid pJP4 (Pemberton et al., 1979), resembles *Pseudomonas* sp. strain B13 in also synthesizing two separate sets of enzymes for the degradation of catechol and halocatechols via *ortho* cleavage. Since the pJP4-free strain JMP222 still grows with benzoate, the genes of the first-mentioned set of enzymes presumably lie on the chromosome (or, less likely, on a megaplasmid that has been detected in this organism by Friedrich et al. [1983]). In contrast, the genes for the halocatechol-degrading enzymes have, except for the MAR gene, been located on pJP4 (Don et al., 1985). This plasmid also codes for the initial enzymes of 2,4-D degradation, that is, for the 2,4-D monooxygenase and for the 2,4-dichlorophenol hydroxylase (Streber et al., 1987; Don et al., 1985). Despite the overall resemblance between *Pseudomonas* sp. strain B13 and *A. eutrophus* JMP134 with respect to the enzymology of halocatechol degradation, closer investigation of some of the enzymes of JMP134 revealed some remarkable differences between the two strains.

FIRST VARIATION: pJP4-ENCODED DIOXYGENASE AND CYCLOISOMERASE, ENZYMES BETTER ADAPTED TO DISUBSTITUTED THAN TO MONOSUBSTITUTED SUBSTRATES

Whereas the catechol 1,2-dioxygenase type I of *Pseudomonas* sp. strain B13, which is induced during growth with benzoate, exhibits low activities with substituted catechols, the type II enzyme, induced during growth with 3CB, shows high turnover rates for these substrates (Table 1). A similar situation is observed in *A. eutrophus* JMP134, the main difference being that the type II enzyme of JMP134 shows the highest V_{max} values with disubstituted substrates, whereas the corresponding enzyme from B13 seems to have a slight preference for monosubstituted compounds.

This distinction between B13 and JMP134 enzymes is more obvious when one examines cycloisomerizing activities (Table 2). The two cycloisomerases of strain B13 differ from each other mainly with respect to their relative V_{max} values for chlorosubstituted muconates, the CMCI showing higher activities than does the ordinary muconate cycloisomerase (MCI). The dichloromuconate cycloisomerase (DMCI) of strain JMP134 can be differentiated from both enzymes on the basis of V_{max} values. More pronounced, however, are the differences in the affinities toward various substrates. The K_m value of the DMCI of JMP134 for *cis,cis*-muconate is so high that it is difficult to assay the activity with this substrate at the concentration commonly used in these tests (100 µM). Whereas the affinity of this enzyme for monosubstituted muconates is lower than that of the B13 enzyme, 2,4-dichloromuconate is bound with high affinity. Thus, although the enzyme

TABLE 1

Substrate specificities of different catechol 1,2-dioxygenases[a]

Substrate	Relative apparent V_{max} value[b]			
	Pseudomonas sp. strain B13		*A. eutrophus* JMP134	
	C12O I	C12O II	C12O I	C12O II
Catechol	100	100	100	100
3-Chlorocatechol	<1	164	2	124
4-Chlorocatechol	11	120	14	122
3-Methylcatechol	(11)	(337)	41	167
3,5-Dichlorocatechol	<1	148	1	181
5-Chloro-3-methylcatechol	ND[c]	ND	38	376

[a] Data are from Reineke and Knackmuss (1980) and Pieper et al. (1988); those in parentheses are from Dorn and Knackmuss (1978).
[b] Expressed as percentage of the value with catechol, taken as 100%. C12O I and C12O II, Catechol 1,2-dioxygenase types I and II.
[c] ND, Not determined.

sequence of strain B13 is able to degrade 3,5-dichlorocatechol (Schwien et al., 1988) and although JMP134 can grow with 3CB (Don and Pemberton, 1981), the cycloisomerases seem to be adapted to the breakdown of different substrates, the enzyme from B13 preferring monosubstituted and that from JMP134 clearly preferring disubstituted muconates.

A remarkable difference between the pAC27- and the pJP4-encoded cycloisomerases lies in the turnover numbers of their respective substrates. Ngai and Ornston (1988), after having purified the pAC27-specified CMCI, observed a K_{cat} of 110 min^{-1}, which is more than 30-fold below the K_{cat} of the MCI of *Pseudomonas putida*. Ngai and Ornston suggested that a loss in catalytic activity accompanied evolutionary acquisition of broad substrate specificity. The pJP4-encoded DMCI, however, exhibits turnover numbers of 3,860 min^{-1} for 2,4-

TABLE 2

Apparent K_m and relative V_{max} values of different cycloisomerizing enzymes[a]

Substrate	*Pseudomonas* sp. strain B13				*A. eutrophus* JMP134, dichloromuconate cycloisomerase	
	Muconate cycloisomerase		Chloromuconate cycloisomerase			
	V_{max} (%)[b]	K_m (μM)	V_{max} (%)	K_m (μM)	V_{max} (%)[c]	K_m (μM)
cis,cis-Muconate	100	55.8	100	92.8	100	4,000
2-Methyl-*cis,cis*-muconate	90	105.0	276	30.9	20	115
3-Methyl-*cis,cis*-muconate	11.7	18.0	232	13.4	120	155
2-Chloro-*cis,cis*-muconate	0.8	415.0	180	60.1	30	540
3-Chloro-*cis,cis*-muconate	7.1	134.8	201	128.6	260	330
2,4-Dichloro-*cis,cis*-muconate	ND[d]	ND	ND	ND	125	20

[a] Data are from Schmidt and Knackmuss (1980) and Kuhm et al. (submitted).
[b] Expressed as percentage of the value with *cis,cis*-muconate, taken as 100%.
[c] Calculated from data of Kuhm et al. (submitted).
[d] ND, Not determined.

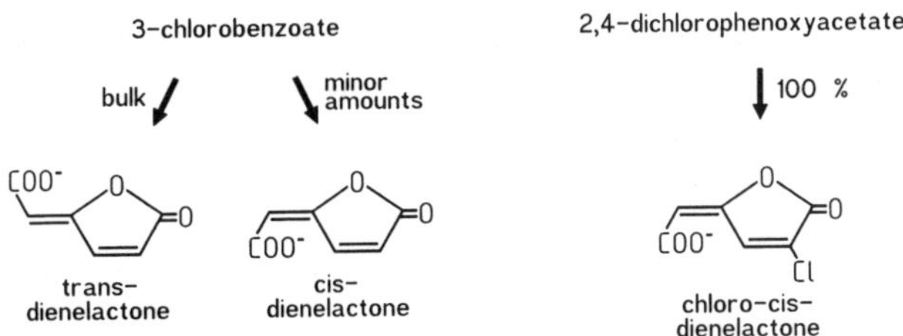

FIGURE 2. Lactonic intermediates in the degradation of 3CB by *Pseudomonas* sp. strain B13 and of 2,4-D by *A. eutrophus* JMP134.

dichloromuconate and 3,090 min^{-1} for *cis,cis*-muconate (A. E. Kuhm et al., *Biochem. J.*, in press). Thus the hypothesis of Ngai and Ornston does not seem to be generally applicable.

Despite these differences in kinetic properties, the DMCI of strain JMP134 resembles other procaryotic cycloisomerases in Mn^{2+} dependence and in the molecular masses of subunits and native enzyme (Kuhm et al., submitted). More detailed insight into the factors determining the remarkable substrate specificity and its evolution will probably result from sequencing and X-ray data. The *tfdD* gene, coding for DMCI, has already been subcloned and partially sequenced by Ghosal and You (1988). This information will offer comparisons with known sequences of the pAC27-encoded CMCI (Frantz and Chakrabarty, 1987) and of the MCI from *P. putida* (Aldrich et al., 1987). In addition, the DMCI has recently been crystallized (A. Hammer et al., unpublished results), possibly offering a chance for X-ray analysis, which might allow comparisons with a model of the *P. putida* MCI (Goldman et al., 1987).

SECOND VARIATION: THE pJP4-ENCODED DLH AND THE CORRESPONDING ENZYME FROM *PSEUDOMONAS* SP. STRAIN B13

Because of the predominance of 1,2-dioxygenation over 1,6-dioxygenation of 3CB (Reineke and Knackmuss, 1978), *Pseudomonas* sp. strain B13 degrades most of its growth substrate via 3-chlorocatechol, 2-chloro-*cis,cis*-muconate, and *trans*-4-carboxymethylenebut-2-en-4-olide (*trans*-dienelactone). Only minor amounts of 3CB are catabolized via the parallel route, including 4-chlorocatechol, 3-chloro-*cis,cis*-muconate, and the *cis* isomer of the dienelactone (Fig. 2). This corresponds to the substrate specificity of the DLH from strain B13, which has a considerably higher affinity for the *trans*-dienelactone (K_m = 15 μM) than for the *cis* isomer (K_m = 400 μM) (Schmidt and Knackmuss, 1980). On the other hand, 2,4-D seems to be almost exclusively degraded by JMP134 via the route 3,5-dichlorocatechol, 2,4-dichloro-*cis,cis*-muconate, *cis*-2-chloro-4-carboxymethylenebut-2-en-4-olide (2-chloro-*cis*-dienelactone in Fig. 2) and not via the *trans* isomer of the chlorodienelactone, as suggested by Schwien et al. (1988) for B13. This appears to be reflected by the substrate specificity of purified pJP4-encoded DLH, which in contrast to the B13 enzyme lacks the preference for the *trans* isomer (K_m = 190 μM for *trans*-dienelactone; K_m = 180 μM for the *cis*-dienelactone [G. Bauer et al., unpublished results]). Since a model of the DLH of B13 based on X-ray crystallographic data has recently been published by Pathak et al. (1988), for comparison efforts are being made to crystallize the pJP4-encoded hydrolase (Bauer et al., unpublished results).

The DLH of B13 and the corresponding pJP4-encoded enzyme show similar molecular masses (26 kilodaltons) and considerable overall similarity. Nevertheless, significant differences with respect to inhibition by *p*-chloromercuribenzoate and amino acid composition have been observed (M. Schlömann, Ph.D. thesis, Universität Stuttgart, Stuttgart, Federal Republic of Germany, 1988). Although amino acid compositions of both enzymes suggest, despite the differences, a common evolutionary origin, Ghosal and You (1988) did not find hybridization between *tfdE* of pJP4 and *clcD* of pAC27, the gene product of which seems to be identical to the B13 DLH (Frantz et al., 1987).

THIRD VARIATION: AN ADDITIONAL DLH OF DIFFERENT SUBSTRATE SPECIFICITY IN *A. EUTROPHUS* JMP134

The above-mentioned pJP4-encoded DLH is induced not only during growth of JMP134 with 2,4-D but also when this strain utilizes 4-fluorobenzoate (4FB) as a carbon source. Interestingly, the cured strain *A. eutrophus* JMP222, lacking pJP4, is still able to grow with 4FB (M. Schlömann, E. Schmidt, and H.-J. Knackmuss, *Syst. Appl. Microbiol.* **5:**259, 1984). The DLH from these cells, however, shows a substrate specificity distinctly different from those of the pJP4-encoded and the B13 enzymes. The *cis* isomer of the dienelactone is not hydrolyzed at a significant rate, suggesting classification of this enzyme as a different type of DLH (type I in Fig. 3).

From the results described above, it had to be concluded that strain JMP134 possesses at least two different DLHs, one encoded by pJP4 and another encoded by the chromosome or the megaplasmid of this strain (Schlömann et al., *Syst. Appl. Microbiol.*, 1984). This hypothesis was supported by ion-exchange chromatography of crude extracts from JMP134 and JMP222 (Schlömann, Ph.D. thesis, 1988). Besides one major peak for DLH activity, chromatography of JMP134 extracts yielded three to four major activity peaks. One of these eluted at the same position as did the DLH of JMP222 and did not show activity for the *cis*-dienelactone. Remarkably, the peak coincided with a maximum for 3-oxoadipate enol-lactone hydrolase activity. One of the other minor DLH activity peaks seemed to represent a form of DLH that was derived from the main form by Mn^{2+}-accelerated processes (Bauer et al., unpublished results). Whether the remaining one or two peaks also represent artifacts or are somehow associated with a second set of chlorocatechol degradation genes, located on pJP4 by Ghosal and You (1988), has not yet been investigated.

Like *A. eutrophus* JMP222, the type strain of this species, *A. eutrophus* 335, is able to utilize 4FB (Schlömann et al., *Syst. Appl. Microbiol.*, 1984). The DLH, which is induced by *A. eutrophus* 335, also hydrolyzes the *trans*-dienelactone and

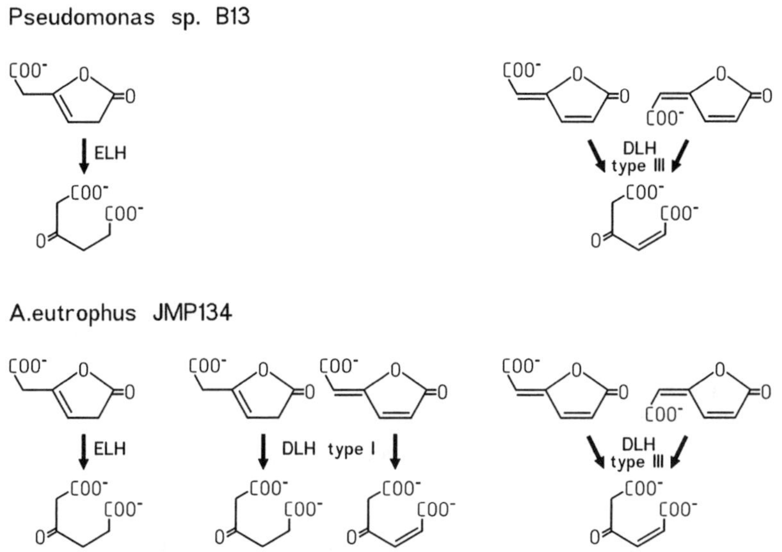

Pseudomonas sp. B13

A.eutrophus JMP134

FIGURE 3. Reactions catalyzed by different types of lactone hydrolases in *Pseudomonas* sp. strain B13 and in *A. eutrophus* JMP134.

3-oxoadipate enol-lactone but not the *cis*-dienelactone. The enzyme was purified ca. 100-fold and was shown to be inactivated by *p*-chloromercuribenzoate and EDTA, whereas it was stabilized in the presence of Mn^{2+} (Schlömann, Ph.D. thesis, 1988). The molecular mass was estimated by gel filtration to be 58 kilodaltons, which is about twice as large as that of the known 3-oxoadipate enol-lactone hydrolases and the DLHs from B13 and from strains carrying pJP4 or pAC27. The substrate specificities of the DLHs of *A. eutrophus* 335 and *A. eutrophus* JMP222 pose interesting questions as to the evolution of this activity.

A VARIATION OF *P. CEPACIA* ON A THEME BY *PSEUDOMONAS* SP. STRAIN B13: A THIRD TYPE OF DLH

Like the *Alcaligenes* strain discussed above, *Pseudomonas cepacia* has the ability to utilize 4FB as a sole carbon and energy source (Schlömann et al., *Syst. Appl. Microbiol.*, 1984). Under these conditions, a DLH that differs from the corresponding enzymes of all other strains investigated is induced. This enzyme is unique in hydrolyzing only the *cis*-dienelactone, not the *trans* isomer or 3-oxoadipate enol-lactone (Fig. 4). In addition, the enzyme does not convert the fluorolactone (4-carboxymethyl-4-fluorobut-2-en-4-olide), which is an essential metabolite of the 4FB degradative pathway (Schlömann, Ph.D. thesis, 1988). Hydrolysis of the fluorolactone to maleylacetate, a reaction without which growth with 4FB would not be feasible, is catalyzed in *P. cepacia* by the 3-oxoadipate enol-lactone hydrolase. Both hydrolases of *P. cepacia* have been purified and partially characterized. The DLH is not inhibited by *p*-chloromercuribenzoate and

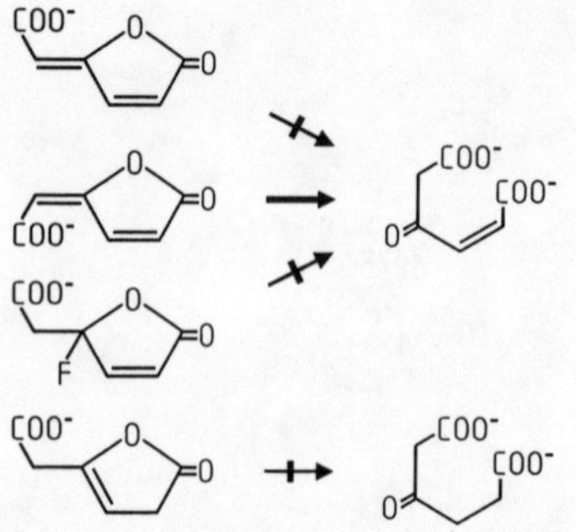

FIGURE 4. Substrate specificity of the DLH from *P. cepacia*.

has an amino acid composition that bears no resemblance to those of the above-mentioned hydrolases, suggesting that these enzymes are not related. The substrate specificities of the different types of DLH are summarized in Table 3.

A NEW THEME BY *ALCALIGENES*: MAR AND ITS ROLE IN THE DEGRADATION OF 2,4-D

Maleylacetate and chloromaleylacetate have long been known as intermediates of haloaromatic degradation (Fig. 1; Tiedje et al., 1969; Evans et al., 1971a; Evans et al., 1971b), and MAR activities have been shown to be present in 3CB-grown cells of strain B13 (Reineke, 1984) as well as in 2,4-D-grown cells of JMP134 (Pieper et al., 1988). Chapman (1979) suggested that the MAR would first reduce chloromaleylacetate to 5-chloro-3-oxoadipate, which by elimination of

TABLE 3
Substrates of different lactone hydrolases

Compound	Substrate[a]			
	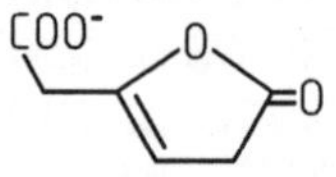	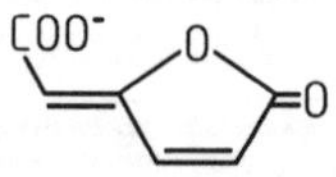	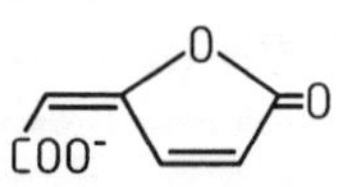	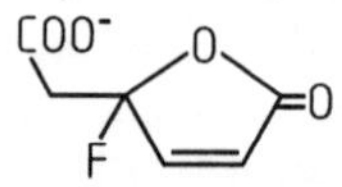
3-Oxoadipate enol-lactone hydrolase (different species)	+	−	−	+
DLH type I *A. eutrophus* JMP134 *A. eutrophus* JMP222 *A. eutrophus* 335	+	+	−	+
DLH type II *P. cepacia*	−	−	+	−
DLH type III *Pseudomonas* sp. strain B13 *A. eutrophus* JMP134	−	+	+	+

[a] +, Significant activity with given substrate; −, no significant activity.

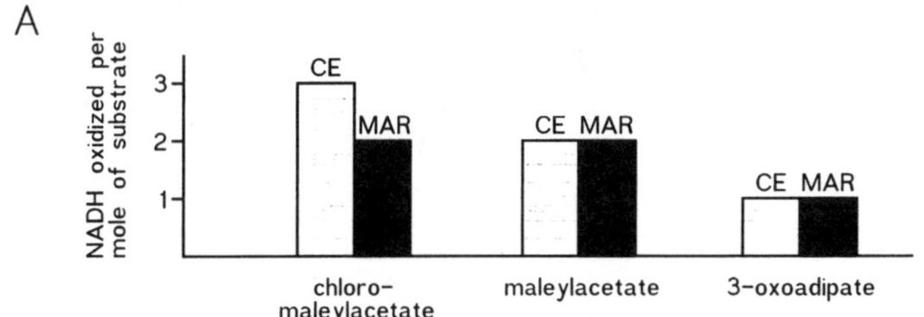

FIGURE 5. Reduction of chloromaleylacetate by crude extracts (CE) and purified MAR of *A. eutrophus* JMP134. (A) Schematic representation of amount of NADH oxidized per mole of substrate; (B) hypothetical interpretation of the results shown in panel A.

HCl would yield maleylacetate, the substrate of a second reduction by MAR (Fig. 1). These proposals were recently supported by Kukor et al. (1989), who showed that a MAR from a nonfluorescent pseudomonad can be recruited to complement the pathway encoded by pJP4. They observed a 18-kilodalton polypeptide in extracts of strains with cloned MAR and suggested that this enzyme might also play a role in tyrosine degradation.

During our investigation of enzymes from strain JMP134, we also partially purified and characterized the MAR of this strain. On the basis of mutagenesis experiments, it was proposed by Don et al. (1985) to be chromosomally encoded. This hypothesis was supported by anion-exchange chromatography, which showed that the MAR activities of JMP134 and JMP222 have the same retention volume (Schlömann, Ph.D. thesis, 1988). Furthermore, it was observed that chloromaleylacetate reductase and MAR activities coeluted from the column. These results are consistent with the findings of Chapman (1979) and Kukor et al. (1989).

However, when total NADH consumption by crude extract and by partially purified MAR was assayed with different substrates, some unexpected observations were made (Fig. 5A). Apparently, 3-oxoadipate is reduced in a possibly gratuitous and nonphysiological reaction to 3-hydroxyadipate (Fig. 5B). Whether this reaction is catalyzed by MAR or by a contaminant not separated from it during the purification procedure has not yet been investigated. The reduction of the oxo group in addition to the reduction of the olefinic double bond would explain the observed consumption of 2 mol of NADH per mol of maleylacetate (Fig. 5A). When chloromaleylacetate was used as substrate, crude extract from

2,4-D-grown cells of JMP134 catalyzed the oxidation of 3 mol of NADH per mol of chloromaleylacetate. These should represent the three reduction steps between chloromaleylacetate and 3-hydroxyadipate (Fig. 5B). Remarkably, partially purified MAR catalyzed the consumption of only 2 mol of NADH per mol of chloromaleylacetate. This result can be explained by assuming that a 5-chloro-3-oxoadipate dehalogenating enzyme was separated from MAR during the purification procedure. The NADH could then be consumed for the two subsequent reductions between chloromaleylacetate and 5-chloro-3-hydroxyadipate. The hypothesis that the dehalogenation of 5-chloro-3-oxoadipate is not or is not only a spontaneous reaction but is accelerated by an enzyme certainly needs further confirmation. If it should prove to be correct, this hypothesis would offer a good explanation for another open question: Don et al. (1985) observed that the gene product of *tfdF* was necessary for growth with 2,4-D but not for 3CB utilization. Their interpretation, based on the data of Schwien et al. (1988), that a chlorodienelactone isomerase activity is encoded by *tfdF* seems to be incorrect, since 2,4-dichloro-*cis*,*cis*-muconate apparently is directly converted to the chloro-*cis*-dienelactone. Frantz and Chakrabarty (1987), when sequencing the *clc* gene cluster of pAC27, also found a fourth open reading frame, to which a function could not be assigned. Further investigations will have to test the hypothesis that *tfdF* as well as the fourth open reading frame on pAC27 encode a protein with a 5-chloro-3-oxoadipate dehalogenating activity.

ACKNOWLEDGMENTS. We thank our colleagues who allowed us to cite their unpublished results. We are grateful to K. Stadler for perfect technical assistance. We also very much appreciate valuable and stimulating discussions with K.-L. Ngai, L. N. Ornston, J. J. Stezowski, K.-H. Engesser, W. Reineke, and E. Schmidt.

LITERATURE CITED

Aldrich, T. L., B. Frantz, J. F. Gill, J. J. Kilbane, and A. M. Chakrabarty. 1987. Cloning and complete nucleotide sequence determination of the *catB* gene encoding *cis*,*cis*-muconate lactonizing enzyme. *Gene* **52**:185–195.

Bollag, J.-M., G. G. Briggs, J. E. Dawson, and M. Alexander. 1968. 2,4-D metabolism. Enzymatic degradation of chlorocatechols. *J. Agric. Food Chem.* **16**:829–833.

Chapman, P. J. 1979. Degradation mechanisms, p. 28–66. *In* A. W. Bourquin and P. H. Pritchard (ed.), *Proceedings of the Workshop: Microbial Degradation of Pollutants in Marine Environments.* U.S. Environmental Protection Agency, Gulf Breeze, Fla.

Chatterjee, D. K., and A. M. Chakrabarty. 1983. Genetic homology between independently isolated chlorobenzoate-degradative plasmids. *J. Bacteriol.* **153**:532–534.

De Bont, J. A. M., M. J. A. W. Vorage, S. Hartmans, and W. J. J. van den Tweel. 1986. Microbial degradation of 1,3-dichlorobenzene. *Appl. Environ. Microbiol.* **52**:677–680.

Don, R. H., and J. M. Pemberton. 1981. Properties of six pesticide degradation plasmids isolated from *Alcaligenes paradoxus* and *Alcaligenes eutrophus*. *J. Bacteriol.* **145**:681–686.

Don, R. H., A. J. Weightman, H.-J. Knackmuss, and K. N. Timmis. 1985. Transposon mutagenesis and cloning analysis of the pathways for degradation of 2,4-dichlorophenoxyacetic acid and 3-chlorobenzoate in *Alcaligenes eutrophus* JMP134(pJP4). *J. Bacteriol.* **161**:85–90.

Dorn, E., M. Hellwig, W. Reineke, and H.-J. Knackmuss. 1974. Isolation and characterization of a 3-chlorobenzoate degrading pseudomonad. *Arch. Microbiol.* **99**:61–70.

Dorn, E., and H.-J. Knackmuss. 1978. Chemical structure and biodegradability of halogenated aromatic compounds. Substituent effects on 1,2-dioxygenation of catechol. *Biochem. J.* **174**:85–94.

Evans, W. C., B. S. W. Smith, H. N. Fernley, and J. I. Davies. 1971a. Bacterial metabolism of 2,4-dichlorophenoxyacetate. *Biochem. J.* **122**:543–551.

Evans, W. C., B. S. W. Smith, P. Moss, and H. N. Fernley. 1971b. Bacterial metabolism of 4-chlorophenoxyacetate. *Biochem. J.* **122:**509–517.

Frantz, B., and A. M. Chakrabarty. 1987. Organization and nucleotide sequence determination of a gene cluster involved in 3-chlorocatechol degradation. *Proc. Natl. Acad. Sci. USA* **84:**4460–4464.

Frantz, B., K.-L. Ngai, D. K. Chatterjee, L. N. Ornston, and A. M. Chakrabarty. 1987. Nucleotide sequence and expression of *clcD*, a plasmid-borne dienelactone hydrolase gene from *Pseudomonas* sp. strain B13. *J. Bacteriol.* **169:**704–709.

Friedrich, B., M. Meyer, and H. G. Schlegel. 1983. Transfer and expression of the herbicide-degrading plasmid pJP4 in aerobic autotrophic bacteria. *Arch. Microbiol.* **134:**92–97.

Ghosal, D., and I.-S. You. 1988. Nucleotide homology and organization of chlorocatechol oxidation genes of plasmids pJP4 and pAC27. *Mol. Gen. Genet.* **211:**113–120.

Goldman, A., D. L. Ollis, and T. A. Steitz. 1987. Crystal structure of muconate lactonizing enzyme at 3 Å resolution. *J. Mol. Biol.* **194:**143–153.

Haigler, B. E., S. F. Nishino, and J. C. Spain. 1988. Degradation of 1,2-dichlorobenzene by a *Pseudomonas* sp. *Appl. Environ. Microbiol.* **54:**294–301.

Knackmuss, H.-J., and M. Hellwig. 1978. Utilization and cooxidation of chlorinated phenols by *Pseudomonas* sp. B13. *Arch. Microbiol.* **117:**1–7.

Kukor, J. J., R. H. Olsen, and J.-S. Siak. 1989. Recruitment of a chromosomally encoded maleylacetate reductase for degradation of 2,4-dichlorophenoxyacetic acid by plasmid pJP4. *J. Bacteriol.* **171:**3385–3390.

Müller, R., and F. Lingens. 1986. Mikrobieller Abbau halogenierter Kohlenwasserstoffe: Ein Beitrag zur Lösung vieler Umweltprobleme? *Angew. Chem.* **98:**778–787.

Ngai, K.-L., and L. N. Ornston. 1988. Abundant expression of *Pseudomonas* genes for chlorocatechol metabolism. *J. Bacteriol.* **170:**2412–2413.

Pathak, D., K. L. Ngai, and D. Ollis. 1988. X-ray crystallographic structure of dienelactone hydrolase at 2.8 Å. *J. Mol. Biol.* **204:**435–445.

Pemberton, J. M., B. Corney, and R. H. Don. 1979. Evolution and spread of pesticide degrading ability among soil micro-organisms, p. 287–299. *In* K. N. Timmis and A. Pühler (ed.), *Plasmids of Medical, Environmental and Commercial Importance.* Elsevier/North-Holland Biochemical Press, Amsterdam.

Pieper, D. H., W. Reineke, K.-H. Engesser, and H.-J. Knackmuss. 1988. Metabolism of 2,4-dichlorophenoxyacetic acid, 4-chloro-2-methylphenoxyacetic acid and 2-methylphenoxyacetic acid by *Alcaligenes eutrophus* JMP134. *Arch. Microbiol.* **150:**95–102.

Reineke, W. 1984. Microbiol degradation of halogenated aromatic compounds, p. 319–360. *In* D. T. Gibson (ed.), *Microbial Degradation of Organic Compounds.* Marcel Dekker, Inc., New York.

Reineke, W., and H.-J. Knackmuss. 1978. Chemical structure and biodegradability of halogenated aromatic compounds. Substituent effects on 1,2-dioxygenation of benzoic acid. *Biochim. Biophys. Acta* **542:**412–423.

Reineke, W., and H.-J. Knackmuss. 1980. Hybrid pathway for chlorobenzoate metabolism in *Pseudomonas* sp. B13 derivatives. *J. Bacteriol.* **142:**467–473.

Reineke, W., and H.-J. Knackmuss. 1984. Microbial metabolism of haloaromatics: isolation and properties of a chlorobenzene-degrading bacterium. *Appl. Environ. Microbiol.* **47:**395–402.

Reineke, W., and H.-J. Knackmuss. 1988. Microbial degradation of haloaromatics. *Annu. Rev. Microbiol.* **42:**263–287.

Rochkind-Dubinsky, M. L., G. S. Sayler, and J. W. Blackburn. 1987. *Microbiological Decomposition of Chlorinated Aromatic Compounds.* Marcel Dekker, Inc., New York.

Schmidt, E., and H.-J. Knackmuss. 1980. Chemical structure and biodegradability of halogenated aromatic compounds. Conversion of chlorinated muconic acids into maleoylacetic acid. *Biochem. J.* **192:**339–347.

Schraa, G., M. L. Boone, M. S. M. Jetten, A. R. W. van Neerven, P. J. Colberg, and A. J. B. Zehnder. 1986. Degradation of 1,4-dichlorobenzene by *Alcaligenes* sp. strain A175. *Appl. Environ. Microbiol.* **52:**1374–1381.

Schwien, U., E. Schmidt, H.-J. Knackmuss, and W. Reineke. 1988. Degradation of chlorosubstituted aromatic compounds by *Pseudomonas* sp. strain B13: fate of 3,5-dichlorocatechol. *Arch. Microbiol.* **150:**78–84.

Streber, W. R., K. N. Timmis, and M. H. Zenk. 1987. Analysis, cloning, and high-level expression of 2,4-dichlorophenoxyacetate monooxygenase gene *tfdA* of *Alcaligenes eutrophus* JMP134. *J. Bacteriol.* **169**:2950–2955.

Surovtseva, E. G., V. S. Ivoilov, and Y. N. Karasevich. 1986. Metabolism of chlorinated anilines by *Pseudomonas diminuta. Mikrobiologiya* **55**:591–595.

Tiedje, J. M., J. M. Duxbury, M. Alexander, and J. E. Dawson. 1969. 2,4-D metabolism: pathway of degradation of chlorocatechols by *Arthrobacter* sp. *J. Agric. Food Chem.* **17**:1021–1026.

Weisshaar, M.-P., F. C. H. Franklin, and W. Reineke. 1987. Molecular cloning and expression of the 3-chlorobenzoate-degrading genes from *Pseudomonas* sp. strain B13. *J. Bacteriol.* **169**:394–402.

Zeyer, J., A. Wasserfallen, and K. N. Timmis. 1985. Microbial mineralization of ring-substituted anilines through an *ortho*-cleavage pathway. *Appl. Environ. Microbiol.* **50**:447–453.

Chapter 21

Metabolic Pathways for Biodegradation of Chlorobenzenes

J. C. Spain

Chlorobenzenes are used extensively as solvents, fumigants, deodorants, pesticides, and synthetic intermediates. Because of their patterns of use, a large fraction of the total production is released into the environment. For example, about 100,000 tons of *p*-dichlorobenzene (*p*-DCB) are released into the atmosphere annually (Rippen et al., 1984). The toxicity of the chlorobenzenes to higher organisms is relatively low, but recent preliminary studies have indicated that *p*-DCB may be a carcinogen (National Toxicology Program, 1987). In addition, detection of chlorobenzenes in groundwater has led to increasing concern about the fate and persistence of such compounds in the environment.

Chlorobenzoates and chlorophenols are degraded by a variety of bacteria, and their biochemistry and metabolic pathways have been studied extensively (Reinecke, 1984). The genetics and regulation of such pathways are understood well enough that strains that degrade chlorophenols or chlorobenzoates can be used as a basis for degradation of other halogenated aromatic compounds. In recent reviews, Chapman (1988) and Timmis et al. (1988) have described a variety of approaches to construction of bacterial strains for biodegradation of chloroaromatic compounds.

Biodegradation of chlorobenzenes has been reported in groundwater (Schwarzenbach et al., 1983), fixed-film columns (Bouwer and McCarty, 1982), and soil columns (Kuhn et al., 1985). However, until recently nothing was known about the pathways used by bacteria for metabolism of chlorobenzenes because strains able to grow on such compounds in pure culture had not been isolated. The toxicity of the chlorobenzenes accounts for much of the difficulty in isolation of bacteria able to degrade them. Recently, extended selected enrichment with the substrate provided at low concentrations in the vapor phase has allowed isolation of bacteria able to grow at the expense of chlorobenzenes. Reinecke and

---

J. C. Spain ● U.S. Air Force Engineering and Services Laboratory, Tyndall Air Force Base, Florida 32403.

Knackmuss (1984) isolated a chlorobenzene-degrading strain designated WR1306 after 9 months of chemostat selection during which benzene was gradually replaced with chlorobenzene as the growth substrate. The original inoculum was obtained from a mixture of soil and sewage. Similar approaches yielded an *Alcaligenes* (Schraa et al., 1986) and a *Pseudomonas* sp. (Spain and Nishino, 1987) able to degrade *p*-DCB; an *Alcaligenes* sp. able to degrade *m*-DCB (de Bont et al., 1986); a *Pseudomonas* sp. that grows on *o*-DCB (Haigler et al., 1988); and a *Pseudomonas* sp. able to grow on all the DCB isomers and 1,2,4-trichlorobenzene (van der Meer et al., 1987).

In addition to the strains isolated from natural systems, several chlorobenzene-degrading strains have been constructed in the laboratory. For example, a mating between a benzene degrader, *Pseudomonas putida* F1 (Gibson et al., 1968), and a chlorobenzoate degrader, *Pseudomonas* sp. strain B13 (Dorn et al., 1974), yielded a strain able to grow on chlorobenzene (Weisshaar et al., 1987). Extended selective enrichment yielded *P. putida* WR1323, which was able to grow on both chlorobenzene and *p*-DCB (Oltmanns et al., 1988). Similarly, Kröckel and Focht (1988) used a novel chemostat selection technique for construction of a strain of *P. putida* able to grow on both chlorobenzene and *p*-DCB. Chapman (1988) used a different approach to construct strains able to degrade chloro- and bromotoluenes by conjugal transfer of the TOL plasmid into a 3-chlorobenzoate-degrading *P. putida*.

METABOLIC PATHWAYS

The aerobic catabolism of each isomer of the chlorobenzenes proceeds by a similar sequence of reactions. In all of the systems studied to date, the initial attack is mediated by a dioxygenase which catalyzes the insertion of molecular oxygen into the aromatic ring to form a chlorosubstituted *cis*-dihydrodiol. The reactions appear to be identical to those catalyzed by toluene dioxygenase from *P. putida* F1, described by Gibson et al. (1968). Subsequent work (Gibson and Subramanian, 1984) showed that toluene dioxygenase could convert all of the DCB isomers to the corresponding *cis*-dihydrodiols. The *cis*-dihydrodiols were converted to the corresponding substituted catechols by a pyridine nucleotide-dependent dihydrodiol dehydrogenase. *P. putida* F1 could not metabolize the chlorocatechols, and they accumulated in the medium. In contrast, each of the chlorobenzene-degrading isolates investigated to date contains not only the dioxygenase enzyme system for initial attack on the chlorobenzenes, but also the enzymes of the modified *ortho* pathway (Evans et al., 1971; Dorn et al., 1974) for conversion of chlorocatechols to tricarboxylic acid cycle intermediates.

CHLOROBENZENE

The pathway described by Reinecke and Knackmuss (1984) for catabolism of chlorobenzene by strain WR1306 is shown in Fig. 1. The evidence for the pathway

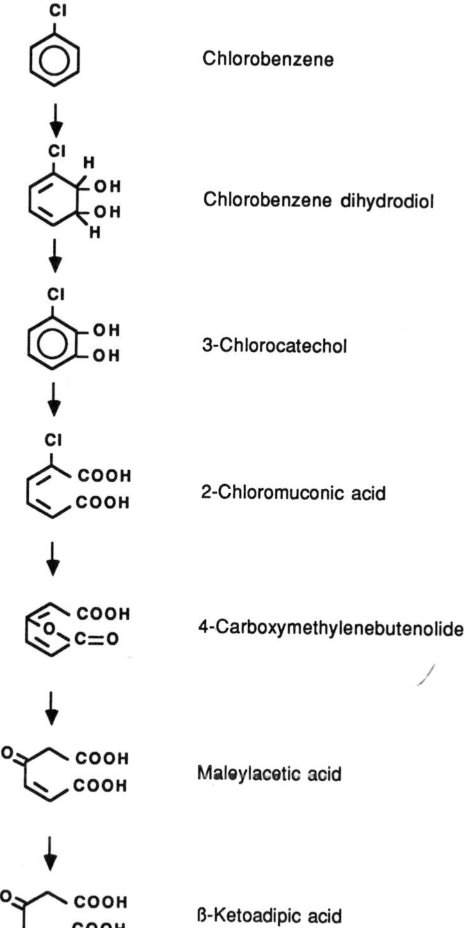

FIGURE 1. Pathway for metabolism of chlorobenzene by strain WR1306. Initial attack by a dioxygenase and dihydrodiol dehydrogenase results in the formation of 3-chlorocatechol. Ring fission by a 1,2-dioxygenase and subsequent lactonization lead to the loss of HCl and formation of a butenolide which is hydrolyzed to form maleylacetic acid. Maleylacetate reductase converts maleylacetate to β-ketoadipate (from Reinecke and Knackmuss, 1984).

is based on the detection in cell extracts of enzymes which catalyze each of the indicated reactions. The enzymes were induced in cells grown on chlorobenzene, but not in acetate-grown cells. The initial dioxygenase was not assayed in cell extracts because such enzymes have been shown in other systems to be unstable multicomponent enzyme systems (Gibson and Subramanian, 1984). The initial attack was carried out with high specificity and resulted in dioxygenation at the 2,3 position only. DCBs and substituted phenols were not oxidized by chlorobenzene-grown cells. Chlorobenzene-grown cells cooxidized toluene by what appeared to be a similar 2,3 attack, but accumulated a dead-end metabolite because they did not have the enzymes necessary for complete metabolism of the methyl-substituted catechol.

The 3-chloro-*cis*-1,2-dihydroxycyclohexa-3,5-diene (chlorobenzene dihydrodiol) presumed to be formed in the initial reaction was not detected, but an authentic sample was readily oxidized by a dihydrodiol dehydrogenase in cell extracts. Soluble enzymes in cell extracts degraded 3-chlorocatechol by a modified *ortho* cleavage pathway (Evans et al., 1971; Dorn and Knackmuss, 1978) in which a 1,2-dioxygenase catalyzed the ring-fission reaction, resulting in formation of 2-chloro-*cis,cis*-muconic acid. Cycloisomerization and concomitant loss of HCl yielded 4-carboxymethylene-but-2-en-4-olide, which was hydrolyzed to form maleylacetate. The maleylacetate was reduced to β-ketoadipic acid by maleylacetate reductase in a reaction requiring NADH.

Chlorobenzene-grown cultures of strain WR1306 contained only one enzyme for fission of the aromatic ring of 3-chlorocatechol. The type I pyrocatechase (Dorn and Knackmuss, 1978) was not present, and the inducible metapyrocatechase in the initial isolate was lost after continued cultivation on chlorobenzene. The induction of only a single enzyme for cleavage of the chlorocatechol was necessary to prevent misrouting of metabolites into unproductive pathways and to allow rapid growth of the isolate.

o-DCB

o-DCB degradation by *Pseudomonas* sp. strain JS100 is initiated by a dioxygenation at the 3,4 position (Haigler et al., 1988). Studies with radiolabeled 1,2-DCB revealed the presence of enzymes in cell extracts that converted *o*-DCB to the corresponding *o*-DCB dihydrodiol (Fig. 2). To date, this has been the only rigorous demonstration of this type of dioxygenation by enzymes in extracts prepared from cells grown on chlorobenzenes. The *o*-DCB dihydrodiol was converted to 3,4-dichlorocatechol by an NAD^+-dependent dihydrodiol dehydrogenase. Ring fission, lactonization, and hydrolysis reactions result in removal of one of the halogens and formation of 2-chloromaleylacetic acid. Subsequent steps for removal of the second halogen have not been determined.

Acetate-grown cells of JS100 contain constitutive levels of the initial dioxygenase and dihydrodiol dehydrogenase enzymes. Thus, when acetate-grown cells are transferred to *o*-DCB, the 3,4-dichlorocatechol accumulates in the medium and induces the synthesis of enzymes of the modified *ortho* ring-fission pathway. It is not clear whether 3,4-dichlorocatechol or a subsequent intermediate in the pathway serves as the actual inducer. The disadvantage of this mode of induction is that if uninduced cells are exposed to high concentrations of *o*-DCB, toxic levels of 3,4-dichlorocatechol can accumulate. Therefore, cells must be induced with low concentrations of *o*-DCB.

The chlorobenzene degrader WR1306 studied by Reinecke and Knackmuss (1984) contained a specific chlorobenzene dioxygenase that was strictly inducible. JS100, in contrast, elaborates a constitutive dioxygenase enzyme system that oxidizes a wide range of substituted benzenes. It is tempting to speculate that the chlorobenzene degrader WR1306 could not grow on *o*-DCB because the substrate and inducer specificity of the initial enzymes were narrow. The evolution necessary for an ancestral chlorobenzene degrader to gain the ability to degrade *o*-DCB might involve (i) loss of substrate specificity by mutation in a structural gene and (ii) loss of inducer specificity or conversion from strictly inducible to partly constitutive synthesis of the initial enzymes.

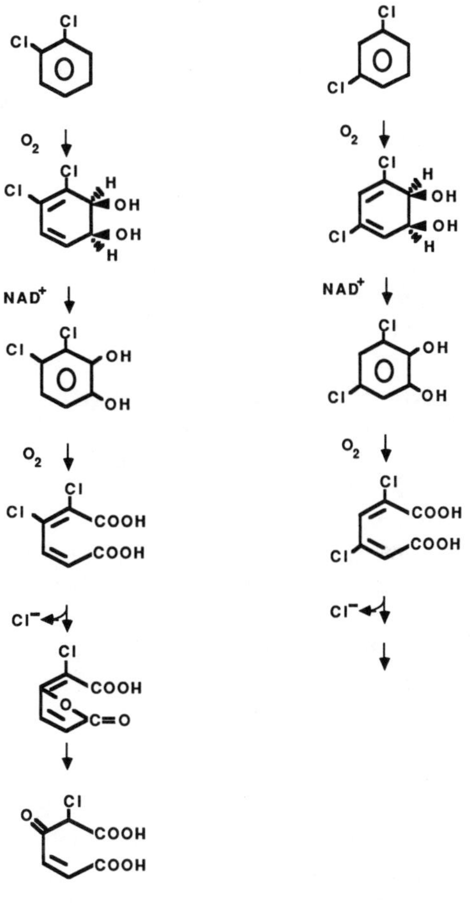

FIGURE 2. Metabolic pathway for degradation of *o*-DCB by *Pseudomonas* sp. strain JS100 (from Haigler et al., 1988) and *m*-DCB by *Alcaligenes* sp. strain OBB65 (from de Bont et al., 1986).

m-DCB

The initial steps in the biodegradation of *m*-DCB by an *Alcaligenes* sp. were described by de Bont et al. (1986). The reactions were analogous to those described for chlorobenzene degradation (Fig. 1) (Reinecke and Knackmuss, 1984). *m*-DCB was converted to the corresponding dichlorodihydrodiol, which was oxidized to 3,5-dichlorocatechol (Fig. 2). The dichlorocatechol was converted to 2,4-dichloromuconate by 1,2-dioxygenase enzymes in cell extracts. The initial enzymes for chlorobenzene degradation were constitutive in *Alcaligenes* sp. strain OBB65. This suggests that OBB65 might also have arisen from an ancestral chlorobenzene degrader with a more stringent inducer specificity.

p-DCB

p-DCB degradation has been studied more extensively than degradation of the other DCB isomers. The metabolic pathways used by *Alcaligenes* sp. (Schraa et al., 1986) and *Pseudomonas* sp. strain JS6 (Spain and Nishino, 1987) appear to be identical (Fig. 2). In *Pseudomonas* sp. strain JS6 the initial attack by a dioxygenase at the 2,3 position results in the formation of *p*-DCB dihydrodiol. The enzyme is very nonspecific and seems to be similar to the toluene dioxygenase system studied by Gibson et al. (D. T. Gibson, G. J. Zylstra, and S. Chauhan, this volume). In JS6, the activity is induced by toluene, chlorobenzene, and *p*-DCB. *p*-DCB dihydrodiol is oxidized to 3,6-dichlorocatechol in an NAD^+-dependent reaction. *p*-DCB-grown cells of JS6 contained both a catechol 1,2-dioxygenase and a 2,3-dioxygenase. The substrate range of the 1,2-dioxygenase indicated that it was a type II pyrocatechase (Dorn and Knackmuss, 1978) with high activity for chlorosubstituted catechols. The 2,3-dioxygenase was inhibited by chlorocatechols, yet it was active toward catechol in extracts of *p*-DCB-grown cells. The activity of the enzyme must somehow be suppressed in cells growing on chloroaromatic compounds, but the mechanism of such suppression is not known. *Alcaligenes* sp. strain A175 grown on *p*-DCB did not contain the 2,3-oxygenase (Schraa et al., 1986), and in this respect it was similar to the chlorobenzene degrader strain WR1306 (Reinecke and Knackmuss, 1984).

The 2,5-dichloromuconic acid formed by the action of the catechol 1,2-dioxygenase on 3,6-dichlorocatechol was assumed to be the *cis,cis* isomer, but the structure has not been rigorously determined. The enzyme that catalyzes lactonization of 2,5-dichloromuconic acid was inhibited by EDTA and seemed to require manganese ions for full activity, as is the case with the lactonizing enzyme studied by Schmidt and Knackmuss (1980). Lactonization and subsequent rearrangements resulted in the elimination of one of the halogens from the lactone. Hydrolysis of the lactone yielded 2-chloromaleylacetic acid, which was further metabolized in the presence of NADH. The mechanism of removal of the halogen from 2-chloromaleylacetic acid has not been proven, but the most likely explanation involves reduction of the double bond, elimination of HCl, and a second reduction to β-ketoadipic acid, all catalyzed by maleylacetic acid reductase as suggested by Chapman (1979).

SUBSTRATE RANGE OF STRAIN JS6

Strain JS6 and its derivatives have shown a very broad substrate range (Table 1) because they can synthesize the enzymes of several pathways for biodegradation of aromatic compounds. Furthermore, many of the enzymes are nonspecific and can accommodate a variety of substitutions on the aromatic substrates.

p-DCB-grown cells of JS6 can mineralize a variety of chlorophenols because the dioxygenase that attacks *p*-DCB can also catalyze the conversion of phenols to the corresponding catechols (Spain and Nishino, 1987; Spain and Gibson, 1988). The reaction seems to be a dihydroxylation of the phenol to form a trihydroxyl intermediate and then a spontaneous elimination of water to form the catechol. The reaction sequence in JS6 appears to be similar to that in *P. putida* F1, which contains toluene dioxygenase (Spain and Gibson, 1988), and to that in a *Pseudomonas* sp. which contains a naphthalene dioxygenase (Brilon et al.,

TABLE 1
Partial list of substituted aromatic compounds degraded by
Pseudomonas sp. strain JS6 or its derivatives[a]

Growth substrate	Compound
Chlorobenzene	*o*-DCB
Bromobenzene	*m*-DCB
Iodobenzene	1,2,4-Trichlorobenzene
p-DCB	Trichloroethylene
4-CT	4-Chlorophenol
2-Chlorobenzoate	2-Chlorophenol
3-Chlorobenzoate	3-Chlorophenol
4-Chlorobenzoate	2,5-Dichlorophenol
Toluene	
Benzene	
Ethylbenzene	
Phenol	
Benzoate	
p-Hydroxybenzoate	
Naphthalene	
Salicylate	

[a] Cooxidation experiments were done with toluene- or *p*-DCB-grown cells.

1981). Thus, the ability to hydroxylate phenols may be a common property in dioxygenase enzyme systems that oxidize nonpolar aromatic compounds.

JS6 grows on benzoate, but not on chlorobenzoates. However, spontaneous mutants able to grow on each of the isomers of chlorobenzoate can be readily isolated (B. E. Haigler and J. C. Spain, unpublished data). This suggests that JS6 can synthesize a benzoate dioxygenase able to oxidize the substituted benzoates. Benzoate-grown cells of JS6 contain the enzymes of the *ortho* pathway for metabolism of catechol (Ornston and Stanier, 1966). The enzymes of this pathway are specific and will not degrade chlorosubstituted catechols. In contrast, strains selected for the ability to grow on chlorobenzoates synthesize enzymes of the modified *ortho* pathway (Haigler and Spain, unpublished) for degradation of the chlorocatechols.

Strain JS6 grows on toluene by the use of toluene dioxygenase and the enzymes of the 2,3-oxygenase pathway for metabolism of 3-methylcatechol (Haigler and Spain, 1989). Preliminary results indicate that the toluene dioxygenase in JS6 is similar to that of *P. putida* F1 (Yeh et al., 1977) and similar to or identical with the dioxygenase induced by growth on *p*-DCB. These enzymes share the ability to oxidize a variety of compounds, including benzene, toluene, chlorobenzenes, trichloroethylene, chlorophenols, and methylphenols (Gibson et al., this volume). JS6 cannot grow on *p*-chlorotoluene (*p*-CT) because *p*-CT causes induction of the enzymes used for growth on toluene, but not the enzymes of the modified *ortho* pathway. The catechol 2,3-oxygenase which acts on 3-methylcatechol is inhibited by 3-chloro-6-methylcatechol formed from *p*-CT. Therefore, the chloromethylcatechol accumulates to toxic levels in the culture fluids. Spontaneous mutants of JS6 have been selected for the ability to grow on *p*-CT. Such mutants are found to have altered induction patterns such that the

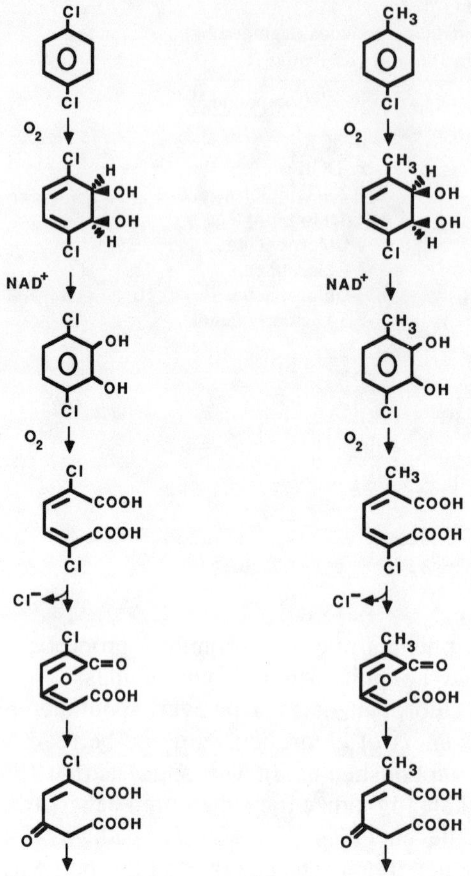

FIGURE 3. Pathway for metabolism of *p*-DCB by *Pseudomonas* sp. strain JS6 (from Spain and Nishino, 1987) and *p*-CT by a spontaneous mutant of JS6, strain JS21 (Haigler and Spain, 1989).

catechol 1,2-oxygenase and other enzymes of the modified *ortho* pathway are induced in response to *p*-CT (Haigler and Spain, 1989). The pathway for *p*-CT metabolism in JS21 (Fig. 3) is analogous to that for *p*-DCB degradation by JS6, except that 2-methyl- rather than 2-chloromaleylacetic acid is the product of hydrolysis of the lactone. The mechanism of 2-methylmaleylacetic acid degradation is not known; however, spontaneous mutants able to grow on 2-methylsuccinate can be readily isolated. This suggests that 2-methylmaleylacetic acid is converted to 3-oxo-5-methyladipic acid, which is hydrolyzed to methylsuccinate and acetate or their coenzyme A esters.

From the above discussion, it is clear that strain JS6 and its derivatives can synthesize a wide array of enzymes for conversion of substituted aromatic compounds to the corresponding catechols. The toluene dioxygenase enzyme system oxidizes toluene, benzene, ethylbenzene, and even trichloroethylene. A benzoate dioxygenase oxidizes benzoates and chlorobenzoates. Phenol hydroxylase can be induced for the oxidation of phenol (unpublished data). JS6 cannot grow on naphthalene, but the parental strain from which it was isolated, JS1, grows readily on both naphthalene and salicylate (C. A. Pettigrew and J. C. Spain, unpublished data). It appears to be able to synthesize two additional oxygenases, naphthalene dioxygenase and salicylate hydroxylase.

Three pathways are available in strain JS6 for the further oxidation of substituted catechols. The modified *ortho* pathway (Evans et al., 1971; Dorn et al., 1974), comprising a catechol 1,2-dioxygenase, chloromuconate cycloisomerase, butenolide hydrolase, and maleylacetate reductase, converts halogenated catechols. The *meta* ring-fission pathway, initiated by a catechol 2,3-dioxygenase (Gibson and Subramanian, 1984), is used for conversion of alkyl-substituted catechols, and the β-ketoadipate pathway (Ornston and Stanier, 1966) is used for degradation of the unsubstituted catechol formed from benzoate or benzene. The availability of a variety of enzymes for conversion of aromatic compounds to catechols, along with the ability to degrade substituted catechols by three different pathways, allows strain JS6 and its derivatives to grow on a wide range of aromatic substrates (Table 1). Furthermore, cells grown on several of these substrates can cooxidize a number of related compounds that cannot induce the appropriate enzymes. Thus, this strain has considerable potential for practical application in biodegradation of hazardous wastes where a variety of aromatic solvents must be removed. Additional work must be done, however, to discover what controls regulate synthesis of the enzymes of these pathways and how misrouting of intermediates is avoided.

LITERATURE CITED

Bouwer, E. J., and P. L. McCarty. 1982. Removal of trace chlorinated organic compounds by activated carbon and fixed-film bacteria. *Environ. Sci. Technol.* **16**:836–843.

Brilon, C., W. Beckmann, and H.-J. Knackmuss. 1981. Catabolism of naphthalenesulfonic acids by *Pseudomonas* sp. A3 and *Pseudmonas* sp. C22. *Appl. Environ. Microbiol.* **42**:44–55.

Chapman, P. J. 1979. Degradation mechanisms, p. 29–69. *In* A. W. Bourquin and P. H. Pritchard (ed.), *Microbial Degradation of Pollutants in Marine Environments.* EPA-600/9-79-012. U.S. Environmental Protection Agency, Washington, D.C.

Chapman, P. J. 1988. Constructing microbial strains for degradation of halogenated aromatic compounds, p. 81–95. *In* G. S. Omenn (ed.), *Environmental Biotechnology: Reducing the Risks from Environmental Pollution through Biotechnology.* Plenum Publishing Corp., New York.

de Bont, J. A. M., M. J. A. Vorage, S. Hartmans, and W. J. J. van den Tweel. 1986. Microbial degradation of 1,3-dichlorobenzene. *Appl. Environ. Microbiol.* **52**:677–680.

Dorn, E., M. Hellwig, W. Reineke, and H.-J. Knackmuss. 1974. Isolation and characterization of a 3-chlorobenzoate degrading pseudomonad. *Arch. Microbiol.* **99**:61–70.

Dorn, E., and H.-J. Knackmuss. 1978. Chemical structure and biodegradability of halogenated aromatic compounds. Two catechol 1,2-dioxygenases from a 3-chlorobenzoate-grown pseudomonad. *Biochem. J.* **174**:73–84.

Evans, W. C., B. S. W. Smith, H. N. Fernley, and J. I. Davies. 1971. Bacterial metabolism of 2,4-dichlorophenoxyacetate. *Biochem. J.* **122**:543–551.

Gibson, D. T., J. R. Koch, and R. E. Kallio. 1968. Oxidative degradation of aromatic hydrocarbons by microorganisms. I. Enzymatic formation of catechol from benzene. *Biochemistry* **7**:2653–2662.

Gibson, D. T., and V. Subramanian. 1984. Microbial degradation of aromatic hydrocarbons, p. 181–252. *In* D. T. Gibson (ed.), *Microbial Degradation of Organic Compounds.* Marcel Dekker, Inc., New York.

Haigler, B. E., S. F. Nishino, and J. C. Spain. 1988. Degradation of 1,2-dichlorobenzene by a *Pseudomonas* sp. *Appl. Environ. Microbiol.* **54**:294–301.

Haigler, B. E., and J. C. Spain. 1989. Degradation of *p*-chlorotoluene by a mutant strain of *Pseudomonas* sp. strain JS6. *Appl. Environ. Microbiol.* **55**:372–379.

Kröckel, L., and D. D. Focht. 1988. Construction of chlorobenzene-utilizing recombinants by progenitive manifestation of a rare event. *Appl. Environ. Microbiol.* **53:**2470–2475.

Kuhn, E. P., P. Colberg, L. Schnoor, O. Wanner, A. J. B. Zehnder, and R. P. Schwarzenbach. 1985. Microbial transformation of substituted benzenes during infiltration of river water to groundwater: laboratory column studies. *Environ. Sci. Technol.* **19:**961–968.

National Toxicology Program. 1987. *National Toxicology Program Technical Report on the Toxicology and Carcinogenesis Studies of 1,4-Dichlorobenzene (CAS no. 106-46-7) in F344/N Rats and B6C3F Mice (Gavage Studies).* National Institutes of Health publication no. 86-2757. Department of Health and Human Services, Research Triangle Park, N.C.

Oltmanns, R. H., H. G. Rast, and W. R. Reineke. 1988. Degradation of 1,4-dichlorobenzene by enriched and constructed bacteria. *Appl. Microbiol. Biotechnol.* **28:**609–616.

Ornston, L. N., and R. Y. Stanier. 1966. The conversion of catechol and protocatechuate to beta ketoadipate by *Pseudomonas putida.* I. Biochemistry. *J. Biol. Chem.* **241:**3776–3786.

Reineke, W. 1984. Microbial degradation of halogenated aromatic compounds, p. 319–360. *In* D. T. Gibson (ed.), *Microbial Degradation of Organic Compounds.* Marcel Dekker, Inc., New York.

Reineke, W., and H.-J. Knackmuss. 1984. Microbial metabolism of haloaromatics: isolation and properties of a chlorobenzene-degrading bacterium. *Appl. Environ. Microbiol.* **47:**395–402.

Rippen, G., W. Klopffer, R. Frische, and K. Gunther. 1984. The environmental model segment approach for estimating potential environmental concentrations. *Exotoxicol. Environ. Safety.* **8:**363–377.

Schmidt, E., and H.-J. Knackmuss. 1980. Chemical structure and biodegradability of halogenated aromatic compounds. Conversion of chlorinated muconic acids into maleoylacetic acid. *Biochem. J.* **192:**339–347.

Schraa, G., M. L. Boone, M. S. M. Jetten, A. R. W. Van-Neerven, P. J. Colberg, and A. J. Zehnder. 1986. Degradation of 1,4-dichlorobenzene by *Alcaligenes* sp. strain A175. *Appl. Environ. Microbiol.* **52:**1374–1381.

Schwarzenbach, R. P., W. Ginger, E. Hoehn, and J. R. Schneider. 1983. Behavior of organic compounds during infiltration of river water to groundwater: field studies. *Environ. Sci. Technol.* **17:**472–479.

Spain, J. C., and D. T. Gibson. 1988. Oxidation of substituted phenols by *Pseudomonas putida* F1 and *Pseudomonas* sp. strain JS6. *Appl. Environ. Microbiol.* **54:**1399–1404.

Spain, J. C., and S. F. Nishino. 1987. Degradation of 1,4-dichlorobenzene by a *Pseudomonas* sp. *Appl. Environ. Microbiol.* **53:**1010–1019.

Timmis, K. N., F. Rojo, and J. L. Ramos. 1988. Prospects for laboratory engineering of bacteria to degrade pollutants, p. 61–79. *In* G. S. Omenn (ed.), *Environmental Biotechnology: Reducing Risks from Environmental Chemicals through Biotechnology.* Plenum Publishing Corp., New York.

van der Meer, J. R., W. Roelofsen, G. Schraa, and A. J. B. Zehnder. 1987. Degradation of low concentrations of dichlorobenzenes and 1,2,4-trichlorobenzene by *Pseudomonas* sp. strain P51 in nonsterile soil columns. *FEMS Microbiol. Ecol.* **45:**333–341.

Weisshaar, M.-P., F. C. H. Franklin, and W. Reineke. 1987. Molecular cloning and expression of the 3-chlorobenzoate-degrading genes from *Pseudomonas* sp. strain B13. *J. Bacteriol.* **169:**394–402.

Yeh, W. K., D. T. Gibson, and E. Liu. 1977. Toluene dioxygenase: a multicomponent enzyme system. *Biochem. Biophys. Res. Commun.* **78:**401–410.

Chapter 22

Subtle Selection and Novel Mutation during Evolutionary Divergence of the β-Ketoadipate Pathway

L. Nicholas Ornston, John Houghton, Ellen L. Neidle, and Leslie A. Gregg

THE β-KETOADIPATE PATHWAY, A WIDELY DISTRIBUTED BIOLOGICAL TRAIT

The generic designation *Pseudomonas* gathers diverse organisms, and one of the challenges of systematics is to find traits that unify taxa within this biological group. A trait that deserves to be examined is the β-ketoadipate pathway, a metabolic mechanism for assimilation of aromatic and hydroaromatic growth substrates (Fig. 1). The pathway is universally shared by fluorescent *Pseudomonas* species (Stanier et al., 1966). Full appreciation of the breadth of the biological distribution of the pathway sometimes requires somewhat indirect observation. For example, discovery that the pathway is utilized by members of the acidovorans group, a major subdivision within *Pseudomonas*, could be described as a series of surprises (Buvinger et al., 1981; Ornston and Ornston, 1972; Robert-Gero et al., 1969) because these organisms were known to degrade aromatic compounds by *meta*-cleavage pathways, metabolic sequences in which β-ketoadipate is not an intermediate (Fig. 2). In these bacteria, the metabolic direction taken at the level of catechol cleavage depends on conditions of growth.

In the laboratory, bacterial growth generally is observed visually, and a substantial amount of growth must take place before colonies on plates or turbidity in tubes becomes apparent. Potential nutrients can prove to be toxic at concentrations that might support such growth, and therefore the nutritional potential of organisms can be masked if they are exposed to substrates at concentrations greatly exceeding those that might be encountered in the natural

---

L. Nicholas Ornston, John Houghton, and Leslie A. Gregg ● Department of Biology, Yale University, New Haven, Connecticut 06511. *Ellen L. Neidle* ● Department of Microbiology, University of Illinois, 407 South Goodwin Avenue, Urbana, Illinois 61801.

environment. By using auxanography to provide a gentle gradient of growth substrate, it was possible to demonstrate that the β-ketoadipate pathway is a universal trait in the members of the family *Rhizobiaceae*. This diverse set of organisms is grouped largely according to their potential to interact with plants, and the ubiquitous presence of the β-ketoadipate pathway in the *Rhizobiaceae* suggests that aromatic compounds may contribute to their interactions with their hosts (Parke and Ornston, 1984).

β-KETOADIPATE IN THE ENVIRONMENT

The β-ketoadipate pathway acquired its name because the compound accumulated transiently in laboratory cultures during growth with an aromatic substrate (Kilby, 1948). What happens in the laboratory may occasionally happen in the environment, and therefore it is possible that β-ketoadipate is formed in niches in which aromatic or hydroaromatic compounds are metabolized. As judged by the physiological preparedness of the bradyrhizobia, this would seem to be the case. These bacteria constitutively respond to β-ketoadipate as a chemoattractant (Parke et al., 1985). Furthermore, the organisms, known for their slow growth, constitutively form the coenzyme A transferase that acts on β-ketoadipate (Parke and Ornston, 1986). Such constitutive expression of genes associated with aromatic metabolism is highly exceptional, and it is noteworthy that the level of coenzyme A transferase expression in the slow growers rivals that found in rapidly growing *Pseudomonas* cultures under conditions causing full enzyme induction (Parke and Ornston, 1986). It would appear that the bradyrhizobia are evolutionarily adapted to be ready to grow with β-ketoadipate.

β-KETOADIPATE TRANSPORT AND STARVATION SURVIVAL

For many years, prevailing evidence indicated that extracellular β-ketoadipate did not make a significant contribution to the physiology of *Pseudomonas* species. Outlines of pathways for aromatic metabolism were established by simultaneous adaptation, a technique that rested on the capacity of physiologically preadapted whole cells to respire growth substrates and metabolites formed therefrom (Stanier, 1951). In studies with the organism that now is the biotype strain for *Pseudomonas putida*, Stanier established that β-ketoadipate, known to be an intermediate in aromatic metabolism, did not permeate the cell membrane at a rate sufficient to permit rapid respiration (Stanier, 1951). On the basis of this and related observations, it seemed likely that the negatively charged metabolites formed after oxygenative ring cleavage (Fig. 1) did not diffuse readily across the cell membrane and therefore that the biological function of the pathway was restricted largely to growth with aromatic or hydroaromatic substrates.

This view was challenged by the observation that selective enrichment from natural samples with muconate, the product of the *ortho* cleavage of catechol (Fig. 2), tended to yield *Pseudomonas* species in the acidovorans group (Robert-Gero

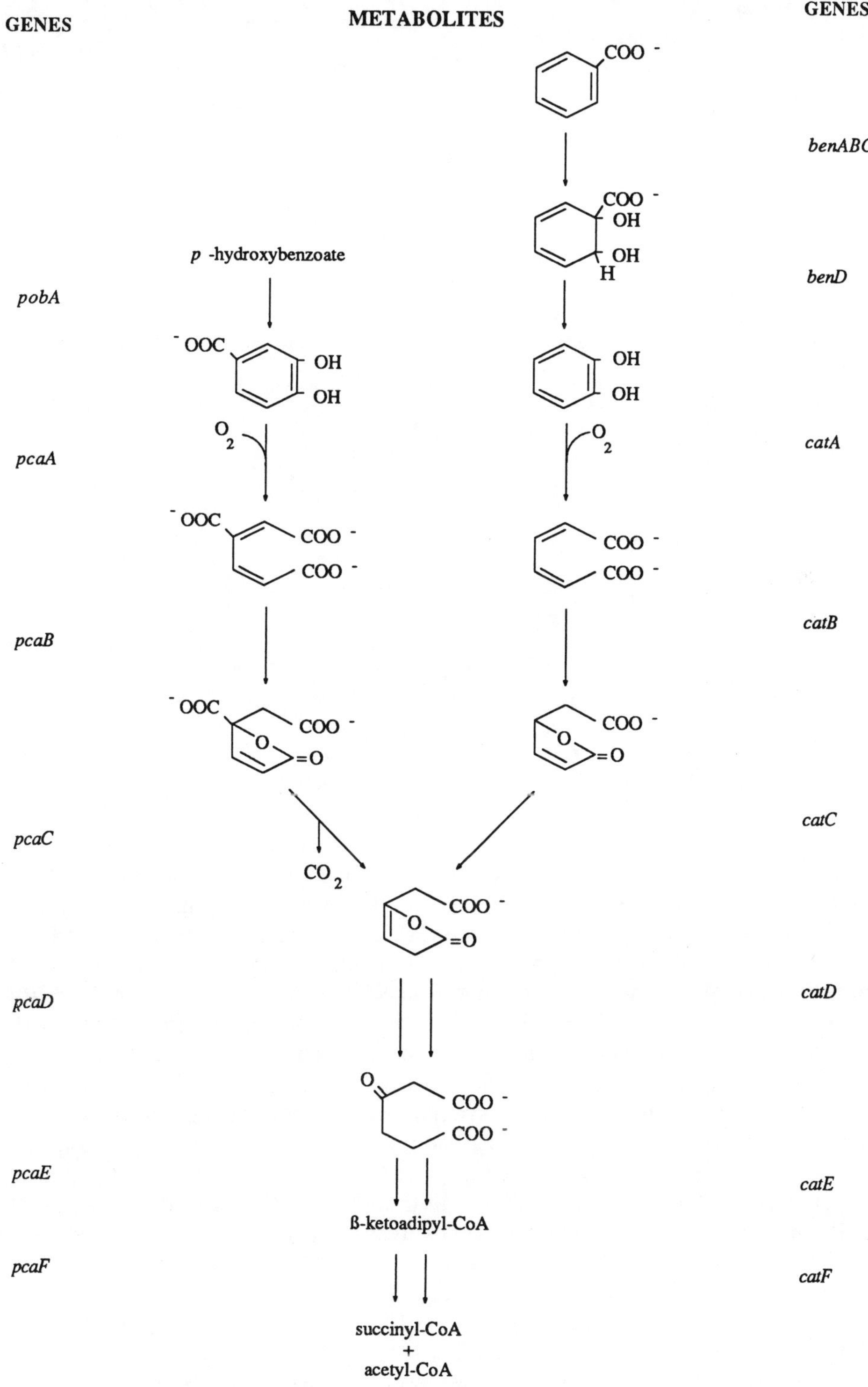

FIGURE 1. Pathways for aromatic catabolism in *Acinetobacter calcoaceticus*.

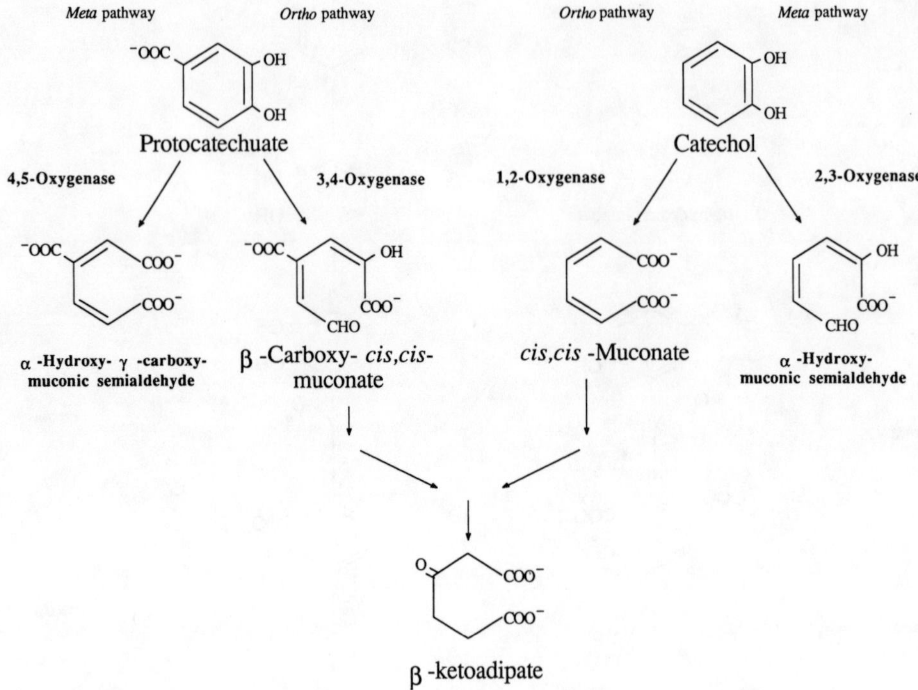

FIGURE 2. Divergent pathways for dissimilation of aromatic compounds via protocatechuate and catechol. Oxygenative ring fission by *ortho* cleavage leads to formation of β-ketoadipate. This metabolite is not formed in pathways initiated by *meta* cleavage of the diphenols.

et al., 1969). Indeed, the capacity to utilize muconate could be acquired by mutation in *P. putida* (Ornston, 1966), although such mutations proved to be genetically unstable (Ornston and Parke, 1976a). The inference that extracellular β-ketoadipate could make a contribution to the physiology of *P. putida* emerged from analysis of mutant strains that had been selected on the basis of their ability to grow relatively rapidly when exposed to β-ketoadipate as the sole growth substrate (Parke and Ornston, 1976). When initially isolated, the mutant organisms were curiosities because they constitutively formed enzymes that gave rise to β-ketoadipate. Constitutive expression of these enzymes cannot have been the direct target of selection with β-ketoadipate; the presumed target of selection, the coenzyme A transferase that acts upon the compound, remained inducible in the mutant strains. An unexpected finding was that the mutations causing constitutive enzyme synthesis also caused high level expression of a transport system that acts on β-ketoadipate, a compound that was presumed not to diffuse readily across the cell membrane of *P. putida* (Ornston and Parke, 1976b).

The β-ketoadipate transport system is formed inducibly, albeit at relatively low levels, in wild-type cells, and similar systems have been found in divergent fluorescent *Pseudomonas* species (Ondrako and Ornston, 1980). Traits that are conserved are likely to have been selected, and it is reasonable to speculate on what the selective benefit of the β-ketoadipate transport system is. One clue emerges from its regulation. The system is expressed optimally in starved cells; it is both repressed and inhibited by compounds that provide cells with energy (Ornston and Parke, 1976b). Endogenous energy reserves are sufficient to maintain the system during several weeks of starvation, and the reserves also provide enough energy to allow starved cells to concentrate adipate, a nonmetabolizable analog of β-ketoadipate in *P. putida* (Harwood and Ornston, 1988). Since the physiological function of the transport system, largely unexpressed in growing cells, is called into play during starvation, it seems most likely that the system makes a contribution during survival by scavenging extracellular β-ketoadipate. A similar interpretation may account for the physiological properties of an inducible system that transports carboxymuconate into *P. putida* (Meagher et al., 1972).

Adipate does not support the growth of *P. putida*, but it invariably serves as a growth substrate for members of the closely related species *Pseudomonas aeruginosa* (Stanier et al., 1966). The biological relatedness of the species raises the possibility that their nutritional niches overlap. If so, adipate is likely to be encountered by *P. putida* in the natural environment, and the cells must control a potentially fatal process: futile transport of adipate during starvation of *P. putida* could deplete energy reserves and thus might threaten survival of the bacteria. This indeed seems to be the case. Mutations causing overexpression of the transport system proved lethal when starved cells were exposed to adipate; cells exerting stringent wild-type control over the β-ketoadipate transport system were unharmed by adipate during starvation (Harwood and Ornston, 1988).

β-KETOADIPATE AS A REGULATORY METABOLITE

The β-ketoadipate transport system poses risks to *P. putida*, and its continued selection suggests that the metabolite plays a significant role in the physiology of the bacteria. This inference is supported by the central function of the compound as an inducer of gene expression (Ornston, 1966). The available evidence indicates that β-ketoadipate exerts its regulatory effect in combination with a transcriptional activator, the *pcaR* gene (Hughes et al., 1988). This gene has been cloned and shown to lie about 15 kilobase pairs (kbp) upstream from the *pcaBDC* operon, which it governs (Fig. 3). Enzymes encoded by this operon give rise to β-ketoadipate (Fig. 1) and are formed constitutively as a consequence of mutations that lead to overexpression of the β-ketoadipate transport system (Parke and Ornston, 1976). The constitutive mutations do not alter the expression of other genes that are governed by *pcaR*. These include the unlinked *pcaE* gene, encoding the enzyme that acts on β-ketoadipate (Hughes et al., 1988), and genes for benzoate chemotaxis (C. Harwood, personal communication).

Perhaps induction of the benzoate chemotactic system (Harwood et al., 1984) is the most remarkable physiological control exerted by β-ketoadipate. Formation of the inducer from benzoate requires six metabolic steps and expression of no less than nine structural genes. The TOL plasmid contains enzymes that direct

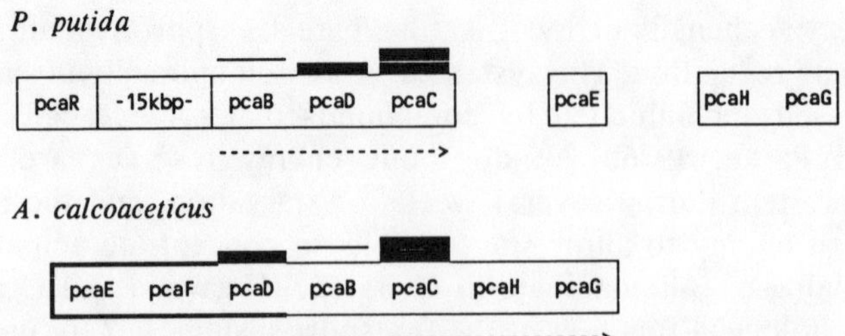

FIGURE 3. Rearrangements that occurred during evolution of *pca* genes in the chromosomes of *P. putida* and *A. calcoaceticus*. Arrows indicate the order of transcription of genes within operons, and contiguous boxes enclose the designations of genes that are known to be clustered. The *pca* genes of *P. putida* are relatively scattered and, except for *pcaHG*, are induced by β-ketoadipate through the intermediacy of the transcriptional activator encoded by *pcaR*. The *A. calcoaceticus pca* structural genes are linked within a single operon that is expressed in response to protocatechuate. Distinctive markings above *pcaB*, *pcaC*, and *pcaD* draw attention to their rearrangement during their evolutionary divergence.

metabolic flow of catechol through *meta* cleavage and thus away from β-ketoadipate formation. Thus, the TOL plasmid, encoding all of the enzymes for metabolism of benzoate via an alternative pathway, prevents induction of the system that attracts the cells to benzoate (Harwood and Ornston, 1984). A similar metabolic system is found in *Azotobacter* spp. (Durham and Ornston, 1980). These organisms metabolize catechol via *meta* cleavage and therefore appear not to give rise to β-ketoadipate during growth with benzoate. On the other hand, they utilize protocatechuate by a metabolic system that seems closely homologous to the β-ketoadipate pathway of *P. putida* and is regulated in a similar manner. If *Azobacter* spp. form an inducible benzoate chemotaxis system, the cells must be regulated by a mechanism divergent from that exercised in *P. putida*.

CONSERVATION OF TRANSCRIPTIONAL CONTROLS IN SOME BACTERIA AND REARRANGEMENT OF STRUCTURAL GENES DURING DIVERGENCE OF TRANSCRIPTIONAL CONTROLS IN OTHER BACTERIA

Patterns of transcriptional control exercised over the *pca* genes are common to fluorescent pseudomonads (Kemp and Hegeman, 1968; Ornston, 1966), *Azotobacter* spp. (Durham and Ornston, 1980), and, with some minor variation, *Pseudomonas cepacia* (Zylstra et al., 1989). In all of these bacteria, the role of β-ketoadipate as an inducer is central. The only other metabolite that acts as an inducer of enzymes associated with protocatechuate metabolism is protocatechuate itself, and the sole genes governed by this metabolite are the *pcaHG* genes that encode protocatechuate oxygenase (Hosokawa, 1970). Distinctive forms of transcriptional control are exercised in gram-positive organisms (Cain, 1980), rhizobia (Parke and Ornston, 1986), *Alcaligenes eutrophus* (Johnson and Stanier, 1971), pseudomonads of the acidovorans group (Ornston and Ornston, 1972), and

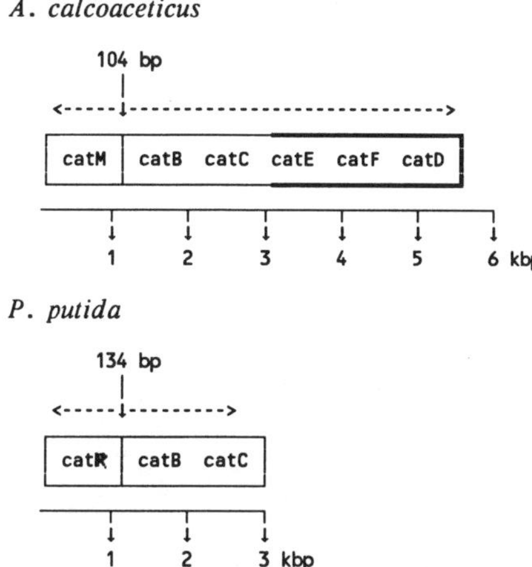

FIGURE 4. Organization of *cat* genes in *A. calco-aceticus* and *P. putida*. Divergently transcribed from *catB* are *catM*, a repressor gene in *A. calco-aceticus*, and *catR*, a transcriptional activator in *P. putida*.

Acinetobacter calcoaceticus (Canovas and Stanier, 1967). Of these, the system most thoroughly characterized at the gene level is the *pca* operon of *A. calcoaceticus* (Doten et al., 1987b); the arrangement of these genes is compared with the organization of *P. putida pca* genes (Hughes et al., 1988) in Fig. 3.

A. calcoaceticus pca genes are linked within a single operon that is expressed in response to a single inducer, protocatechuate (Fig. 3). β-Ketoadipate, a cardinal inducer of independently transcribed genes in *P. putida*, has no known inducing function in *A. calcoaceticus*; evidently, these bacteria have no requirement for a functional equivalent of the *pcaR* transcriptional activator gene. Isofunctional *pca* genes from *A. calcoaceticus* and *P. putida* share common ancestors (Durham et al., 1980; Yeh et al., 1980a, 1980b; Yeh and Ornston, 1981), so the differences in gene organization shown in Fig. 3 were achieved in part by rearrangement of structural genes during evolutionary divergence. Perhaps the most remarkable rearrangement shifted the order of *pca* genes that are transcribed consecutively in the two bacterial species. The transcriptional order of the *pcaB* and *pcaD* genes, part of the *pcaBDC* operon in *P. putida* (Hughes et al., 1988), is reversed within the *pcaEFDBCHG* operon of *A. calcoaceticus* (Doten et al., 1987b; Fig. 3).

A further indication of gene rearrangement during evolution is revealed by examination of the *cat* genes of *A. calcoaceticus* (Fig. 4). The *catEFD* genes encode enzymes isofunctional with the respective *pcaEFD* genes, and the two regions of *A. calcoaceticus* DNA share regions of close sequence homology (Doten et al., 1987b; Shanley et al., 1986). The *pcaEFD* genes are transcribed at the beginning of the *pcaEFDBCHG* operon (Fig. 3), and the homologous *catEFD* genes are transcribed at the end of the *catBCEFD* operon (Fig. 4). The *catEFD* genes have no counterpart in *P. putida*, in which their physiological function is fulfilled by the apparently unlinked *pcaD*, *pcaE*, and *pcaF* genes.

EVOLUTIONARY DIVERGENCE OF A REGULATORY GENE PRODUCED POSITIVE TRANSCRIPTIONAL CONTROL IN *P. PUTIDA* AND NEGATIVE TRANSCRIPTIONAL CONTROL IN *A. CALCOACETICUS*

A similarity between the *A. calcoaceticus catBCEFD* and *P. putida catBC* operons is that they are governed by regulatory genes each of which, directly upstream from *catB*, is transcribed divergently from this gene (Fig. 4). Both regulatory gene products respond to the inducer muconate, and the regulatory genes, designated *catM* in *A. calcoaceticus* (Neidle et al., 1989) and *catR* in *P. putida* (Wu et al., 1972; J. E. Houghton, E. J. Hughes, J. S. Williamson, and L. N. Ornston, *Abstr. Annu. Meet. Am. Soc. Microbiol. 1988*, K-4, p. 207), share common ancestry (Fig. 5). The genes are members of the *lysR* evolutionary family of regulatory proteins (Henikoff et al., 1988). Most of these proteins are transcriptional activators, and *P. putida catR* is no exception. Inactivation of this gene by spontaneous mutation (Wheelis and Ornston, 1972) or by insertion of Tn5 (E. J. Hughes, J. E. Houghton, and L. N. Ornston, unpublished data) prevents expression of either the *catBC* operon or the separately transcribed *catA* gene. In contrast to *P. putida catR*, *A. calcoaceticus catM* encodes a repressor: mutations in *catM* result in constitutive expression of *cat* structural genes (Neidle et al., 1989). Thus the regulatory proteins, evolutionarily homologous and similar in many respects, differ in that *catR* exercises positive control and *catM* exerts negative control.

EVOLUTION SELECTED FOR CLUSTERING OF INDEPENDENTLY TRANSCRIBED GENES

Numerous gene rearrangements occurred during evolutionary divergence of the β-ketoadipate pathway, and if unconstrained by selection, these events might have led to the scattering of independently transcribed genes to distant chromosomal positions. Contrary to this expectation, independently transcribed genes for physiologically related metabolic functions often are clustered in the chromosome. This phenomenon, first suggested by transductional analysis of *P. putida* (Wheelis and Stanier, 1970) and *P. aeruginosa* (Rosenberg and Hegeman, 1969), has been fully documented by cloning and sequencing of 16 kbp of DNA encompassing the 12 structural genes associated with benzoate utilization in *A. calcoaceticus* (Neidle et al., 1987; Shanley et al., 1986). The clustered genes appear to be organized in four separate transcriptional units (Fig. 6), and with the possible exception of three open reading frames of unknown function, this region of DNA appears to be associated solely with benzoate and catechol utilization.

One interpretation for the clustering of *ben* and *cat* genes is that this form of organization allows them to fall under some kind of global regulatory control. Possibilities for physiological interactions among the genes are accentuated by knowledge that a single gene may be expressed in response to structurally dissimilar metabolites (Neidle and Ornston, 1987). Evidently, the genes fall under several layers of transcriptional control, as illustrated by the fact that the *catA*

```
                                10                    20                    30                    40
Acinetobacter repressor  MetGluLeuArgHisLeuArgTyrPheValThrValValGluGluGlnSerIleSerLysAlaAlaGluLysLeuCysIleAlaGlnProProLeuSerArgGlnIleGlnLysLeuGlu
                         ||||||||||||||||||||||||||       |||        |||||||||    |||    |||||||||||||||||||||||||||||||||||||||       ||||||
Pseudomonas activator    MetGluLeuArgHisLeuArgTyrPheLysValLeuAlaGluThrLeuAsnPheThrArgAlaAlaGluLeuLeuHisIleAlaGlnProProLeuSerArgGlnIleSerGlnLeuGlu
                                10                    20                    30                    40

                           .         .        30         .         .        60         .         .        90         .         .       120
Acinetobacter catM       ATGGAACTAAGACACCTCAGATATTTTGTGACCGTGGTTGAAGAGCAAAGCATTTCCAAAGCTGCTGAAAAGTTGTGTATTGCCCAGCCGCCCCTCAGCCGACAAATTCAAAAACTCGAA
                         |||||       ||||||                                                        ||||||||| ||||||||| |||||           ||||||
Pseudomonas catR         ATGGAGCTGCGCCACCTGCGTTACTTCAAGGTCTTGGCCGAGACCCTGAACTTCACCCGCGCCGCCGAGCTGCTGCACATTGCCCAACCGCCCCTGAGCCGGCAGATCAGCCAGCTGGAG
                           .         .        30         .         .        60         .         .        90         .         .       120
```

FIGURE 5. Homologous sequences corresponding to the NH$_2$-terminal amino acid region of *cat* regulatory gene products from *A. calcoaceticus* and *P. putida*. Vertical lines connect amino acids that are identical in the aligned sequences. Vertical lines connect aligned DNA nucleotides where sequence identities of four or more contiguous bases appear. This relatively stringent measure of sequence homology calls attention to high DNA sequence similarity in the region between nucleotides 79 and 101 of the aligned genes. The same measure of DNA sequence homology is used in Fig. 7 and 8.

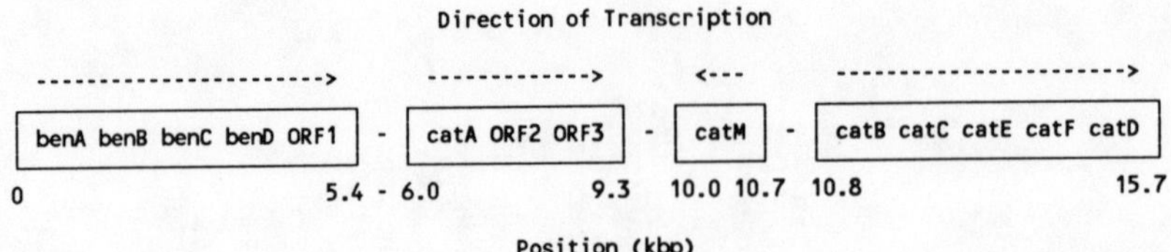

FIGURE 6. Clustering of separately transcribed sets of genes in *A. calcoaceticus*. The cluster contains all of the structural genes required for metabolism of benzoate via catechol. It is noteworthy that the *catA* gene, carried on a plasmid, remains subject to some inducible control in *A. calcoaceticus* strains from which the depicted chromosomal region has been deleted.

structural gene, introduced on a plasmid into an *A. calcoaceticus* strain from which all known *ben* and *cat* genes had been deleted, exhibited 10-fold induction in response to either benzoate or muconate (Neidle et al., 1989).

EXCHANGE OF DNA SEQUENCES AS SOURCES OF STABILITY OR INSTABILITY AMONG COEVOLVING GENES

Genetic stability is another selective force that might contribute to the clustering of functionally related genes. According to this hypothesis, DNA sequences may be maintained by exchange of DNA sequences among coevolving genes; the sequence transfers could maintain genetic integrity by eliminating mutations (Ornston et al., 1990). These notions gather some strength in light of recent evidence obtained with an *A. calcoaceticus Sal*I restriction fragment containing *catC* and most of *catE* in 1.5 kbp of DNA. Deletion of this fragment from the *A. calcoaceticus* chromosome increases the stability of a *pcaE* mutation 300-fold (Doten et al., 1987a). This evidence suggests that *catE* DNA may serve as a template for repair of the mutation within the homologous *pcaE* gene. The inference that legitimate genetic exchange could contribute to repair of the mutation is fortified by demonstration that the repair process depends on a functional *recA*-like gene (L. A. Gregg and L. N. Ornston, *Abstr. Annu. Meet. Am. Soc. Microbiol. 1989*, H-259, p. 212).

A large fraction of strains that have undergone apparent *catE*-mediated repair of the *pcaE* mutation are genetically unstable and undergo mutations that delete *pca* genes and, in some cases, delete *cat* genes as well (Doten et al., 1987a). Intriguingly, the genetic events underlying the deletions appear to be nonreciprocal in that deletions eliminating *cat* genes while leaving the *pca* genes intact were not recovered. Evidently, some of the repair events heightened homology between the *cat* and *pca* regions, and the increased DNA sequence similarity triggered genetic instability that appeared to emanate from the *pca* region. Possible significance of such nonreciprocal genetic events is that they may provide clues about how wild-type template sequences and modified mutant sequences might be distinguished from each other during repair by sequence-directed nucleotide substitution.

Events associated with apparent *catE*-mediated repair represent a biological paradox that warrants further exploration. On one hand, repair of the *pcaE* mutation seems to buffer against genetic variation. On the other hand, the repair process occasionally can trigger further mutations and thus has the potential to stimulate rapid genetic divergence. Genetic systems that are poised against change and yet can, on occasion, diversify rapidly have been grouped by I. C. Gunsalus as the basis for the biology of anticipation (Ornston et al., 1990). Representatives of the group are the immune system, detoxification processes, and the mind. They are characterized by a rapid, seemingly structured response to a stimulus and by a memory of the response. As noted by Gunsalus, the catabolic pathways of bacteria represent the biology of anticipation and are particularly amenable to experimental analysis.

An example of the experimentation envisioned by Gunsalus is transposition of the 1.5-kbp *Sal*I fragment carrying the *catC* gene from its evolutionarily selected position within the *A. calcoaceticus ben-cat* cluster to a new locus within the *pcaH* region. The transposition brings *catE* DNA into relative proximity with the *pcaE* region, with which it has shown a propensity for interaction. Strains that have undergone such transposition prove to be genetically unstable, as determined by loss of *catC* function (L. A. Gregg and L. N. Ornston, unpublished data). Yet to be explored are the genetic basis for the loss and the nature of further mutations that might stabilize the transposed DNA. Conclusions that can be drawn are that the genetic stability of a DNA segment can be determined by its position in the chromosome and that genetic transposition can trigger additional mutations.

DNA SEQUENCE EXCHANGE AS A GENETIC MECHANISM FOR EVOLUTIONARY DIVERGENCE: EVIDENCE FROM AMINO ACID SEQUENCES

A preexisting gene provides much of the information selected in a newly evolved gene, and a major question in molecular evolution is the nature of the information that is initially selected. One of the first efforts to address this question was presented by Horowitz (1945), who, noting that consecutively formed metabolic intermediates often possess similar chemical structures, suggested that substrate binding might be the first function selected in newly evolving enzymes. According to this view, enzymes catalyzing consecutive reactions in a metabolic pathway might be expected to share similar amino acid sequences conserved from a common ancestor. In a later review, Hegeman and Rosenberg (1970) concluded that the weight of the evidence favored the interpretation that structures contributing to the catalytic activity of enzymes tended to be selected and that evolution of new metabolic pathways was achieved by borrowing genetic information for catalytically analogous enzymes associated with other pathways. Their prediction that similar amino acid sequences would be found in enzymes catalyzing analogous chemical reactions in different metabolic pathways has been supported by identification of evolutionary families of catalytically similar enzymes and, more recently, by recognition of the *lysR* regulatory gene family (Henikoff et al., 1988), which contains *catM* and *catR* (Fig. 5).

A possible exception to the general lineage of families with similar catalytic activities emerged when similar amino acid sequences were identified in enzymes encoded by the *catC* and *catD* (or the homologous *pcaD*) genes (Yeh et al., 1978). The enzymes catalyze consecutive metabolic transformations, isomerization and hydrolysis, respectively, of biochemically unusual lactones in the β-ketoadipate pathway (Fig. 1). At first, it seemed possible that the amino acid sequence similarities represented residues conserved because they contributed to binding of the lactone substrates. A seemingly bizarre alternative interpretation, that the genes arose from different ancestors and acquired similar sequences as they coevolved, could not be excluded and indeed gained strength as additional sequence information on enzymes from different biological sources became available (McCorkle et al., 1980; Ornston and Yeh, 1979; Yeh et al., 1980a, 1980b). Amino acid sequences shared in some isomerase-hydrolase comparisons diverged within the isomerase or the hydrolase enzyme family. Therefore, it was difficult to maintain that the sequence similarities were the consequence of selection for lactone binding, a property shared by all the enzymes (Ornston and Yeh, 1981). Furthermore, sequence similarities in isomerase-hydrolase comparisons emerged from different alignments (Yeh et al., 1980a). This evidence was most consistent with multiple genetic events superimposing sequences from differently aligned templates (Ornston and Yeh, 1979).

Any possibility that observed amino acid sequence similarities were attributable to conservation of substrate-binding sites in enzymes with different activities was eliminated when such similarities emerged from comparison of a lactone decarboxylase, product of the *pcaC* gene, and a coenzyme A transferase, product of the *pcaE* gene (Yeh and Ornston, 1982; Fig. 1). The primary characteristic shared by these enzymes, catalyzing different transformations of unlike substrates, is an evolutionary history brought into common as they were selected as components of a single metabolic pathway. It is difficult to escape the conclusion that the coselected genes have exchanged sequence information (Yeh and Ornston, 1980). Genetic mechanisms causing sequence exchange also are likely to have contributed to distinctive patterns of internal sequence repetition that were acquired as genes diverged from a common ancestor (McCorkle et al., 1980; Ornston and Yeh, 1979; Yeh et al., 1980b; Yeh et al., 1981).

SEQUENCE-DIRECTED MUTATION AS A FORCE FOR GENETIC CHANGE

The conclusion that sequence repetitions, either within genes or shared by different genes, were acquired during evolution demanded characterization of mutations that might create such repetitions. Relevant evidence accrued as an outgrowth of the study of sequence-directed mutagenesis. It had long been known that DNA contained hot spots for deletion (Benzer, 1961), and sequence analysis revealed that the hot spots frequently were flanked by short, direct (Farabaugh et al., 1978), or inverted (Albertini et al., 1982) DNA sequence repetitions. In some cases, sets of sequence repetitions appeared to have the potential ability to reinforce each other in the formation of structures in which slipped DNA strands might hybridize before mutation (Albertini et al., 1982; Glickman and Ripley, 1984; Schaaper et al., 1986). Other genetic investigations characterized mutations that perfect partial sequence repetitions (de Boer and Ripley, 1984; Drake et al., 1983; Fix et al., 1987). Thus, sequence-directed mutation (Golding and Glickman, 1985) could lead to nucleotide substitution as well as deletion. This evidence provides a mechanistic framework that might account for our observations and those of others who have documented the acquisition of sequence repetitions in diverging genes (Golding and Glickman, 1985; Levinson and Gutman, 1987; Tautz et al., 1986).

DNA SEQUENCE EXCHANGE AS A GENETIC MECHANISM FOR EVOLUTIONARY DIVERGENCE: EVIDENCE FROM DNA SEQUENCES

Amino acid sequence comparisons leave open the question of the extent to which observed similarities will be evident at the level of DNA. In principle, convergent evolution could produce similar peptides in different alignments. Convincing evidence for common ancestry requires knowledge of the degree to which encoding nucleotide triplets have been conserved in DNA. Furthermore, DNA sequences offer opportunities to observe additional similarities that might not be observed at the level of protein because of differences in phase of translation or because inverted repetitions, evident in nucleotide sequence, are not apparent in amino acid sequences.

Systematic surveys have indicated that slippagelike mechanisms have contributed to evolutionary divergence, but a problem with DNA sequence evidence by itself is that slipped alignments give no indication of which alignment was ancestral. In the absence of knowledge about protein structure, it is difficult to know what portions of sequence were conserved and which portions diverged. Crystal structures have now been established for protocatechuate 3,4-dioxygenase (Ohlendorf et al., 1988), muconate cycloisomerase (Goldman et al., 1985), and muconolactone isomerase (Katti et al., 1988; Katz et al., 1985) from *P. putida*, and this information provides a valuable frame of reference for sequence comparisons. Perhaps the clearest examples are offered by the amino acid sequences of intradiol oxygenases, which can be aligned with the amino acid sequence of *P. putida* protocatechuate oxygenase (Iwaki et al., 1979; Kohlmiller and Howard, 1979). Highly conserved within all of the oxygenase sequences are regions encompassing pairs of histidyl and tyrosyl residues that ligate ferric ion within the proteins (Ohlendorf et al., 1988); these regions provide an outline of an ancestral sequence from which dioxygenases diverged (Neidle et al., 1988; Hartnett et al., 1990).

An example is shown in Fig. 7, in which amino acid sequences directly preceding the iron-binding region of *A. calcoaceticus* catechol (Neidle et al., 1988) and protocatechuate (Hartnett et al., 1990) dioxygenases are compared. Considerable conservation of amino acid sequence (Fig. 7A) is reflected in DNA sequence conservation (Fig. 7B). There is no way to be certain how divergence of DNA sequence was achieved in this region, but the extent to which divergent

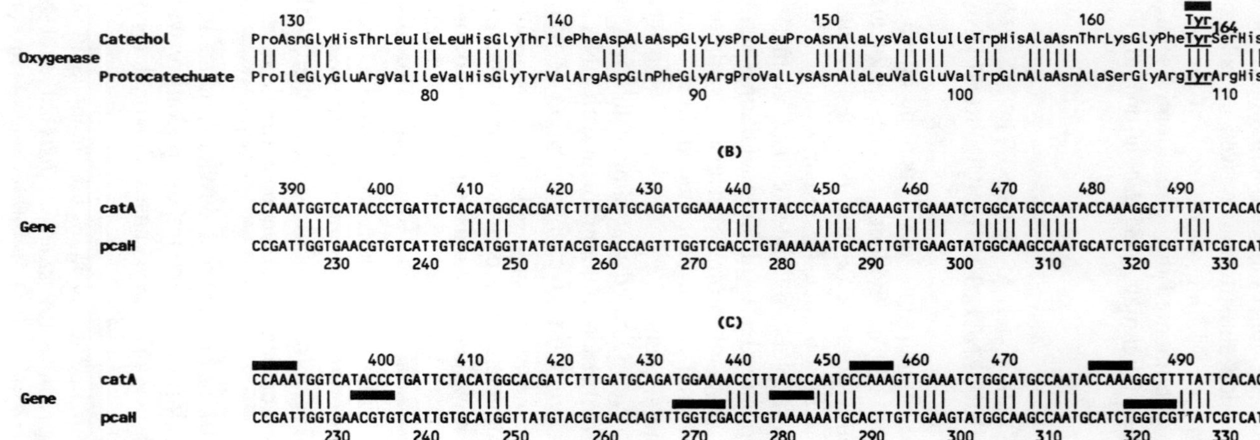

FIGURE 7. Divergence of genes by acquisition of DNA sequence repetitions. (A) The compared regions of *A. calcoaceticus* catechol and protocatechuate oxygenase precede a conserved tyrosyl residue (Tyr-164 in the catechol oxygenase sequence) that ligates iron. (B) DNA sequences encoding the conserved regions exhibit a high level of sequence identity. (C) Bars above and below the DNA sequences mark oligonucleotide repetitions that appear to have been introduced as the genes diverged.

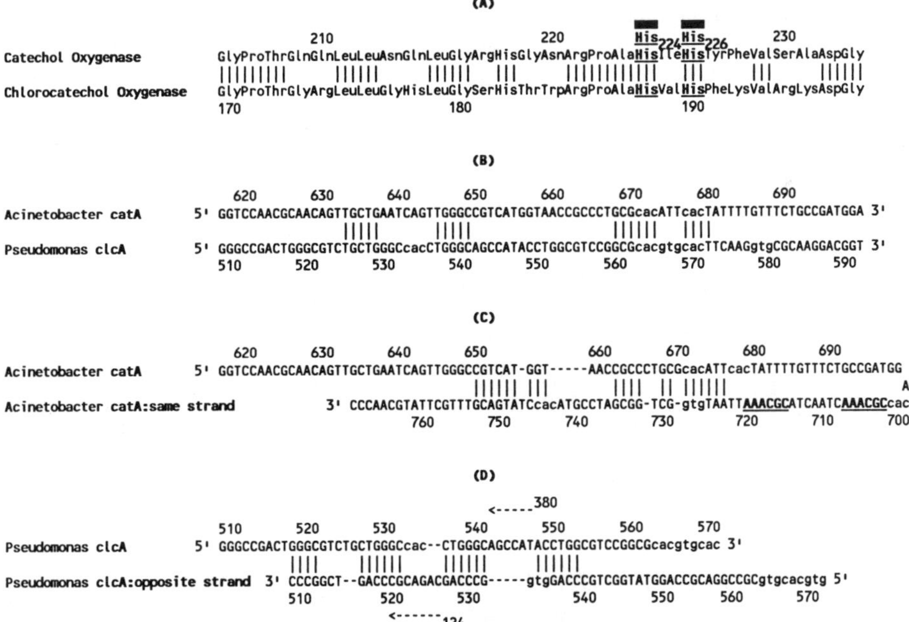

FIGURE 8. Slippage structures acquired as *Acinetobacter* catechol oxygenase and *Pseudomonas* chlorocatechol oxygenase diverged. (A) The compared region encodes two conserved histidyl residues (His-224 and His-226 in the catechol oxygenase sequence) that ligate iron. (B) Regions of sequence identity are evident in the aligned regions of the respective oxygenase genes. The nucleotide triplet cac and its complement gtg are distinguished by representation in lowercase because they frequently flank regions in which DNA strand slippage is likely to occur. (C) The 5' strand of the *Acinetobacter* DNA sequence contains an inverted repetition that might allow it to form an internal loop. Within the loop, the underlined sequence repetition AAACGC might afford opportunity for hybridization with the 3' strand after slippage. (D) An entirely different slippage structure was acquired as the *Pseudomonas* gene diverged. Direct DNA sequence repetition is so extensive that the gene resembles itself, after slippage, as closely as it resembles its homolog from *A. calcoaceticus*. Hybridization between 5' and 3' strands after slippage pinches into single strandedness from the *Pseudomonas* DNA oligonucleotides that have the potential ability to hybridize with inverted repetitions upstream in the gene. These potential hybridization sites are indicated by the numbers accompanying the dashed arrows.

sequences are repeated (Fig. 7C) strongly suggests that mutations causing sequence repetition made a major contribution.

In some cases, repeated sequences confer on DNA the potential ability to form slippage structures characterized by hybridization between misaligned strands. Examples are shown in Fig. 8, which depicts a region in which the amino acid sequences near the pair of iron-binding histidyl residues have been conserved in *Acinetobacter* catechol oxygenase (Neidle et al., 1988) and *Pseudomonas* chlorocatechol oxygenase (Frantz and Chakrabarty, 1987; Fig. 8A). Some short elements of DNA sequence have been conserved in this region of genes for the oxygenases, genes that differ by more than 15% in G+C content (Fig. 8B). Different patterns of internal sequence repetition were acquired as dioxygenase genes diverged, and these are reflected in differences in the dominant slippage structure that emerges within a single region of comparison. The major possibility for hybridization within the compared region of the *Acinetobacter catA* gene is based on inverted repetitions that could hybridize within a strand to form a loop (Fig. 8C). The presence of direct repetitions within the strand might allow for additional hybridization between strands (Fig. 8C).

Figure 8D depicts an alternative hybridization pattern for the *Pseudomonas clcA* sequence, which encodes chlorocatechol oxygenase. After slippage of 11 to 14 residues, the *clcA* sequence resembles itself as closely as it resembles the homologous DNA sequence from *Acinetobacter catA*. The sequence similarity would allow for extensive hybridization between slipped 5′ and 3′ strands within the *clcA* gene (Fig. 8D). The depicted slippage structure contains gaps, and these are of interest because DNA strands opposite the gaps would be pinched into single strandedness by the slippage structure. Such DNA has the potential ability to initiate formation of alternative slippage patterns by hybridizing with DNA upstream within the same strand (Fig. 8D). Thus, one slippage pattern might help to give rise to others.

SEQUENCE-DIRECTED MUTATION AND POSSIBILITIES FOR GENETIC REPAIR

We have described DNA that has demonstrated a capacity for dramatic change, as evidenced by gene transposition and by the shuffling of oligonucleotide sequences during evolutionary history. The same DNA has exhibited extraordinary constancy in the continued selection of supraoperonic clusters and the conservation of sequence repetitions within genes. In addition, we have noted that a transposition, a radical change in DNA structure, can elicit further genetic events. It is tempting to speculate that genetic mechanisms that confer stability to DNA in an established chromosomal environment can contribute to rapid divergence of the same DNA after its transposition. The premise is that sequence-directed mutation, a putative source of repair in established DNA slippage structures, can serve as a basis for change as novel slippage structures are established after gene rearrangement. One avenue for exploring these possibilities is to examine the genetic consequences of transposition. A potential difficulty with this approach is that events which occurred over geological time may be difficult to reproduce in the laboratory. An alternative approach that may yield more rapid insight is to explore the mechanism by which unstable mutations are repaired. Ironically, investigation of the basis for genetic instability might reveal sources of constancy in evolution.

ACKNOWLEDGMENTS. Our results were made possible by support from Celgene Corp., the United States Army Research Office, and the National Institutes of Health.

LITERATURE CITED

Albertini, A. M., M. Hofer, M. P. Calos, and J. H. Miller. 1982. On the formation of spontaneous deletions: the importance of short sequence homologies in the generation of large deletions. *Cell* **29**:319–328.

Benzer, S. 1961. On the topography of genetic fine structure. *Proc. Natl. Acad. Sci. USA* **47**:403–415.

Buvinger, W. E., L. C. Stone, and H. E. Heath. 1981. Biochemical genetics of tryptophan synthesis in *Pseudomonas acidovorans. J. Bacteriol.* **147**:62–68.

Cain, R. B. 1980. The uptake and catabolism of lignin-related aromatic compounds and their regulation in microorganisms, p. 21–60. *In* T. Kent Kirk, T. Higuchi, and H. Chang (ed.), *Lignin Biodegradation: Microbiology, Chemistry and Potential Applications*, vol. 1. CRC Press, Inc., Boca Raton, Fla.

Canovas, J. L., and R. Y. Stanier. 1967. Regulation of the enzymes of the β-ketoadipate pathway in *Moraxella calcoaceticus. Eur. J. Biochem.* **1**:289–300.

de Boer, J. G., and L. S. Ripley. 1984. Demonstration of the production of frameshift and base-substitution mutations by quasipalindromic DNA sequences. *Proc. Natl. Acad. Sci. USA* **81**:5528–5531.

Doten, R. C., L. A. Gregg, and L. N. Ornston. 1987a. Influence of the *catBCE* sequence on the phenotypic reversion of a *pcaE* mutation in *Acinetobacter calcoaceticus. J. Bacteriol.* **169**:3175–3180.

Doten, R. C., K.-L. Ngai, D. J. Mitchell, and L. N. Ornston. 1987b. Cloning and genetic organization of the *pca* gene cluster from *Acinetobacter calcoaceticus. J. Bacteriol.* **169**:3168–3174.

Drake, J. W., B. W. Glickman, and L. S. Ripley. 1983. Updating the theory of mutation. *Am. Sci.* **71**:621–630.

Durham, D. R., and L. N. Ornston. 1980. Homologous structural genes and similar induction patterns in *Azotobacter* and *Pseudomonas. J. Bacteriol.* **143**:834–840.

Durham, D. R., L. A. Stirling, L. N. Ornston, and J. J. Perry. 1980. Intergeneric evolutionary homology revealed by the study of protocatechuate 3,4-dioxygenase from *Azotobacter vinelandii. Biochemistry* **19**:149–155.

Farabaugh, P. J., U. Schmeissner, M. Hofer, and J. H. Miller. 1978. Genetic studies of the *lac* repressor. VII. On the molecular nature of spontaneous hotspots in the *lacI* gene of *Escherichia coli. J. Mol. Biol.* **126**:847–863.

Fix, D. F., P. A. Burns, and B. W. Glickman. 1987. DNA sequence analysis of spontaneous mutation in a PolA1 strain of *Escherichia coli* indicates sequence specific effects. *Mol. Gen. Genet.* **207**:267–272.

Frantz, B., and A. M. Chakrabarty. 1987. Organization and nucleotide sequence determination of a gene cluster involved in 3-chlorocatechol degradation. *Proc. Natl. Acad. Sci. USA* **84**:4460–4464.

Glickman, B. W., and L. S. Ripley. 1984. Structural intermediates of deletion mutagenesis: a role for palindromic DNA. *Proc. Natl. Acad. Sci. USA* **81**:512–516.

Golding, G. B., and B. W. Glickman. 1985. Sequence directed mutagenesis: evidence from a phylogenetic history of human α-interferon. *Proc. Natl. Acad. Sci. USA* **82**:8577–8581.

Goldman, A., D. L. Ollis, K.-L. Ngai, and T. A. Steitz. 1985. Crystal structure of muconate lactonizing enzyme at 6.5Å resolution. *J. Mol. Biol.* **182**:353–355.

Hartnett, C., E. L. Neidle, K.-L. Ngai, and L. N. Ornston. 1990. DNA sequence of genes encoding *Acinetobacter calcoaceticus* protocatechuate 3,4-dioxygenase: evidence indicating shuffling of genes and DNA sequences within genes during their evolutionary divergence. *J. Bacteriol.*, in press.

Harwood, C. S., and L. N. Ornston. 1984. TOL plasmid can prevent induction of chemotactic responses to aromatic acids. *J. Bacteriol.* **160**:797–800.

Harwood, C. S., and L. N. Ornston. 1988. Futile high-level transport activity impairs starvation-survival of *Pseudomonas putida. J. Gen. Microbiol.* **134**:2421–2/427.

Harwood, C. S., M. Rivelli, and L. N. Ornston. 1984. Aromatic acids are chemoattractants for *Pseudomonas putida. J. Bacteriol.* **160**:622–628.

Hegeman, G. D., and S. L. Rosenberg. 1970. The evolution of bacterial enzyme systems. *Annu. Rev. Microbiol.* **24**:429–462.

Henikoff, S., G. W. Haughn, J. M. Calco, and J. C. Wallace. 1988. A large family of activator proteins. *Proc. Natl. Acad. Sci. USA* **85**:6602–6606.

Horowitz, N. H. 1945. On the evolution of biochemical syntheses. *Proc. Natl. Acad. Sci. USA* **31**:153–157.

Hosokawa, K. 1970. Regulation of synthesis of early enzymes of the *p*-hydroxybenzoate pathway in *Pseudomonas putida. J. Biol. Chem.* **245**:5304–5308.

Hughes, E. J., M. Shapiro, J. E. Houghton, and L. N. Ornston. 1988. Cloning and expression of *pca* genes from *Pseudomonas putida* in *Escherichia coli*. *J. Gen. Microbiol.* **134:**2877–2887.

Iwaki, M., H. Kagamiyama, and M. Nozaki. 1979. The complete amino acid sequence of the α-subunit of protocatechuate 3,4-dioxygenase from *Pseudomonas aeruginosa*. *J. Biochem.* **86:**1159–1162.

Johnson, B. F., and R. Y. Stanier. 1971. Regulation of the β-ketoadipate pathway in *Alcaligenes eutrophus*. *J. Bacteriol.* **107:**476–485.

Katti, S. K., B. Katz, and H. W. Wyckoff. 1988. Crystal structure of muconolactone isomerase at 3.3 angstrom resolution. *J. Mol. Biol.* **205:**557–571.

Katz, B., D. L. Ollis, and H. W. Wyckoff. 1985. Low resolution crystal structure of muconolactone isomerase. *J. Mol. Biol.* **184:**311–318.

Kemp, M. B., and G. D. Hegeman. 1968. Genetic control of the β-ketoadipate pathway in *Pseudomonas aeruginosa*. *J. Bacteriol.* **96:**1488–1499.

Kilby, B. A. 1948. The bacterial oxidation of phenol to β-ketoadipic acid. *Biochem. J.* **43:**v–vi.

Kohlmiller, N. A., and J. B. Howard. 1979. The primary structure of the β-unit of protocatechuate 3,4-dioxygenase. II. Isolation and sequence of overlapping peptides and complete sequence. *J. Biol. Chem.* **254:**7309–7315.

Levinson, G., and G. A. Gutman. 1987. Slipped-strand mispairing: a major mechanism for DNA sequence evolution. *Mol. Biol. Evol.* **4:**203–221.

McCorkle, G. M., W. K. Yeh, P. Fletcher, and L. N. Ornston. 1980. Repetitions in the NH$_2$-terminal amino acid sequence of β-ketoadipate enol-lactone hydrolase from *Pseudomonas putida*. *J. Biol. Chem.* **255:**6335–6341.

Meagher, R. B., G. M. McCorkle, and L. N. Ornston. 1972. Inducible uptake system for carboxy-*cis,cis*-muconate in a permeability mutant of *Pseudomonas putida*. *J. Bacteriol.* **111:**465–473.

Neidle, E. L., C. Hartnett, S. Bonitz, and L. N. Ornston. 1988. DNA sequence of the *Acinetobacter calcoaceticus* catechol 1,2-dioxygenase I structural gene *catA*: evidence for evolutionary divergence of intradiol dioxygenases by acquisition of DNA repetitions. *J. Bacteriol.* **170:**4874–4880.

Neidle, E. L., C. Hartnett, and L. N. Ornston. 1989. Characterization of *Acinetobacter calcoaceticus catM*, a repressor gene homologous in sequence to transcriptional activator genes. *J. Bacteriol.* **171:**5410–5421.

Neidle, E. L., and L. N. Ornston. 1987. Benzoate and muconate, structurally dissimilar metabolites, induce expression of *catA* in *Acinetobacter calcoaceticus*. *J. Bacteriol.* **169:**414–415.

Neidle, E. L., M. Shapiro, and L. N. Ornston. 1987. Cloning and expression in *Escherichia coli* of *Acinetobacter calcoaceticus* genes for benzoate degradation. *J. Bacteriol.* **169:**5496–5503.

Ohlendorf, D. H., J. D. Lipscomb, and P. C. Weber. 1988. Structure and assembly of protocatechuate 3,4-dioxygenase. *Nature* (London) **336:**403–405.

Ondrako, J. M., and L. N. Ornston. 1980. Biological distribution and physiological role of the β-ketoadipate transport system. *J. Gen. Microbiol.* **120:**199–209.

Ornston, L. N. 1966. The conversion of catechol and protocatechuate to β-ketoadipate by *Pseudomonas putida*. IV. Regulation. *J. Biol. Chem.* **241:**3800–3810.

Ornston, L. N., E. L. Neidle, and J. E. Houghton. 1990. Gene rearrangements, a force for evolutionary change; DNA sequence arrangements, a source of genetic constancy, p. 325–334. *In* M. Riley and K. Drlica (ed.), *The Bacterial Chromosome*. American Society for Microbiology, Washington, D.C.

Ornston, L. N., and D. Parke. 1976a. Evolution of catabolic pathways. *Biochem. Soc. Trans.* **4:**468–473.

Ornston, L. N., and D. Parke. 1976b. Properties of an inducible uptake system for β-ketoadipate in *Pseudomonas putida*. *J. Bacteriol.* **125:**475–488.

Ornston, L. N., and W. K. Yeh. 1979. Origins of metabolic diversity: evolutionary divergence by sequence repetition. *Proc. Natl. Acad. Sci. USA* **76:**3996–4000.

Ornston, L. N., and W. K. Yeh. 1981. Toward molecular natural history, p. 140–143. *In* D. Schlessinger (ed.), *Microbiology—1981*. American Society for Microbiology, Washington, D.C.

Ornston, M. K., and L. N. Ornston. 1972. The regulation of the β-ketoadipate pathway in *Pseudomonas acidovorans* and *Pseudomonas testosteroni*. *J. Gen. Microbiol.* **73:**455–464.

Parke, D., and L. N. Ornston. 1976. Constitutive synthesis of enzymes of the protocatechuate pathway and of the β-ketoadipate uptake system in mutant strains of *Pseudomonas putida*. *J. Bacteriol.* **126:**272–281.

Parke, D., and L. N. Ornston. 1984. Nutritional diversity of Rhizobiaceae revealed by auxanography. *J. Gen. Microbiol.* **130:**1743–1750.

Parke, D., and L. N. Ornston. 1986. Enzymes of the β-ketoadipate pathway are inducible in *Rhizobium* and *Agrobacterium* spp. and constitutive in *Bradyrhizobium* spp. *J. Bacteriol.* **165:**288–292.

Parke, D., M. Rivelli, and L. N. Ornston. 1985. Chemotaxis to aromatic and hydroaromatic acids: comparison of *Bradyrhizobium japonicum* and *Rhizobium trifolii*. *J. Bacteriol.* **163:**417–422.

Robert-Gero, M., M. Poiret, and R. Y. Stanier. 1969. The function of the β-ketoadipate pathway in *Pseudomonas acidovorans*. *J. Gen. Microbiol.* **57:**207–214.

Rosenberg, S. L., and G. D. Hegeman. 1969. Clustering of functionally related genes in *Pseudomonas aeruginosa*. *J. Bacteriol.* **108:**1270–1276.

Schaaper, R. M., B. N. Danforth, and B. W. Glickman. 1986. Mechanisms of spontaneous mutagenesis: an analysis of the spectrum of spontaneous mutation in the *E. coli lacI* gene. *J. Mol. Biol.* **189:**273–284.

Shanley, M. S., E. L. Neidle, R. E. Parales, and L. N. Ornston. 1986. Cloning and expression of *Acinetobacter calcoaceticus catBCDE* genes in *Pseudomonas putida* and *Escherichia coli*. *J. Bacteriol.* **165:**557–563.

Stanier, R. Y. 1951. Enzymatic adaptation in bacteria. *Annu. Rev. Microbiol.* **5:**35–56.

Stanier, R. Y., N. J. Palleroni, and M. Doudoroff. 1966. The aerobic pseudomonads: a taxonomic study. *J. Gen. Microbiol.* **43:**159–271.

Tautz, D., M. Trick, and G. A. Dover. 1986. Cryptic simplicity in DNA is a major source of genetic variation. *Nature* (London) **322:**652–656.

Wheelis, M. L., and L. N. Ornston. 1972. Genetic control of enzyme induction in the β-ketoadipate pathway of *Pseudomonas putida*: deletion mapping of *cat* mutations. *J. Bacteriol.* **108:**790–795.

Wheelis, M. L., and R. Y. Stanier. 1970. The genetic control of dissimilatory pathways in *Pseudomonas putida*. *Genetics* **66:**245–266.

Wu, C. H., M. K. Ornston, and L. N. Ornston. 1972. Genetic control of enzyme induction in the β-ketoadipate pathway of *Pseudomonas putida*: two-point crosses with a regulatory mutant strain. *J. Bacteriol.* **109:**796–802.

Yeh, W. K., G. Davis, P. Fletcher, and L. N. Ornston. 1978. Homologous amino acid sequences in enzymes mediating sequential metabolic reactions. *J. Biol. Chem.* **253:**4920–4923.

Yeh, W. K., D. R. Durham, P. Fletcher, and L. N. Ornston. 1981. Evolutionary relationships among γ-carboxymuconolactone decarboxylases. *J. Bacteriol.* **146:**233–238.

Yeh, W. K., P. Fletcher, and L. N. Ornston. 1980a. Evolutionary divergence of coselected β-ketoadipate enol-lactone hydrolases in *Acinetobacter calcoaceticus*. *J. Biol. Chem.* **255:**6342–6346.

Yeh, W. K., P. Fletcher, and L. N. Ornston. 1980b. Homologies in the NH$_2$-terminal amino acid sequence of γ-carboxymuconolactone decarboxylases and muconolactone isomerases. *J. Biol. Chem.* **255:**6347–6354.

Yeh, W. K., and L. N. Ornston. 1980. Origins of metabolic diversity: substitution of homologous sequences into genes for enzymes with different catalytic activities. *Proc. Natl. Acad. Sci. USA* **77:**5365–5369.

Yeh, W. K., and L. N. Ornston. 1981. Evolutionarily homologous α$_2$β$_2$ oligomeric structures in β-ketoadipate succinyl CoA transferases from *Acinetobacter calcoaceticus* and *Pseudomonas putida*. *J. Biol. Chem.* **256:**1565–1569.

Yeh, W. K., and L. N. Ornston. 1982. Similar structures in γ-carboxymuconolactone decarboxylase and β-ketoadipate coenzyme A transferase. *J. Bacteriol.* **149:**374–377.

Zylstra, G. J., R. H. Olsen, and D. P. Ballou. 1989. Genetic organization and sequence of the *Pseudomonas cepacia* genes for the alpha and beta subunits of protocatechuate 3,4-dioxygenase. *J. Bacteriol.* **171:**5915–5921.

Part IV

PLASMIDS, VECTORS, GENE MAPPING, AND CLONING

Promiscuous Plasmids of the IncQ Group: Mode of Replication and Use for Gene Cloning in Gram-Negative Bacteria

Victor Morales, Mira M. Bagdasarian, and Michael Bagdasarian

In vitro gene manipulation is among the most effective methods to study the metabolic activities of living cells, particularly those of microorganisms. In the overwhelming majority of cases, *Escherichia coli* hosts and their plasmid or bacteriophage vectors are used for these studies. These host-vector systems, however, exhibit serious limitations. (i) The transcription-translation machinery of *E. coli* does not recognize well the transcription-translation signals from many other species. In consequence, heterologous genes are expressed poorly in this host unless they are placed under regulatory signals that are functional in *E. coli*. (ii) Studies of heterologous operons, regulons, or individual genes, whose function is dependent of, or related to, other biological properties of the original host, are often impossible in *E. coli* because this organism does not encode the ancillary functions required for expression of these properties (e.g., degradation of hydrocarbons, photosynthesis, pathogenicity, and interaction with plants). (iii) Products of certain heterologous genes are toxic to the new host, which results in the inability to maintain the cloned genes in *E. coli*. This is often the case for genes encoding secretable proteins or membrane components. However, selection of an appropriate host may allow stable maintenance of a heterologous gene and expression of its product. This was demonstrated by Elleman and co-workers (1986), who have successfully overproduced the pili of *Bacteroides nodosus* in *Pseudomonas aeruginosa*. (iv) Many vectors currently used in *E. coli* are based on narrow-host-range replicons or bacteriophages specific for *E. coli*. They cannot be introduced and stably maintained in other bacterial species that are not closely related to the original host (for reviews, see Bagdasarian et al. [1981], Bagdasarian and Timmis [1982], Mermod et al. [1986a], and Schmidhauser et al. [1987]).

Victor Morales, Mira M. Bagdasarian, and Michael Bagdasarian ● Department of Microbiology, Michigan State University and Michigan Biotechnology Institute, 3900 Collins Road, Lansing, Michigan 48909.

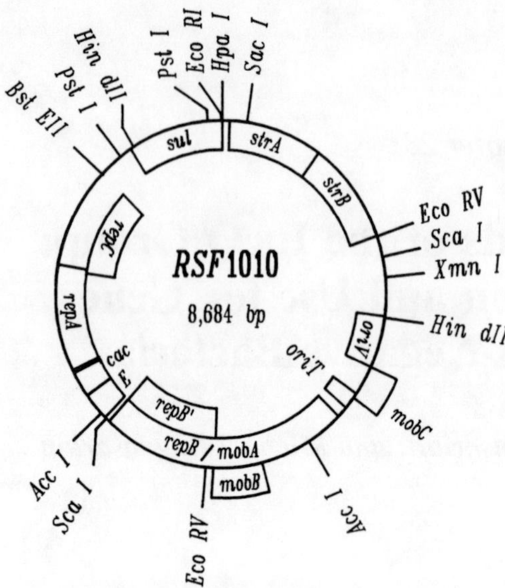

FIGURE 1. Physical and genetic map of RSF1010. The map is based on the nucleotide sequence data (Scholz et al., 1989) and results from biochemical studies (Haring and Scherzinger, 1989). See Table 3 for explanation of genetic organization. Abbreviations: *sul*, sulfonamide resistance; *strA* and *strB*, genes coding for streptomycin resistance. bp, Base pairs.

Considerations outlined above explain why it is difficult, and often impossible, to screen for cloned heterologous genes in the *E. coli* system by complementation of mutations. Instead, it is necessary to resort to more elaborate methods such as activity determination, hybridization to probes, or immunodetection.

Clearly, it is of great scientific interest as well as of considerable practical advantage to have versatile cloning systems available for different microbial species. Several strategies are currently being used for gene cloning in microorganisms other than *E. coli*: (i) double-replicon shuttle vectors that can replicate in both *E. coli* and another organism, which have been developed for cloning in *Bacillus subtilis* (for a review, see Errington [1987]), *Saccharomyces* sp. (for a review, see West [1987]), and higher eucaryotic cells (for a review, see Ridgway [1987]); (ii) narrow-host-range vectors able to replicate in the desired host (such vectors have been constructed for *Pseudomonas aeruginosa* [Itoh et al., 1984]); and (iii) broad-host-range vectors that are able to replicate in many different microbial species (for reviews, see Bagdasarian and Timmis [1982], Mermod et al. [1986a], and Schmidhauser et al. [1987]).

Of these three approaches, the use of broad-host-range vectors seems to be the most appealing because it allows the use of different species, including *E. coli*, as intermediary hosts, provides plasmid vectors that are generally smaller than double-replicon vehicles, and avoids possible complications resulting from multiple origins and replication genes in the same replicating unit.

Despite some efforts put into the construction of wide-host-range cloning systems, reflected in several review articles cited above, only two replicons have been studied and manipulated extensively enough to produce cloning vehicles of satisfactory performance. These are the replicons from RK2 and of RSF1010 plasmids. The use of vectors constructed from other replicons, such as that of the

TABLE 1
Host range of RSF1010-derived cloning vectors

Species	Reference
Acetobacter xylinum	Valla et al., 1986
Actinobacillus pleuropneumoniae	J. Perrin, personal communication
Aerobacter aerogenes	Mermod et al., 1986a, 1986b
Aeromonas hydrophila	Frey and Krisch, 1985
Agrobacterium tumefaciens	Hille and Schilperoort, 1981
Alcaligenes eutrophus	F. C. H. Franklin, personal communication
Azotobacter vinelandii	David et al., 1983
Azospirillum sp.	C. Elmerich, personal communication
Caulobacter crescentus	Ely, 1979
Desulfovibrio desulfuricans	Powell et al., 1989
Erwinia carotovora	M. Chippaux, personal communication
Escherichia coli	Barth and Grinter, 1974
Gluconobacter sp.	H. F. Kung, personal communication
Hyphomicrobium sp.	Mermod et al., 1986a, 1986b
Klebsiella aerogenes	Fürste et al., 1986
Methylophilus methylotrophus	Windass et al., 1980
Moraxella sp.	Mermod et al., 1986a, 1986b
Paracoccus denitrificans	Frey and Krisch, 1985
Proteus mirabilis	Fürste et al., 1986
Pseudomonas aeruginosa	Nagahari and Sakaguchi, 1978
Pseudomonas putida	Nagahari and Sakaguchi, 1978
Rhizobium leguminosarum	Windass et al., 1980
Rhizobium meliloti	David et al., 1983
Rhodobacter sphaeroides	Fornari and Kaplan, 1982
Serratia marcescens	Fürste et al., 1986
Xanthomonas campestris	M. Daniels, personal communication
Xanthomonas maltophilia	M. Sandkvist, personal communication
Vibrio (8 species)	M. Sandkvist and M. Bagdasarian, unpublished data
Yersinia enterocolitica	J. Heesmann, personal communication
Zymomonas mobilis	Buchholz and Eveleigh, 1986

IncW (Tait et al., 1983; Valentine and Kado, 1989) or IncN (Iyer, 1989) plasmids, has been limited since not enough information on their structures and host ranges is available.

RK2, similar or identical to RP1, RP4, and R68 (Burkhardt et al., 1979), is a large, low-copy-number, self-transferable plasmid that required extensive engineering before user-friendly vectors could be generated from it. However, reduction in size of the RK2 replicon resulted in the loss of functions that, although nonessential, are apparently required for the stability and maintenance of correct copy number of the plasmid. In consequence, RK2-based cloning vectors are often unstable in certain bacteria such as *Pseudomonas* spp. (Schmidhauser and Helinski, 1985). A recent review by Schmidhauser et al. (1987) contains an exhaustive coverage of cloning vectors derived from RK2 and other wide-host-range replicons. We will therefore limit this chapter to a description of vectors based on the RSF1010 plasmid and to discussion of the replication mode that allows this extrachromosomal element to be stably maintained in a wide range of different bacterial hosts.

TABLE 2

Properties of IncQ-derived broad-host-range vectors

Vector	Size (kilobase pairs)	Markers	Cloning site(s)	Insertional change	Reference
General-type cloning					
pKT210	11.8	Cm, Sm	*Sst*I	Sm^r → Sm^s	Bagdasarian
		mob$^+$	*Eco*RI	Sm^r → Sm^s	et al., 1979
			*Hin*dIII	None	
pKT231	13.0	Sm, Km	*Sst*I, *Sst*II	Sm^r → Sm^s	Bagdasarian
		mob$^+$	*Eco*RI, *Hpa*I	Sm^r → Sm^s	et al., 1981
			*Hin*dIII, *Xho*I	Km^r → Km^s	
			*Cla*I, *Xma*I, *Pvu*I	Km^r → Km^s	
			*Bam*HI, *Bgl*II	None	
pKT248	12.4	Cm, Sm	*Eco*RI	Sm^r → Sm^s	Bagdasarian
		mob$^+$	*Sst*I, *Sst*II	Sm^r → Sm^s	et al., 1981
			*Sal*I	Cm^r → Cm^s	
pDSK509	9.1	Km, Sm	*Pst*I, *Sal*I, *Xba*I	Sm^r → Sm^s	Keen et al.,
		mob$^+$	*Bam*HI, *Kpn*I	Sm^r → Sm^s	1988
			*Sst*I, *Eco*RI	Sm^r → Sm^s	
Joint replicon					
pKT230	11.9	Km, Sm	*Bam*HI	None	Bagdasarian
		mob$^+$	*Eco*RI, *Sst*I, *Sst*II	Sm^r → Sm^s	et al., 1981
		pACYC177	*Hin*dIII, *Sma*I, *Xho*I	Km^r → Km^s	
pFG7	13.3	Ap, Sm	*Sst*I, *Sst*II	Sm^r → Sm^s	Gautier and Bone-
		Su, Tc	*Sst*I, *Sst*II	Sm^r → Sm^s	wald, 1980
		mob$^+$	*Bam*HI, *Cla*I	Tc^r → Tc^s	
		pBR322	*Hin*dIII, *Sal*I	Tc^r → Tc^s	
pUI81	13.3	Sm, Su, Tc	*Sst*I, *Sst*II	Sm^r → Sm^s	Fornari and
		mob$^+$	*Bam*HI, *Cla*I	Tc^r → Tc^s	Kaplan, 1982
		pBR322	*Hin*dIII, *Sal*I	Tc^r → Tc^s	
pMW79	13.3	Ap, Sm, Tc	*Sst*I	Sm^r → Sm^s	Wood et al.,
		mob$^+$	*Sst*II	Sm^r → Sm^s	1981
		pBR322	*Bam*HI, *Cla*I	Tc^r → Tc^s	
			*Hin*dIII, *Sal*I	Tc^r → Tc^s	
pSUP104	9.5	Cm, Tc	*Eco*RI	Cm^r → Cm^s	Priefer et al.,
		mob$^+$	*Bam*HI, *Hin*dIII, *Sal*I	Tc^r → Tc^s	1985
		pACYC184	*Pst*I	None	
Cosmid					
pMMB33,	13.8	Km, *cos*	*Bam*HI, *Eco*RI	None	Frey et al., 1983
pMMB34		*mob*$^+$	*Hpa*I, *Sst*I, *Sst*II	None	
pFG6	15.3	Ap, Tc	*Bam*HI, *Cla*I	Tc^r → Tc^s	Gautier and Bone-
		mob$^+$, *cos*	*Hin*dIII, *Sal*I	Tc^r → Tc^s	wald, 1980
pSUP106	9.9	Cm, Tc	*Eco*RI	Cm^r → Cm^s	Priefer et al.,
		mob$^+$, *cos*	*Bam*HI, *Hin*dIII	Tc^r → Tc^s	1985
		pACYC184	*Sal*I	Tc^r → Cm^s	
pJRD215	10.2	Km, Sm	*Bam*HI, *Kpn*I, *Mlu*I,	None	Davison et al.,
			*Hpa*I, *Nde*I, *Stu*I,		1987
			*Xba*I, *Spe*I, *Eco*RI		

TABLE 2—*Continued*

Vector	Size (kilobase pairs)	Markers	Cloning site(s)	Insertional change	Reference
Promoter probe					
pKT240	12.9	Km, Ap *mob*[+]	*Eco*RI, *Hpa*I	Sm[s] → Sm[r]	Bagdasarian et al., 1983
pCF32	15.1	Km, Ap *mob*[+]	*Hin*dIII	*xylE* → *xylE*[+]	Spooner et al., 1987
pUI523A, pUI533A	9.7	Tc, *mob*[+], *lacZ*	*Kpn*I, *Dra*I, *Stu*I, *Sma*I	Fusion to *lacZ*	Tai et al., 1988
Controlled expression					
pMMB66EH	8.8	Ap, P_{tac}	*Eco*RI, *Sma*I, *Bam*HI	None	Fürste et al., 1986
		mob[+], *lacI*[q]	*Sal*I, *Pst*I, *Hin*dIII	None	
pMMB67EH	8.8	Ap, P_{tac}, *mob*[+]	*Eco*RI, *Sst*I, *Kpn*I, *Sma*I, *Bam*HI, *Xba*I	None	Fürste et al., 1986
		lacI[q]	*Sal*I, *Pst*I, *Sph*I, *Hin*dIII	None	
pMMB207	9.0	Cm, P_{tac}, *mob*[+]	Same as pMMB67EH	None	Morales et al., submitted
pMMB206	9.3	Cm, *mob*[+], *lacI*[q], P_{tac}-P_{lac}, *lacZ*α	Same as pMMB67EH	*lacZ*α[+] → *lacZ*α	Morales et al., in preparation
pNM185	14.0	Km, *mob*[+], Pm, *xylS*	*Eco*RI, *Sst*I, *Sst*II	None	Mermod et al., 1986b
pERD21	13.8	Km, *mob*[+] Pm, *xylS*	*Eco*RI, *Sst*I, *Sst*II *Kpn*I, *Sal*I, *Hpa*I, *Bcl*I	None None	Ramos et al., 1988
pPLGN1		Km, P_L *mob*[+], *c*I857	*Eco*RI	None	Leemans et al., 1987

IncQ PLASMIDS

The incompatibility group IncQ (also referred to as IncP4) is a distinct group of plasmids characterized by small size, relatively low copy number, and very broad host range among gram-negative bacteria. The sources for isolation and the basic properties of the best known IncQ plasmids have recently been reviewed (Frey and Bagdasarian, 1989).

The most extensively studied representatives of the IncQ/IncP4 plasmids are R1162 (Meyer et al., 1982) and RSF1010 (Guerry et al., 1974). They are very similar or identical to R300B, the first representative of the group to be described (Barth and Grinter, 1974). A simplified physical and genetic map of RSF1010 is shown in Fig. 1. The complete nucleotide sequence of this plasmid and the organization of its genome have been determined recently (Scholz et al., 1989).

RSF1010 is a relatively small (8,684-base-pair) plasmid that carries genes for streptomycin resistance (*strA* and *strB*; aminoglycoside phosphotransferase C) and for sulfonamide resistance (*sul*; dihydropteroate synthase). It is harbored by *E. coli* and *Pseudomonas putida* hosts at an intermediate copy number of 13 copies per cell (Frey and Bagdasarian, 1989), a concentration maintained under strict genetic control. Its host range seems to be as wide as that of RK2. Table 1 lists those species in which RSF1010, or one of its derivatives, has been shown to replicate. However, the actual host range of this plasmid may be wider. Indeed, the only gram-negative genus reported to date in which RSF1010 replicon could not be established is *Bacteroides* (Guiney et al., 1985; Smith et al., 1985).

GENERAL-TYPE CLONING VECTORS

Initially, general-type cloning vectors were constructed from RSF1010 by insertion of different DNA fragments that encoded a variety of antibiotic resistance genes into the drug resistance region of the plasmid. This introduced convenient selection markers, unique cloning sites, and the possibility of screening for recombinant clones by insertional inactivation. Examples of these vectors, the ones that have found the widest application, are presented in Table 2. For a more complete list of broad-host-range vectors, the reader is referred to the recent review by Schmidhauser et al. (1987). These earlier constructions suffered from the disadvantage of carrying DNA fragments on which little information was available about nucleotide sequence and encoded genetic functions. However, these cloning tools have been, and still are, quite useful for simple gene cloning and for introduction of genes into a wide range of hosts.

Several joint-replicon cloning plasmids have been constructed from RSF1010 and recommended as broad-host-range vectors. At present, the introduction of another replicon into RSF1010 does not appear to carry any advantage for the vector. RSF1010 is quite stably maintained in many species, and its derivatives have been used successfully in cloning and controlled expansion of genes in different species, including *E. coli* (Bailone et al., 1988).

SPECIAL-PURPOSE CLONING VECTORS WITH WIDE HOST RANGE

Vectors encoding the bacteriophage λ *cos* site (cosmid vectors) are particularly useful for cloning large fragments of DNA (over 35 kilobase pairs) and generation of gene banks (Hohn and Collins, 1980). Several cosmid vectors have been constructed on the basis of RSF1010 (Table 2). However, the method still requires that an *E. coli* strain be used as an intermediary host for the initial introduction into bacterial cells of recombinant plasmids, packaged in vitro into bacteriophage λ heads. Efficient introduction of λ receptors into species of another genus, such as *Pseudomonas*, may resolve this difficulty in the future and allow direct cosmid cloning without the use of *E. coli* as an intermediary. At present, RSF1010-based cosmid vectors are particularly useful because recombi-

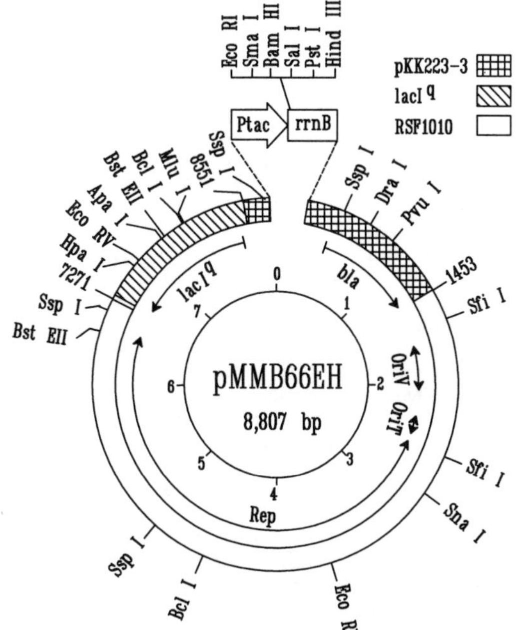

FIGURE 2. Physical and genetic map of controlled-expression vector pMMB66EH. The map is based on nucleotide sequence of the DNA fragments used for construction of the plasmid (Fürste et al., 1986; Scholz et al., 1989; V. Morales and M. Bagdasarian, unpublished data). See Table 3 for explanation of genetic organization. Abbreviations: *bla*, β-lactamase; *rrnB*, transcriptional termination sequence from the *E. coli rrnB* gene, P*tac*, *tac* promoter; *lacI*q, *lac* repressor gene specifying high levels of repressor protein. bp, Base pairs.

nant plasmids may be efficiently transferred from the intermediary host into other species by mobilization (Frey et al., 1983).

To clone and quantitatively study the functions of promoters in different gram-negative species, vectors containing a promoterless *aphC* gene of RSF1010 or the *xylE* gene of the TOL plasmid have been constructed (Table 2). The first type of vector allows the positive selection for insertion of DNA fragments containing promoters by plating of transformants on streptomycin media (Bagdasarian et al., 1983). The second type permits rapid screening by spraying colonies growing on agar plates with a solution of catechol. A quick and simple method for quantitative determination of the *xylE* gene product, catechol 2,3-oxygenase, makes the study of promoter function and regulation with *xylE*-containing vectors particularly convenient (Spooner et al., 1987). Vectors for translational fusions to *lacZ* gene have also been constructed on the basis of RSF1010 replicon and used to study gene expression in *Rhodobacter sphaeroides* (Tai et al., 1988).

CONTROLLED-EXPRESSION VECTORS

Three different regulatory systems have been introduced into the RSF1010 replicon to achieve controlled expression of cloned genes in gram-negative bacteria other than *E. coli* (Table 2). The nucleotide sequence and genome organization of vectors that utilized the *tac* promoter and the *lacI*q repressor have now been determined. The genetic and physical map of one of these vectors, pMMB66EH, is presented in Fig. 2, and its complete nucleotide sequence is

```
   1 TTCCCGGGGA TCCGTCGACC TGCAGCCAAG CTTGGCTGTT TTGGCGGATG AGAGAAGATT TTCAGCCTGA TACAGATTAA
  81 ATCAGAACGC AGAAGCGGTC TGATAAAACA GAATTTGCCT GGCGGCAGTA GCGCGGTGGT CCCACCTGAC CCCATGCCGA
 161 ACTCAGAAGT GAAACGCCGT AGCGCCGATG GTAGTGTGGG GTCTCCCCAT GCGAGAGTAG GGAACTGCCA GGCATCAAAT
 241 AAAACGAAAG GCTCAGTCGA AAGACTGGGC CTTTCGTTTT ATCTGTTGTT TGTCGGTGAA CGCTCTCCTG AGTAGGACAA
 321 ATCCGCCGGG AGCGGATTTG AACGTTGCGA AGCAACGGCC CGGAGGGTGG CGGGCAGGAC GCCCGCCATA AACTGCCAGG
 401 CATCAAATTA AGCAGAAGGC CATCCTGACG GATGGCCTTT TTGCGTTTCT ACAAACTCTT TTGTTTATTT TTCTAAATAC
 481 ATTCAAATAT GTATCCGCTC ATGAGACAAT AACCCTGATA AATGCTTCAA TAATATTGAA AAAGGAAGAG TATGAGTATT
 561 CAACATTTCC GTGTCGCCCT TATTCCCTTT TTTGCGGCAT TTTGCCTTCC TGTTTTTGCT CACCCAGAAA CGCTGGTGAA
 641 AGTAAAAGAT GCTGAAGATC AGTTGGGTGC ACGAGTGGGT TACATCGAAC TGGATCTCAA CAGCGGTAAG ATCCTTGAGA
 721 GTTTTCGCCC CGAAGAACGT TTTCCAATGA TGAGCACTTT TAAAGTTCTG CTATGTGGCG CGGTATTATC CCGTGTTGAC
 801 GCCGGGCAAG AGCAACTCGG TCGCCGCATA CACTATTCTC AGAATGACTT GGTTGAGTAC TCACCAGTCA CAGAAAAGCA
 881 TCTTACGGAT GGCATGACAG TAAGAGAATT ATGCAGTGCT GCCATAACCA TGAGTGATAA CACTGCGGCC AACTTACTTC
 961 TGACAACGAT CGGAGGACCG AAGGAGCTAA CCGCTTTTTT GCACAACATG GGGGATCATG TAACTCGCCT TGATCGTTGG
1041 GAACCGGAGC TGAATGAAGC CATACCAAAC GACGAGCGTG ACACCACGAT GCCTGTAGCA ATGGCAACAA CGTTGCGCAA
1121 ACTATTAACT GGCGAACTAC TTACTCTAGC TTCCCGGCAA CAATTAATAG ACTGGATGGA GGCGGATAAA GTTGCAGGAC
1201 CACTTCTGCG CTCGGCCCTT CCGGCTGGCT GGTTTATTGC TGATAAATCT GGAGCCGGTG AGCGTGGGTC TCGCGGTATC
1281 ATTGCAGCAC TGGGGCCAGA TGGTAAGCCC TCCCGTATCG TAGTTATCTA CACGACGGGG AGTCAGGCAA CTATGGATGA
1361 ACGAAATAGA CAGATCGCTG AGATAGGTGC CTCACTGATT AAGCATTGGT AACTGTCAGA CCAAGTTTAC TCATATATAC
1441 TTTAGATTGA TTTCTGAAAG CGACCAGGTG CTCGGCGTGG CAAGACTCGC AGCGAACCCG TAGAAAGCCA TGCTCCAGCC
1521 GCCCGCATTG GAGAAATTCT TCAAATTCCC GTTGCACATA GCCCGGCAAT TCCTTTCCCT GCTCTGCCAT AAGCGCAGCG
1601 AATGCCGGGT AATACTCGTC AACGATCTGA TAGAGAAGGG TTTGCTCGGG TCGGTGGCTC TGGTAACGAC CAGTATCCCG
1681 ATCCCGGCTG GCCGTCCTGG CCGCCACATG AGGCATGTTC CGCGTCCTTG CAATACTGTG TTTACATACA GTCTATCGCT
1761 TAGCGGAAAG TTCTTTTACC CTCAGCCGAA ATGCCTGCCG TTGCTAGACA TTGCCAGCCA GTGCCCGTCA CTCCCGTACT
1841 AACTGTCACG AACCCCTGCA ATAACTGTCA CGCCCCCCTG CAATAACTGT CACGAACCCC TGCAATAACT GTCACGCCCC
1921 CAAACCTGCA AACCCAGCAG GGGCGGGGGC TGGCGGGGTG TTGGAAAAAT CCATCCATGA TTATCTAAGA ATAATCCACT
2001 AGGCGCGGTT ATCAGCGCCC TTGTGGGGCG CTGCTGCCCT TGCCCAATAT GCCCGGCCAG AGGCCGGATA GCTGGTCTAT
2081 TCGCTGCGCT AGGCTACACA CCGCCCCACC GCTGCGCGGC AGGGGGAAAG GCGGGCAAAG CCCGCTAAAC CCCACACCAA
2161 ACCCCGCAGA AATACGCTGG AGCGCTTTTA GCCGCTTTAG CGGCCTTTCC CCCTACCCGA AGGGTGGGGG CGCGTGTGCA
2241 GCCCCGCAGG GCCTGTCTCG GTCGATCATT CAGCCCGGCT CATCCTTCTG GCGTGGCGGC AGACCGAACA AGGCGCGGTC
2321 GTGGTCGCGT TCAAGGTACG CATCCATTGC CGCCATGAGC CGATCCTCCG GCCACTCGCT GCTGTTCACC TTGGCCAAAA
2401 TCATGGCCCC CACCAGCACC TTGCGCCTTG TTTCGTTCTT GCGCTCTTGC TGCTGTTCCC TTGCCCGCTC CCGCTGAATT
2481 TCGGCATTGA TTCGCGCTCG TTGTTCTTCG AGCTTGGCCA GCCGATCCGC CGCCTTGTTG CTCCCCTTAA CCATCTTGAC
2561 ACCCCATTGT TAATGTGCTG TCTCGTAGGC TATCATGGAG GCACAGCGGC GGCAATCCCG ACCCTACTTT GTAGGGGAGG
2641 GCGCACTTAC CGGTTTCTCT TCGAGAAACT GGCCTAACGG CCACCCTTCG GCGGTGCGC TCTCCGAGGG CCATTGCATG
2721 GAGCCGAAAA GCAAAAGCAA CAGCGAGGCA GCATGGCGAT TTATCACCTT ACGGCGAAAA CCGGCAGCAG GTCGGGCGGC
2801 CAATCGGCCA GGGCCAAGGC CGACTACATC CAGCGCGAAG GCAAGTATGC CCGCGACATG GATGAAGTCT TGCACGCCGA
2881 ATCCGGGCAC ATGCCGGAGT TCGTCGAGCG GCCCGCCGAC TACTGGGATG CTGCCGACCT GTATGAACGC GCCAATGGGC
2961 GGCTGTTCAA GGAGGTCGAA TTTGCCCTGC CGGTCGAGCT GACCCTCGAC CAGCAGAAGG CGCTGGCGTC CGAGTTCGCC
3041 CAGCACCTGA CCGGTGCCGA GCGCCTGCCG TATACGCTGG CCATCCATGC CGGTGGCGGC GAGAACCCGC ACTGCCACCT
3121 GATGATCTCC GAGCGGATCA ATGACGGCAT CGAGCGGCCC GCCGCTCAGT GGTTCAAGCG GTACAACGGC AAGACCCCGG
3201 AGAAGGGCGG GGCACAGAAG ACCGAAGCGC TCAAGCCCAA GGCATGGCTT GAGCAGACCC GCGAGGCATG GGCCGACCAT
3281 GCCAACCGGG CATTAGAGCG GGCTGGCCAC GACGCCCGCA TTGACCACAG AACACTTGAG GCGCAGGGCA TCGAGCGCCT
3361 GCCCGGTGTT CACCTGGGGC CGAACGTGGT GGAGATGGAA GGCCGGGGCA TCCGCACCGA CCGGGCAGAC GTGGCCCTGA
3441 ACATCGACAC CGCCAACGCC CAGATCATCG ACTTACAGGA ATACCGGGAG GCAATAGACC ATGAACGCAA TCGACAGAGT
3521 GAAGAAATCC AGAGGCATCA ACGAGTTAGC GGAGCAGATC GAACCGCTGG CCCAGAGCAT GGCGACACTG GCCGACGAAG
3601 CCCGGCAGGT CATGAGCCAG ACCAAGCAGG CCAGCGAGGC GCAGGCGGCG GAGTGGCTGA AAGCCCAGCG CCAGACAGGG
3681 GCGGCATGGG TGGAGCTGGC CAAAGAGTTG CGGGAGGTAG CCGCCGAGGT GAGCAGCGCC GCGCAGAGCG CCCGGAGCGC
3761 GTCGCGGGGG TGGCACTGGA AGCTATGGCT AACCGTGATG CTGGCTTCCA TGATGCCTAC GGTGGTGCTG CTGATCGCAT
3841 CGTTGCTCTT GCTCGACCTG ACGCCACTGA CAACCGAGGA CGGCTCGATC TGGCTGCGCT TGGTGGCCCG ATGAAGAACG
3921 ACAGGACTTT GCAGGCCATA GGCCGACAGC TCAAGGCCAT GGGCTGTGAG CGCTTCGATA TCGGCGTCAG GACGCACCCC
4001 ACCGGCCAGA TGATGAACCG GGAATGGTCA GCCGCCGAAG TGCTCCAGAA CACGCCATGG CTCAAGCGGA TGAATGCCCA
4081 GGGCAATGAC GTGTATATCA GGCCCGCCGA GCAGGAGCGG CATGGTCTGG TGCTGGTGGA CGACCTCAGC GAGTTTGACC
4161 TGGATGACAT GAAAGCCGAG GGCCGGGAGC CTGCCCTGGT AGTGGAAACC AGCCCGAAGA ACTATCAGGC ATGGGTCAAG
4241 GTGGCCGACG CCGCAGGCGG TGAACTTCGG GGGCAGATTG CCCGGACGCT GGCCAGCGAG TACGACGCCG ACCCGGCCAG
4321 CGCCGACAGC CGCCACTATG GCCGCTTGGC GGGCTTCACC AACCGCAAGG ACAAGCACAC CACCCGCGCC GGTTATCAGC
4401 CGTGGGTGCT GCTGCGTGAA TCCAAGGGCA AGACCGCCAC CGCTGGCCCG GCGCTGGTGC AGCAGGCTGG CCAGCAGATC
```

FIGURE 3. Complete nucleotide sequence of the vector pMMB66EH. Nucleotides are numbered starting from the unique *Eco*RI site. Only the mRNA-like strand, coding for all replication genes, is shown in the 5′-to-3′ direction. See Table 3 for exact positions of genes in the sequence. The sequence was established from the data on the component DNA (Fürste et al., 1986) and on determination of sequences in the junction regions (Morales and Bagdasarian, unpublished data).

```
4481 GAGCAGGCCC AGCGGCAGCA GGAGAAGGCC CGCAGGCTGG CCAGCCTCGA ACTGCCCGAG CGGCAGCTTA GCCGCCACCG
4561 GCGCACGGCG CTGGACGAGT ACCGCAGCGA GATGGCCGGG CTGGTCAAGC GCTTCGGTCA TGACCTCAGC AAGTGCGACT
4641 TTATCGCCGC GCAGAAGCTG GCCAGCCGGG GCCGCAGTGC CGAGGAAATC GGCAAGGCCA TGGCCGAGGC CAGCCCAGCG
4721 CTGGCAGAGC GCAAGCCCGG CCACGAAGCG GATTACATCG AGCGCACCGT CAGCAAGGTC ATGGGTCTGC CCAGCGTCCA
4801 GCTTGCGCGG GCCGAGCTGG CACGGGCACC GGCACCCCGC CAGCGAGGCA TGGACAGGGG CGGGCCAGAT TTCAGCATGT
4881 AGTGCTTGCG TTGGTACTCA CGCCTGTTAT ACTATGAGTA CTCACGCACA GAAGGGGGTT TTATGGAATA CGAAAAAAGC
4961 GCTTCAGGGT CGGTCTACCT GATCAAAAGT GACAAGGGCT ATTGGTTGCC CGGTGGCTTT GGTTATACGT CAAACAAGGC
5041 CGAGGCTGGC CGCTTTTCAG TCGCTGATAT GGCCAGCCTT AACCTTGACG GCTGCACCTT GTCCTTGTTC CGCGAAGACA
5121 AGCCTTTCGG CCCCGGCAAG TTTCTCGGTG ACTGATATGA AAGACCAAAA GGACAAGCAG ACCGGCGACC TGCTGGCCAG
5201 CCCTGACGCT GTACGCCAAG CGCGATATGC CGAGCGCATG AAGGCCAAAG GGATGCGTCA GCGCAAGTTC TGGCTGACCG
5281 ACGACGAATA CGAGGCGCTG CGCGAGTGCC TGGAAGAACT CAGAGCGGCG CAGGGCGGGG GTAGTGACCC CGCCAGCGCC
5361 TAACCACCAA CTGCCTGCAA AGGAGGCAAT CAATGGCTAC CCATAAGCCT ATCAATATTC TGGAGGCGTT CGCAGCAGCG
5441 CCGCCACCGC TGGACTACGT TTTGCCCAAC ATGGTGGCCG GTACGGTCGG GGCGCTGGTG TCGCCCGGTG GTGCCGGTAA
5521 ATCCATGCTG GCCCTGCAAC TGGCCGCACA GATTGCAGGC GGGCCGGATC TGCTGGAGGT GGGCGAACTG CCCACCGGCC
5601 CGGTGATCTA CCTGCCCGCC GAAGACCCGC CCACCGCCAT TCATCACCGC CTGCACGCCC TTGGGGCGCA CCTCAGCGCC
5681 GAGGAACGGC AAGCCGTGGC TGACGGCCTG CTGATCCAGC CGCTGATCGG CAGCCTGCCC AACATCATGG CCCCGGAGTG
5761 GTTCGACGGC CTCAAGCGCG CCGCCGAGGG CCGCCGCCTG ATGGTGCTGG ACACGCTGCG CCGGTTCCAC ATCGAGGAAG
5841 AAAACGCCAG CGGCCCCATG GCCCAGGTCA TCGGTCGCAT GGAGGCCATC GCCGCCGATA CCGGGGTGCTC TATCGTGTTC
5921 CTGCACCATG CCAGCAAGGG CGCGGCCATG ATGGGCGCAG GCGACCAGCA GCAGGCCAGC CGGGGCAGCT CGGTACTGGT
6001 CGATAACATC CGCTGGCAGT CCTACCTGTC GAGCATGACC AGCGCCGAGG CCGAGGAATG GGGTGTGGAC GACGACCAGC
6081 GCCGGTTCTT CGTCCGCTTC GGTGTGAGCA AGGCCAACTA TGGCGCACCG TTCGCTGATC GGTGGTTCAG GCGGCATGAC
6161 GGCGGGGTGC TCAAGCCCGC CGTGCTGGAG AGGCAGCGCA AGAGCAAGGG GGTGCCCCGT GGTGAAGCCT AAGAACAAGC
6241 ACAGCCTCAG CCACGTCCGG CACGACCCGG CGCACTGTCT GGCCCCCGGC CTGTTCCGTG CCCTCAAGCG GGGCGAGCGC
6321 AAGCGCAGCA AGCTGGACGT GACGTATGAC TACGGCGACG GCAAGCGGAT CGAGTTCAGC GGCCCGGAGC CGCTGGGCGC
6401 TGATGATCTG CGCATCCTGC AAGGGCTGGT GGCCATGGCT GGGCCTAATG GCCTAGTGCT TGGCCCGGAA CCCAAGACCG
6481 AAGGCGGACG GCAGCTCCGG CTGTTCCTGG AACCCAAGTG GGAGGCCGTC ACCGCTGAAT GCCATGTGGT CAAAGGTAGC
6561 TATCGGGCGC TGGCAAAGGA AATCGGGGCA GAGGTCGATA GTGGTGGGGC GCTCAAGCAC ATACAGGACT GCATCGAGCG
6641 CCTTTGGAAG GTATCCATCA TCGCCCAGAA TGGCCGCAAG CGGCAGGGGT TTCGGCTGCT GTCGGAGTAC GCCAGCGACG
6721 AGGCGGACGG GCGCCTGTAC GTGGCCCTGA ACCCCTTGAT CGCGCAGGCC GTCATGGGTG GCGGCCAGCA TGTGCGCATC
6801 AGCATGGACG AGGTGCGGGC GCTGGACAGC GAAACCGCCC GCCTGCTGCA CCAGCGGCTG TGTGGCTGGA TCGACCCCGG
6881 CAAAACCGGC AAGGCTTCCA TAGATACCTT GTGCGGCTAT GTCTGGCCGT CAGAGGCCAG TGGTTCGACC ATGCGCAAGC
6961 GCCGCAAGCG GGTGCGCGAG GCGTTGCCGG AGCTGGTCGC GCTGGGCTGG ACGGTAACCG AGTTCGCGGC GGGCAAGTAC
7041 GACATCACCC GGCCCAAGGC GGCAGGCTGA CCCCCCCCAC TCTATTGTAA ACAAGACATT TTTATCTTTT ATATTCAATG
7121 GCTTATTTTC CTGCTAATTG GTAATACCAT GAAAAATACC ATGCTCAGAA AAGGCTTAAC AATATTTTGA AAAATTGCCT
7201 ACTGAGCGCT GCCGCACAGC TCCATAGGCC GCTTTCCTGG CTTTGCTTCC AGATGTATGC TCTTCTGCTC CCGAACGCCA
7281 GCAAGACGTA GCCCAGCGCG TCGGCCAGCT TGCAATTCGC GCTAACTTAC ATTAATTGCG TTGCGCTCAC TGCCCGCTTT
7361 CCAGTCGGGA AACCTGTCGT GCCAGCTGCA TTAATGAATC GGCCAACGCG CGGGGAGAGG CGGTTTGCGT ATTGGGCGCC
7441 AGGGTGGTTT TTCTTTTCAC CAGTGAGACG GGCAACAGCT GATTGCCCTT CACCGCCTGG CCCTGAGAGA GTTGCAGCAA
7521 GCGGTCCACG TGGTTTGCCC CAGCAGGCGA AAATCCTGTT TGATGGTGGT TAACGGCGGG ATATAACATG AGCTGTCTTC
7601 GGTATCGTCG TATCCCACTA CCGAGATATC CGCACCAACG CGCAGCCCGG ACTCGGTAAT GGCGCGCATT GCGCCCAGCG
7681 CCATCTGATC GTTGGCAACC AGCATCGCAG TGGGAACGAT GCCCTCATTC AGCATTTGCA TGGTTTGTTG AAAACCGGAC
7761 ATGGCACTCC AGTCGCCTTC CCGTTCCGCT ATCGGCTGAA TTTGATTGCG AGTGAGATAT TTATGCCAGC CAGCCAGACG
7841 CAGACGCGCC GAGACAGAAC TTAATGGGCC CGCTAACAGC GCGATTTGCT GGTGACCCAA TGCGACCAGA TGCTCCACGC
7921 CCAGTCGCGT ACCGTCTTCA TGGGAGAAAA TAATACTGTT GATGGGTGTC TGGTCAGAGA CATCAAGAAA TAACGCCGGA
8001 ACATTAGTGC AGGCAGCTTC CACAGCAATG GCATCCTGGT CATCCAGCGG ATAGTTAATG ATCAGCCCAC TGACGCGTTG
8081 CGCGAGAAGA TTGTGCACCG CCGCTTTACA GGCTTCGACG CCGCTTCGTT CTACCATCGA CACCACCACG CTGGCACCCA
8161 GTTGATCGGC GCGAGATTTA ATCGCCGCGA CAATTTGCGA CGGCGCGTGC AGGGCCAGAC TGGAGGTGGC AACGCCAATC
8241 AGCAACGACT GTTTGCCCGC CAGTTGTTGT GCCACGCGGT TGGGAATGTA ATTCAGCTCC GCCATCGCCG CTTCCACTTT
8321 TTCCCGCGTT TTCGCAGAAA CGTGGCTGGC CTGGTTCACC ACGCGGGAAA CGGTCTGATA AGAGACACCG GCATACTCTG
8401 CGACATCGTA TAACGTTACT GGTTTCACAT TCACCACCCT GAATTGACTC TCTTCCGGGC GCTATCATGC CATACCGCGA
8481 AAGGTTTTGC ACCATTCGAT GGTGTCAACG TAAATGCCGC TTCGCCTTCG CGCGCGAATT GCAAGCTGAT CCGGGCTTAT
8561 CGACTGCACG GTGCACCAAT GCTTCTGGCG TCAGGCAGCC ATCGGAAGCT GTGGTATGGC TGTGCAGGTC GTAAATCACT
8641 GCATAATTCG TGTCGCTCAA GGCGCACTCC CGTTCTGGAT AATGTTTTTT GCGCCGACAT CATAACGGTT CTGGCAAATA
8721 TTCTGAAATG AGCTGTTGAC AATTAATCAT CGGCTCGTAT AATGTGTGGA ATTGTGAGCG GATAACAATT TCACACAGGA
8801 AACAGAA
```

FIGURE 3. Continued

TABLE 3

Gene organization of the vector pMMB66EH

Gene	Position of coding sequence (base pairs)	Function
bla	552–1412	β-Lactamase
oriV	1850–2245	Origin of vegetative replication
mobC	2554–2270[a]	Conjugative DNA transfer
oriT	2585–2672	Origin of conjugative DNA transfer
repB/mobA	2753–4882	Primase
mobB	3501–3914	Conjugative DNA transfer
repB'	3911–4882	Primase
Gene E	4943–5155	Unknown
cac	5157–5363	Control of *repA* and *repC*
repA	5393–6232	DNA helicase
repC	6219–7070	Replication initiator
lacI[a]	8428–7347[a]	*lac* repressor gene

[a] Numbering reflects the direction of transcription.

shown in Fig. 3. Information on the essential genes identified on this plasmid is summarized in Table 3. The orientation of the cloning site cassette with respect to the *tac* promoter is indicated by the designation EH (*tac-Eco*RI-*Hin*dIII) or HE (the reverse, *tac-Hin*dIII-*Eco*RI). Plasmids of the pMMB67 series are identical to pMMB66, but they contain an extended cloning-site cassette derived from plasmids pUC18 and pUC19, respectively (Fürste et al., 1986).

BROAD-HOST-RANGE MODE OF REPLICATION

Studies of RSF1010 DNA replication in vivo and in vitro (Haring et al., 1985; Haring and Scherzinger, 1989; Frey and Bagdasarian, 1989) have determined that three genes encoded on this plasmid are essential for its replication. These are *repC*, coding for an initiator protein that recognizes the origin of vegetative replication (*oriV*), *repA*, coding for a DNA helicase similar in function but not homologous to the DnaB protein of *E. coli*, and *repB*, coding for a primase also analogous in function but not homologous to the DnaG protein of *E. coli* (Table 3). These genes are transcribed from two promoter regions, P1/P3 and P4, and are organized into two operonlike regulatory units as shown in Fig. 4. Preliminary results indicate that stringent negative regulation at both promoter regions is exerted by gene products encoded downstream of the promoters (Frey and Bagdasarian, 1989).

Replication proteins of RSF1010 provide the most essential functions of the DNA replication complex, the primosome, such as recognition of the origin, unwinding of the DNA duplex, and synthesis of the initiation primer. The replication of RSF1010 is therefore independent from initiation functions encoded on the host chromosome. This has been shown experimentally at least in *E. coli* (Scholz et al., 1984). This independence is presumably the main factor that allows RSF1010 to replicate in such a wide range of bacterial hosts.

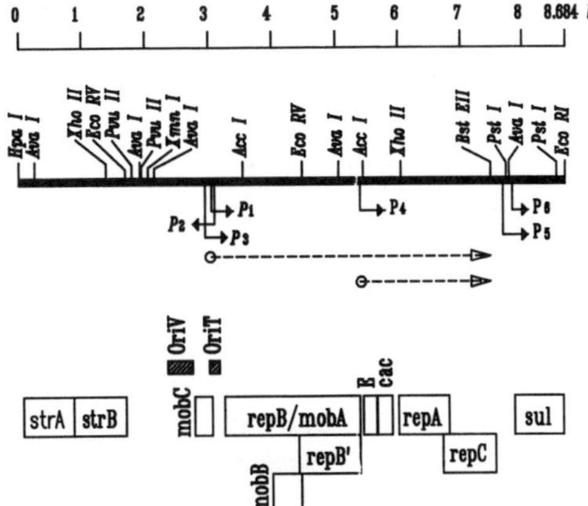

FIGURE 4. Transcriptional units within the *rep* operon of RSF1010. P1 through P6 represent promoters identified by RNA polymerase-binding studies, direct analysis of promoter activity, and nucleotide sequence analysis. The dotted lines represent transcriptional and regulatory units. Abbreviations are as in Table 3 and Fig. 1. kb, Kilobase pairs.

ACKNOWLEDGMENTS. This work was supported by grants from the U.S. Department of Agriculture (grant 89-01053 to the Michigan Biotechnology Institute) and the Research Excellence Fund from the State of Michigan (to M.B.).

LITERATURE CITED

Bagdasarian, M., M. M. Bagdasarian, S. Coleman, and K. N. Timmis. 1979. New vectors for cloning in Pseudomonas, p. 411–422. *In* K. N. Timmis and A. Pühler (ed.), *Plasmids of Environmental, Commercial and Medical Importance.* Elsevier/North-Holland Publishing Co., Amsterdam.

Bagdasarian, M., R. Lurz, B. Rückert, F. C. H. Franklin, M. M. Bagdasarian, and K. N. Timmis. 1981. Specific purpose cloning vectors. II. Broad host range, high copy number RSF1010-derived vectors and a host vector system for gene cloning in *Pseudomonas. Gene* **16:**237–247.

Bagdasarian, M., and K. N. Timmis. 1982. Host vector system for gene cloning in *Pseudomonas. Curr. Top. Microbiol. Immunol.* **96:**47–67.

Bagdasarian, M. M., E. Aman, R. Lurz, B. Rückert, and M. Bagdasarian. 1983. Activity of the hybrid *trp-lac* (*tac*) promoter of *Escherichia coli* in *Pseudomonas putida.* Construction of broad host range, controlled-expression vectors. *Gene* **26:**273–282.

Bailone, A., A. Bäckman, S. Sommer, J. Céleérier, M. M. Bagdasarian, M. Bagdasarian, and R. Devoret. 1988. PsiB polypeptide prevents activation of RecA protein in *Escherichia coli. Mol. Gen. Genet.* **214:**389–395.

Barth, P. T., and N. J. Grinter. 1974. Comparison of the deoxyribonucleic acid molecular weights and homologies of plasmids conferring linked resistance to streptomycin and sulfonamides. *J. Bacteriol.* **120:**618–630.

Buchholz, S. E., and D. E. Eveleigh. 1986. Transfer of plasmids to an antibiotic-sensitive mutant of *Zymomonas mobilis. Appl. Environ. Microbiol.* **52:**366–370.

Burkhardt, H. J., G. Riess, and A. Pühler. 1979. Relationship of group P1 plasmids revealed by heteroduplex experiments: RP1, RP4, R68 and RK2 are identical. *J. Gen. Microbiol.* **114:**341–348.

David, M., M. Vielma, and J. S. Julliot. 1983. Introduction of IncQ plasmids into *Rhizobium meliloti.* Isolation of a host range mutant of RSF1010 plasmid. *FEMS Microbiol. Lett.* **16:**2–3.

Davison, J., M. Heusterspeute, and F. Brunel. 1987. Restriction site bank vectors for cloning in Gram-negative bacteria and yeast. *Methods Enzymol.* **153:**34–54.

Elleman, T. C., P. A. Hoyne, J. D. Stewart, N. M. McKern, and J. D. Peterson. 1986. Expression of pili from *Bacteroides nodosus* in *Pseudomonas aeruginosa. J. Bacteriol.* **168:**574–580.

Ely, B. 1979. Transfer of drug resistant factors to the dimorphic bacterium *Caulobacter crescentus. Genetics* **91:**371–380.

Errington, J. 1987. Generalized cloning vectors for *Bacillus subtilis,* p. 345–362. *In* R. L. Rodriguez and D. T. Denhardt (ed.), *Vectors: a Survey of Molecular Cloning Vectors and Their Uses.* Butterworths, Boston.

Fornari, C. S., and S. Kaplan. 1982. Genetic transformation of *Rhodopseudomonas sphaeroides* by plasmid DNA. *J. Bacteriol.* **152:**89–97.

Frey, J., and M. Bagdasarian. 1989. The molecular biology of IncQ plasmids, p. 79–94. *In* C. M. Thomas (ed.), *Promiscuous Plasmids of Gram-Negative Bacteria.* Academic Press, Inc., New York.

Frey, J., M. Bagdasarian, D. Feiss, F. C. H. Franklin, and J. Deshusses. 1983. Stable cosmid vectors that enable the introduction of cloned fragments into a wide range of Gram-negative bacteria. *Gene* **24:**299–308.

Frey, J., and H. M. Krisch. 1985. Mutagenesis in Gram-negative bacteria: a selectable interposon which is strongly polar in a wide range of bacterial species. *Gene* **36:**143–150.

Fürste, J. P., W. Pansegrau, R. Frank, H. Blöcker, P. Scholz, M. Bagdasarian, and E. Lanka. 1986. Molecular cloning of the plasmid RP4 primase region in a multi-host-range *tac*P expression vector. *Gene* **48:**119–131.

Gautier, F., and R. Bonewald. 1980. The use of plasmid R1162 and derivatives for gene cloning in the methanol utilizing *Pseudomonas* AM1. *Mol. Gen. Genet.* **178:**375–380.

Guerry, P., J. van Embden, and S. Falkow. 1974. Molecular nature of two non-conjugative plasmids carrying drug resistance genes. *J. Bacteriol.* **117:**619–630.

Guiney, D. G., G. Chikami, C. Deiss, and E. Yacobson. 1985. The origin of plasmid DNA transfer during bacterial conjugation, p. 521–534. *In* D. R. Helinski, S. N. Cohen, D. B. Clewell, D. A. Jackson, and A. Hollaender (ed.), *Plasmids in Bacteria.* Plenum Publishing Corp., New York.

Haring, V., and E. Scherzinger. 1989. Replication proteins of IncQ plasmids, p. 95–124. *In* C. M. Thomas (ed.), *Promiscuous Plasmids of Gram-Negative Bacteria.* Academic Press, Inc., New York.

Haring, V., P. Scholz, E. Scherzinger, J. Frey, K. Derbyshire, G. Hatfull, N. S. Willetts, and M. Bagdasarian. 1985. Protein RepC is involved in copy number control of the broad host range plasmid RSF1010. *Proc. Natl. Acad. Sci. USA* **82:**6090–6094.

Hille, J., and R. Schilperoort. 1981. Behaviour of IncQ plasmids in *Agrobacterium tumefaciens. Plasmid* **6:**360–362.

Hohn, B., and J. Collins. 1980. A small cosmid for efficient cloning of large DNA fragments. *Gene* **11:**291–298.

Itoh, Y., J. H. Watson, D. Haas, and T. Leisinger. 1984. Genetic and molecular characterization of the *Pseudomonas* plasmid pVS1. *Plasmid* **11:**206–220.

Iyer, V. N. 1989. IncN group plasmids and their genetic systems, p. 165–184. *In* C. M. Thomas (ed.), *Promiscuous Plasmids of Gram-Negative Bacteria.* Academic Press, Inc., New York.

Keen, N. T., S. Tamaki, D. Kobayashi, and D. Trollinger. 1988. Improved broad-host-range plasmids for DNA cloning in Gram-negative bacteria. *Gene* **70:**191–197.

Leemans, R., E. Remaut, and W. Fiers. 1987. A broad-host-range expression vector based on the p_L promoter of coliphage λ: regulated synthesis of human interleukin 2 in *Erwinia* and *Serratia* species. *J. Bacteriol.* **169:**1899–1904.

Mermod, N., P. R. Lehrbach, R. H. Don, and K. N. Timmis. 1986a. Gene cloning and manipulation in *Pseudomonas*, p. 325–355. *In* I. C. Gunsalus, J. R. Sokatch, and L. N. Ornston (ed.), *The Bacteria*, vol. 10. *The Biology of Pseudomonas.* Academic Press, Inc., Orlando, Fla.

Mermod, N., J. L. Ramos, P. R. Lehrbach, and K. N. Timmis. 1986b. Vector for regulated expression of cloned genes in a wide range of gram-negative bacteria. *J. Bacteriol.* **167:**447–454.

Meyer, R., M. Hinds, and M. Brasch. 1982. Properties of R1162, a broad-host-range, high copy number plasmid. *J. Bacteriol.* **150:**552–562.

Nagahari, K., and K. Sakaguchi. 1978. RSF1010 plasmid as potentially useful vector in *Pseudomonas* species. *J. Bacteriol.* **133:**1527–1529.

Powell, B., M. Mergeay, and N. Christofi. 1989. Transfer of broad host range plasmids to sulfate-reducing bacteria. *FEMS Lett.* **59:**269–274.

Priefer, U. B., R. Simon, and A. Pühler. 1985. Extension of the host range of *Escherichia coli* vectors by incorporation of RSF1010 replication and mobilization functions. *J. Bacteriol.* **163:**324–330.

Ramos, J. L., M. Gonzales-Carrero, and K. N. Timmis. 1988. Broad-host range expression vectors containing manipulated *meta*-cleavage pathway regulatory elements of the TOL plasmid. *FEBS Lett.* **226:**241–246.

Ridgway, A. A. G. 1987. Mammalian expression vectors, p. 467–492. *In* R. L. Rodriguez and D. T. Denhardt (ed.), *Vectors: a Survey of Molecular Cloning Vectors and Their Uses*. Butterworths, Boston.

Schmidhauser, T. J., G. Ditta, and D. R. Helinski. 1987. Broad-host-range plasmid cloning vectors for Gram-negative bacteria, p. 287–332. *In* R. L. Rodriguez and D. T. Denhardt (ed.), *Vectors: a Survey of Molecular Cloning Vectors and Their Uses*. Butterworths, Boston.

Schmidhauser, T. J., and D. R. Helinski. 1985. Regions of broad-host-range plasmid RK2 involved in replication and stable maintenance in nine species of gram-negative bacteria. *J. Bacteriol.* **164:**446–455.

Scholz, P., V. Haring, E. Scherzinger, R. Lurz, M. M. Bagdasarian, H. Schuster, and M. Bagdasarian. 1984. Replication determinants of the broad-host-range plasmid RSF1010, p. 243–259. *In* D. R. Helinski, S. N. Cohen, D. B. Clewell, D. A. Jackson, and A. Hollaender (ed.), *Plasmids in Bacteria*. Plenum Publishing Corp., New York.

Scholz, P., V. Haring, B. Wittmann-Liebold, K. Ashman, M. Bagdasarian, and E. Scherzinger. 1989. Complete nucleotide sequence and gene organization of the broad host range plasmid RSF1010. *Gene* **75:**271–288.

Smith, J. C., M. C. Liechty, J. L. Rasmussen, and F. L. Macrina. 1985. Genetics of clindomycin resistance in *Bacteroides*, p. 555–570. *In* D. R. Helinski, S. N. Cohen, D. B. Clewell, D. A. Jackson, and A. Hollaender (ed.), *Plasmids in Bacteria*. Plenum Publishing Corp., New York.

Spooner, R. A., M. Bagdasarian, and F. C. H. Franklin. 1987. Activation of the *xylDLEGF* promoter of the TOL toluence-xylene degradation pathway by overproduction of the *xylS* regulatory gene product. *J. Bacteriol.* **169:**3581–3586.

Tai, T. N., W. A. Havelka, and S. Kaplan. 1988. A broad-host-range vector system for cloning and translational *lacZ* fusion analysis. *Plasmid* **19:**175–188.

Tait, R. C., T. J. Close, R. C. Lundquist, M. Hagiya, R. L. Rodriguez, and C. Kado. 1983. Construction and characterization of a versatile broad host range DNA cloning system for Gram-negative bacteria. *Bio/Technology* **1:**269–275.

Valentine, C. R. I., and C. I. Kado. 1989. Molecular genetics of IncW plasmids, p. 125–164. *In* C. M. Thomas (ed.), *Promiscuous Plasmids of Gram-Negative Bacteria*. Academic Press, Inc., New York.

Valla, S., D. H. Coucheron, and J. Kjosbakken. 1986. Conjugative transfer of the naturally occurring plasmids of *Acetobacter xylinum* by IncP-plasmid-mediated mobilization. *J. Bacteriol.* **165:**336–339.

West, R. W., Jr. 1987. Molecular cloning vectors of *Saccharomyces*: generalized cloning vectors, p. 387–404. *In* R. L. Rodriguez and D. T. Denhardt (ed.), *Vectors: a Survey of Molecular Cloning Vectors and Their Uses*. Butterworths, Boston.

Windass, J. D., M. J. Worsey, E. M. Pioli, D. Pioli, P. T. Barth, K. T. Atherton, E. C. Dart, D. Byrom, K. Powell, and P. J. Senior. 1980. Improved conversion of methanol to single-cell protein by *Methylophilus methylotrophus*. *Nature* (London) **287:**396–401.

Wood, D. O., M. F. Hollinger, and M. B. Tindol. 1981. Versatile cloning vector for *Pseudomonas aeruginosa*. *J. Bacteriol.* **145:**1448–1452.

Chapter 24

Recombinant DNA Vectors for *Pseudomonas*

John Davison, Françoise Brunel, Kone Kaniga,
and Nathalie Chevalier

Recombinant DNA technology in gram-negative soil bacteria, such as *Pseudomonas* and *Rhizobium* spp., has lagged behind that for the enteric bacteria, such as *Escherichia coli*. One reason for this was the lack of suitable plasmid vectors, since the typical *E. coli* vectors are unable to replicate in *Pseudomonas* spp. A second problem is that many gram-negative bacteria are very difficult to transform with naked DNA. To solve these problems, wide-host-range plasmids that can be transferred by conjugation have been used. The IncQ plasmid RSF1010 has proven particularly useful, since the minimal replicon, though somewhat large, contains few unique restriction sites and includes the mobilization functions and origin of conjugal transfer (Nagahari and Sakaguchi, 1978; Bagdasarian et al., 1981).

WIDE-HOST-RANGE COSMID VECTOR

To improve the characteristics of RSF1010 as a cloning vector, several modifications were made. The sulfonamide gene was replaced by the kanamycin resistance gene of Tn5, and the streptomycin resistance gene was equipped with a promoter from the tetracycline resistance gene of pBR322. A restriction nuclease site bank was added from pJRD184, a small *E. coli* vector having 50 unique restriction nuclease sites (Heusterspreute et al., 1985), resulting in pJRD215, which has 23 unique restriction sites (Fig. 1; Davison et al., 1987a; Davison et al., 1987c). The large number of unique restriction sites facilitates subsequent subcloning and deletion analysis to localize the gene of interest. To permit the incorporation of large (35- to 40-kilobase-pair) DNA fragments, the new vector was equipped with a 403-base-pair fragment containing the *cos* region

John Davison ● Transgène s.a., Rue de Molsheim 11, 67000 Strasbourg, France. *Françoise Brunel* ● European Patent Office, Erhardtstrasse 27, D-8000 Munich, Federal Republic of Germany. *Kone Kaniga and Nathalie Chevalier* ● Unit of Molecular Biology, International Institute of Cellular and Molecular Pathology, 75 Avenue Hippocrate, 1200 Brussels, Belgium.

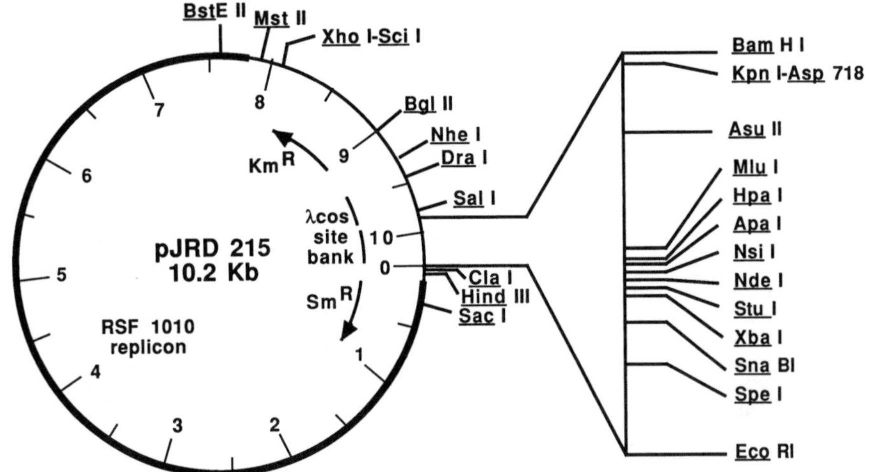

FIGURE 1. Physical map of restriction site bank vector pJRD215. Only unique restriction nuclease sites are shown. The numbers divide the vector into 1-kilobase segments.

of bacteriophage λ. This permits in vitro packaging of a gene bank into λ phage particles (Meyerowitz et al., 1980), which can then be used to infect *E. coli* S17-1, a specially constructed strain in which the conjugative transfer functions of plasmid RP4 are integrated into the chromosome (Simon et al., 1983). From this strain, individual clones from the gene bank can be transferred to *Pseudomonas* spp. by virtue of the mobilization functions and origin of transfer carried by the RSF1010 plasmid.

The utility of pJRD215 for cloning and identifying *Pseudomonas* genes from a shotgun library has been demonstrated by cloning the genes coding for aspartase and asparaginase (Ursi et al., 1987), vanillate demethylase (Brunel and Davison, 1988), and alkyl sulfatase (A. Phanopoulos, F. Brunel, D. Prozzi, N. Chevalier, and J. Davison, manuscript in preparation; J. Davison, F. Brunel, and A. Phanopoulos, this volume). The complete nucleotide sequence of pJRD215 can now be compiled from the published sequences (Davison et al., 1987c; Scholz et al., 1989).

EXPRESSION VECTOR

Although *E. coli* genes can be easily expressed in *Pseudomonas* spp., it is difficult to express *Pseudomonas* genes in *E. coli*. *Pseudomonas* promoters do not follow the typical −10/−35 consensus pattern of *E. coli* promoters (Deretic et al., 1987). In contrast, *E. coli* and *Pseudomonas* ribosome-binding sites are similar so that *Pseudomonas* genes can be expressed in *E. coli* when a suitable *E. coli* type promoter is provided (Frantz and Chakrabarty, 1986).

To develop a system for regulated gene expression that will function both in *E. coli* and in *Pseudomonas* spp., an expression cassette containing the ther-

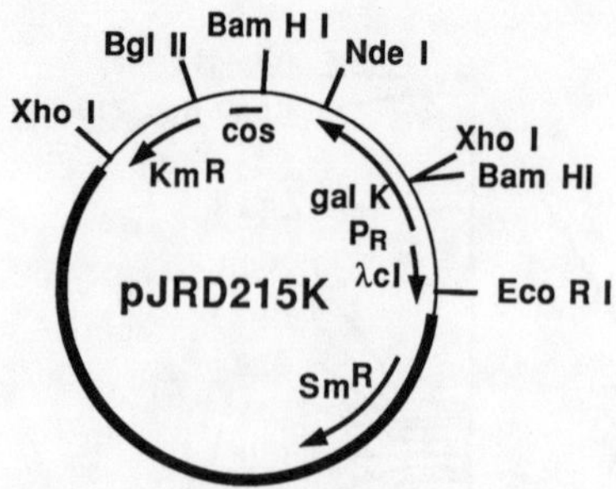

FIGURE 2. λ cI regulated galactokinase expression plasmid. Expression of the *galK* target gene is negatively regulated by the λ cI thermosensitive λ cI857 gene at 32°C.

mosensitive λ cI857 repressor, the λ p_R promoter, and a λ *cro-galK* translational fusion was transferred to pJRD215. The *galK* gene codes for *E. coli* galactokinase, which served as an easily measured indicator enzyme in *Pseudomonas* spp., which does not encode its own galactokinase (Heusterspreute et al., 1984). The resulting plasmid, pJRD215K (Fig. 2), was able to express galactokinase in a number of gram-negative bacteria after temperature induction to inactivate the λ repressor. One example, showing thermoinducible galactokinase expression in the obligate methylotroph *Pseudomonas insueta*, is shown in Fig. 3. These results show that both the λ p_{RM} and p_R promoters are active in *Pseudomonas* spp. and that the λ repressor can correctly interact with the rightward operator to prevent transcription (Davison et al., 1987b). Similar observations have been made for the *E. coli lacI* repressor in *Pseudomonas* (Bagdasarian et al., 1983; Deretic et al., 1987).

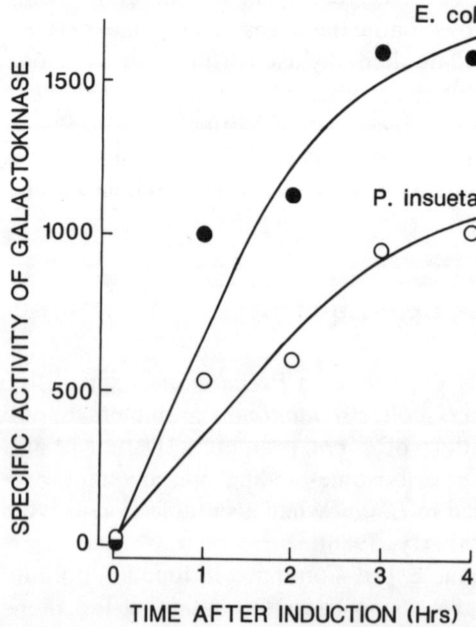

FIGURE 3. Induction of galactokinase in *P. insueta*. Bacteria growing at 32°C were transferred to 42°C, and galactokinase synthesis was monitored by enzyme assay (Davison et al., 1987b). *P. insueta* is an obligate methylotroph and was grown with methanol as a carbon source.

VECTOR FOR GENE PRODUCT CHARACTERIZATION

Present techniques for the exclusive expression and radiolabeling of cloned gene products are confined to *E. coli*, as the host, as a consequence of the need for specific mutants of *E. coli* that result either in minicell production (Reeve, 1977) or in UV-sensitive maxicells (Sancar et al., 1979). Various factors influence expression of the final gene product, including the nature of the ribosome-binding site, codon utilization, processing of signal sequences, protein cleavage, protein folding, and synthesis or incorporation of prosthetic groups. Thus, a system for monitoring gene expression in the different bacterial species, including the original host, would be useful.

A novel type of gene product identification system has been developed for *E. coli* and uses the phage T7 RNA polymerase, which specifically recognizes the $\Phi10$ promoter of phage T7. Since the T7 RNA polymerase functions in the presence of rifampin (whereas most bacterial RNA polymerases do not), specific labelling of the polypeptide product of a target gene (cloned downstream of the $\Phi10$ promoter) can be obtained (Tabor and Richardson, 1985). The T7 RNA polymerase system operates only in *E. coli* and related bacteria, since it is based on *E. coli*-specific plasmids.

To investigate the possible use of the T7 RNA polymerase system in gram-negative bacteria other than *E. coli*, the functional components were transferred to two compatible plasmids, pJRD215 (Fig. 1; Davison et al., 1987a) and pVDZ'2 (Deretic et al., 1987). Plasmid pT7pol has an RK2 replicon and carries the T7 RNA polymerase gene expressed from the λ p_{L} promoter and controlled by the λ *c*I857 repressor (Fig. 4). Thermoinduction permits synthesis of the T7 RNA polymerase, which acts in *trans* on a second plasmid, pJRD251, which contains the *E. coli galK* gene cloned, as an indicator gene, downstream of the T7 $\Phi10$ promoter. Addition of rifampin (to inhibit *E. coli* or *Pseudomonas* RNA polymerase), followed by [^{35}S]methionine, results in specific labeling of the 44-kilodalton galactokinase polypeptide (Debouck et al., 1985) both in *E. coli* and in *Pseudomonas* sp. strain ATCC 19151 (Fig. 5; Davison et al., 1989). In *Pseudomonas* sp. strain ATCC 19151, two other proteins (60 and 14 kilodaltons) are also labeled. These proteins are not plasmid encoded, since they can also be detected in plasmid-free cells. They seem to result from translation of stable mRNA species.

The construction of these new plasmids extends the use of the T7 RNA polymerase expression system to other gram-negative bacteria. It has recently been used for the overexpression of alkyl sulfatase in *Pseudomonas* sp. strain ATCC 19151 (Davison et al., this volume).

TRANSPOSON VECTOR

The plasmid vectors described above are very useful in laboratory manipulations, since their high copy number enhances gene expression and facilitates recovery of the recombinant DNA. However, at present there is considerable

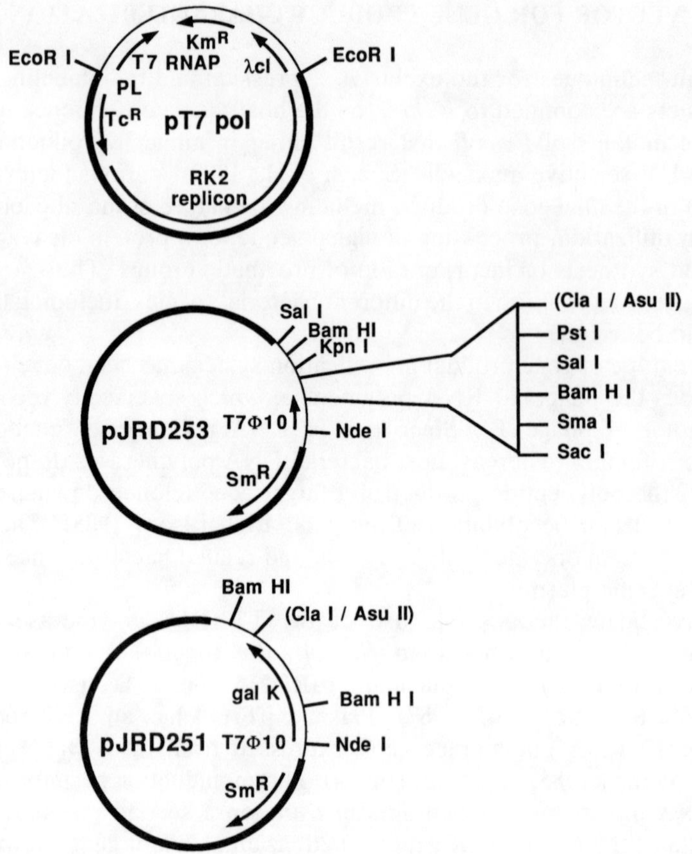

FIGURE 4. T7 RNA polymerase expression system. Plasmid pT7pol is a wide-host-range, RK2-based plasmid that permits the temperature-inducible synthesis of T7 RNA polymerase in *Pseudomonas* spp. Plasmid pJRD253 is an RSF1010-based plasmid containing multiple restriction sites located downstream of the phage T7 Φ10 promoter. Plasmid pJRD251 uses the *E. coli galK* gene as a model system for T7 RNA polymerase-controlled gene expression in *Pseudomonas* spp.

interest in the improvement of bacteria for pollution control (Chakrabarty et al., 1984), agricultural purposes (nitrogen fixation and phytopathogen control [Davison, 1988]), and live vaccines. For these purposes, the wide-host-range vectors available to date are unsuitable for several reasons. First, they are unstable in the absence of continued antibiotic selection. Second, they can be mobilized in the presence of a self-conjugative plasmid, and this would facilitate undesirable horizontal transfer to other bacteria. Third, they have antibiotic resistance genes as selective markers, and it is undesirable to facilitate the spread of these in the environment.

As an alternative to plasmids, the use of transposons as recombinant vector systems has the advantages of enhanced stability and reduced (though not zero) horizontal transfer. Transposon Tn5 has been used, for example, to clone the insecticidal δ-toxin of *Bacillus thuringiensis* into rhizosphere pseudomonads

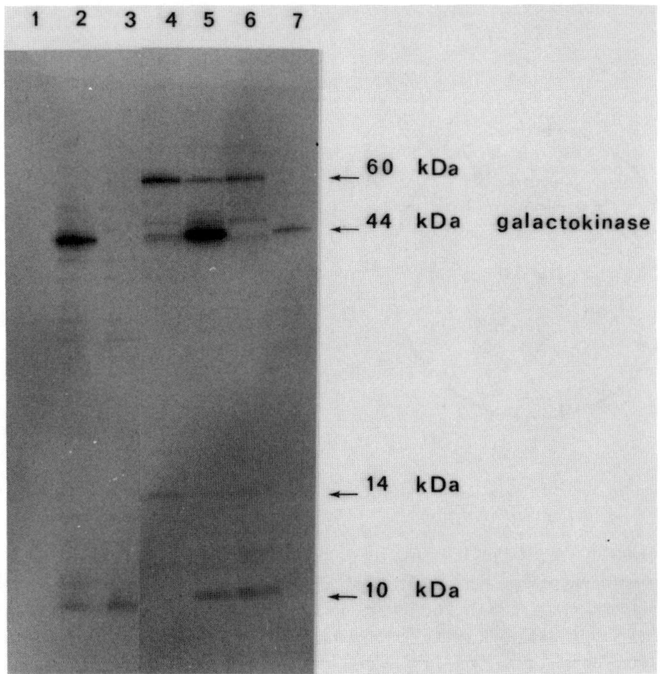

FIGURE 5. Polypeptides synthesized in *E. coli* and *Pseudomonas* sp. strain ATCC 19151 under control of the T7 Φ10 promoter. Cultures containing combinations of plasmids (Fig. 4) were induced at 42°C, treated with rifampin, and labeled with [^{35}S]methionine. The radioactive polypeptides were analyzed by polyacrylamide gel electrophoresis and autoradiography. Lanes 1 to 3 contain extracts of *E. coli* MM294; lanes 4 to 6 contain extracts of *Pseudomonas* sp. strain ATCC 19151. The *E. coli* or *Pseudomonas* cultures contained the following plasmids: pJRD251 (lanes 1 and 4), pJRD251 plus pT7pol (lanes 2 and 5), and a *galK* deletion derivative of pJRD251 plus pT7pol (lanes 3 and 6). Lane 7 serves as a control for authentic galactokinase synthesized in *E. coli*, using the standard plasmid system of Tabor and Richardson (1985). The 10-kilodalton polypeptide, present in lanes 2, 3, 5, and 6, is encoded by the RSF1010 part of the T7 promoter vectors.

(Obukowicz et al., 1987). However, transposon Tn*5* is not ideal as a cloning vector, since it is large and contains only few useful unique cloning sites. The problem is compounded by the fact that Tn*5* must be carried by a suitable delivery vehicle (usually a phage or suicide plasmid), which increases the genetical and physical complexity. We have constructed an improved transposon cloning vector, Tn*5*-K24, using a modified Tn*5* derivative, by increasing the number of unique cloning sites within the transposon (Fig. 6; K. Kaniga, F. Brunel, and J. Davison, manuscript in preparation). At the same time, the complexity of the suicide delivery plasmid has been decreased so that useful cloning sites within the transposon are not duplicated. This delivery vehicle, pDK8, is based on a pMB9 replicon and cannot replicate in *Pseudomonas* spp. However, in the presence of a self-transmissible RP4 plasmid, it can be transferred to *Pseudomonas* spp. with high efficiency by virtue of the mobilization region (*mob*) of plasmid RP4 that it contains (Fig. 6). This transient transfer permits the transposon, accompanied by

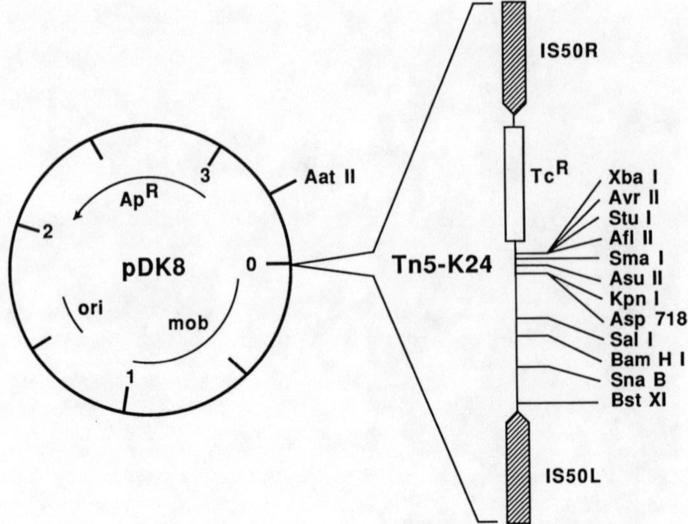

FIGURE 6. Transposon vector Tn5-K24 and its delivery vehicle. The circular module represents the plasmid delivery vehicle, pDK8, derived from pIC20H (Marsh et al., 1984) and containing the *mob* region of RP4 (Selvaraj et al., 1984). The linear module represents the modified transposon Tn5-K24 derived from Tn5-Tc1 (Sasakawa and Yoshikawa, 1987) containing the restriction site bank of pJRD184 (Heusterspreute et al., 1985).

any DNA cloned into it, to jump to the *Pseudomonas* chromosome at low frequency (10^{-6} per recipient cell).

The transposon vectors are still in the developmental stages and suffer two disadvantages. First, they still contain at least one antibiotic resistance gene; for environmental use, this should be replaced by a different selective marker, preferably having application to a wide variety of bacteria such as plant-beneficial pseudomonads and rhizobia (Davison, 1988). Second, the transposons are usually integrated as a single copy per chromosome so that the advantage of the copy number effect on gene expression, seen in plasmid vectors, is lost. On the other hand, it has been shown previously that high expression can be obtained, even with a single, chromosomally integrated copy, when strong transcription and translation signals are provided (Davison et al., 1974). In contrast to wide-host-range plasmid vectors, the integrated transposon vectors are highly stable in the absence of continued selection. No transposon-free segregants were found in a strain grown, in the absence of antibiotic, with daily subculture for one week.

Figure 7 shows the strategy for cloning in transposon Tn5-K24, using the *xylE* gene, from the TOL plasmid of *P. putida* as an example. The *xylE* genes codes for catechol 2,3-dioxygenase; when sprayed with catechol, recipient colonies become bright yellow because of the formation of 2-hydroxymuconic semialdehyde (Zukowski et al., 1983). The *xylE* transposon has been successfully transferred to several gram-negative bacteria and may thus be a useful marker to tag bacteria destined for environmental release.

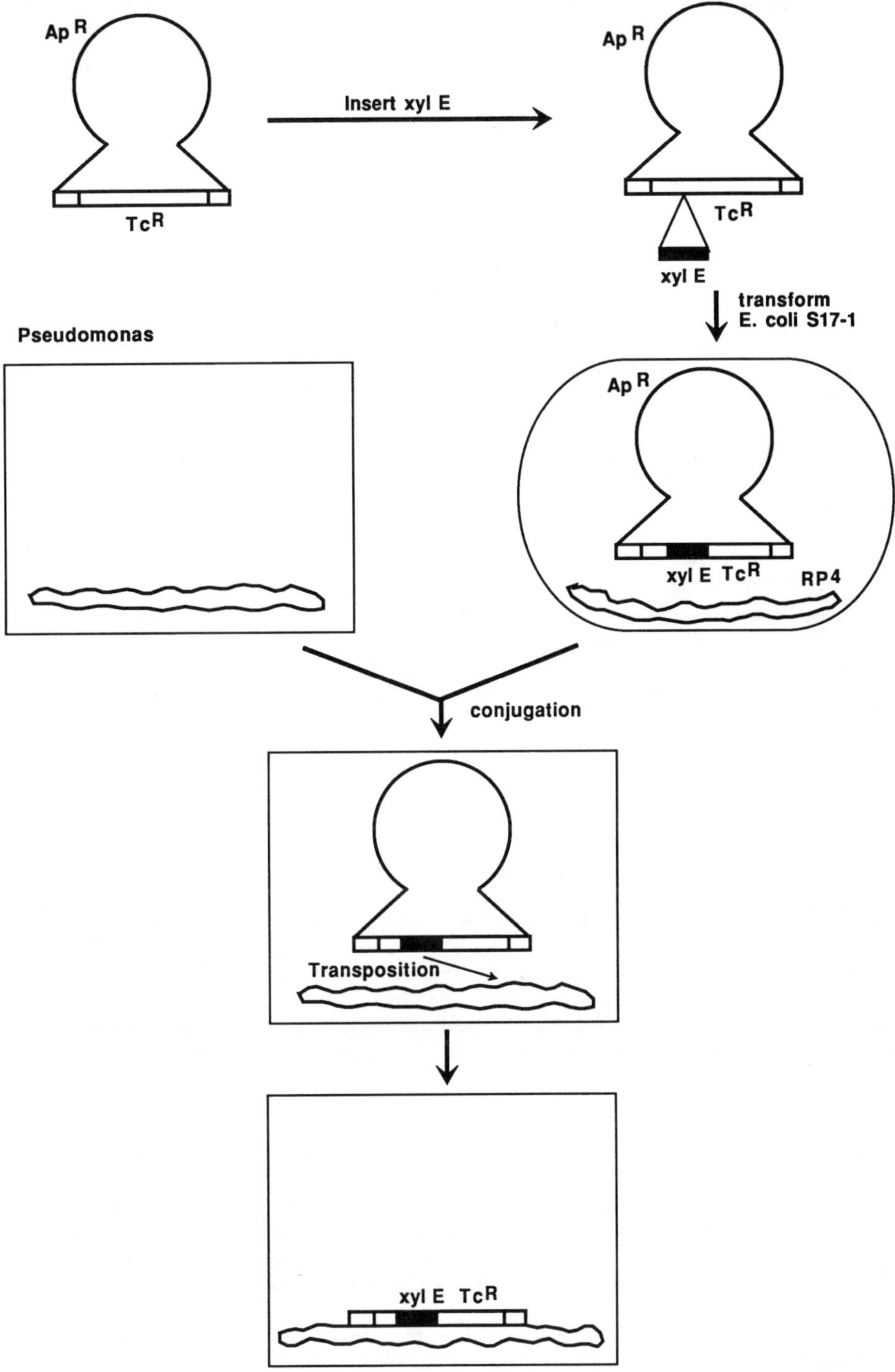

FIGURE 7. Delivery of recombinant transposon to *Pseudomonas* sp. The pBR322-based plasmid is unable to replicate after transfer to *Pseudomonas* sp. Transposition to the *Pseudomonas* chromosome occurs at low frequency ($\pm 10^{-7}$ per recipient cell).

ACKNOWLEDGMENTS. This research was carried out under research contracts BAP-0048-B and BAP-0358 (GBF) of the Commission of the European Communities. We are grateful for extensive discussions with A. M. Chakrabarty during the tenure of North Atlantic Treaty Organization grant 0177/87.

We thank P. Mulder for nucleotide sequence analysis and for typing the manuscript.

LITERATURE CITED

Bagdasarian, M., R. Lurz, B. Rückert, F. C. H. Franklin, M. M. Bagdasarian, J. Frey, and K. N. Timmis. 1981. Specific-purpose plasmid cloning vectors. II. Broad-host-range, high copy number, RSF1010 derived vectors, and a host-vector system for gene cloning in *Pseudomonas*. *Gene* **16:**237–247.

Bagdasarian, M. M., E. Amann, R. Lurz, B. Rückert, and M. Bagdasarian. 1983. Activity of the hybrid *trp-lac* (*tac*) promoter of *Escherichia coli* in *Pseudomonas putida*. Construction of broad-host-range, controlled-expression vectors. *Gene* **26:**273–282.

Brunel, F., and J. Davison. 1988. Cloning and sequencing of *Pseudomonas* genes encoding vanillate demethylase. *J. Bacteriol.* **170:**4924–4930.

Chakrabarty, A. M., J. S. Karns, J. J. Kilbane, and D. K. Chatterjee. 1984. Selective evolution of genes for enhanced degradation of persistent, toxic chemicals, p. 43–54. *In* W. Arber, W. J. Peacock, K. Illmensee, and P. Starlinger (ed.), *Genetic Manipulation, Impact on Man and Society*. International Committee of Scientific Unions Press, Miami.

Davison, J. 1988. Plant beneficial bacteria. *Bio/Technology* **6:**282–286.

Davison, J., W. J. Brammar, and F. Brunel. 1974. Quantitative aspects of gene expression in a λ-*trp* fusion operon. *Mol. Gen. Genet.* **130:**9–20.

Davison, J., N. Chevalier, and F. Brunel. 1989. Bacteriophage T7 RNA polymerase-controlled specific gene expression in *Pseudomonas*. *Gene* **83:**371–375.

Davison, J., M. Heusterspreute, and F. Brunel. 1987a. Restriction site bank vectors for cloning in Gram-negative bacteria and yeast. *Methods Enzymol.* **153:**34–54.

Davison, J., M. Heusterspreute, N. Chevalier, and F. Brunel. 1987b. A phase-shift fusion system for the regulation of foreign gene expression by λ repressor in Gram-negative bacteria. *Gene* **60:**227–235.

Davison, J., M. Heusterspreute, N. Chevalier, V. Ha-Thi, and F. Brunel. 1987c. Vectors with restriction site banks. V. pJRD215, a wide host range cosmid vector with multiple cloning sites. *Gene* **51:**275–280.

Debouck, C., A. Riccio, D. Schumperli, K. McKenney, J. Jeffers. C. Hughes, M. Rosenberg, M. Heusterspreute, F. Brunel, and J. Davison. 1985. Structure of the galactokinase gene of *Escherichia coli*, the third and last (?) gene of the *gal* operon. *Nucleic Acids Res.* **13:**1841–1853.

Deretic, V., S. Chandrasekharappa, J. F. Gill, D. K. Chatterjee, and A. M. Chakrabarty. 1987. A set of cassettes and improved vectors for genetic and biochemical characterization of *Pseudomonas* genes. *Gene* **57:**61–72.

Frantz, B., and A. M. Chakrabarty. 1986. Degradative plasmids in *Pseudomonas*, p. 295–325. *In* I. C. Gunsalus, J. R. Sokatch, and L. N. Ornston (ed.), *The Bacteria*, vol. 10. *The Biology of Pseudomonas*. Academic Press, Inc., Orlando, Fla.

Heusterspreute, M., V. Ha Thi, and J. Davison. 1984. Expression of galactokinase as a fusion protein in *Escherichia coli* and *Saccharomyces cerevisiae*. *DNA* **3:**377–386.

Heusterspreute, M., V. Ha-Thi, S. Emery, S. Tournis-Gamble, N. Kennedy, and J. Davison. 1985. Vectors with restriction site banks. IV. pJRD184, a 3793bp plasmid vector having 43 unique cloning sites. *Gene* **39:**299–304.

Marsh, J. L., M. Erfle, and E. J. Wykes. 1984. The pIC plasmid and phage vectors with versatile cloning sites for recombinant selection by insertional inactivation. *Gene* **32:**481–485.

Meyerowitz, E. M., G. M. Guild, L. S. Prestidge, and D. S. Hogness. 1980. A new cosmid vector and its use. *Gene* **11:**271–282.

Nagahari, K., and K. Sakaguchi. 1978. RSF1010 plasmid as a potentially useful vector in *Pseudomonas* species. *J. Bacteriol.* **134:**1527–1529.

Obukowicz, M. G., F. J. Perlak, S. L. Bolten, K. Kusano-Kretzmer, E. J. Mayer, and L. S. Watrud. 1987. IS50L as a non-self transposable vector used to integrate the *Bacillus thuringiensis* delta-endotoxin gene into the chromosome of root-colonizing Pseudomonads. *Gene* **51**:91–96.

Reeve, J. N. 1977. Bacteriophage infection of mini-cells. A general method for identification of in vivo bacteriophage directed polypeptide biosynthesis. *Mol. Gen. Genet.* **158**:73–79.

Sancar, A., A. M. Hack, and W. D. Rupp. 1979. Simple method for identification of plasmid-coded proteins. *J. Bacteriol.* **137**:692–693.

Sasakawa, C., and M. Yoshikawa. 1987. A series of Tn5 variants with drug-resistance markers and suicide vector for transposon mutagenesis. *Gene* **56**:283–288.

Scholz, P., V. Haring, B. Wittmann-Liebold, K. Ashman, M. Bagdasarian, and E. Scherzinger. 1989. Complete nucleotide sequence and gene organization of the broad-host-range plasmid RSF1010. *Gene* **75**:271–288.

Selvaraj, G., Y. C. Fong, and V. N. Iyer. 1984. A portable DNA sequence carrying the cohesive site (*cos*) of bacteriophage λ and the *mob* (mobilization) region of the broad-host-range plasmid RK2: a module for the construction of new cosmids. *Gene* **32**:235–241.

Simon, R., U. Priefer, and A. Pühler. 1983. A broad host range mobilization system for *in vivo* genetic engineering: transposon mutagenesis in Gram-negative bacteria. *Bio/Technology* **1**:784–791.

Tabor, S., and C. C. Richardson. 1985. A bacteriophage T7 RNA polymerase/promoter system for controlled exclusive expression of specific genes. *Proc. Natl. Acad. Sci. USA* **82**:1074–1078.

Ursi, D., D. Prozzi, J. Davison, and F. Brunel. 1987. Cloning and expression of aspartase and asparaginase from *Pseudomonas* P07111. *J. Biotechnol.* **5**:221–225.

Zukowski, M. M., D. F. Gafney, D. Speck, M. Kaufmann, A. Findeli, A. Wisecup, and J. P. Lecocq. 1983. Chromogenic identification of genetic regulatory signals in *Bacillus subtilis* based on expression of a cloned *Pseudomonas* gene. *Proc. Natl. Acad. Sci. USA* **80**:1101–1105.

Chapter 25

Environmental and Molecular Characterization of Systems Which Affect Genome Alteration in *Pseudomonas aeruginosa*

Robert V. Miller, Tyler A. Kokjohn, and Gary S. Sayler

With the recent advances of genetic engineering have come new questions about genetic stability and exchange among microbes in natural ecosystems. The proposed release of genetically engineered microorganisms (GEMs) to attack problems of environmental pollution and for agricultural uses has raised concerns over the ultimate fate of these organisms and their engineered genes. Only recently have investigators begun to combine the tools of molecular biology and microbial ecology to address questions of genome stability in natural communities of free-living bacteria.

We have been using *Pseudomonas aeruginosa* as a model organism to study genome alteration in freshwater microbial populations and have demonstrated horizontal gene transmission by both transduction and conjugation. Our studies have also provided data which suggest that intracellular genome instability may be increased in the aquatic environment as a result of stresses encountered by the cell in this habitat.

In *Escherichia coli*, the RecA protein is central to many of the molecular processes that control genome alteration. It has been generally accepted that inclusion of a RecA$^-$ mutation in a GEM would reduce genome alteration in natural environments, yet little is known about the functions of the RecA protein in environmentally significant genera. We have therefore addressed the question of the roles of the *P. aeruginosa recA* analog in regulating genome instability in this natural member of the aquatic microbiota.

Robert V. Miller and Tyler A. Kokjohn ● Department of Biochemistry and The Program in Molecular Biology, Loyola University of Chicago, Maywood, Illinois 60153.   ***Gary S. Sayler*** ● Department of Microbiology and The Program in Ecology, University of Tennessee, Knoxville, Tennessee 37932.

INTERCELLULAR GENOME ALTERATION THROUGH HORIZONTAL GENE TRANSFER

The majority of studies on genetic transfer in aquatic environments have been epidemiological (Saye and Miller, 1989). The spread of specific phenotypes (most often associated with extrachromosomal DNA elements) has been followed in a specific environmental situation without regard for the mechanism of transfer. Most of these studies have assumed that the only fertile method of intracellular transfer of these elements in nature is conjugation. This is not the case.

Our investigations have been directed at identifying the mechanisms of gene exchange among populations of *P. aeruginosa* in freshwater ecosystems. In our protocols, laboratory investigations, using sterile and natural lake water microcosms, are used to evaluate systems to be tested in the field. Field investigations are then carried out in a freshwater lake to validate our laboratory studies. For these field trials, we use biological containment chambers that restrict the movement of bacteria and bacteriophages. These chambers are filled with either sterilized or natural lake water and incubated at the field site. Using these protocols, we have documented transduction of both chromosomal and extrachromosomal DNA (Morrison et al., 1978; Saye et al., 1987; D. J. Saye, O. Ogunseitan, G. S. Sayler, and R. V. Miller, *Appl. Environ. Microbiol.*, in press) as well as the conjugal transfer of plasmids (O'Morchoe et al., 1988).

Conjugation

We carried out crosses between a donor strain that contained one of the self-transmissible plasmids R68.45 (Haas and Holloway, 1976) or FP5 (Matsumoto and Tazaki, 1973) and a genetically identifiable recipient strain under environmentally relevant conditions (10^4 recipient cells per ml). Presumptive transconjugants were confirmed by screening for the presence of plasmid DNA with the appropriate restriction endonuclease cleavage pattern.

In microcosms and in the field, conjugal transfer of both plasmids was detected at moderate frequencies in the absence of the natural microbial community inhabiting the field site and at low frequencies in their presence (Table 1). Similar effects of natural microbes on conjugation were observed by Bale et al. (1987) in a freshwater river. Transfer of the broad-host-range plasmid R68.45 to organisms other than the introduced recipient was not observed in the field but was detected in laboratory simulations when organisms isolated from the field site were used as recipients.

The natural microbial community also exerted an influence on the number of recoverable donor and recipient cells. Both populations decreased more rapidly when the natural community was present than when it was absent. Thus, it is likely that the presence of the indigenous population primarily affects the recovery of introduced bacteria (whether parental or recombinant) and not the potential for conjugal transfer. Grazing protozoa have been implicated in the decline in the number of introduced bacteria in seawater and in soil (Alexander, 1981) and may exert a similar influence in fresh water. The effects of the indigenous population

TABLE 1

Comparison of the frequencies of conjugation in standard, microcosm, and field matings[a]

Plasmid	Condition		Mating frequency (transconjugants/CFU)[b]		
	Donor/recipient ratio	Natural community[c]	Standard mating	Microcosm	Field
FP5	1:1	Absent	10^{-4}	10^{-4}	10^{-5}
		Present	—[d]	10^{-8}	10^{-9}
	1,000:1	Absent	—	10^{-6}	10^{-6}
		Present	—	10^{-7}	10^{-9}
R68.45	1:1	Absent	10^{-3}	10^{-3}	10^{-4}
		Present	—	10^{-4}	10^{-9}
	1,000:1	Absent	—	10^{-4}	10^{-5}
		Present	—	10^{-4}	10^{-8}

[a] See O'Morchoe et al. (1988) for experimental details.
[b] Total CFU at initiation of incubation.
[c] In experiments reported as natural community absent, sterilized water collected from the field site was used (O'Morchoe et al., 1988).
[d] —, Not done.

were most pronounced in matings carried out in the field, where transconjugants were detected only during the first 24 h of incubation. This may be an example of nonbiological factors acting synergistically with the indigenous microbial population. The survival of introduced organisms in nature is likely affected by competition with the indigenous microbial population for available nutrients. Conditions supporting the growth of an organism may only be transient under our experimental conditions. Bacteria need to be capable of exploiting nutrients when they are abundantly available and need strategies for survival when nutrients are very limited. These strategies are yet to be characterized, and the physical and biological factors affecting them remain to be elucidated.

The effects of several additional factors on the frequency of conjugation were evaluated in laboratory simulations (O'Morchoe et al., 1988). No significant effect was observed on the frequency of transfer as a function of donor cell population when the temperature of the mating (16 to 37°C) or total cell density (10^9 to 10^3 CFU/ml) in the mating mixture was varied. The most significant effects were observed in response to alteration in the donor-to-recipient ratio. Recovery of transconjugants was significantly increased, as much as 100-fold, when recipient cells were in excess in comparison with results obtained when donor cells were in excess (Table 1). Similar results were observed in the field. Clearly, conjugal transfer of Tra$^+$ plasmids can and does occur under conditions found in freshwater environments and must be considered in evaluating the potential for horizontal gene transmission in natural habitats.

Transduction

Transduction, genetic transfer mediated by bacteriophages, has been demonstrated in many bacterial species (Kokjohn, 1989) but has been largely ignored as a method for gene transfer in the environment. We explored the potential for chromosomal (Morrison et al., 1978; Saye et al., in press) and plasmid (Saye et al., 1987) transduction in freshwater *P. aeruginosa* populations, using a variant of the generalized transducing phage F116 (Krishnapillai, 1971; Miller et al., 1974; Miller et al., 1977) originally designated DS1 (D. J. Saye, T. A. Kokjohn, and R. V. Miller, *Abstr. Annu. Meet. Am. Soc. Microbiol. 1987*, M11, p. 238). For studies of plasmid transfer, we utilized the Tra$^-$ Mob$^-$ plasmid Rms149 (Hedges and Jacoby, 1980). Again, plasmid transduction was confirmed by analysis of the restriction endonuclease digestion patterns of extrachromosomal DNA isolated from the presumptive transductants.

Initially, we explored three models for the source of transducing particles in freshwater environments: (i) cell-free lysates of bacteriophages grown on an appropriate DNA donor, (ii) environmental induction of bacteriophages from a lysogenic DNA donor bacterium, and (iii) environmental induction of bacterio-phages from a lysogenic recipient bacterium. In laboratory simulations and in field trials at high cell densities, transduction of both plasmid and chromosomal DNA was observed in each of these models. The highest number of transductants was routinely recovered from systems in which the recipient bacterium was a lysogen and the DNA donor was a nonlysogen (Saye et al., 1987, in press), probably because of the immunity imparted by the resident F116 prophage to superinfection and killing by phage virions (Benedik et al., 1977). In field trials in which cell concentrations were reduced to environmentally appropriate cell densities (10^4 CFU/ml), transduction of plasmid DNA was detected only when the recipient bacterium was a lysogen (Saye et al., 1987).

For transduction to take place in this system, a unique sequence of events must take place. (i) Phage virions must be produced through spontaneous or stress-stimulated induction of the prophage from the lysogen. (ii) These viral particles must infect, propagate, and lyse the plasmid-containing donor. (iii) Transducing particles produced during the lytic infection of the donor must absorb and transfer DNA to the lysogen. Hence, environmental lysogens serve both as efficient sources of transducing phages and as viable recipients for transduced DNA.

The donor-to-recipient ratio was found to affect the level of transductants recovered (Table 2). The frequency of transduction was independent of donor cell concentration, suggesting that the efficiency of lytic infection and production of phages remained constant over a relatively wide range of cell densities. The frequency of transduction was dependent on the relative abundance of recipient cells and was maximized at an intermediate donor-to-recipient ratio (20:1). This relationship may result from differences in the phage-to-bacterium ratio in the various test chambers due to the relative concentrations of lysogens (recipients) and nonlysogens (donors). Optimal transduction efficiency is most likely achieved only at an optimal phage-to-bacterium ratio.

Transduction was observed in both the absence and presence of the natural microbial community (Saye et al., 1987). The presence of the natural community resulted in a rapid decrease in the recovery of both transductants and introduced donors and recipients. Where observed, the ratio of transductants to parental

TABLE 2

Effects of donor-to-recipient ratio on the frequency of transduction observed in field trials[a]

Natural community	Donor/recipient ratio	Transductants[b]		
		Per 100 ml	Per 10^6 recipients	Per 10^6 donors
Absent	2:1	50	1.41	0.24
	20:1	170	14.85	0.37
	200:1	90	11.01	0.45
Present	2:1	NO[c]	NO	NO
	20:1	2	16.0	0.4
	200:1	NO	NO	NO

[a] See Saye et al. (1987) for experimental details.

[b] Values are reported as maximum number of transductants recovered per 100-ml sample during the incubation period, average number of transductants per donor cells recovered at sampling time, and average number of transductants per recipient cell recovered at sampling time.

[c] NO, Not observed; below level of detection (1 transductant per 100 ml).

strains was similar in sterile and natural lake water (Table 2). As observed with conjugation, the natural community appears to reduce our ability to detect transductants and not the absolute potential for gene transfer by this mechanism.

Chromosomal transduction was measured in microcosms and field trials between (i) a lysogenic donor and nonlysogenic recipient, (ii) a nonlysogenic donor and lysogenic recipient, and (iii) two lysogens (Saye et al., in press). Transduction of single chromosomal alleles was observed at frequencies of 10^{-8} to 10^{-6} transductants per CFU in all systems. In chambers containing a lysogenic and a nonlysogenic strain, each strain could act as both a donor and a recipient of transduced DNA. In general, more transductants of the lysogenic parent than of the nonlysogen were recovered. Reciprocal exchange of alleles was also observed in chambers inoculated with two lysogens. Apparently, both primary infection of a nonlysogen and prophage induction from a lysogen can generate sufficient numbers of transducing particles to allow gene exchange to be observed.

Cotransduction of linked chromosomal markers was observed at frequencies similar to those obtained in standard laboratory transduction protocols (Saye et al., in press). However, coinheritance of unlinked markers was not observed, indicating that multiple transduction events in a single cell are too infrequent in natural environments to be detected by our methods.

Lysogeny may lead to increased fitness in natural ecosystems. It has been suggested that the frequency of lysogeny in natural populations of *P. aeruginosa* approaches 100% (Holloway and Krishnapillai, 1979). We found that approximately 45% of *Pseudomonas* isolates from our field site tested positive in colony hybridization when probed with DNA of a naturally occurring phage from that site (O. Ogunseitan, G. S. Sayler, and R. V. Miller, *Microb. Ecol.*, in press). Our studies have demonstrated the ability of lysogens in freshwater habitats to serve as a source of phages capable of mediating transduction as well as recipients of transduced plasmid and chromosomal DNA. It would appear that the lysogenic state increases the size and flexibility of the gene pool available to natural populations of bacteria by increasing the potential for horizontal gene transmission. The diversity generated by the phage-mediated exchange of DNA may be significant in the face of a continually changing, complex environment. We must consider transduction to be far more significant as a mechanism of genetic exchange in natural habitats than has traditionally been envisioned.

ENVIRONMENTAL POTENTIAL FOR INTRACELLULAR GENOME ALTERATION

The estimation of intracellular genome alteration through recombination, transposition, and mutation may be as important as the estimation of intercellular gene transmission in the evaluation of risk associated with the environmental release of GEMs. Such genome alterations may, on the one hand, inactivate the engineered sequence, rendering the GEM ineffectual in carrying out its intended function. On the other hand, they may activate new, and otherwise cryptic, genetic elements within the host organism genome that change the level of hazard associated with the presence of the GEM in the environment. Current practices for assessing the frequency of intracellular genome alteration are based on data obtained under idealized laboratory conditions. During our environmental studies, we have obtained preliminary evidence suggesting that the rates of reassortment and modification of genetic material in natural ecosystems may far exceed those which we have observed in the laboratory setting.

Increased Mutation Frequency

During our studies on horizontal gene transfer, mutation frequencies of several chromosomal loci were increased 50- to 1,000-fold in the field over frequencies observed in microcosms (Bennett et al., 1988; Saye et al., in press). Even though these microcosms were designed to mimic the field site, environmental factors appear to be inducing elevated rates of mutation that are not at present modeled in our microcosms. These factors must be identified.

Increased Frequency of DNA Rearrangements

Rearrangements in plasmid R68.45 DNA after conjugation were 50-fold higher in experiments carried out in the field than in microcosms (O'Morchoe et al., 1988). Approximately 50% of the transconjugants recovered in field trials showed at least one rearrangement or deletion in the transferred plasmid DNA, whereas less than 1% of the transconjugants recovered from microcosms had such alterations. These rearrangements were detected by nonconformity to antibiotic resistance patterns and confirmed by restriction analysis of plasmid DNA from the transconjugants. Various patterns of loss were observed. Either one or both of the nonselected antibiotic resistance phenotypes were lost. Transfer functions were also lost in some transconjugants, either in conjunction with or separately from loss of antibiotic resistance. Similar increases in the frequency of deletion of the

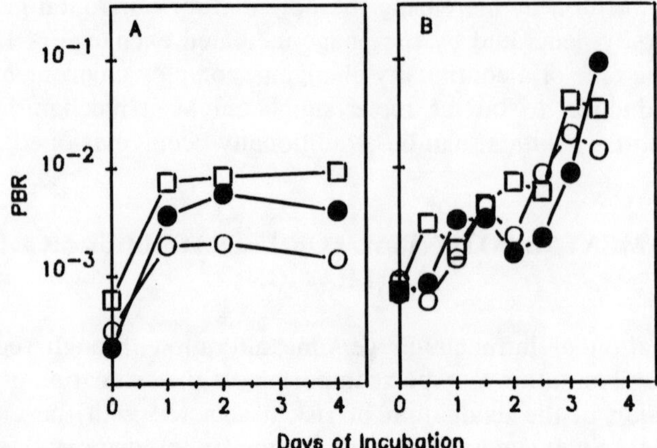

FIGURE 1. Induction of bacteriophages during long-term incubation in microcosms (A) or in the field (B). The phage-to-bacterium ratio (PBR) was calculated from the bacteriophage titers and total cell counts determined at each sampling time. Symbols: ○ and ●, chambers containing a lysogenic and a nonlysogenic strain, respectively; □, chamber containing only lysogens.

primary-selected antibiotic resistance phenotype may explain the apparent reduced conjugation frequency of this plasmid in the field (Table 1). Increased deletion frequency during gene transfer by transformation has also been observed in terrestrial habitats (Bennett et al., 1988). By increasing the frequency of recombination or transposition or both, environmental stress imposed by biological or physical factors may be acting to accelerate genetic evolution to levels that would not be anticipated from laboratory studies.

Increased Frequency of Prophage Induction

Our studies indicate that a major environmental source of phages capable of mediating transduction is the induction of prophages from lysogens present in the natural microbial community. In addition to stimulating gene exchange, the induction of certain prophages, such as the Mu-like *P. aeruginosa* phage D3112, results in transposition and mutagenesis of the host (Rehmat and Shapiro, 1983; Darzins and Casadaban, 1989). The concentrations of *P. aeruginosa*-specific bacteriophages in fresh water often reach 10^2 to 10^3 PFU/ml (J. Replicon and R. V. Miller, unpublished data). Since their half-lives in these environments are calculated to be between 12 and 24 h (Saye et al., 1987; Ogunseitan et al., submitted), phage particles must be continually produced to maintain these levels. By altering the frequencies of the establishment or termination of lysogeny, factors influencing the rate of phage production in natural microbial populations could significantly affect not only horizontal gene transmission but intracellular genome stability as well.

In microcosms, monitoring of phage produced from lysogens showed that after an initial rise, the level of phage remained constant over extended periods of incubation (Fig. 1). In field trials, however, dramatic and periodic increases in phage production were observed during the entire incubation period. Stresses encountered in the environment apparently are capable of increasing the frequency of prophage induction above that observed in the laboratory. These factors may be responsible for the high levels of bacterial viruses observed in aquatic environments (Bergh et al., 1989).

MOLECULAR CONTROL OF GENOME ALTERATION

Many of the molecular mechanisms underlying intracellular genetic instability of the types we observed in the environment have been shown to correlate with the induction of expression of the SOS network after exposure to DNA-damaging stress (Walker, 1984). These include increased rates of mutation, recombination, and prophage induction. In *E. coli*, the product of the *recA* gene is essential to the molecular events that control these processes. It is a positive regulator of the expression of the SOS network, it is essential for homologous recombination, and it has a mechanistic role in several DNA repair pathways (Sedgwick, 1986).

Data from *E. coli* indicate that use of *recA* mutants as hosts for genetically engineered DNA sequences has the potential for reducing genome alteration after release of these organisms into the environment. Since a *Pseudomonas* species is often the host of choice in construction of GEMs for environmental release, we felt it important to investigate the molecular mechanisms that affect genetic stability in this genus and the role of the *recA* gene product in regulating them. Our initial studies have been carried out in *P. aeruginosa*, since the genetics of this naturally occurring aquatic organism are the best understood of any *Pseudomonas* species.

IDENTIFICATION AND CHARACTERIZATION OF THE *P. AERUGINOSA* *recA* GENE

When we initiated our studies, the response of *P. aeruginosa* to DNA-damaging stress either in the natural environment or in the laboratory was virtually unknown. The *recA* gene was yet to be unequivocally identified, and its role in recombination and repair of stress-induced DNA damage had not been elucidated. Therefore, we initiated our studies by using the technique of interspecies complementation (Eitner et al., 1982) to identify the *P. aeruginosa recA* gene. A genomic library of *P. aeruginosa* PAO was constructed and introduced into *E. coli* HB101 (*recA13*). Clones that complemented the methyl methanesulfonate sensitivity associated with the *recA13* allele were selected (Kokjohn and Miller, 1985). After localizing the *P. aeruginosa recA* gene to a 1.5-kilobase *Pvu*II-*Hind*III chromosomal fragment (Kokjohn and Miller, 1987), we characterized the potential of the gene to restore various functions associated with the pleiotropic effects of *E. coli recA* mutations (Table 3). The *P. aeruginosa recA* gene, when introduced into RecA⁻ strains of *E. coli*, is capable of complementing defects in (i) homologous recombination, (ii) induction of the SOS network, and (iii) the

TABLE 3
Functions of *E. coli recA* mutants complemented by the cloned *P. aeruginosa recA* gene

Function	Evidence	Reference(s)
Homologous recombination	Incorporation of exogenote after Hfr-mediated conjugation	Kokjohn and Miller, 1985, 1987; Ohman et al., 1985; Zaitsev et al., 1986
	Replication of Fec⁻ λ phages	Kokjohn and Miller, 1985; Zaitsev et al., 1986
Mechanistic role in DNA repair	Restoration of UV resistance	Kokjohn and Miller, 1985, 1987; Ohman et al., 1985; Sano and Kageyama, 1987; Zaitsev et al., 1986
	Restoration of methyl methanesulfonate resistance	Kokjohn and Miller, 1985, 1987; Ohman et al., 1985; Sano and Kageyama, 1987
	Restoration of nitrofurantoin resistance	Kokjohn and Miller, 1987
	Restoration of UV mutagenesis	
Induction of expression of the SOS network	Spontaneous induction of λ prophages	Kokjohn and Miller, 1985, 1987; Zaitsev et al., 1986
	Mitomycin C-stimulated induction of λ prophages	Kokjohn and Miller, 1985, 1987
	UV and mitomycin C stimulation of UV mutagenesis	Simonson et al., submitted
	UV-stimulated expression of *dinB*	Kokjohn and Miller, 1987

TABLE 4
Characteristics of *P. aeruginosa* Rec⁻ complemented by the *P. aeruginosa recA* clone

Characteristic	Allele[a]	Reference
Homologous recombination	*recA1*	Sano and Kageyama, 1987
	recA7	Horn and Ohman, 1988a; Ohman et al., 1985
	recA102	Kokjohn and Miller, 1987; Horn and Ohman, 1988a; Sano and Kageyama, 1987
	recA908	Kokjohn and Miller, 1987
UV resistance	*recA1*	Sano and Kageyama, 1987
	recA7	Horn and Ohman, 1988a; Ohman et al., 1985
	recA102	Kokjohn and Miller, 1987; Horn and Ohman, 1988a; Sano and Kageyama, 1987
	recA908	Kokjohn and Miller, 1988
Methyl methanesulfonate resistance	*recA7*	Horn and Ohman, 1988a
	recA102	Kokjohn and Miller, 1987; Horn and Ohman, 1988a
Induction of prophages (spontaneous and UV induced)	*recA102*	Kokjohn and Miller, 1987
	recA908	Kokjohn and Miller, 1988
Establishment of lysogeny	*recA908*	Kokjohn and Miller, 1988

[a] *recA1*, *recA102*, and *recA908* are well-characterized alleles isolated in strain PAO. *recA7* was isolated in strain FRD1.

mechanistic roles of the RecA protein in DNA repair (Kokjohn and Miller, 1985, 1987; C. S. Simonson, T. A. Kokjohn, and R. V. Miller, submitted for publication). Similar results have been obtained by Zaitsev et al. (1986) and Sano and Kageyama (1987), using clones of the PAO *recA* gene, and by Ohman et al. (1985), using a *recA* clone obtained from *P. aeruginosa* FRD1.

MUTATIONS OF THE *P. AERUGINOSA recA* GENE

Various mutations of *P. aeruginosa* have been isolated which reduce recombinational proficiency (Holloway, 1966; Chandler and Krishnapillai, 1974; Miller and Ku, 1978; Früh et al., 1983; Ohman et al., 1985). The pleiotropic phenotypes associated with several of these alleles are complemented by the *P. aeruginosa recA* clone (Table 4).

RESPONSE OF *P. AERUGINOSA* TO DNA-DAMAGING STRESS

One of the most striking consequences of the loss of RecA function in *E. coli* is a dramatic increase in sensitivity to far (254 nm) UV radiation (UVC). This not only is the consequence of the inability to induce the SOS activities involved in the repair of UV-induced damage to DNA but is also due to the loss of mechanistic functions of the RecA protein in both the recombinational and *umuDC*-dependent (mutagenic) repair pathways (Sedgwick, 1986). The *P. aeruginosa recA* gene product can complement each of these functions (Table 4).

RecA$^-$ strains of *P. aeruginosa* are more sensitive to irradiation with far-UV radiation than are their Rec$^+$ parents (Miller and Ku, 1978; Früh et al., 1983; Kokjohn and Miller, 1987, 1988). To determine whether this sensitivity is due to the loss of the ability of the mutated protein to carry out its functional roles in DNA repair or to its inability to induce an SOS-like network in *P. aeruginosa* or both, it was necessary to investigate the role of the RecA protein in the response of *P. aeruginosa* to DNA-damaging stress in more detail.

Regulation of Lysogeny by the *P. aeruginosa* RecA Protein

In *E. coli*, the maintenance of lysogeny by prophage λ is regulated by the concentration of the phage-encoded *c*I repressor in the host cell (Ptashne, 1986). Part of the SOS response in λ lysogens is an increased frequency of the termination of lysogeny as a result of the cleavage of *c*I due to activation of a proteaselike activity of the RecA protein in response to UVC exposure. Several *P. aeruginosa* prophages, including the prophages of D3 and F116, are induced to lytic growth after exposure of lysogens to UVC radiation (Cavenagh and Miller, 1986; Miller and Kokjohn, 1987, 1988; Saye et al., *Abstr. Annu. Meet. Am. Soc. Microbiol. 1987*). Both spontaneous and UV-stimulated levels of induction of these prophages require a functional *recA* gene (Kokjohn and Miller, 1987, 1988). Whereas UV-stimulated release is eliminated in *recA908* and *recA102* mutants, the level of spontaneous release of virions is affected differentially by the two alleles. The cloned *P. aeruginosa recA* gene restores the UVC inducibility of these prophages. The identification of the *recA* dependence of UV stimulation of prophage induction was the first clear indication that at least a subset of *recA*-dependent, DNA-damage-inducible functions exists in *P. aeruginosa*.

Several recombination-deficient mutations of *P. aeruginosa*, including *recA908*, significantly reduce the efficiency of the establishment of lysogeny (Les$^-$ phenotype) by various temperate phages, such as D3, F116, and G101 (Holloway, 1966; Miller and Ku, 1978). Lysogeny can be established only at high multiplicities of infection in these mutants. The presence of the cloned *recA* gene restores the ability of *recA908* mutants to be lysogenized at lower multiplicities of infection (Kokjohn and Miller, 1988). In addition, when a clone of the *c1* repressor of phage D3 (Miller and Kokjohn, 1987) was introduced into a *recA908* mutant, the Les$^-$ phenotype was also suppressed (Kokjohn and Miller, 1988). In this case, suppression was phage specific. Lysogeny establishment in *P. aeruginosa* appears to be controlled by the rate of accumulation of phage repressor during the early stages of infection (Kokjohn and Miller, 1988). If the inherent proteolytic activity of the RecA protein is enhanced through mutation, the rate of repressor accumulation is reduced and the Les$^-$ phenotype is produced. The Les$^-$ phenotype associated with *recA908* indicates that this mutation produces a form of the RecA protein that has lost both synaptase activity (Rec$^-$) and functional activity in UV repair (UV^r) but possesses constitutive protease activity even in

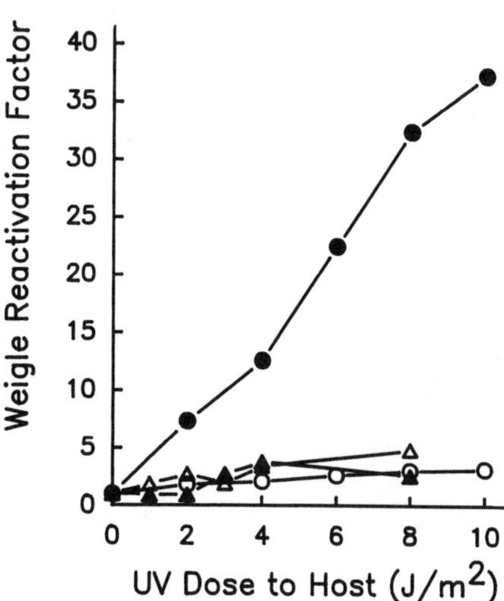

FIGURE 2. UV-inducible repair of UV-irradiated bacteriophage D3 DNA. Lysates of phage D3 were irradiated with a dose of 254-nm UV radiation, which gave approximately 0.01% survival on the unirradiated host. Bacteria were exposed to various low doses of UV radiation. Samples of treated bacteria were infected with either UV-irradiated or unirradiated bacteriophages. The Weigle reactivation factor is a measure of the amount of DNA repair induced in the host after exposure to UV irradiation and is calculated from the formula WRF = [(PFU$_{UV\phi}$/PFU$_{0\phi}$) on irradiated cells]/ [(PFU$_{UV\phi}$/PFU$_{0\phi}$) on unirradiated cells], where PFU$_{UV\phi}$ is the titer of irradiated phages and PFU$_{0\phi}$ is the titer of the unirradiated lysate. Symbols: O, PAO25 (Rec$^+$); ●, PAO25 plus R2; △, RM265 (*recA102*); ▲, RM265 plus R2.

the absence of DNA damage (Prt^c). In this mutant, the appropriate rate of repressor synthesis can be established by either (i) altering the ratio of activated to unactivated RecA protein in the cell (as seen in *recA908* merodiploids containing the cloned wild-type gene) or (ii) increasing the transcription rate of repressor protein by increasing the copy number of the phage repressor gene (as seen when the *cI* clone is introduced into *recA908* cells).

The form of the *P. aeruginosa recA* gene product present within a prospective host cell can influence the establishment, maintenance, and termination of lysogeny. This gene product has the potential for significantly affecting the dynamics of phage-host interactions in natural population of *P. aeruginosa*. Whether *recA* mutations will eliminate the increased rates of production of phage from lysogens observed in the field (Fig. 1) is currently being investigated.

Stress-Inducible DNA Repair in *P. aeruginosa*

To determine whether DNA repair functions are induced in *P. aeruginosa* after UVC irradiation, we used UV-irradiated bacteriophages to infect RecA$^+$ and RecA$^-$ host cells that had been irradiated with increasing but low doses of UVC (Simonson et al., submitted). If a UV-inducible repair system is present in *P. aeruginosa*, the level of repair of the UV-damaged phage DNA will increase as the UV dose to the host increases (Walker, 1984). If the induced repair system is mutagenic, the frequency of mutants among the progeny phages will also increase. Little or no UV-induced increase in the levels of repair of UV-irradiated D3 bacteriophage DNA was detected in Rec$^+$ strains, and the low level that was detected did not appear to be RecA dependent (Fig. 2). No increase in the frequency of mutation was observed. Similar results were obtained with bacteriophage F116L. McBeth (1989) has also observed that the frequency of mutation of various chromosomal genes in *P. aeruginosa* PAC does not increase after UVC irradiation.

Quinolone antimicrobial agents such as nalidixic acid and norfloxacin are also capable of inducing the SOS network in *E. coli* (Walker, 1984). When we assayed the capacity of norfloxacin-treated cells to repair UV-damaged bacteriophages, no increase in repair capacity or mutation frequency was observed (Benbrook and Miller, 1985).

It appears that unlike *E. coli*, *P. aeruginosa* does not contain a UVC-inducible, mutagenic repair system. RecA⁻ mutants of *P. aeruginosa* must therefore be more sensitive to UVC radiation primarily because of the loss of a mechanistic function of the RecA protein in one or more DNA repair pathways. The most obvious of these would be loss of recombinational repair capacity.

We have shown that the *P. aeruginosa* RecA protein is capable of regulating expression of the SOS network in *E. coli* (Kokjohn and Miller, 1985, 1987; Simonson et al., submitted). Since the *recA* gene is autoregulated in *E. coli* as part of the SOS network (Sedgwick, 1986; Smith and Wang, 1989), we wished to determine whether the *P. aeruginosa* RecA protein is induced after exposure to DNA-damaging stresses. Western (immunoblot) analysis was used to identify the *P. aeruginosa* RecA protein in cell lysates. Its concentration increased in RecA⁺ but not RecA⁻ strains after exposure to either UVC radiation or norfloxacin (Miller and Kokjohn, 1988). In addition, Horn and Ohman (1988a, 1988b) demonstrated increased expression of the *P. aeruginosa recA* gene after exposure of Rec⁺ cells to methyl methanesulfonate. Therefore, it appears that the RecA protein of *P. aeruginosa* is capable of regulating gene expression after exposure to DNA-damaging agents and that the lack of inducible, mutagenic DNA repair in this species is due to a lack of functional activities other than those ascribed to the RecA protein.

UV Resistance Associated with Naturally Occurring Plasmids

Many naturally occurring plasmids of *Pseudomonas* species, including the IncP9 plasmid R2, have been shown to increase the UVC resistance of their hosts (Jacoby, 1977; Lehrbach et al., 1979; Jacoby et al., 1983) and are found abundantly in aquatic habitats (Bale et al., 1987). Since expression of similar systems associated with *E. coli* plasmids is controlled by the SOS regulatory system (Strike and Lodwick, 1987), we asked whether R2-augmented UV resistance in *P. aeruginosa* was inducible and dependent on a functional RecA protein (Fig. 2). Introduction of R2 into RecA⁺ strains of *P. aeruginosa* allowed UVC-inducible repair which was accompanied by an increase in mutation frequency. No increase in UV resistance or mutation rate was observed in R2-containing RecA⁻ strains.

For organisms such as *P. aeruginosa* which lack significant levels of UV-inducible, mutagenic repair, UV resistance plasmids may be very important to the natural ecology of their host bacteria. They have the potential for significantly increasing the fitness of their hosts in numerous and varied environments. Many contain genes for the catabolism of unusual carbon sources or resistance to heavy metals and antibiotics (Jacoby, 1977; Jacoby et al., 1983). Since many plasmid-encoded repair systems are mutagenic, they may also significantly increase the genetic diversity of natural bacterial populations. The role of plasmids such as R2 in the population biology and ecology of *P. aeruginosa* is currently under investigation in our laboratories.

STRESS-INDUCED GENOME INSTABILITY IN THE FRESHWATER ENVIRONMENT

Higher levels of several types of genetic instability in populations of RecA$^+$ *P. aeruginosa* were observed during incubations at field sites on a freshwater lake than were observed during microcosm incubation. Could these increases be due to the effects of solar radiation? Certainly it is one of the most pervasive of the numerous stresses encountered by the bacterial cell in natural environments (Fletcher, 1979) and is one factor that was not controlled in our microcosm studies.

Our investigations of the ways in which *P. aeruginosa* responds to exposure to UVC radiation suggest that this stress may contribute to at least some types of instability that we observed. Prophage induction is stimulated by UVC exposure, as is the potential for homologous recombination through increased synthesis of the RecA protein. However, the response of *P. aeruginosa* to exposure to UVC cannot account for the increases observed in mutation frequency. DNA repair and mutagenesis are not significantly increased in this species after UVC irradiation. Our studies suggest that the use of *recA* mutants, at least of *P. aeruginosa*, in the construction of GEMs will not significantly reduce risk associated with their release into the environment. The steps in horizontal gene transfer (i.e., intercellular genome alteration) that the RecA protein can control (e.g., recombination and prophage induction) are functions most important to the recipient bacterium. Functions ascribed to the donor (e.g., transducing-particle formation and mobilization of plasmids for transfer) are, in general, RecA-independent processes. In the environmental community, the GEM assumes the role of genetic donor, and its RecA phenotype is unimportant. In *P. aeruginosa* at least, many of the factors controlling intracellular genome stability (e.g., mutation and transposition) do not appear to be controlled by the RecA protein, and use of *recA* mutants is unlikely to increase the genetic stability of GEMs released into the environment. In addition, the use of *recA* mutants as hosts for genetically engineered DNA may act to reduce the environmental fitness of the GEM by increasing its sensitivity to environmental stress factors. In this case, the use of *recA* mutants may be counterproductive, since the survival of the GEM may be reduced to a level that will not allow it to carry out its desired function. The validity of these conclusions is now being tested in field trials using isogenic RecA$^+$ and RecA$^-$ strains of *P. aeruginosa*. In any case, it is clear from our studies that assumptions concerning the efficacy of using *recA* mutants in the construction of GEMs cannot be blindly extrapolated from data obtained in other species. Efficacy must be evaluated in the specific species to be used.

The solar UV spectrum does not contain UVC wavelengths (<290 nm). A slight amount of UVB (290 to 320 nm) is present, and the flux rapidly increases as the wavelength increases into the UVA (>320 nm) region (Larson and Berenbaum, 1988). Whereas the primary damage to DNA caused by UVC is the formation of pyrimidine dimers, the types of damage most commonly produced by UVA exposure are strand breaks, formation of alkali-labile sites, and formation of DNA-to-protein cross-links (Peak and Peak, 1989). The little that is known about the ways in which microorganisms deal with damage caused by exposure to UVA and UVB radiation suggests that the molecular mechanisms for repair of this damage and their regulation are very different from those used to repair pyrimidine dimers (Jagger, 1985). Whether RecA has a role in the repair of UVA- and UVB-induced DNA damage is not yet certain (Sammartano et al., 1986).

Increased concern over the stability of engineered genetic sequences in the environment as well as the possible consequences of alteration in the solar spectrum due to decreases in the atmospheric ozone layer make it imperative for us to understand the potentials of free-living organisms to deal with natural DNA-damaging stresses. The ways in which *P. aeruginosa* and other environmentally significant species respond to stresses such as exposure to UVB and UVA radiation must be understood if we are to predict and perhaps eliminate the consequences of anthropogenic changes to our environment. Such investigations are now being pursued in our laboratories.

ACKNOWLEDGMENTS. We thank O. A. Ogunseitan for assistance in the environmental studies, C.-M. C. Ku for isolating our Les⁻ mutants, C. S. Simonson for help with the R2 experiments, and S. B. O'Morchoe and D. J. Saye for technical assistance.

These studies were supported in part by cooperative agreements CR12494, CR815234, and CR815282 from the Gulf Breeze Laboratory of the U.S. Environmental Protection Agency and by grants from the Potts Foundation, Chicago, Ill.

LITERATURE CITED

Alexander, M. 1981. Why microbial predators and parasites do not eliminate their prey and hosts. *Annu. Rev. Microbiol.* **35:**113–133.

Bale, M. J., J. C. Fry, and M. J. Day. 1987. Plasmid transfer between strains of *Pseudomonas aeruginosa* on membrane filters attached to river stones. *J. Gen. Microbiol.* **133:**3099–3107.

Benbrook, D. M., and R. V. Miller. 1985. Effects of norfloxacin on DNA metabolism in *Pseudomonas aeruginosa. Antimicrobial. Agents Chemother.* **29:**1–6.

Benedik, M., M. Fennewald, and J. Shapiro. 1977. Transposition of a beta-lactamase locus from RP1 into *Pseudomonas putida* degradative plasmids. *J. Bacteriol.* **129:**809–814.

Bennett, P. M., S. Baumberg, P. M. Barth, C. Sanchez-Rivas, and R. V. Miller. 1988. Round table 4: genetic stability and expression, p. 239–244. *In* M. Sussman, C. H. Collins, F. A. Skinner, and D. B. Tull (ed.), *The Release of Genetically-Engineered Micro-Organisms.* Academic Press, Inc. (London), Ltd., London.

Bergh, Ø., K. Y. Børsheim, G. Bratbak, and M. Heldal. 1989. High abundance of viruses found in aquatic environments. *Nature* (London) **340:**467–468.

Cavenagh, M. M., and R. V. Miller. 1986. Specialized transduction of *Pseudomonas aeruginosa* PAO by bacteriophage D3. *J. Bacteriol.* **165:**448–452.

Chandler, P. M., and V. Krishnapillai. 1974. Isolation and properties of recombination-deficient mutants of *Pseudomonas aeruginosa. Mutat. Res.* **23:**15–23.

Darzins, A., and M. J. Casadaban. 1989. Mini-D3112 bacteriophage transposable elements for genetic analysis of *Pseudomonas aeruginosa. J. Bacteriol.* **171:**3909–3916.

Eitner, G., B. Adler, V. A. Lanzov, and J. Hoemeister. 1982. Interspecies *recA* protein substitution in *Escherichia coli* and *Proteus mirabilis. Mol. Gen. Genet.* **185:**481–486.

Fletcher, M. 1979. The aquatic environment, p. 92–114. *In* J. M. Lynch and N. J. Poole (ed.), *Microbial Ecology: a Conceptual Approach*. John Wiley & Sons, Inc., New York.

Früh, R., J. M. Watson, and D. Haas. 1983. Construction of recombination-deficient strains of *Pseudomonas aeruginosa*. *Mol. Gen. Genet.* **191**:334–337.

Haas, D., and B. W. Holloway. 1976. R factor variants with enhanced sex factor activity. *Mol. Gen. Genet.* **144**:243–251.

Hedges, R. W., and G. A. Jacoby. 1980. Compatibility and molecular properties of plasmid Rms149 in *Pseudomonas aeruginosa* and *Escherichia coli*. *Plasmid* **3**:1–6.

Holloway, B. W. 1966. Mutants of *Pseudomonas aeruginosa* with reduced recombinational ability. *Mutat. Res.* **3**:452–455.

Holloway, B. W., and V. Krishnapillai. 1979. Bacteriophages and bacteriocins, p. 99–132. *In* P. H. Clark and M. H. Richmond (ed.), *Genetics and Biochemistry of Pseudomonas*. John Wiley & Sons, Inc., New York.

Horn, J. M., and D. E. Ohman. 1988a. Transcriptional and translational analyses of *recA* mutant alleles in *Pseudomonas aeruginosa*. *J. Bacteriol.* **170**:1637–1650.

Horn, J. M., and D. E. Ohman. 1988b. Autogenous regulation and kinetics of induction of *Pseudomonas aeruginosa recA* transcription as analyzed with operon fusions. *J. Bacteriol.* **170**:4699–4705.

Jacoby, G. A. 1977. Classification of plasmids in *Pseudomonas aeruginosa*, p. 119–126. *In* D. Schlessinger (ed.), *Microbiology—1977*. American Society for Microbiology, Washington, D.C.

Jacoby, G. A., L. Sutton, L. Knobel, and P. Mammen. 1983. Properties of IncP-2 plasmids of *Pseudomonas* spp. *Antimicrob. Agents Chemother.* **24**:168–175.

Jagger, J. 1985. *Solar-UV Actions on Living Cells*. Praeger Publishing Co., New York.

Kokjohn, T. A. 1989. Transduction: mechanism and potential for gene transfer in the environment, p. 73–97. *In* S. B. Levy and R. V. Miller (ed.), *Gene Transfer in the Environment*. McGraw-Hill Publishing Co., New York.

Kokjohn, T. A., and R. V. Miller. 1985. Molecular cloning and characterization of the *recA* gene of *Pseudomonas aeruginosa* PAO. *J. Bacteriol.* **163**:568–572.

Kokjohn, T. A., and R. V. Miller. 1987. Characterization of the *Pseudomonas aeruginosa recA* analog and its protein product: *rec 102* is a mutant allele of the *P. aeruginosa* PAO *recA* gene. *J. Bacteriol.* **169**:1499–1508.

Kokjohn, T. A., and R. V. Miller. 1988. Characterization of the *Pseudomonas aeruginosa recA* gene: the Les⁻ phenotype. *J. Bacteriol.* **170**:578–582.

Krishnapillai, V. 1971. A novel transducing phage. Its role in recognition of a possible new host controlled modification system in *Pseudomonas aeruginosa*. *Mol. Gen. Genet.* **114**:134–143.

Larson, R. A., and M. R. Berenbaum. 1988. Environmental phototoxicity. Solar ultraviolet radiation affects the toxicity of natural and man-made chemicals. *Environ. Sci. Technol.* **22**:354–360.

Lehrbach, P. R., B. T. O. Lee, and C. D. Dirckze. 1979. Effect of repair deficiency and R plasmids on spontaneous and radiation-induced mutability in *Pseudomonas aeruginosa*. *J. Bacteriol.* **139**:953–960.

Matsumoto, M., and T. Tazaki. 1973. FP5 factor, an undescribed sex factor of *Pseudomonas aeruginosa*. *Jpn. J. Microbiol.* **17**:409–417.

McBeth, D. L. 1989. Effect of degradative plasmid CAM-OCT on responses of *Pseudomonas aeruginosa* bacteria to UV light. *J. Bacteriol.* **171**:975–982.

Miller, R. V., and T. A. Kokjohn. 1987. Cloning and characterization of the *cI* repressor of *Pseudomonas aeruginosa* bacteriophage D3: a functional analog of phage lambda cI protein. *J. Bacteriol.* **169**:1847–1852.

Miller, R. V., and T. A. Kokjohn. 1988. Expression of the *recA* gene of *Pseudomonas aeruginosa* PAO is inducible by DNA-damaging agents. *J. Bacteriol.* **170**:2385–2387.

Miller, R. V., and C.-M. C. Ku. 1978. Characterization of *Pseudomonas aeruginosa* mutants deficient in the establishment of lysogeny. *J. Bacteriol.* **134**:875–883.

Miller, R. V., J. M. Pemberton, and A. J. Clark. 1977. Prophage F116: evidence for extrachromosomal location in *Pseudomonas aeruginosa* strain PAO. *J. Virol.* **22**:844–847.

Miller, R. V., J. M. Pemberton, and K. E. Richards. 1974. F116, D3, and G101: temperate bacteriophages of *Pseudomonas aeruginosa*. *Virology* **59**:566–569.

Morrison, W. D., R. V. Miller, and G. S. Sayler. 1978. Frequency of F116-mediated transduction of *Pseudomonas aeruginosa* in a freshwater environment. *Appl. Environ. Microbiol.* **36**:724–730.

Ohman, D. E., M. A. West, J. L. Flynn, and J. B. Goldberg. 1985. Method for gene replacement in *Pseudomonas aeruginosa* used in construction of *recA* mutants: *recA*-independent instability of alginate production. *J. Bacteriol.* **162**:1068–1074.

O'Morchoe, S. B., O. Ogunseitan, G. S. Sayler, and R. V. Miller. 1988. Conjugal transfer of R68.45 and FP5 between *Pseudomonas aeruginosa* strains in a freshwater environment. *Appl. Environ. Microbiol.* **54**:1923–1929.

Peak, M. J., and J. G. Peak. 1989. Solar-ultraviolet-induced damage to DNA. *Photodermatology* **6**:1–15.

Ptashne, M. 1986. *A Genetic Switch. Gene Control and Phage* λ. Cell Press and Blackwell Scientific Publications, Cambridge, Mass.

Rehmat, S., and J. A. Shapiro. 1983. Insertion and replication of the *Pseudomonas aeruginosa* mutator phage D3112. *Mol. Gen. Genet.* **192**:416–423.

Sammartano, L. J., R. W. Tuveson, and R. Davenport. 1986. Control of sensitivity to inactivation by H_2O_2 and broad-spectrum near-UV radiation by the *Escherichia coli katF* locus. *J. Bacteriol.* **168**:13–21.

Sano, Y., and M. Kageyama. 1987. The sequence and function of the *recA* gene and its protein in *Pseudomonas aeruginosa* PAO. *Mol. Gen. Genet.* **208**:412–419.

Saye, D. J., and R. V. Miller. 1989. The aquatic environment: consideration of horizontal gene transmission in a diversified habitat, p. 223–259. *In* S. B. Levy and R. V. Miller (ed.), *Gene Transfer in the Environment*. McGraw-Hill Publishing Co., New York.

Saye, D. J., O. Ogunseitan, G. S. Sayler, and R. V. Miller. 1987. Potential for transduction of plasmids in a natural freshwater environment: effect of plasmid donor concentration and a natural microbial community on transduction in *Pseudomonas aeruginosa*. *Appl. Environ. Microbiol.* **53**:987–995.

Sedgwick, S. G. 1986. Inducible DNA repair in microbes. *Microbiol. Sci.* **3**:76–83.

Smith, K. C., and T. V. Wang. 1989. *recA*-Dependent DNA repair processes. *BioEssays* **10**:12–16.

Strike, P., and D. Lodwick. 1987. Plasmid genes affecting DNA repair and mutation. *J. Cell Sci. Suppl.* **6**:303–321.

Walker, G. C. 1984. Mutagenesis and inducible responses to deoxyribonucleic acid damage in *Escherichia coli*. *Microbiol. Rev.* **48**:60–93.

Zaitsev, E. N., E. M. Zaitseva, I. V. Bakhlanova, V. I. Gorelov, N. P. Kuz'min, V. M. Kryukov, and V. A. Lantsov. 1986. Cloning and characterization of gene *recA* from *Pseudomonas aeruginosa*. *Genetika* **22**:2721–2727.

Chapter 26

Chromosome Organization in *Pseudomonas aeruginosa* and *Pseudomonas putida*

*B. W. Holloway, S. Dharmsthiti, C. Johnson, A. Kearney,
V. Krishnapillai, A. F. Morgan, E. Ratnaningsih, R. Saffery,
M. Sinclair, D. Strom, and C. Zhang*

The availability of physical methods of analyzing large fragments of DNA has stimulated interest in the comprehensive description of whole genomes, ranging from human to bacterial. Our knowledge of the chromosome maps of two species of *Pseudomonas*, *P. aeruginosa* and *P. putida*, has revealed common features of gene arrangement as well as significant differences which have led us to propose mechanisms by which the chromosomes of these organisms have originated (Holloway and Morgan, 1986). The combination of traditional mapping techniques together with cosmid clone-mediated interspecific complementation and the technique of pulsed-field gel electrophoresis (PFGE) has enabled us to make a comparison of the chromosome organization of these two species.

LINKAGE RELATIONSHIPS IN *P. AERUGINOSA* AND *P. PUTIDA*

Circular chromosome maps of each species have been constructed by using time-of-entry data combined with transduction. In *P. aeruginosa* PAO, a temperature-sensitive replication-defective (*trfA*) derivative of the IncP1 plasmid R68 loaded with the transposon Tn*2521* has been used to construct donors in which this plasmid is integrated into the chromosome. Such donors have marker transfer frequencies up to 10^{-1} per donor parent (O'Hoy and Krishnapillai, 1987). Using data obtained from this and other chromosome-mobilizing plasmids (FP2, FP5, and R68.45) and the transducing bacteriophages F116L and G101, a map with over 250 markers is now available (Holloway et al., 1990).

For *P. putida*, plasmid R91-5, or various transposon-loaded derivatives, have

---

B. W. Holloway, S. Dharmsthiti, C. Johnson, A. Kearney, V. Krishnapillai, A. F. Morgan, E. Ratnaningsih, R. Saffery, M. Sinclair, D. Strom, and C. Zhang • Department of Genetics and Developmental Biology, Monash University, Clayton, Victoria 3168, Australia.

been shown to integrate at various sites, creating Hfr donors. A wide range of Hfrs with predetermined chromosome transfer origins and mobilizing chromosome in either direction can be constructed by first isolating Tn*5* inserts in the *P. putida* chromosome and then introducing R91-5 loaded with Tn*5*, which will insert in either orientation at the same site as the original Tn*5* insertion. About 70 markers have been mapped on the *P. putida* PPN map (Holloway et al., 1990).

Cosmid libraries of both *P. aeruginosa* PAO and *P. putida* PPN have been constructed by using the wide-host-range vector pLA2917 (Allen and Hanson, 1985). *Escherichia coli* S17-1 (Simon et al., 1983) is used as the cloning host organism to facilitate complementation tests for isofunctionality. This strain has the *mob* gene functions of the wide-host-range plasmid RP4 integrated into the *E. coli* chromosome, enabling transfer of the cosmid from *E. coli* to *Pseudomonas* spp. By using banks of between 1,500 and 2,000 individual cosmids, 15% of the *P. aeruginosa* PAO cosmids have been found to complement one or more known markers; the comparable figure for *P. putida* PPN is 12%.

The distinctive features of gene arrangement in these two species of *Pseudomonas* include the following. (i) Genes of a biosynthetic pathway are not contiguous in *Pseudomonas* spp. (ii) There is clustering for genes of catabolic pathways, although contiguity has not been demonstrated for all clusters. (iii) Catabolic structural genes on degradative plasmids show clustering. (iv) Auxotroph-rich regions occur on the chromosomes of *P. aeruginosa* and *P. putida*. For example, in *P. putida* PPN, 84% of known auxotrophic markers are restricted to 36% of the genetic map. (v) In *P. aeruginosa* there are two catabolic-rich regions, together containing 82% of the known markers of this type in 27% of the chromosomal map. (vi) Pyocinogenic determinants of *P. aeruginosa* are integrated into the chromosome, unlike in enterobacteria, where bacteriocins are autonomous plasmids (Shinomiya et al., 1983; Sano and Kageyama, 1984).

CONSTRUCTION OF A PHYSICAL MAP

As pointed out by Smith et al. (1987) in their work on *E. coli* K-12, construction of a physical map is an essential stage in the complete characterization of the genome of any organism. Using an approach similar to that used by these authors, namely, a combination of PFGE, procedures to identify contiguous fragments produced by selected restriction enzyme digestion, and location of individual genes in fragments by probing with cosmid clones carrying known genes, we have constructed a partial physical map of *P. aeruginosa* PAO. The high G+C content of pseudomonad genomes has meant that the enzymes *Not*I and *Sfi*I, which proved so useful for the analysis of *E. coli*, are not suitable. However, *Spe*I, which recognizes a sequence containing the rare (in procaryotes) tetranucleotide CTAG, gives sufficiently few fragments to allow their separation.

In *P. aeruginosa* PAO, 30 *Spe*I fragments have been identified, ranging in size from 10 to 525 kilobases (kb) and giving a total genome size of 5,850 kb. This figure is larger than the figure of 5,300 kb obtained by Bautsch et al. (1988), who used two-dimensional field inversion gel electrophoresis and *Spe*I. However, while our size estimate of large *Spe*I fragments is in close agreement with that obtained by these workers, they apparently have not resolved all of the smaller fragments, reporting only 20 to 25 in total.

*Dra*I, *Ssp*I, and *Xba*I all give too many small (<50-kb) fragments to permit successful resolution and hence cannot be used to determine genome size. However, they will be of considerable value in the mapping of additional sites within *Spe*I fragments.

The order of *Spe*I fragments on the chromosome has been determined primarily by probing Southern blots of PFGE gels with cosmid clones carrying known markers. So far 26 fragments, representing 93% of the genome, have been assigned in this way. However, scarcity of suitable markers in the 50- to 65-min region of the genetic map means that several fragments in that region remain to be identified.

Five of the cosmid clones hybridized to two *Spe*I fragments, indicating the presence of a *Spe*I site within the clone. This proves contiguity of the two fragments involved and also provides a precise point of correlation between the physical and genetic maps.

To demonstrate circularity of the physical map (and to show that all identified *Spe*I fragments are chromosomal and not plasmid), we have constructed a junction fragment library containing *Spe*I sites, using the plasmid pGEM5Zf(+). To date, 12 additional pairs of fragments have been shown to be contiguous by this method.

The physical-genetic map of *P. aeruginosa* PAO is shown in Fig. 1. As a few small (<30-kb) *Spe*I fragments remain unassigned, it is possible that some of them will be located between fragments shown as adjacent in the figure.

For *P. putida* PPN, 27 *Spe*I fragments, ranging in size from 25 to 710 kb and totaling 5,620 kb, have been identified. A combined physical and genetic map is being constructed in a manner similar to that used for *P. aeruginosa* PAO.

COMPARISON OF CHROMOSOME MAPS OF *P. AERUGINOSA* AND *P. PUTIDA*

Our mapping of these two species, and the ability to do isofunctional tests of individual markers by R-prime or cosmid complementation tests, permits a comparison of gene distribution on the chromosomes of these organisms. As a result, it is possible to identify chromosomal rearrangements that have taken place since divergence from a presumed common ancestor (Holloway et al., 1990).

Figure 2 shows the chromosome maps of the two species superimposed one on the other, with the centers of the auxotroph-rich regions aligned. For convenience, the isofunctional markers are identified by numbers. The similarity in map positions of some is clearly evident, whereas others show evidence of past rearrangements. For example, markers 7 to 13 in *P. putida* can be rearranged to give the order found in *P. aeruginosa* by means of two successive inversions of about 6 and 2 min. The five groups of markers standing out from each map are those with markedly different map positions. These differences could have arisen by chromosomal translocation events.

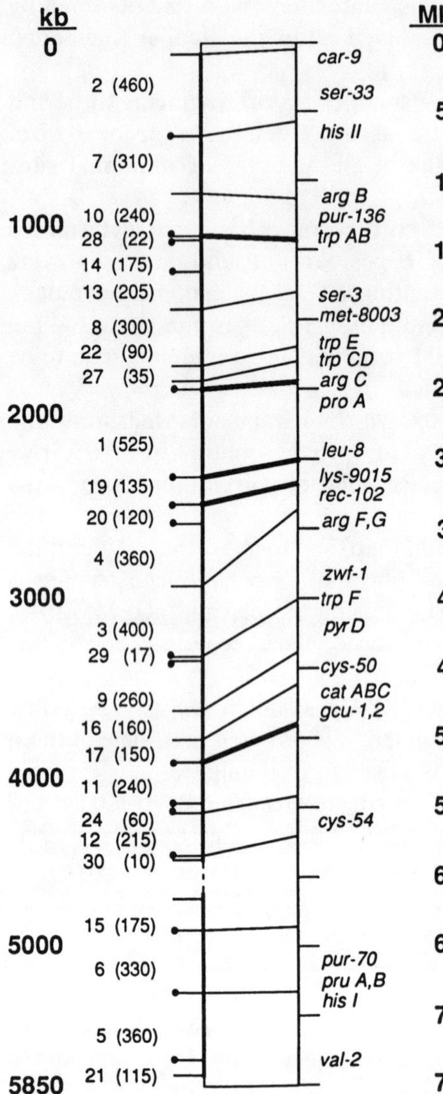

FIGURE 1. Partial physical-genetic map of *P. aeruginosa* PAO. Twenty-six *Spe*I fragments are shown, numbered in descending order of size and representing 93% of the genome. They are ordered according to position on the chromosome, determined by probing with cosmid clones carrying known genes, although only those markers defining the genetic limits of a fragment are shown. For the 17 pairs of fragments separated by a line ending in a circle, contiguity has been established from the existence of a linking clone (see text). Five of these linking clones also carry known markers, allowing exact correlation of the maps at those points. These are shown by bold lines linking the two maps.

Data from specific regions of both the *P. aeruginosa* PAO and *P. putida* PPN chromosomes have confirmed the existence of regions that have undergone rearrangement. The distance between the isofunctional *hisV* and *ser* markers (*ser-3* and *hisV* in PAO; *ser-400* and *his-810* in PPN) has been measured in both species by means of Tn*5* mutagenesis of overlapping recombinant cosmids from the respective *P. aeruginosa* PAO and *P. putida* PPN libraries. In *P. aeruginosa* PAO the distance between the two markers is 8.0 kb, whereas in *P. putida* PPN these markers are 14.2 kb apart, indicating that either genetic material has been inserted between the two markers or there has been a chromosomal rearrangement. The same measurements with a group of four other isofunctional markers

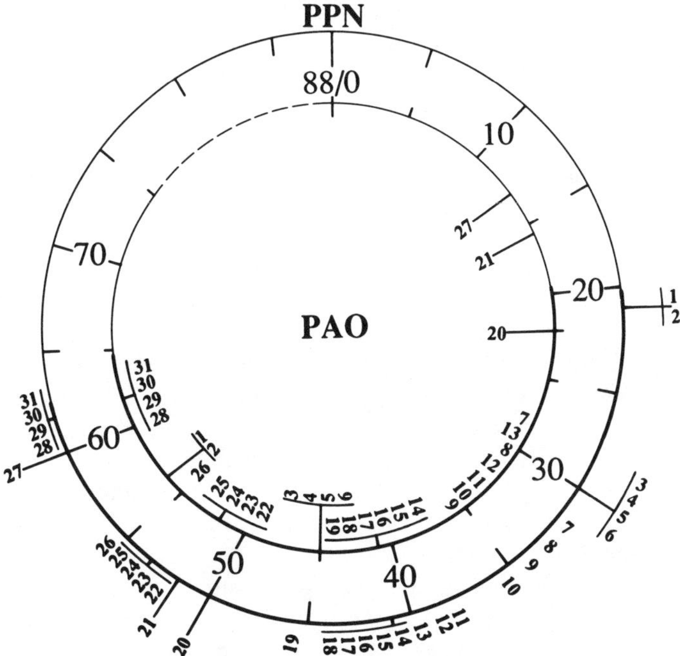

FIGURE 2. Comparison of the *P. aeruginosa* PAO (inner circle) and *P. putida* PPN (outer circle) chromosome maps, except that the *P. aeruginosa* PAO map has been rotated 22 min clockwise in order to align the centers of the auxotroph-rich regions of each map. These are denoted by thickened lines and have been taken to extend from *val-2* (73 min) to *pyrF* (42 min) for *P. aeruginosa* PAO and from *argG* (21 min) to *met-801* (62 min) for *P. putida* PPN. The following *P. aeruginosa* PAO and *P. putida* PPN loci are included: 1, *argG*; 2, *argF*; 3, *argC*; 4, *trpC*; 5, *trpD*; 6, *trpE*; 7, *hisII/his-401*; 8, *argH*; 9, *trpB*; 10, *pur-136/pur-804*; 11, *argB*; 12, *lysA*; 13, *argA*; 14, *ser-3/ser-400*; 15, *hisV/(his)*; 16, *ilvD*; 17, *met-28/met-400*; 18, *proC*; 19, *pyrB*; 20, *ilvB,C/ilv-400*; 21, *hisD*; 22, *leu-8/leu-802*; 23, *pur-66/pur-400*; 24, *thr-48/thr-400*; 25, *thr-59/(thr)*; 26, *rec-102/recA800*; 27, *pur-70/pur-410*; 28, *leu-10/leu-803*; 29, *trpF*; 30, *pur-9013/(pur)*; 31, *met-9011/met-801*. Markers immediately adjacent to the circles are those whose map position is in close agreement in the two species after rotation of the *P. aeruginosa* PAO map (Holloway et al., 1990).

(*leu-10*, *trpF*, *pur-9013*, and *met-9011* in *P. aeruginosa* PAO and *leu-803*, *trpF802*, *pur*, and *met-801* in *P. putida* PPN) showed no difference in the distances between these markers, confirming that this region has been genetically conserved in the two species.

A comparison of the *P. aeruginosa* PAO and *P. putida* PPN maps suggests that the marker *argA* has been translocated or been involved in an inversion during the evolution of these two species. The mechanism of such a rearrangement possibly involved copies of reiterated DNA such as rRNA or tRNA genes or ancestral insertion sequences. Overlapping cosmids for the region containing *argA* and both flanking regions from both the *P. aeruginosa* PAO and *P. putida* PPN cosmid libraries have been identified, restriction maps for the *argA* region in both species have been constructed, and the location of the *argA* gene has been identified by Tn5 mutagenesis. Homology between *P. aeruginosa* PAO and *P.*

putida PPN has been detected to one side of *argA* within an *Eco*RI fragment of about 10 kb. This fragment could well contain sequences that have contributed to the rearrangement and that may occur in other regions of the *P. aeruginosa* PAO and *P. putida* PPN chromosomes.

With the caveat that it has not yet been established that all identified *Spe*I fragments are chromosomal and not from some previously undetected plasmid(s), our genome sizes of 5,850 and 5,620 kb for *P. aeruginosa* PAO and *P. putida* PPN, respectively, indicate that these species have chromosomes of similar size. Although on the face of it this supports our conclusion from a comparison of the genetic maps that each chromosome has an auxotroph-rich region of similar size (Holloway et al., 1990), there is in fact an anomaly. Assuming that DNA is conjugally transferred at the same rate for all regions of the chromosome (and for *P. aeruginosa* PAO, this is supported by the data in Fig. 1), the transfer rate for *P. aeruginosa* PAO (75-min genetic map) is 78 kb/min, and that for *P. putida* PPN (88-min genetic map) is 64 kb/min. Given the difference in optimum growth temperatures (37 versus 28°C), this difference is not surprising, but it translates to an auxotroph-rich region of nearly 3,300 kb in length for *P. aeruginosa* PAO but only 2,600 kb for *P. putida* PPN.

Although the ill-defined boundaries of the auxotroph-rich regions may be responsible for this apparent difference, a specific discrepancy can be shown to exist for a 21-min chromosomal region of each species shown in Fig. 3. While translocation events have been postulated for this region in both species (Morgan and Dean, 1985), and a specific difference has been identified as described above for the *ser-3/hisV* and *ser-400/his-810* markers, the good correlation in map position for 14 of the 15 isofunctional markers depicted suggests that this region has been genetically stable since the two species diverged from a common ancestor. However, on the basis of the DNA transfer rates estimated above, the size of this region is 1,640 kb for *P. aeruginosa* PAO but only 1,340 kb for *P. putida* PPN. If the data shown in the combined genetic-physical map are included, the 19- to 40-min region for *P. aeruginosa* is 1,940 kb, increasing the difference with *P. putida* to a total of 600 kb.

ACCRETION OF NEW GENES IN *PSEUDOMONAS* SPP.

We have previously suggested that modern-day pseudomonads have acquired new genes and new metabolic functions by integration into an historically smaller chromosome of fragments of plasmids carrying genes for metabolic functions. Such accretion would possibly be less disruptive if it occurred in regions of the chromosome other than the auxotroph-rich, essential-function region.

We have identified an experimental system for studying the integration of plasmid-borne metabolic genes into the *Pseudomonas* chromosome. *P. putida* MW was found to carry 56 kb of DNA almost identical with a part of the well-characterized TOL plasmid integrated into the chromosome (Sinclair et al., 1986). This strain can grow on toluene and xylene and carries the structural genes of the TOL dissimilation pathway (Franklin et al., 1981). This 56-kb segment has

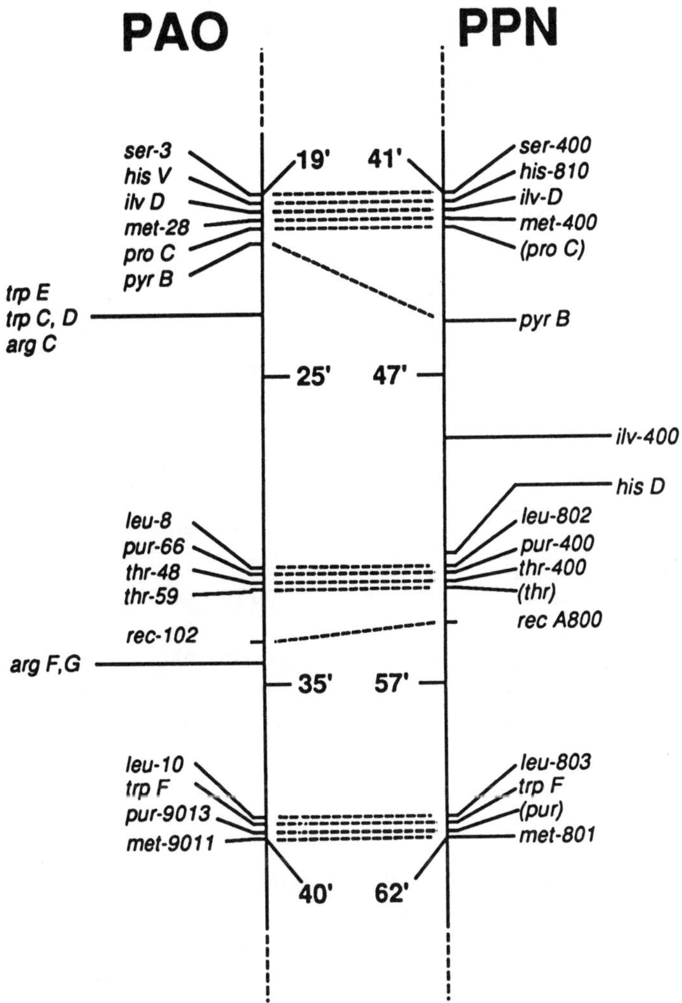

FIGURE 3. Comparison of a 21-min region of the *P. aeruginosa* PAO chromosome map extending from *ser-3* (19 min) to *met-9011* (40 min) with the corresponding region of the *P. putida* PPN chromosome map extending from *ser-400* (41 min) to *met-801* (62 min). Only markers representing genes for which isofunctionality has been established have been included, and such pairs of markers are joined as indicated. The *trpC,D,E-/argC,F,G* markers for PAO and *ilv-400-/hisD* markers for PPN have been shown to have isofunctional equivalents elsewhere on the map of the other species. Holloway et al. (1990) have proposed that these markers could have undergone translocation since *P. putida* and *P. aeruginosa* diverged from a common ancestor.

been mapped on the *P. putida* MW chromosome at the 85-min mark, between *ben-8000* and *vil-801* (Holloway et al., 1990) in the region where *ben* and *cat* genes are clustered. It appears to be equivalent to the transposon Tn*4651* as described by Tsuda and Iino (1987).

A cosmid library of *P. putida* MW has been constructed, and by hybridization, homology has been shown between the chromosomal *ben* gene cluster in *P.*

putida MW, the chromosomal *ben* gene cluster in *P. aeruginosa* PAO, the *xylD* gene region of the 56-kb insert in *P. putida* MW, and the *xylD* gene of the pWWO TOL plasmid, suggesting a common origin for these genes (Holloway et al., 1990). The present arrangement of the *P. putida* MW genome may reflect two inserts of plasmid material, an ancestral insertion that has resulted in what we now call *ben* genes in a common ancestor of *P. putida* and *P. aeruginosa* and the more recent insertion of a larger segment of the TOL plasmid into the *P. putida* MW genome.

Examination of derivatives of the MW wild-type isolate has shown that further rearrangements of the TOL DNA continue to occur in these strains, probably resulting from the transposon functions of the 56-kb segment. The termini of the TOL DNA segment have also been demonstrated to promote deletions of chromosomal DNA when these regions are cloned into a cosmid vector.

The *ben* gene cluster of *P. aeruginosa* PAO has been localized on a 4.6-kb *Kpn*I fragment, and four complementation groups have been identified among *ben* mutants; however, the correspondence of these to the *xylD* cistrons of the TOL plasmid pWWO described by Harayama et al. (1986) has not yet been determined. The functional and genetic relationships of these plasmid and chromosomal gene clusters are being further investigated by complementation testing and DNA sequence analysis.

A selection procedure has been developed that allows the isolation of TOL DNA inserts from pWWO into the *P. aeruginosa* PAO chromosome. Among five insertions examined by PFGE, four different insertion sites have been identified. Two of these sites are located in catabolic-rich regions of the chromosome; the remaining two insert sites are yet to be completely characterized.

DISCUSSION

Our physical and genetic analysis of these two species of *Pseudomonas* has posed a variety of questions on genome size and structure, chromosomal rearrangements, the acquisition of new material, and the mechanisms by which such changes occur.

The combined techniques of PFGE, cosmid library characterization, complementation, and transposon mutagenesis have shown a new approach to bacterial genome mapping which should be applicable to any bacterium. From experience gained in this laboratory over many years, it has been found that traditional techniques are not always readily transferable across generic boundaries.

The genome sizes of the two *Pseudomonas* species examined are more than 20% greater than that of *E. coli*, and the higher rate of chromosome transfer during conjugation has implications for the rate of DNA replication in pseudomonads.

From the data available, it appears that *P. aeruginosa* and *P. putida* differ by more than numerous but simple chromosomal rearrangements, possibly, for example, by the introduction of several hundred kilobases of DNA into the 21-min chromosomal region of *P. aeruginosa* depicted in Fig. 3 while conserving the spacing of existing genes. If confirmed, this raises interesting questions as to exactly how the chromosomes of the two species have evolved from a common ancestor. However, such questions cannot be posed until accurate physical and genetic maps of both species have been generated. It will also be necessary, as pointed out by Haas et al. (1987), to identify the map locations of more essential genes. To this end, we are attempting to identify such genes in *Pseudomonas* spp. by complementation of characterized mutants in *E. coli* for DNA replication and repair, RNA function, and related macromolecular functions or by using cloned *E. coli* genes as probes.

Plasmids have undoubtedly played a crucial role in the evolution of the pseudomonad genome. The demonstration that a portion of the TOL plasmid can integrate into both the *P. putida* and *P. aeruginosa* chromosomes and the relationship of TOL structural genes to existing chromosomal genes provides a model by which the origins of genes and their accretion can be studied.

There is still no evidence for sequences in the pseudomonad chromosome analogous to insertion sequences in the chromosomes of other bacteria. Although it is clear from the available data that acquisition and rearrangements of DNA have occurred in the past and may well be still occurring, there is an urgent need to identify the mechanisms by which future evolution could take place.

ACKNOWLEDGMENTS. Work in our laboratory is supported by the Australian Research Council, the National Health and Medical Research Council, and Celgene Corp.

LITERATURE CITED

Allen, L. N., and R. S. Hanson. 1985. Construction of broad-host-range cosmid cloning vectors: identification of genes necessary for growth of *Methylobacterium organophilum* on methanol. *J. Bacteriol.* **161:**955–962.

Bautsch, W., D. Grothines, and B. Tummler. 1988. Genome fingerprinting of *Pseudomonas aeruginosa* by two dimensional field inversion gel electrophoresis. *FEMS Lett.* **52:**255–258.

Franklin, F. C. H., M. Bagdasarian, M. M. Bagdasarian, and K. N. Timmis. 1981. Molecular and functional analysis of the TOL plasmid pWWO from *Pseudomonas putida* and cloning of genes for the entire regulated aromatic ring meta cleavage pathway. *Proc. Natl. Acad. Sci. USA* **78:**7458–7462.

Haas, D., A. Jann, C. Reimmann, E. Luthi, and T. Leisinger. 1987. Chromosome organization in *Pseudomonas aeruginosa*. *Antibiot. Chemother.* **39:**256–263.

Harayama, S., M. Rekik, and K. N. Timmis. 1986. Genetic analysis of a relaxed substrate specificity aromatic ring dioxygenase, toluate 1,2-dioxygenase, encoded by TOL plasmid pWWO of *Pseudomonas putida*. *Mol. Gen. Genet.* **202:**226–234.

Holloway, B. W., S. Dharmsthiti, V. Krishnapillai, A. Morgan, V. Obeyesekere, E. Ratnaningsih, M. Sinclair, D. Strom, and C. Zhang. 1990. Patterns of gene linkages in *Pseudomonas* species, p. 97–105. *In* M. Riley and K. Drlica (ed.), *The Bacterial Chromosome*. American Society for Microbiology, Washington, D.C.

Holloway, B. W., and A. F. Morgan. 1986. Genome organization in *Pseudomonas*. *Annu. Rev. Microbiol.* **40:**79–105.

Morgan, A. F., and H. F. Dean. 1985. Chromosome map of *Pseudomonas putida* PPN and a comparison of gene order with the *Pseudomonas aeruginosa* PAO chromosome map. *J. Gen. Microbiol.* **131:**885–896.

O'Hoy, K., and V. Krishnapillai. 1987. Recalibration of the *Pseudomonas aeruginosa* strain PAO chromosome map in time units using high frequency of recombination donors. *Genetics* **115:**611–618.

Sano, Y., and M. Kageyama. 1984. Genetic determinant of pyocin AP41 as an insert in the *Pseudomonas aeruginosa* chromosome. *J. Bacteriol.* **158**:562–570.

Shinomiya, T., S. Shiga, and M. Kageyama. 1983. Genetic determinant of pyocin R2 in *Pseudomonas aeruginosa* PAO. I. Localization of the pyocin R2 gene cluster between *trpCD* and *trpE* genes. *Mol. Gen. Genet.* **189**:375–381.

Simon, R., U. Priefer, and A. Puhler. 1983. A broad host range mobilization system for *in vivo* genetic engineering: transposon mutagenesis in gram negative bacteria. *Bio/Technology* **1**:784–791.

Sinclair, M. I., P. C. Maxwell, B. R. Lyon, and B. W. Holloway. 1986. Chromosomal location of TOL plasmid DNA in *Pseudomonas putida*. *J. Bacteriol.* **168**:1302–1308.

Smith, C. L., J. G. Econome, A. Schutt, S. Klco, and C. P. Cantor. 1987. A physical map of the *Escherichia coli* K12 genome. *Science* **236**:1448–1453.

Tsuda, M., and T. Iino. 1987. Genetic analysis of a transposon carrying toluene degrading gene on a TOL plasmid pWWO. *Mol. Gen. Genet.* **210**:270–274.

Chapter 27

Transposable Gene-Activating Elements in *Pseudomonas cepacia*

T. G. Lessie, M. S. Wood, A. Byrne, and A. Ferrante

CHARACTERISTICS OF *P. CEPACIA*

The taxonomic study of the aerobic pseudomonads by Stanier et al. (1966) delineated a group of nonfluorescent, polyhydroxybutyrate-accumulating pseudomonads that were designated *Pseudomonas multivorans* because of their extraordinary nutritional versatility. Subsequently, it was recognized that this species was identical to the onion-rotting phytopathogen *Pseudomonas cepacia* (Ballard et al., 1970; Palleroni and Doudoroff, 1972; Palleroni and Holmes, 1981). Recently, *P. cepacia* has emerged as a frequent cause of respiratory tract infections in patients with cystic fibrosis (Isles et al., 1984; Goldmann and Klinger, 1986). Ability to produce exopolysaccharide may, as in the case of *Pseudomonas aeruginosa* (Ohman, 1986; Deretic et al., 1987; DeVault et al., 1989), be an important determinant of pathogenicity. *P. cepacia* forms large amounts of an exopolymer consisting of galactose, glucose, mannose, rhamnose, and glucuronic acid (A. Sage, A. Linker, L. R. Evans, and T. G. Lessie, *Curr. Microbiol.*, in press).

Most studies of *P. cepacia* have focused on its unusual degradative potential (Stanier et al., 1966; Ballard et al., 1970; Palleroni and Doudoroff, 1972; Lessie and Phibbs, 1984; Lessie and Gaffney, 1986), which makes it a highly suitable bacterium for studies of the evolution of catabolic pathways and of the mechanisms by which they are regulated (Lessie and Gaffney, 1986). Particular strains have been shown to degrade such ordinarily recalcitrant compounds as the herbicide 2,4,5-T (Kilbane et al., 1982; Sangodkar et al., 1988) and the environmental pollutant trichloroethylene (Nelson et al., 1987). The majority of strains are able to utilize penicillin G as a sole source of carbon and energy (Beckman and Lessie, 1979). Many *P. cepacia* strains contain plasmids of various sizes, but the unusual nutritional versatility of this species appears not to depend upon their

T. G. Lessie, M. S. Wood, A. Byrne, and A. Ferrante • Department of Microbiology, University of Massachusetts, Amherst, Massachusetts 01003.

TABLE 1

Characteristics of selected insertion elements in *P. cepacia* 249

Element	Size (kb)	No. of genomic copies[a]	Comments
IS*401*	1.0	1–6	2 copies on pTGL6, none on pTGL1; promoted fusion of pTGL6 and pMR5 (Gaffney and Lessie, 1987)
IS*402*	0.9	2–4	1 copy on pTGL6, none on pTGL1; promoted fusion of pTGL6 and pMR5; activated Tn*1 bla* gene in both orientations (see Fig. 2; Barsomian and Lessie, 1986; Lessie and Gaffney, 1986; Robinson et al., 1980; Scordilis et al., 1987)
IS*403*	0.8	9	Activated *bla* gene of Tn*1* from >500 bp away (Lessie and Gaffney, 1986; Scordilis et al., 1987)
IS*405*	1.5	12–13	1 copy on pTGL1 and pTGL6; *bla* gene activating (Lessie and Gaffney, 1986; Scordilis et al., 1987)
IS*406*	1.3	5	Activated *lac* gene expression by inserting into $lacP_{Tn951}$ (see Fig. 5; Lessie and Gaffney, 1986)
IS*407*	1.2	3–5	Activated *lac* gene expression by inserting into $lacO_{Tn951}$ (see Fig. 5; Lessie and Gaffney, 1986)
IS*408*	2.7	4	1 copy on pTGL1 and pTGL6; activated *lacY* expression by inserting into *lacZ* of Tn*951* (Gaffney and Lessie, 1987)
IS*411*	2.0	7	1 copy on pTGL1 and pTGL6 (Gaffney and Lessie, 1987)
IS*415*	3.0	6–8	Activated Tn*951 lac* gene expression by inserting upstream of *lacI* of Tn*951* (see Fig. 3)

[a] Total of plasmid and chromosomal copies.

presence (Beckman and Lessie, 1979; Beckman et al., 1982; Gonzalez and Vidaver, 1979; Lessie and Gaffney, 1986).

P. cepacia 249 (ATCC 17616), which has been subjected to the most extensive biochemical analysis and in which the majority of insertion sequences have been identified, was isolated by Norberto Palleroni in 1961 by selection for growth on anthranilate at 41°C. This strain had a higher G+C content of its DNA than did the other strains examined (Stanier et al., 1966). It is one of a minority of strains that grow on phthalate. We recently isolated phthalate utilization genes from strain 249 by using the cosmid vector pLAFR (Friedman et al., 1982; T. G. Lessie, unpublished observation). The enzymes involved in phthalate degradation have been described in a different strain (Batie et al., 1987).

PREVALENCE OF INSERTION ELEMENTS IN *P. CEPACIA*

The single most important factor underlying the extraordinary adaptability and catabolic potential of *P. cepacia* may be the prevalence of insertion elements in its genome (Lessie and Gaffney, 1986). A large number of insertion sequences have been identified in this bacterium on the basis of their ability to promote genomic rearrangements (Gaffney and Lessie, 1987) and to recruit foreign genes by replicon fusion and insertional activation (Barsomian and Lessie, 1986; Lessie and Gaffney, 1986; Scordilis et al., 1987). Certain of these are listed in Table 1.

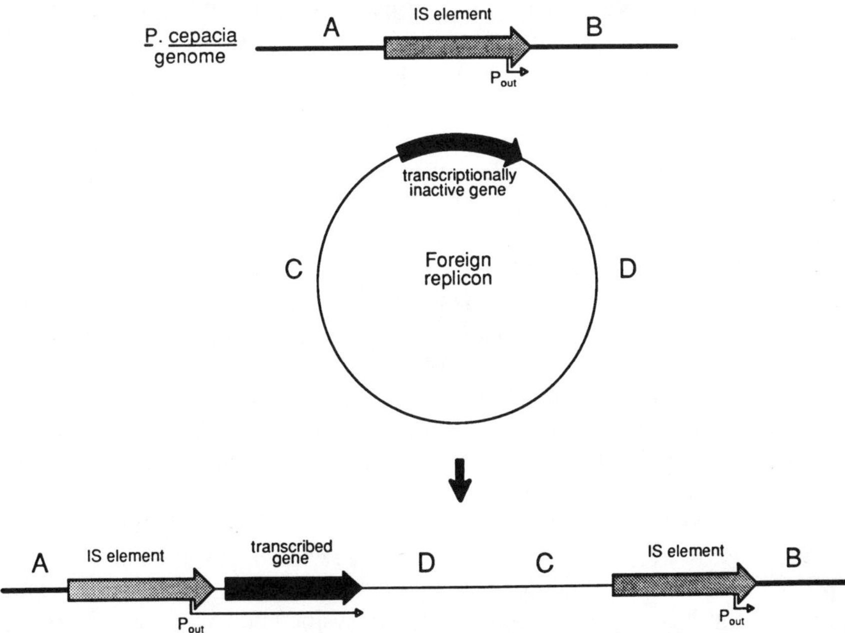

FIGURE 1. Insertion-sequence (IS)-dependent activation and incorporation into the *P. cepacia* genome of foreign genes. The schematic shows how transposable gene-activating elements within the *P. cepacia* genome might recruit genes on a foreign replicon for a novel catabolic pathway. The dark arrows represents such a gene; lighter arrows represent copies of the insertion sequence. Capture of the foreign DNA by replicon fusion would assure its maintenance. Transcription of the activated gene would depend on the upstream outwardly directed promoter (P_{out}) at the end of the element. The same or other elements might be involved subsequently in rearrangements of the incorporated DNA (i.e., inversions, deletions, or additional transposition events), leading to more efficient regulation of the new gene.

Tomasek et al. (1989) identified a 1.5-kilobase-pair (kb) element, RS1100, in a 2,4,5-T-utilizing strain of *P. cepacia* (AC1100). Their analysis has raised the possibility that RS1100, which was not detected in other *P. cepacia* strains, may have been implicated in the recruitment of genes related to 2,4,5-T degradation from another bacterium. RS1100 has also been shown to activate gene expression (R. A. Haugland, U. M. X. Sangodkar, and A. M. Chakrabarty, *Mol. Gen. Genet.*, in press). Figure 1 shows how a foreign gene might be recruited by a process of simultaneous replicon fusion and insertional activation.

DISCOVERY OF INSERTION ELEMENTS IN *P. CEPACIA* 249

The discovery of insertion sequences in strain 249 stemmed from studies of the role of beta-lactamase in penicillin utilization. Two different enzymes of 29 and 34 kilodaltons were induced during growth of this bacterium on penicillin G (W. S. Beckman, Ph.D. thesis, University of Massachusetts, Amherst, 1982;

Lessie and Gaffney, 1986; Prince et al., 1988). Analysis of several Lys$^-$ derivatives of this strain revealed that they were deficient in both beta-lactamase species and had become highly sensitive to beta-lactam antibiotics in addition to losing their ability to utilize penicillin as a carbon and energy source (Beckman and Lessie, 1979; Lessie and Gaffney, 1986). We were unable to isolate Lys$^+$ revertants or strains in which ability to utilize penicillin had been restored. The lysine auxotrophs exhibited a loss of other functions, including the capacity to utilize trehalose and ribitol. This finding suggested that the pleiotropy might have been due to elimination of a plasmid. Comparison of the plasmid contents of various strains indicated that this was not the case but did reveal the presence of a 170-kb cryptic plasmid in strain 249, which was designated pTGL6 (Beckman and Lessie, 1979). Curing Lys$^+$ strains of pTGL6 did not result in a Lys$^-$ or a Bla$^-$ phenotype, indicating that the genes related to lysine biosynthesis and penicillin dissimilation were located on the chromosome. Other attempts to identify genes associated with pTGL6 have been unsuccessful despite the availability of strains cured of this plasmid (Lessie and Gaffney, 1986).

We used the broad-host-range vector pLAFR (Friedman et al., 1982) to isolate cosmids carrying fragments of the *P. cepacia* chromosome that could complement the *lys* or the *bla* defects of strain 249-2. None of the isolates conferred the ability to grow in the absence of lysine and to utilize penicillin. The recombinant cosmids were used in Southern hybridization experiments to probe for homologous sequences in chromosomal digests of the Lys$^+$ and Lys$^-$ strains. The results indicated that the Lys$^-$ mutants were missing more than 40 kb of DNA present in Lys$^+$ strains (M. S. Wood, unpublished observations). We conclude that the pleiotropic loss of function in the Lys$^-$ mutants was a consequence of deletion of a significant segment of the chromosome. The gene encoding the major *P. cepacia* beta-lactamase was subsequently subcloned from one of the pLAFR recombinants that complemented the *bla* defect of strain 249-2 (Prince et al., 1988).

The first evidence for the existence of insertion elements in *P. cepacia* 249 came from efforts to explain rearrangements of the 170-kb plasmid detected in this strain. The majority of the mutant strains in our collection contained variants of pTGL6, the plasmid in our laboratory prototroph (Beckman et al., 1982). Most of the mutants were auxotrophs. The fact that strains could be cured of pTGL6 without causing similar auxotrophy indicated that the pertinent genes were not located on the plasmid (Lessie and Gaffney, 1986). The plasmid rearrangements were shown subsequently to result from transposition events involving insertion sequences present on the chromosome or to represent inversions or deletions mediated by elements already present on the plasmid (Gaffney and Lessie, 1987). The fact that plasmid alterations are common among auxotrophs is in part due to the sorting of single bacteria from the population during mutant selection. It might also reflect increased rates of transposition associated with the UV treatment used during mutant isolation. This might have resulted in a coincidence of plasmid alterations and insertional inactivation of chromosomal genes.

An important insight into the nature of the plasmid alterations came from the observation that the plasmid in the prototrophic stock of *P. cepacia* 249 maintained in the American Type Culture Collection (ATCC 17616) differed from the one present in our laboratory strain (249-UM). Both strains originated from the same stock at the University of California, Berkeley. The pTGL1 plasmid in the ATCC strain contained three insertion elements, IS*405*, IS*408*, and IS*411* (Gaffney and Lessie, 1987). In the course of being transferred in our laboratory at the University of Massachusetts, pTGL6, the plasmid in strain 249-UM, acquired two new insertion sequences, IS*401* and IS*402*, and suffered a deletion of 5.4 kb of plasmid DNA (Gaffney and Lessie, 1987). The deletion of plasmid DNA resulted from recombination between two of the three copies of IS*401* that had transposed to pTGL1. One of the copies of IS*401* on pTGL6 inserted immediately adjacent to the IS*408* element on pTGL1 and was implicated in the formation of cointegrate plasmids by a process of replicative transposition (Fig. 1; Barsomian and Lessie, 1986; Haas and Reimmann, 1989). The chromosomes of strains harboring pTGL6 contained between two and four copies of IS*401*, in contrast to the single copy of this element present in the ATCC strain. IS*408* was found subsequently to activate *lac* gene expression when it inserted into the broad-host-range plasmid pGC91.14 (Cornelis et al., 1978, 1979; Lessie and Gaffney, 1986). It therefore is possible that the increased copy number of IS*401* in pTGL6-containing strains reflects increased transposition of IS*401* due to its proximity to IS*408*. For example, IS*408* might promote increased transcription of a transposase gene on IS*401*, as has been reported for the interaction between the two copies of IS*21* on pR68.45 (Schurter and Holloway, 1985; Reimmann et al., 1989). An Ilv⁻ derivative of strain 249-UM was isolated subsequently that contained a 27-kb derivative of pTGL6 missing all insertion sequences except IS*411* (Lessie and Gaffney, 1986; Gaffney and Lessie, 1987). This plasmid, pTGL25, may have arisen in a deletion event promoted by IS*411*. The availability of pTGL25 should facilitate the identification of regions of pTGL1 and pTGL6 important for replication.

INSERTIONAL ACTIVATION OF FOREIGN GENES IN *P. CEPACIA*

The capacity of *P. cepacia* insertion sequences to increase the expression of neighboring genes was discovered in the course of experiments carried out to determine the extent of blockage of the penicillin dissimilation pathway in the aforementioned Lys⁻ mutants. We reasoned that if penicillin utilization was blocked solely because of the loss of beta-lactamase activity, introducing the *bla* gene of the broad-host-range plasmid pRP1 (Guiney and Lanka, 1989) into Lys⁻ strains should restore the ability to grow on this antibiotic. This proved not to be true. Although the *bla* gene of pRP1 was expressed in *P. cepacia* and did confer resistance to penicillin, the level of expression was too low to support growth with penicillin as a carbon source (Beckman and Lessie, 1979). The RP1-containing transconjugants, although themselves unable to utilize penicillin, gave rise to variants which did. These expressed the Tn*1 bla* gene on pRP1 at 20- to 40-fold-higher levels as a consequence of the upstream insertion of insertion sequence elements from the *P. cepacia* genome (Lessie and Gaffney, 1986; Scordilis et al., 1987).

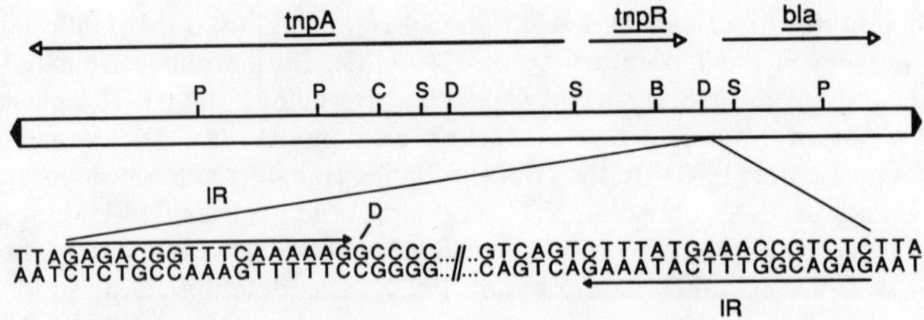

FIGURE 2. Insertion of IS*402* into Tn*1* (5.0 kb). The *bla* gene-activating element IS*402* (914 bp) inserted between the *Dra*II and *Ssp*I sites in the region between the *tnpR* and *bla* genes of this element. The inserted element contains 17-bp terminal inverted repeats (IR) and caused a duplication of 3 bp of target DNA. IS*404* and IS*405* inserted in the same general region as did IS*402*. Another element, IS*403*, inserted upstream of the unique *Bam*HI site in Tn*1*. Abbreviations for restriction sites: P, *Pst*I; C, *Cla*I; S, *Ssp*I; B, *Bam*HI; D, *Dra*II.

The first transposable gene-activating element identified was isolated in our laboratory by Young Nam Lee in the course of screening for RP1-containing derivatives of strain 249-2 cured of pTGL6. Lee identified a larger than normal pRP1 variant, pTGL51, in which a 13.7-kb element had inserted into Tn*1* immediately upstream of its *bla* gene. This strain was found subsequently to grow on penicillin as a consequence of increased expression of the Tn*1 bla* gene (Lessie and Gaffney, 1986; Scordilis et al., 1987). A more extensive search for such elements resulted in the identification of several insertion sequences that were reiterated in the chromosome and on pTGL6 (Lessie and Gaffney, 1986; Gaffney and Lessie, 1987; Scordilis et al., 1987). One of these, IS*402*, has recently been sequenced and shown to possess features characteristic of insertion elements in other bacteria (A. Ferrante and T. G. Lessie, manuscript in preparation; Galas and Chandler, 1989). Figure 2 shows the region of Tn*1* into which IS*402* inserted, the 3-base-pair (bp) duplication of target DNA generated at the site of insertion, and the 17-bp inverted repeats at the ends of the element.

ACTIVATION OF THE *lac* GENES OF Tn*951* IN *P. CEPACIA*

Despite their ability to adapt to grow on numerous exotic compounds, most *P. cepacia* strains have not evolved the ability to utilize lactose as a sole carbon source (Lessie and Phibbs, 1984). Furthermore, when the *lac* genes of the transposable element Tn*951* were introduced on the broad-host-range plasmids pGC91.14 and pGC210 (Cornelis et al., 1979), they failed to confer the ability to utilize lactose (Lessie and Gaffney, 1986). The *lac* genes of Tn*951*, which originated from *Yersinia enterolitica* (Cornelis et al., 1978), were poorly expressed in *P. cepacia*. Other investigators reported similar results after transferring pGC91.14 to *Pseudomonas fluorescens* and *P. aeruginosa* (Baumberg et al., 1980), *Rhodopseudomonas sphaeroides* (Nano and Kaplan, 1982), and *Zymomonas mobilis* (Carey et al., 1983). We exploited the failure of pGC91.14 and pGC210

TABLE 2

IS*406*- and IS*407*-dependent expression of the *lacZ* gene of Tn*951* in different bacteria

Strain[a]	β-Galactosidase specific activity[b]		
	No element	IS*406*	IS*407*
Pseudomonas cepacia 249-42-3 (*arg-1 ileA4*)	20	336	848
Pseudomonas fluorescens 13525	15	400	630
Acetobacter xylinum 3413	62	21	645
Acinetobacter calcoaceticus ADP-1	8	1,335	32

[a] *A. xylinum* was grown in medium consisting of 1% yeast extract, 1% glycerol, and 0.3% KH_2PO_4 plus 1 mg of cellulase per ml. The other bacteria were grown in inorganic salts medium (Gaffney and Lessie, 1987) containing 1% yeast extract.

[b] Nanomoles of *o*-nitrophenyl-β-D-galactopyranoside (ONPG) cleaved per minute per milligram of protein.

to confer the ability to utilize lactose to select for insertions into Tn*951* of *P. cepacia* elements able to increase *lac* gene expression (Lessie and Gaffney, 1986). Bacteria in which such insertions had occurred grew rapidly on lactose. The increase in gene expression was due to increased formation of *lac* mRNA (M. S. Wood, C. Lory, and T. G. Lessie, submitted for publication). The isolation of broad-host-range plasmids carrying activated *lac* genes afforded an opportunity to examine the influence of *P. cepacia* insertion sequence elements on gene expression in other bacteria (M. Wood, C. Lory, and T. G. Lessie, *Abstr. Annu. Meet. Am. Soc. Microbiol. 1987*, H-23, p. 143). Certain insertion sequences were more effective in turning on *lac* gene expression in other bacteria than they were in *P. cepacia* (Table 2). The elements exhibited some differences in specificity. For example, IS*406* promoted constitutive formation of β-galactosidase in *Acinetobacter calcoaceticus* but not in the cellulose-forming bacterium *Acetobacter xylinum*. In contrast, IS*407* activated *lac* gene expression in *Acetobacter xylinum* but not in *Acinetobacter calcoaceticus*.

Figure 3 is a schematic representation of plasmid pGC91.14 showing the location of the *lacI*, *lacZ*, and *lacY* genes of Tn*951* as well as *Pvu*II fragments within this transposon into which the *P. cepacia* elements IS*406*, IS*407*, IS*408*, and IS*415* inserted. These genes and fragments were contained within a 10-kb *Bam*HI fragment internal to Tn*951*. Not shown in Fig. 3 is the distribution of *Hin*dIII sites on pGC91.14, two of which are near the two *Bam*HI sites in Tn*951* and provide the option of recovering the aforementioned *lac* genes and *Pvu*II fragments on a 10-kb *Hin*dIII fragment. Analysis of the sites of insertion of various *P. cepacia* elements was facilitated by cloning the *lac* gene-containing *Bam*HI and *Hin*dIII fragments of pGC91.14, as well as the corresponding fragments of various activated plasmids, into the multicopy *Escherichia coli* vector pBR329.

Figure 4 compares the complement of *Pvu*II fragments in digests of pTGL260 and pTGL269, two pBR329 recombinants carrying, respectively, the *lac* gene-containing *Bam*HI and *Hin*dIII fragments of pGC91.14 and of pTGL75 (pGC91.14::IS*415*). IS*415* inserted into the 1.1-kb *Pvu*II fragment of Tn*951*, which was present in pTGL260, but missing from pTGL269 (Fig. 4A). In its place there were four new fragments of 0.4, 0.5, 1.5, and 1.7 kb. The net gain of DNA was 3

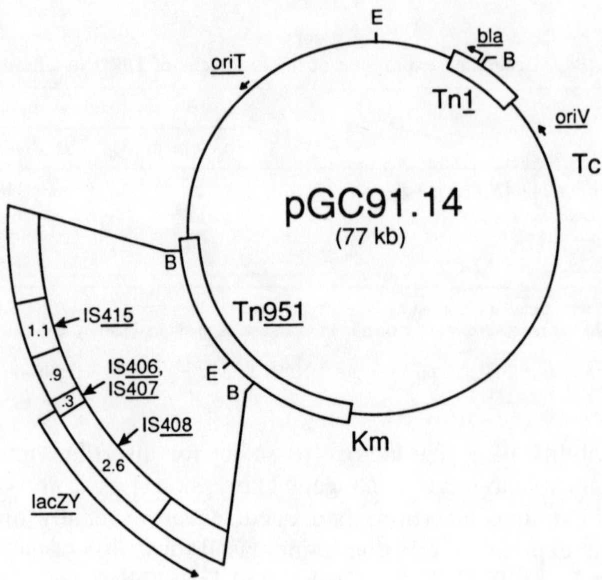

FIGURE 3. Pertinent features of pGC91.14. The schematic shows the location of Tn*951* and of the *Pvu*II fragments within this transposon into which the *lac* gene-activating elements IS*406*, IS*407*, IS*408*, and IS*415* transposed. Also indicated are the positions of Tn*1*, the kanamycin (Km) and tetracycline (Tc) resistance determinants, the origins of replication (*oriV*) and transfer (*oriT*), and restriction enzyme cleavage sites for *Eco*RI (E) and *Bam*HI (B).

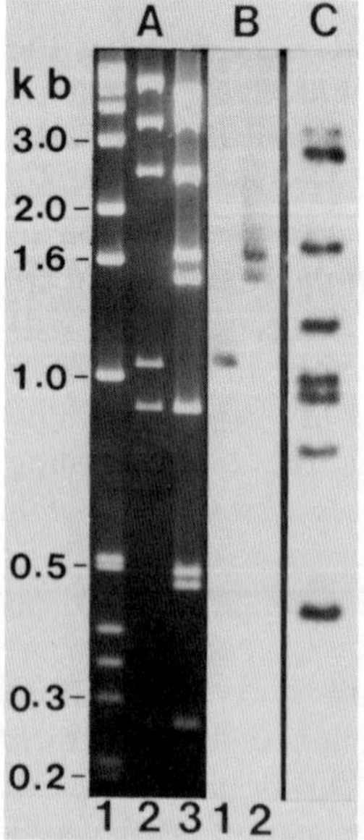

FIGURE 4. Site of insertion IS*415* into Tn*951*. (A) Electrophoretic resolution on a 2.5% agarose gel of *Pvu*II fragments from digests of pTGL260 and pTGL269, pBR329 derivatives carrying the *lac* genes of Tn*951*. Lanes: 1, kilobase-ladder size markers; 2 and 3, digests of pTGL260 and of the corresponding IS*415*-containing derivative, pTGL69, respectively. The 1.1-kb *Pvu*II fragment of pTGL260 was replaced in pTGL269 by four fragments of 1.7, 1.5, 0.5, and 0.4 kb (IS*415* contains three *Pvu*II sites). (B) Results of a Southern hybridization experiment in which the 1.1-kb fragment of pTGL260 was used as a probe to show that the 1.5- and 1.7-kb fragments of pTGL269 contained the disrupted segments of the 1.1-kb fragment. (C) Results of another Southern hybridization experiment in which the internal 0.4- and 0.5-kb fragments of IS*415* from pTL269 were used as a probe to estimate the number of copies of this element in the chromosome. Chromosomal DNA was digested with *Pst*I, and the radiolabeled IS*415* DNA was used to probe for homologous chromosomal fragments.

kb, representing the size of the inserted element. The relationship between pTGL260 and pTGL269 fragments was established by a Southern hybridization experiment in which a ^{32}P-labeled preparation of the 1.1-kb fragment of pTGL260 was used to probe fragments of pTGL269 (Fig. 4B). Only the 1.7- and 1.5-kb fragments of pTGL269 exhibited homology. They represented segments of the disrupted 1.1-kb fragment fused to the ends of IS*415*. The 0.4- and 0.5-kb fragments of pTGL269 were internal fragments of IS*415*. The latter two fragments were recovered by electroelution and used in a Southern hybridization experiment (Fig. 4C) to estimate the number of copies of IS*415* in the genome of strain 249-2 (pTGL6$^-$). Chromosomal DNA from this strain was digested with *Pst*I, which did not cut within IS*415*. On the basis of the number of homologous *Pst*I fragments, we estimated that the chromosome contains six copies of IS*415*.

The results indicated that IS*415* had inserted upstream of *lacI*, which was located mostly in the 0.9-kb *Pvu*II fragment of Tn*951* (Fig. 3). How this contributed to increased expression of downstream *lacZ* and *lacY* genes remains to be clarified. Another element, IS*408*, inserted into the 2.8-kb *Pvu*II fragment, containing the bulk of the *lacZ* gene, and increased expression of the downstream *lacY* gene, thereby conferring ability to utilize lactulose as a carbon source (Lessie and Phibbs, 1984; Lessie and Gaffney, 1986).

The sites of insertion of two other *lac* gene-activating elements, IS*406* and IS*407*, have been defined more precisely than those of IS*415* and IS*408*. Both of these elements inserted into the 0.3-kb *Pvu*II fragment of Tn*951*, generating new fragments of 1.6 and 1.5 kb. The latter two fragments were subcloned from pTGL265 and pTGL266, pBR329 recombinants carrying the ca. 11-kb *Bam*HI fragments of pTGL66 (pGC91.14::IS*406*) and pTGL67 (pGC91.14::IS*407*), into the Bluescript phagemid KS$^+$ (Stratagene Cloning Systems, La Jolla, Calif.). This facilitated the construction of sets of nested deletions extending into each element that were used for nucleotide sequence analysis (M. S. Wood, A. Ferrante, A. Byrne, and T. G. Lessie, *Abstr. Annu. Meet. Am. Soc. Microbiol. 1989*, H143, p. 193). Pertinent features of the sequence analysis are summarized in Fig. 5.

IS*407* inserted into the *lac* operator, separating the downstream *lac* genes from their normal promoter. IS*406* inserted immediately upstream of the -10 region of the Tn*951 lac* promoter ($lacP_{Tn951}$). As in the case of IS*402*, both elements contained inverted repeat sequences at their ends, and each insertion event caused a short duplication of target DNA. The terminal inverted repeat of IS*406* contained a sequence TTTACA, identical to the -35 region of $lacP_{Tn951}$. The spacing between the substituted -35 region and the -10 region of $lacP_{Tn951}$ was 20 bp, compared with 18 bp in the case of Tn*951*. If the putative hybrid promoter is responsible for the observed increase in *lac* gene expression, then one or more of the following might account for its activity: increased spacing between the -35 and -10 regions, the removal of upstream sequences within Tn*951*, or the presence of upstream sequences in IS*406*. It should be noted that IS*2* has been reported to activate gene expression in *E. coli* by generating new promoters (Jaurin and Normark, 1983; Brosius and Walz, 1982).

IS*407* inserted into Tn*951* 10 bp downstream of the normal *lac* transcription start site (Fig. 5). This element carried an outwardly directed *E. coli*-like promoter

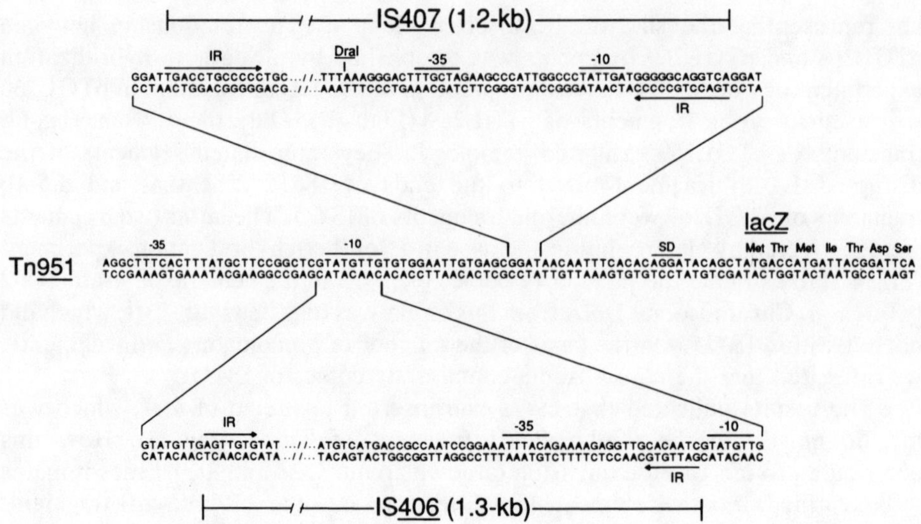

FIGURE 5. Nucleotide sequences of the target regions of Tn*951* into which IS*406* and IS*407* transposed and of the ends of the inserted elements. The middle sequence shows the region of Tn*951* into which IS*406* and IS*407* inserted. Shown are the −35 and −10 regions of the *lac* promoter, the Shine-Dalgarno (SD) sequence, and first seven codons of *lacZ*. The upper and lower sequences show respective 12- and 7-bp inverted repeats (IR) at the ends of IS*407* and IS*406*. IS*406* inserted immediately upstream of *lac*P_{Tn951}, generating an 8-bp target duplication that encompassed the entire −10 region. IS*406* supplied a new −35 region identical to that of *lac*P_{Tn951}. The spacing between the −10 and −35 regions of the resulting hybrid promoter was 20 bp (as compared with 18 bp in *lac*P_{Tn951}). IS*407* inserted into *lac*O_{Tn951}, generating a 4-bp target duplication. IS*407* contained an *E. coli*-like outwardly directed promoter adjacent to the inverted repeat upstream of the activated *lac* genes.

adjacent to the inverted repeat near the activated *lac* genes. We are in the process of carrying out S1 nuclease protection and primer extension experiments to define the site at which IS*407*-dependent transcription initiates and establish whether this promoter is active in vivo. Comparable data will also be obtained for IS*406*, IS*408*, and IS*415*. Our working hypothesis is that the majority of the transposable gene-activating elements carry strong outwardly directed promoters, as has been shown for IS*3* in *E. coli* (Charlier et al., 1982). However, we anticipate that other mechanisms of gene activation may also be uncovered. For example, some elements might carry enhancer sequences of the type identified recently in *E. coli* (Gralla, 1989).

FUTURE DIRECTIONS

Although there is a significant amount of information about promoter structure in *Pseudomonas* species (Frantz and Chakrabarty, 1986; Thomas and Franklin, 1989), essentially nothing is known about *P. cepacia* promoters. As with other pseudomonads, it is clear that there are differences in transcription specificity between *P. cepacia* and *E. coli*. For example, the *ilvA* gene of *P.*

cepacia was expressed at high constitutive levels in this bacterium but poorly in *E. coli* (Barsomian and Lessie, 1987), whereas the *bla* gene of pRP1 was more efficiently expressed in *E. coli* than in *P. cepacia* (Lessie and Gaffney, 1986; Scordilis et al., 1987). In contrast, elements such as IS*407* may carry promoters that are recognized in a variety of gram-negative bacteria. The availability of broad-host-range plasmids carrying various *P. cepacia* transposable gene-activating elements should afford an opportunity to define features of promoter structure that account for such differences in transcription specificity.

A corollary goal is to attempt to identify *P. cepacia* gene-activating elements with the capacity to transpose as well as activate gene expression in other bacteria. Broad-host-range plasmids carrying such elements would be valuable tools for manipulating the expression of foreign genes in bacteria lacking well developed systems of genetic analysis.

Because of the large number of gene-activating elements in the *P. cepacia* genome, it has not been possible to arrive at meaningful estimates of transposition frequency based on the insertional activation of the *bla* or *lac* genes of plasmids such as pGC91.14. Now that nucleotide sequence information is available for several *P. cepacia* insertion sequence elements, it will be possible to construct derivatives bearing drug resistance markers and use these to obtain such estimates. An important question that remains to be addressed is whether transpositional activity in *P. cepacia* is subject to regulation. For example, it seems reasonable that transposition might increase under conditions of physiological stress. Information about the frequency of transposition under different conditions of growth should provide insight into mechanisms balancing the genomic plasticity conferred by insertion sequences and the maintenance of the relatively stable phenotypes characteristic of *P. cepacia*.

ACKNOWLEDGMENTS. The work described here was supported by the U.S. Environmental Protection Agency (project CR-815308-01-0), in cooperation with the Gulf Breeze Laboratory, and in part by a grant from the National Science Foundation (DMB-8415028).

LITERATURE CITED

Ballard, R. W., N. J. Palleroni, M. Doudoroff, R. Y. Stanier, and M. Mandel. 1970. Taxonomy of the aerobic pseudomonads: *Pseudomonas cepacia*, *P. marginata*, *P. alliicola* and *P. caryophylli*. *J. Gen. Microbiol.* **60**:199–214.

Barsomian, G., and T. G. Lessie. 1986. Replicon fusions promoted by insertion sequences on *Pseudomonas cepacia* plasmid pTGL6. *Mol. Gen. Genet.* **204**:273–280.

Barsomian, G., and T. G. Lessie. 1987. IS2 activates the *ilvA* gene of *Pseudomonas cepacia* in *Escherichia coli*. *J. Bacteriol.* **169**:1777–1779.

Batie, C. J., E. LaHaie, and D. P. Ballou. 1987. Purification and characterization of phthalate oxygenase and phthalate oxygenase reductase from *Pseudomonas cepacia*. *J. Biol. Chem.* **262**: 1510–1518.

Baumberg, S., G. Cornelis, M. Panagiotakopoulos, and M. Roberts. 1980. Expression of the lactose transposon Tn*951* in *Escherichia coli*, *Proteus* and *Pseudomonas*. *J. Gen. Microbiol.* **119**:257–262.

Beckman, W., T. Gaffney, and T. G. Lessie. 1982. Correlation between auxotrophy and plasmid alteration in mutant strains of *Pseudomonas cepacia*. *J. Bacteriol.* **149**:1154–1158.

Beckman, W., and T. G. Lessie. 1979. Response of *Pseudomonas cepacia* to beta-lactam antibiotics: utilization of penicillin G as the carbon source. *J. Bacteriol.* **140**:1126–1128.

Brosius, J., and A. Walz. 1982. DNA sequences flanking an *E. coli* insertion element IS*2* in a cloned yeast *TRP5* gene. *Gene* **17**:223–228.

Carey, V. C., S. K. Walia, and L. O. Ingram. 1983. Expression of a lactose transposon (Tn*951*) in *Zymomonas mobilis*. *Appl. Environ. Microbiol.* **46**:1163–1168.

Charlier, D., J. Piette, and N. Glansdorf. 1982. IS*3* can function as a mobile promoter in *E. coli*. *Nucleic Acids Res.* **10**:5935–5948.

Cornelis, G., D. Ghosal, and H. Saedler. 1978. Tn*951*: a new transposon carrying a lactose operon. *Mol. Gen. Genet.* **160**:215–224.

Cornelis, G., D. Ghosal, and H. Saedler. 1979. Multiple integration sites for the lactose transposon Tn*951* on plasmid RP1 and establishment of a coordinate system for Tn*951*. *Mol. Gen. Genet.* **168**:61–67.

Deretic, V., J. F. Gill, and A. M. Chakrabarty. 1987. Alginate biosynthesis: a model system for gene regulation and function in *Pseudomonas*. *Bio/Technology* **5**:469–477.

DeVault, J. D., A. Berry, T. K. Misra, A. Darzins, and A. M. Chakrabarty. 1989. Environmental sensory signals and microbial pathogenesis: *Pseudomonas aeruginosa* infection in cystic fibrosis. *Bio/Technology* **7**:352–357.

Frantz, B., and A. M. Chakrabarty. 1986. Degradative plasmids in *Pseudomonas*, p. 295–323. *In* J. R. Sokatch and L. N. Ornston (ed.), *The Bacteria*, vol. 10. *The Biology of Pseudomonas*. Academic Press, Inc., Orlando, Fla.

Friedman, A. M., S. R. Long, S. E. Brown, W. J. Buikema, and F. M. Ausubel. 1982. Construction of a broad host range cosmid cloning vector and its use in the genetic analysis of *Rhizobium* mutants. *Gene* **18**:289–296.

Gaffney, T. D., and T. G. Lessie. 1987. Insertion-sequence-dependent rearrangements of *Pseudomonas cepacia* plasmid pTGL1. *J. Bacteriol.* **169**:224–230.

Galas, D. J., and M. Chandler. 1989. Bacterial insertion sequences, p. 109–162. *In* D. E. Berg and M. M. Howe (ed.), *Mobile DNA*. American Society for Microbiology, Washington, D.C.

Goldmann, D. A., and J. D. Klinger. 1986. *Pseudomonas cepacia*: biology, mechanisms of virulence, epidemiology. *J. Pediatr.* **108**:806–812.

Gonzalez, C. F., and A. K. Vidaver. 1979. Bacteriocin, plasmid, and pectolytic diversity in *Pseudomonas cepacia* of clinical and plant origin. *J. Gen. Microbiol.* **110**:161–170.

Gralla, J. D. 1989. Bacterial gene regulation from distant DNA sites. *Cell* **57**:193–195.

Guiney, D. G., and E. Lanka. 1989. Conjugative transfer of IncP plasmids, p. 27–56. *In* C. M. Thomas (ed.), *Promiscuous Plasmids of Gram-Negative Bacteria*. Academic Press, Inc., New York.

Haas, D., and C. Reimmann. 1989. Use of IncP plasmids in chromosomal genetics of gram-negative bacteria, p. 185–206. *In* C. M. Thomas (ed.), *Promiscuous Plasmids of Gram-Negative Bacteria*. Academic Press, Inc., New York.

Isles, A., I. Maclusky, M. Corey, R. Gold, C. Prober, P. Fleming, and H. Levison. 1984. *Pseudomonas cepacia* infection in cystic fibrosis: an emerging problem. *J. Pediatr.* **104**:206–210.

Jaurin, B., and S. Normark. 1983. Insertion of IS*2* creates a novel *ampC* promoter in *Escherichia coli*. *Cell* **32**:809–816.

Kilbane, J. J., D. K. Chatterjee, J. S. Karns, S. T. Kellogg, and A. M. Chakrabarty. 1982. Biodegradation of 2,4,5-trichlorophenoxyacetic acid by a pure culture of *Pseudomonas cepacia*. *Appl. Environ. Microbiol.* **44**:72–78.

Lessie, T. G., and T. Gaffney. 1986. Catabolic potential of *Pseudomonas cepacia*, p. 439–481. *In* J. R. Sokatch and L. N. Ornston (ed.), *The Bacteria*, vol. 10. *The Biology of Pseudomonas*. Academic Press, Inc., Orlando, Fla.

Lessie, T. G., and P. V. Phibbs, Jr. 1984. Alternative pathways of carbohydrate utilization in pseudomonads. *Annu. Rev. Microbiol.* **38**:359–387.

Nano, F. E., and S. Kaplan. 1982. Expression of the transposable *lac* operon Tn*951* in *Rhodopseudomonas sphaeroides*. *J. Bacteriol.* **152**:924–927.

Nelson, M. J. K., S. O. Montgomery, W. R. Mahaffey, and P. H. Pritchard. 1987. Biodegradation of trichloroethylene and involvement of an aromatic biodegradative pathway. *Appl. Environ. Microbiol.* **53**:949–954.

Ohman, D. E. 1986. Molecular genetics of exopolysaccharide production by mucoid *Pseudomonas aeruginosa*. *Eur. J. Clin. Microbiol.* **5**:6–10.

Palleroni, N. J., and M. Doudoroff. 1972. Some properties and taxonomic subdivisions of the genus *Pseudomonas. Annu. Rev. Phytopathol.* **10:**73–100.

Palleroni, N. J., and B. Holmes. 1981. *Pseudomonas cepacia* sp. nov., nom. rev. *Int. J. Syst. Bacteriol.* **31:**479–481.

Prince, A., M. S. Wood, G. S. Cacalano, and N. X. Chin. 1988. Isolation and characterization of a penicillinase from *Pseudomonas cepacia* 249. *Antimicrob. Agents Chemother.* **32:**838–843.

Reimmann, C., R. Moore, S. Little, A. Savioz, N. S. Willetts, and D. Haas. 1989. Genetic structure, function and regulation of the transposable element IS*21. Mol. Gen. Genet.* **215:**416–424.

Robinson, M. K., P. M. Bennett, S. Falkow, and H. M. Dodd. 1980. Isolation of a temperature-sensitive derivative of RP1. *Plasmid* **3:**343–349.

Sangodkar, U. M. X., P. J. Chapman, and A. M. Chakrabarty. 1988. Cloning, physical mapping and expression of chromosomal genes specifying degradation of the herbicide 2,4,5-T by *Pseudomonas cepacia. Gene* **71:**267–277.

Schurter, W., and B. W. Holloway. 1985. Genetic analysis of promoters on the insertion sequence IS*21* of plasmid R68.45. *Plasmid* **15:**8–18.

Scordilis, G. E., H. Ree, and T. G. Lessie. 1987. Identification of transposable elements which activate gene expression in *Pseudomonas cepacia. J. Bacteriol.* **169:**8–13.

Stanier, R. Y., N. J. Palleroni, and M. Doudoroff. 1966. The aerobic pseudomonads: a taxonomic study. *J. Gen. Microbiol.* **43:**159–271.

Thomas, C. M., and F. C. H. Franklin. 1989. Gene expression signals in gram-negative bacteria, p. 229–246. *In* C. M. Thomas (ed.), *Promiscuous Plasmids of Gram-Negative Bacteria*. Academic Press, Inc., New York.

Tomasek, P. H., B. Frantz, U. M. X. Sangodkar, R. A. Haugland, and A. M. Chakrabarty. 1989. Characterization and nucleotide sequence determination of a repeat element isolated from a 2,4,5-T degrading strain of *Pseudomonas cepacia. Gene* **76:**227–238.

Chapter 28

Diverse Regulation of the Tryptophan Genes in Fluorescent Pseudomonads

Ming Chang, David W. Essar, and Irving P. Crawford[†]

The *trp* genes of the enteric bacteria are a paradigm of economical organization and efficient control of a bacterial operon (Yanofsky and Crawford, 1987). It is not generally appreciated that this form of organization and regulation of *trp* genes is rare outside members of the family *Enterobacteriaceae*, though the reactions of the pathway and its enzymatic details are apparently universal (Crawford, 1989). Pseudomonads, and the fluorescent subgroup in particular, are especially different and interesting in their *trp* gene organization. Despite their phylogenetic proximity to enteric bacteria and vibrios (Woese, 1987), the pseudomonads exhibit no gene fusions (*Escherichia coli* and *Salmonella typhimurium* have two), have their *trp* genes distributed to four chromosomal locations instead of the single one characteristic of enteric bacteria, and show three distinctly different regulatory mechanisms (Crawford, 1986) rather than the coordinate control by repression-attenuation that has been so well studied in *E. coli*.

Figure 1 shows the tryptophan pathway, the distribution of the *Pseudomonas* structural genes into four clusters (operons), and the mode of regulation of each group. This scheme is well established for *Pseudomonas putida* and *Pseudomonas aeruginosa*, and there is some reason to believe that it will hold for other species in the fluorescent subgroup as well. Pseudomonads in the β subdivision of the purple bacteria, such as *Pseudomonas acidovorans* (Buvinger et al., 1981) and *Pseudomonas cepacia*, do not conform to this pattern.

The most striking deviation in Fig. 1 from the monolithic behavior of the *E. coli trp* genes is a feature that, so far, is unique to *Pseudomonas* spp., an inducible tryptophan synthase. In this chapter, we summarize recent results obtained in the study of this substrate induction mechanism and then consider the two gene

[†] Deceased 8 October 1989.

Ming Chang and Irving P. Crawford • Department of Microbiology, University of Iowa, Iowa City, Iowa 52242. *David W. Essar* • Agricultural Research Service, U.S. Department of Agriculture, Root Disease and Biological Control Research Unit, Washington State University, Pullman, Washington 99164-6430.

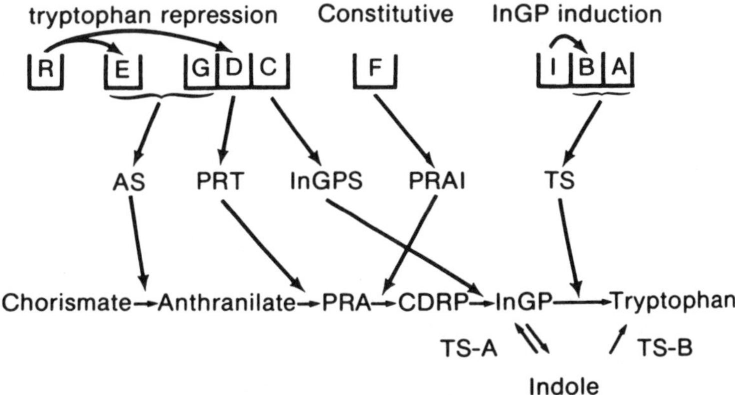

FIGURE 1. Tryptophan synthetic pathway. In *P. aeruginosa* and *P. putida*, the genes responsible for tryptophan synthesis are located in four chromosomal clusters. The proposed *trpR* gene encodes a repressor acting on *trpE* and the *trpGDC* cluster. The *trpI* gene encodes an activator inducing the *trpBA* gene pair. *trpE* and *trpG* encode the large and small subunits of anthranilate synthase, and *trpA* and *trpB* encode the α and β subunits of tryptophan synthase. The gene products and their participation in biosynthetic reactions are indicated by arrows. Abbreviations: AS, anthranilate synthase; PRT, anthranilate phosphoribosyltransferase; InGPS, indoleglycerol phosphate synthase; PRAI, *N*-phosphoribosylanthranilate isomerase; TS, tryptophan synthase; PRA, *N*-phosphoribosylanthranilate; CDRP, 1-(*o*-carboxyphenylamino)-1-deoxyribulose phosphate; InGP, indoleglycerol phosphate; TS-A, tryptophan synthase A reaction; TS-B, tryptophan synthase B reaction.

clusters (*trpE* and *trpGDC*) encoding most of the early enzymes of the pathway, describing some puzzling results we encountered while studying them.

Of the seven *trp* structural genes in *Pseudomonas* spp., six have been sequenced from *P. aeruginosa* PAO1, the same six have been sequenced from *P. putida* PPG1, and two have been sequenced from *P. aeruginosa* PAC174. *trpI*, the divergently transcribed activator gene for *trpBA*, has been sequenced in all three organisms. *trpF*, the structural gene for the midpathway isomerase, and *trpR*, the proposed repressor gene for the *trpE* and *trpGDC* clusters, have yet to be cloned and sequenced. Map positions for the *trp* structural genes on the chromosomes of *P. aeruginosa* and *P. putida* have been determined by Holloway et al. (B. W. Holloway, S. Dharmsthiti, C. Johnson, A. Kearney, V. Krishnapillai, A. F. Morgan, E. Ratnaningsih, R. Saffery, M. Sinclair, D. Strom, and C. Zhang, this volume). Their results show that there has been a transposition during evolution, reversing the order of the *trpBA* and *trpE/trpGDC* clusters on the chromosomes of these organisms. Moreover, the *trpE* and *trpGDC* clusters are separated by about 25 kilobase pairs on the *P. aeruginosa* chromosome, a space occupied by the pyocin B gene cluster (Shinomiya et al., 1983), whereas the same genes in *P. putida* are separated by only 2 kilobase pairs. This space is occupied by a single gene of unknown function on the opposite strand (D. W. Essar et al., manuscript in preparation).

In those cases where genes from the two *P. aeruginosa* strains were sequenced, the amino acids were 98.7% identical and the DNA sequences in the coding regions were 99.7% identical. In those cases where homologous genes from *P. putida* and *P. aeruginosa* were sequenced, the amino acids were 76.0% identical and the DNA sequences were 77.0% identical. The sequences of the two *Pseudomonas* species were always more similar to each other than to sequences of any other of the gram-negative species that have been studied. Among the strains studied, there was in general greater similarity to *Acinetobacter calcoaceticus* and *Caulobacter crescentus* than to the enteric bacteria (Crawford, 1989).

TRYPTOPHAN SYNTHASE INDUCIBILITY

If blocked in the first step of the pathway, tryptophan auxotrophs of most species will grow quite readily when provided with either anthranilate or indole in place of tryptophan. Our first indication of unusual regulation in the tryptophan pathway of *P. putida* came when we observed that such auxotrophs grew much better on low levels of anthranilate than on comparable levels of indole. Mutants blocked later in the pathway and accumulating the intermediate indoleglycerol phosphate grew very well on low levels of indole, however, indicating that the organism has no problems in taking up or tolerating indole. Subsequently, we learned that double mutants, blocked both before anthranilate and after indoleglycerol phosphate, would grow readily on indole only if simultaneously provided anthranilate. Moreover, growth on indole, which accurately reflected the level of tryptophan synthase in the cell, was independent of the levels of other *trp* gene products and depended only on the amount of indoleglycerol phosphate the cells contained (Crawford and Gunsalus, 1966). Later we showed that mutations leading to constitutively high levels of tryptophan synthase always occurred in close proximity to the *trpBA* genes (Gunsalus et al., 1968). Calhoun et al. (1973) obtained similar results with auxotrophs of *P. aeruginosa*.

A few years later, Hedges and co-workers used the wide-host-range plasmid R68.44 to clone the tryptophan synthase genes from *P. aeruginosa* PAC174 into *E. coli*. When moved into appropriate auxotrophic *E. coli* strains, this construct retained the inducible regulation characteristic of its species of origin (Hedges et al., 1977). Subsequent work by Manch and co-workers on subclones of this plasmid revealed the existence of a regulatory gene just upstream of the *trpBA* operon that exerted a positive effect on the transcription of *trpBA* in the presence of indoleglycerol phosphate (Manch and Crawford, 1981, 1982). The gene for this activator was given the designation *trpI*. It is now known to be divergently transcribed from the operon it controls, separated from it by about 100 base pairs (bp) containing its own and the *trpBA* promoter (Fig. 2), and capable of producing an activator molecule having a subunit size of near 32 kilodaltons (Chang et al., 1989).

The sequence of TrpI, the product of the activator gene, has been deduced from the DNA sequence in two *P. aeruginosa* strains and in *P. putida* (Chang et al., 1989 and unpublished results). It shows considerable similarity to a group of bacterial regulatory proteins called the LysR family (Henikoff et al., 1988), many of which are activators of divergently transcribed genes or operons. This similarity is most pronounced in the N-terminal third of the sequence, where a helix-turn-helix DNA-binding motif has been identified.

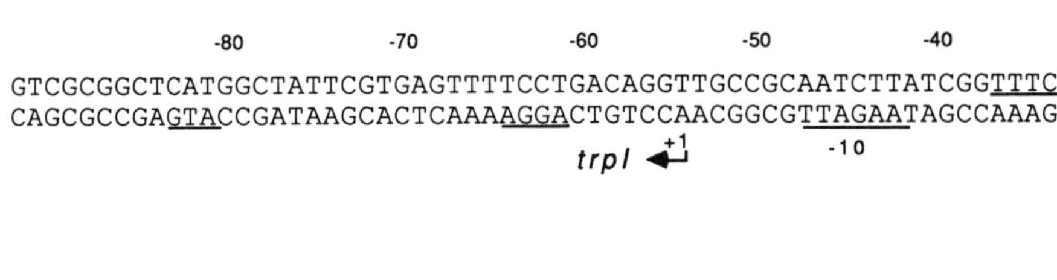

FIGURE 2. Transcription of *trpI* and *trpBA*. *trpI* and *trpBA* are transcribed divergently, and in *P. aeruginosa* their promoters reside in a 103-bp intergenic region between the two translational start codons (underlined). The transcription initiation sites for *trpI* and *trpBA*, determined by S1 nuclease mapping, are numbered +1 on each strand. The predicted −10 and −35 regions for the promoters and the presumed ribosome-binding sites are underlined.

We wished to examine whether TrpI, like several other members of the family, binds to DNA in the vicinity of the promoter of the genes it activates, and if so, what effect the inducer molecule might have on this binding. Our first objective was to identify the promoters of *trpBA* and *trpI* located on opposite strands of the ca. 100-bp segment of DNA separating the coding sequences. This was accomplished by S1 nuclease experiments using crude mRNA preparations from induced cells (Chang et al., manuscript in preparation). The results indicated that the −35 regions of the promoter were nearly overlapping (Fig. 2), that they had −10 regions in reasonable conformity to the *E. coli* σ^{70} consensus promoter sequence, though the –35 regions were not in such close conformity, and that the amount of *trpI* mRNA was much less than the amount of *trpBA* mRNA. To obtain appreciable amounts of the activator protein, its gene was subcloned into the *E. coli* expression vector ptacterm. (In this construction, the promoterless *trpI* gene was cloned between the regulatable *tac* promoter and a strong terminator.) Fortunately, the TrpI protein could be amplified very well in this system and the protein product remained soluble. The TrpI protein has now been purified to near homogeneity, and the first 15 residues of its amino acid sequence agree with those predicted from the DNA sequence. The native protein migrates in sizing columns at the position expected for a tetramer.

DNA-binding studies and protection from both DNase I and hydroxyl radicals indicate strong binding by TrpI near the *trpI* end of the intergenic space, both in the absence and in the presence of the inducer, indoleglycerol phosphate. The location of the TrpI footprint is shown as site I in Fig. 3. In the presence of indoleglycerol phosphate, the protected area is extended considerably in the *trpBA* direction, touching the −35 region of the *trpBA* promoter (site II in Fig. 3). This extension of the footprint agrees with results of gel retardation experiments indicating that indoleglycerol phosphate shifts DNA from the position of an

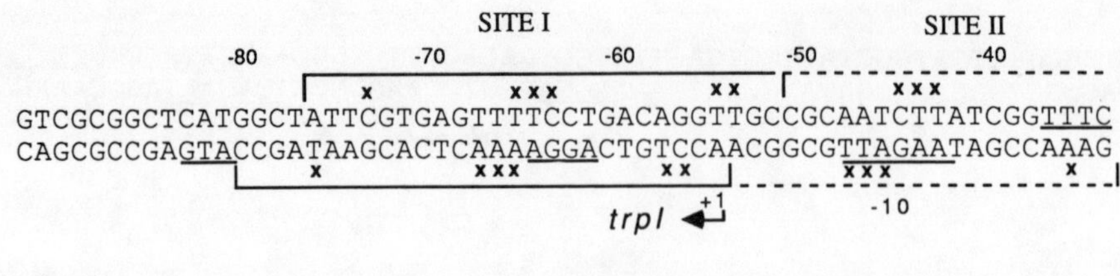

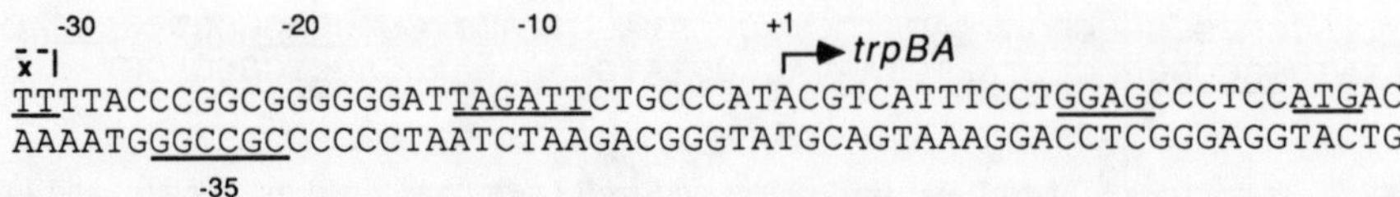

FIGURE 3. *trpI* and *trpBA* promoters and the TrpI-binding sites in the 103-bp intergenic region between the two translational start codons (underlined). The transcription initiation sites for *trpI* and *trpBA*, determined by S1 nuclease mapping, are numbered +1 on each strand. The region indicated by solid brackets, designated site I, is protected by the TrpI protein from DNase I digestion in the absence of indoleglycerol phosphate. The additional region covered by dashed brackets, designated site II, is protected in the presence of indoleglycerol phosphate. The regions protected from hydroxyl radical cleavage by the TrpI protein are indicated by crosses. The predicted −10 and −35 regions for the promoters and the presumed ribosome-binding sites are underlined.

equimolar complex to one that apparently has two TrpI molecules bound to it (Fig. 4).

The foundations have now been laid for more detailed mechanistic studies of this activation system. We would like to know how the inducer modifies the DNA-binding properties of TrpI, whether it induces a conformational change affecting RNA polymerase initiation as well as site II occupation, and how this process can be modified by mutation to make *trpBA* expression constitutive. We also would like to determine whether, as seems likely from the binding of uninduced TrpI to site I, the *trpI* gene is autoregulated at low levels. These experiments might be made easier by comparing the situation in *P. aeruginosa* with that in other fluorescent pseudomonads to see what has been conserved in evolution. The sequence of the entire *trpIBA* region of *P. putida* is now on hand, and we have established that *P. putida* TrpI is quite effective at activating the *P.*

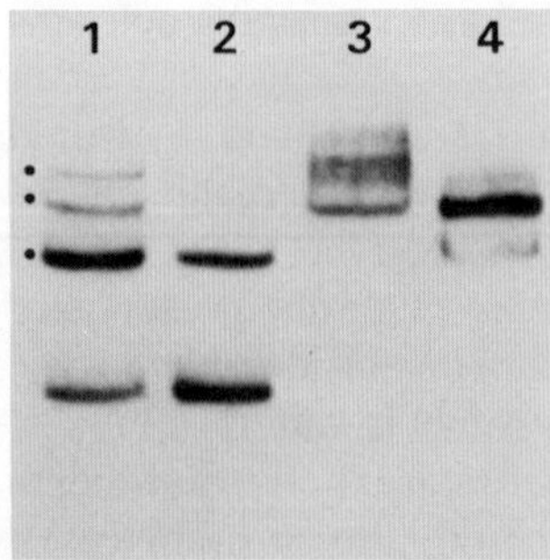

FIGURE 4. DNA-binding assay. The TrpI protein was tested for DNA-binding activity by the gel retardation assay. The TrpI protein used here was 95% pure. The DNA fragment used in the assay was the 172-bp *Bss*HII-*Eco*0109 fragment, comprising the intergenic region and the first portions of *trpI* and *trpB*, labeled by radioactive deoxynucleotide triphosphates. Ten times more of the TrpI protein was used in lanes 1 and 3 than in lanes 2 and 4. In lanes 3 and 4, the reactions included 10^{-3} M indoleglycerol phosphate. Protein-DNA complexes are indicated by dots.

```
                          SITE I                              SITE II  -35
P. aeruginosa PAO1  CATGGCTATTCGTGAGTTTTCCTGACAGGTTGCCGCAATCTTATCGGTTTC
P. putida PPG1        CAT-TTTACCTGTGAGTTTTTCTGACAAGTTTGCGCAATCTTATCGGTTTT
                         TGTNAGNNNNNCTNACA


                     -10              +1
TTTTACCCGGCGGGGGGGATTAGATT-CTGCCCAT-ACG---TCATTT---CCTGGAGCCCTCCATG
CAGCCGGGCTTGCCGTGGTTAGAGTAAAGCCCATCACTCATTCATTTACGCCTGGAGCGCCCATG
```

FIGURE 5. Alignment of the intergenic regions from *P. aeruginosa* PAO1 and *P. putida* PPG1. Site I is underlined, and site II is marked with a dashed line. The transcriptional initiation site for *trpBA* is indicated by +1. Start codons for *trpB* are boxed. The putative consensus sequence for the TrpI-binding site is shown below site I.

aeruginosa trpBA promoter. There are many conserved elements in the operator-promoter regions of these two species (Fig. 5). It is possible to suggest a consensus sequence for TrpI binding at site I, and perhaps even at site II, that they share. This points to one focus for directed and random mutagenesis studies in the future.

REGULATION OF EARLY STEPS IN THE PATHWAY

At about the same time the *trpIBA* region was cloned, Bob Hedges obtained, under similar conditions, an R-prime plasmid from *P. aeruginosa* capable of complementing *E. coli trpE* mutants. At that time it was not clear that *trpE* and *trpG*, the genes for the two subunits of the first enzyme in the tryptophan pathway, were well separated on the chromosome. After subcloning and sequencing, we found open reading frames corresponding to the large and small subunits of anthranilate synthase in a variety of organisms (Crawford et al., 1986; Crawford and Eberly, 1986). The coding regions of these two genes actually overlap by 23 bp (Crawford and Eberly, 1986). The clues that Hedges had actually cloned the genes for a second anthranilate synthase in *P. aeruginosa* came: when the deduced amino acid sequence of the small subunit proved to be more like the sequence of small subunits from other genera than like the *P. putida* small-subunit sequence obtained from the purified protein (Kawamura et al., 1978); when the enzyme activity generated proved not to be feedback inhibited by tryptophan; and when insertionally inactivated mutants transplaced by reverse genetics to the chromosome of *P. aeruginosa* did not require tryptophan for growth (Essar et al., in preparation).

Subsequently, using the cloned small subunit as a probe in low-stringency Southern hybridization, the authentic *trpG* of *P. aeruginosa* was recognized, cloned, and sequenced. We then were able to clone and sequence the *trpE* and *trpGDC* regions of both *P. aeruginosa* and *P. putida* (Fig. 6). In these cases, we confirmed that we had the correct genes by sequence (the deduced *P. aeruginosa* TrpG sequence was very similar to that of Kawamura et al. [1978], and the one

P. <u>aeruginosa</u> PAC chromosome ——— R68.44 prime ———▶ <u>phnAphnB</u>

P. <u>aeruginosa</u> PAO1 chromosome ——— <u>phnB</u> probe / low strin. ———▶ trpG(trpDtrpC)

P. <u>putida</u> PPG1 chromosome ——— P. <u>aer. trpG</u> probe / low strin. ———▶ trpG(trpDtrpC)

P. <u>putida</u> PPG1 chromosome ——— walk ———▶ trpE

P. <u>aeruginosa</u> PAO1 chromosome ——— P. <u>put. trpE</u> probe / low strin. ———▶ trpE

FIGURE 6. Outline of the cloning of *P. aeruginosa* and *P. putida* anthranilate synthase genes. Each line indicates the DNA source, the source of the probe used in Southern hybridizations, the stringency level used, and the designation of the gene(s) recovered.

from *P. putida* was identical to it), by insertional inactivation of the chromosomal versions of the genes (*trp* auxotrophs of the expected phenotype were obtained in each case), and by showing that extracts of cells containing these insertional inactivations were devoid of activity in the first- or second-pathway enzymes, as expected (Essar et al., in preparation).

If the first anthranilate synthase gene pair cloned plays no role in tryptophan synthesis and cannot supply an activity that substitutes for that of *Pseudomonas* TrpE and TrpG, what might its function be? A clue lay in the phenotype of the strains containing insertionally inactivated forms of the first genes isolated. Although prototrophic, these all had defects in the production of pyocyanin, the characteristic blue-green phenazine pigment of the organism. Phenazines are known to be synthesized from two molecules of chorismate plus the amide groups of glutamine, and anthranilate has been proposed but not proved to be an early intermediate in their synthesis. Figure 7 shows the pathway of phenazine synthesis as it is presently understood. The intermediate between chorismate and phenazine-1,6-dicarboxylate appears to be anthranilate, the hypothetical first step being catalyzed by anthranilate synthase. Phenazines are not usually produced in the exponential growth phase, so a difference in time of expression could account for the inability of the phenazine enzyme to complement the tryptophan biosynthetic enzyme. We decided to name the genes for the large and small subunits of the first anthranilate synthase we had cloned *phnA* and *phnB*, for their likely participation in phenazine synthesis. No comparable *phn* genes for a second anthranilate synthase have been detected on the *P. putida* chromosome.

Table 1 shows the amounts of pyocyanin detected in culture supernatants of the wild type and several mutant derivatives of *P. aeruginosa*. In the absence of either *trpE* or *phnA*, pyocyanin synthesis was diminished but not absent. When both anthranilate synthases were missing, however, only negligible amounts of pyocyanin were found. When large quantities of *P. putida trpE* insertionally

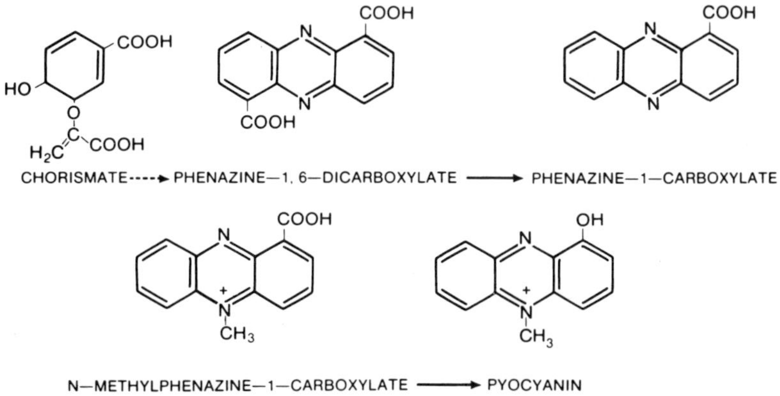

CHORISMATE ----▶ PHENAZINE—1, 6—DICARBOXYLATE ⟶ PHENAZINE—1—CARBOXYLATE

N—METHYLPHENAZINE—1—CARBOXYLATE ⟶ PYOCYANIN

FIGURE 7. Hypothetical scheme for pyocyanin synthesis. In this pathway, phenazine-1,6-dicarboxylate is the common precursor of the phenazines. Phenazine-1,6-dicarboxylate is decarboxylated to yield phenazine-1-carboxylate. *N*-methylation of phenazine-1-carboxylate yields 5-methylphenazine-1-carboxylate. Oxidative decarboxylation of 5-methylphenazine-1-carboxylate yields pyocyanin (1-hydroxy-5-methylphenazine).

inactivated cells were plated on minimal medium without tryptophan, no spontaneous reversion to *trp* prototrophy was observed. Similarly inactivated *trpE* mutants of *P. aeruginosa* reverted quite readily, however, even though they were missing a significant portion of the *trpE* coding sequence. Suspecting that in these "revertants" the anthranilate synthase being used for tryptophan synthesis might be coming from the *phnAB* gene pair, we tested it for feedback inhibition by tryptophan. It showed no inhibition. A probe specific for *phnA* mRNA was isolated from the 5′-terminal portion of the gene, and a similar probe was made for *trpGDC* mRNA. Crude mRNA preparations were made from cells in various phases of the growth cycle and tested by slot blot analysis with these specific probes (Fig. 8). As expected, in the wild type the *trpGDC* message was most abundant in the exponential phase and decreased during stationary phase. *phnA* mRNA, on the other hand, was present sparingly in the exponential phase but more abundantly after growth slowed. *trpE* revertants, however, contained large amounts of *phnA* mRNA even at the earliest time tested. Under these circumstances, the *phnAB* gene products apparently produce all of the anthranilate

TABLE 1

Pyocyanin production by *P. aeruginosa* PAO1 and its derived mutants[a]

Strain	Pyocyanin production (µg/ml of culture)	% of wild-type production
PAO1	6.30	100
PADE *trpE1*	5.44	86
PADE *phnA47*	2.13	34
PADE *phnA48*	1.45	22
PADE *phnA47 trpE1*	0.02	2

[a] Cells were grown for 16 to 20 h in 5 ml of complex broth at 37°C with aeration.

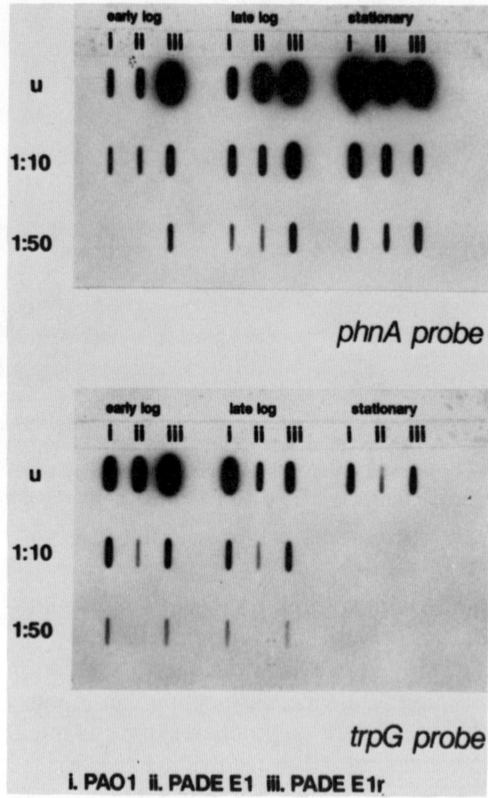

FIGURE 8. Slot blot hybridization analysis of mRNA from *P. aeruginosa* PAO1, its *trpE* mutant PADE E1, and the subsequent Trp⁺ revertant PADE E1r. The top slot blot series was hybridized with a *phnA*-specific probe; the bottom one was hybridized with a *trpG*-specific probe. The first block of samples contains early log-phase RNA, the middle block contains late-log-phase RNA, and the last block contains RNA prepared from cells in stationary phase. The top row of each block is the undiluted sample, the middle row is a 1:10 dilution, and the bottom row is a 1:50 dilution. PAO1 RNA is in lanes i, PADE E1 is in lanes ii, and PADE E1r is in lanes iii of each block.

needed for both tryptophan and pyocyanin synthesis. Perhaps not unexpectedly, these revertants make more pyocyanin per milliliter of culture than wild-type cells do.

We hypothesize that *P. aeruginosa* has one anthranilate synthase used primarily to make tryptophan in the exponential growth phase plus another for use in secondary metabolism in the synthesis of phenazines. Some anthranilate made by the TrpE-TrpG enzyme does apparently find its way into the phenazine pathway, but for the PhnA-PhnB enzyme to produce anthranilate for tryptophan synthesis, it must be transcribed earlier, and perhaps in greater amounts, than normal. An alternative hypothesis, that the anthranilate made by the PhnA-PhnB enzyme is channeled exclusively to phenazine synthesis by the existence of a macromolecular complex containing most or all of the phenazine synthetic enzymes, is not really ruled out by any of our data, and it might help to explain the difficulty in converting externally supplied anthranilate into phenazines. In that case, one might imagine that production of the PhnA-PhnB enzyme earlier and in greater amounts than normal allows the enzyme to exist free in the cytoplasm, independent of the phenazine synthetic complex, and to furnish anthranilate to the tryptophan pathway enzymes.

FUTURE STUDIES

The direction of future studies on the activation of the tryptophan synthase genes by TrpI has been discussed above. The situation with respect to the regulation of the early-pathway enzymes is not so straightforward. Despite the availability of considerable sequence data upstream from *trpE* and *trpGDC* in *P. aeruginosa* and *P. putida*, it is not immediately clear how these genes are regulated. No sequences reminiscent of the attenuator ahead of the *trp* operon in enteric bacteria were found, even though attenuators of this type have been seen ahead of *trp* genes in other, less closely related bacteria such as *Rhizobium meliloti* (Bae et al., 1989), *Brevibacterium lactofermentum* (Matsui and Sano, 1987), and *Thermus thermophilus* (Sato et al., 1988). Neither can one see clear indications of a promoter-operator to be acted on by the product of the unlinked *Pseudomonas trpR* gene, for which there is good genetic evidence (Maurer and Crawford, 1971). There is a rather well-conserved 40-bp sequence a variable distance ahead of the four early gene operons studied, but we have yet to obtain evidence that it serves a regulatory function. Obviously, S1 nuclease studies and fusions to promoterless indicator genes must be used to establish the regulated transcription start points. It would then be desirable to learn whether regulation occurs by repression mediated through the proposed *trpR* gene product, by attenuation of the unusual type found in *Bacillus* species (Kuroda et al., 1988), or by a combination of methods.

When we understand the regulation of the early *trp* genes in pseudomonads, we should compare this with the regulation of the *phnAB* anthranilate synthase. Little is known about the control of secondary metabolism in the genus. These genes may require novel sigma subunits for their transcription, the appearance of specific activators, either proteins or small molecules, or still other unsuspected methods for control of their expression. There is no indication from the flanking sequences that the *phnAB* genes are part of a large operon of genes of secondary metabolism, so they could represent a target of opportunity for investigation of this kind of regulation. As a first step, we intend to locate the mutations that can override this regulation in our *trpE* revertants. More mRNA studies and use of reporter gene fusions would be obvious ways to follow up this serendipitous discovery of a second anthranilate synthase in *Pseudomonas* spp. Similar genes in other bacteria that elaborate phenazine pigments and antibiotics should be sought.

ACKNOWLEDGMENTS. This work was supported by Public Health Service grant AI20279 from the National Institutes of Health and by grant DMB 8606653 from the National Science Foundation.

LITERATURE CITED

Bae, Y. M., E. Holmgren, and I. P. Crawford. 1989. *Rhizobium meliloti* anthranilate synthase: cloning, sequence and expression in *Escherichia coli*. *J. Bacteriol.* **171:**3471–3478.

Buvinger, W. E., L. C. Stone, and H. E. Heath. 1981. Biochemical genetics of tryptophan synthesis in *Pseudomonas acidovorans*. *J. Bacteriol.* **147:**62–68.

Calhoun, D. H., D. L. Pierson, and R. A. Jensen. 1973. The regulation of tryptophan biosynthesis in *Pseudomonas aeruginosa*. *Mol. Gen. Genet.* **121:**117–132.

Chang, M., A. Hadero, and I. P. Crawford. 1989. Sequence of the *Pseudomonas aeruginosa trpI* activator gene and relatedness of *trpI* to other procaryotic regulatory genes. *J. Bacteriol.* **171:**172–183.

Crawford, I. P. 1986. Regulation of tryptophan synthesis in *Pseudomonas*, p. 251–263. *In* J. R. Sokatch and L. N. Ornston (ed.), *The Bacteria*, vol. 10. *The Biology of Pseudomonas*. Academic Press, Inc., Orlando, Fla.

Crawford, I. P. 1989. Evolution of a biosynthetic pathway: the tryptophan paradigm. *Annu. Rev. Microbiol.* **43:**567–600.

Crawford, I. P., and L. Eberly. 1986. Structure and regulation of the anthranilate synthase genes in *Pseudomonas aeruginosa*. I. Sequence of *trpG* encoding the glutamine amidotransferase subunit. *Mol. Biol. Evol.* **3:**436–448.

Crawford, I. P., and I. C. Gunsalus. 1966. Inducibility of tryptophan synthase in *Pseudomonas putida*. *Proc. Natl. Acad. Sci. USA* **56:**717–724.

Crawford, I. P., A. Wilde, E. M. Yelverton, D. Figurski, and R. W. Hedges. 1986. Structure and regulation of the anthranilate synthase genes in *Pseudomonas aeruginosa*. II. Cloning and expression in *Escherichia coli*. *Mol. Biol. Evol.* **3:**449–458.

Gunsalus, I. C., C. F. Gunsalus, A. M. Chakrabarty, S. Sikes, and I. P. Crawford. 1968. Fine structure mapping of the tryptophan genes in *Pseudomonas putida*. *Genetics* **60:**419–435.

Hedges, R. W., A. E. Jacob, and I. P. Crawford. 1977. Wide ranging plasmid bearing the *Pseudomonas aeruginosa* tryptophan synthase genes. *Nature* (London) **267:**283–284.

Henikoff, S., G. W. Haughn, J. M. Calvo, and J. C. Wallace. 1988. A large family of bacterial activator proteins. *Proc. Natl. Acad. Sci. USA* **85:**6602–6606.

Kawamura, M., P. S. Keim, Y. Goto, H. Zalkin, and R. L. Heindrikson. 1978. Anthranilate synthetase component II from *Pseudomonas putida*: covalent structure and identification of the cysteine residue involved in catalysis. *J. Biol. Chem.* **253:**4659–4668.

Kuroda, M. I., D. Henner, and C. Yanofsky. 1988. *cis*-Acting sites in the transcript of the *Bacillus subtilis trp* operon regulate expression of the operon. *J. Bacteriol.* **170:**3080–3088.

Manch, J. N., and I. P. Crawford. 1981. Ordering tryptophan synthase genes of *Pseudomonas aeruginosa* by cloning in *Escherichia coli*. *J. Bacteriol.* **146:**102–107.

Manch, J. N., and I. P. Crawford. 1982. Genetic evidence for a positive-acting regulatory factor mediating induction in the tryptophan pathway of *Pseudomonas aeruginosa*. *J. Mol. Biol.* **156:**67–77.

Matsui, K., and K. Sano. 1987. Structure and function of the trp operon control regions of *Brevibacterium fermentum*, a glutamic-acid-producing bacterium. *Gene* **53:**191–200.

Maurer, R., and I. P. Crawford. 1971. New regulatory mutation affecting some of the tryptophan genes in *Pseudomonas aeruginosa*. *J. Bacteriol.* **106:**331–338.

Sato, S., Y. Nakada, S. Kanaya, and T. Tanaka. 1988. Molecular cloning and nucleotide sequence of *Thermus thermophilus* HB8 *trpE* and *trpG*. *Biochim. Biophys. Acta* **950:**303–312.

Shinomiya, T., S. Shiga, and M. Kageyama. 1983. Genetic determinant of pyocin R2 in *Pseudomonas aeruginosa* PAO. I. Localization of the pyocin R2 gene cluster between the *trpCD* and *trpE* genes. *Mol. Gen. Genet.* **189:**375–381.

Woese, C. R. 1987. Bacterial evolution. *Microbiol. Rev.* **51:**221–271.

Yanofsky, C., and I. P. Crawford. 1987. The tryptophan operon, p. 1453–1472. *In* F. C. Neidhardt, J. L. Ingraham, B. Magasanik, K. B. Low, M. Schaechter, and H. E. Umbarger (ed.), *Escherichia coli and Salmonella typhimurium: Cellular and Molecular Biology*, vol. 2. American Society for Microbiology, Washington, D.C.

Chapter 29

Arginine Network of *Pseudomonas aeruginosa*: Specific and Global Controls

Dieter Haas, Marc Galimand, Marianne Gamper, and Axel Zimmermann

The metabolic versatility of the pseudomonads has several facets. These bacteria utilize a large number of organic compounds as carbon, nitrogen, or sulfur sources (Clarke, 1982), they degrade a wide variety of xenobiotics (Haas, 1983; Frantz and Chakrabarty, 1986), and they also produce a range of secondary metabolites (Leisinger and Margraff, 1979).

To accomplish these metabolic transformations, the pseudomonads possess an amazing repertoire of peripheral pathways encoded by chromosomal or plasmid-borne genes. In addition to the peripheral pathways, the pseudomonads also have an elaborate organization of central metabolism. We wish to illustrate this point by describing the metabolism of the amino acid arginine in *Pseudomonas aeruginosa* PAO.

ARGININE NETWORK OF *P. AERUGINOSA* PAO

Arginine biosynthesis proceeds from glutamate in eight steps (enzymes 1 through 8 in Fig. 1). The acetyl group is recycled by ornithine acetyltransferase (enzyme 5') in the first part of the pathway. This transacetylation, which is not found in *Escherichia coli* or *Bacillus subtilis*, helps to minimize the amount of acetyl-coenzyme A (CoA) consumed by the enzyme 1, *N*-acetylglutamate synthase. The genetic organization and the enzymes of arginine biosynthesis have been reviewed and will not be discussed here (Haas et al., 1977; Cunin et al., 1986).

Most pseudomonads, including *P. aeruginosa*, degrade arginine rapidly under aerobic conditions and during oxygen limitation in sealed culture vessels (Sherris et al., 1959; Thornley, 1960). Since arginine breakdown produces large amounts of ammonia, the growth medium becomes alkaline. Therefore, media

---

Dieter Haas, Marc Galimand, Marianne Gamper, and Axel Zimmermann ● Mikrobiologisches Institut, Eidgenössische Technische Hochschule, CH-8092 Zurich, Switzerland.

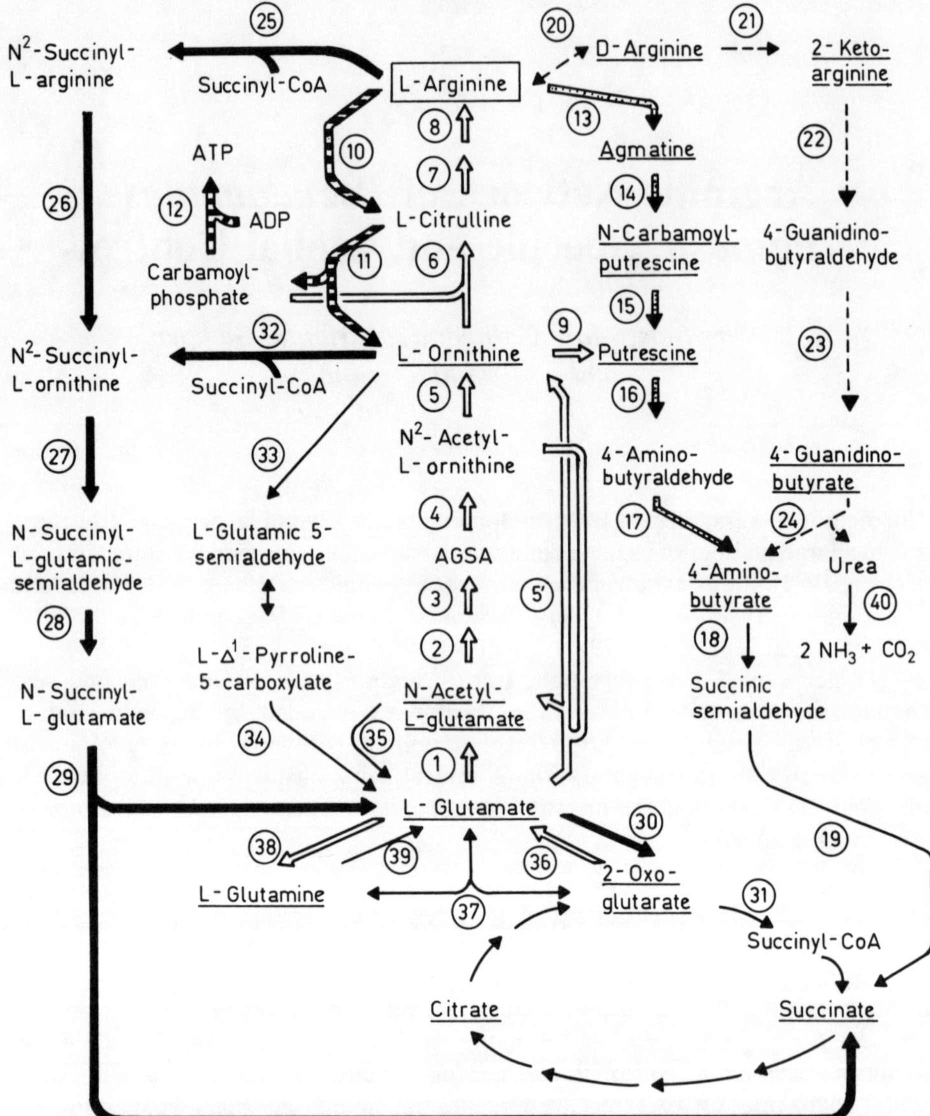

FIGURE 1. Arginine metabolism in *P. aeruginosa*. AGSA, *N*-Acetylglutamic 5-semialdehyde. ▷, Biosynthetic reactions; ⇒, arginine deiminase pathway; ⇒, arginine decarboxylase pathway; --→, D-arginine dehydrogenase pathway, →, arginine succinyltransferase pathway; →, other reactions. Compounds underlined can be used as sole carbon sources by *P. aeruginosa*. Important enzymes (referred to by circled numbers) are mentioned in the text and in Tables 1 to 3. The complete enzymatic reactions and the names of all enzymes can be found in Cunin et al. (1986) and Jann et al. (1988). For simplicity, the reactions of proline synthesis and degradation (Meile et al., 1982), those of spermidine synthesis and degradation (Padmanabhan and Tchen, 1969), and carbamoylphosphate synthetase are not shown.

containing L-arginine and a pH indicator allow a simple test for arginine degradation; they are useful in the taxonomic classification of pseudomonads (Stolp and Gadkari, 1981). *P. aeruginosa* is strongly attracted to L-arginine (Shoesmith and Sherris, 1960). Chemotaxis toward L-arginine occurs at a threshold of <1 μM (Moench and Konetzka, 1978). Active arginine uptake occurs via at least two different routes which have been analyzed in *Pseudomonas putida*, i.e., an arginine-specific ($K_m = 0.05$ μM) and a general basic amino acid ($K_m = 5$ μM) transport system (Fan et al., 1972). The arginine deiminase pathway (sometimes referred to as the arginine dihydrolase pathway) was the first arginine catabolic pathway established in *Pseudomonas* (Shoesmith and Sherris, 1960; Ramos et al., 1967). This pathway converts L-arginine to L-ornithine and carbamoylphosphate, which serves to generate ATP from ADP (Fig. 1). Three enzymes (no. 10 through 12 in Fig. 1) participate in this route: arginine deiminase, catabolic ornithine carbamoyltransferase, and carbamate kinase. Since *P. aeruginosa* can transaminate ornithine to glutamic 5-semialdehyde (Voellmy and Leisinger, 1975, 1976), and since the latter compound can be reduced to glutamate by Δ^1-pyrroline 5-carboxylate dehydrogenase (Meile et al., 1982), it was originally thought that these reactions (33 and 34 in Fig. 1), together with the enzymes of the arginine deiminase pathway, would constitute the major arginine catabolic pathway (Voellmy and Leisinger, 1976; Rahman et al., 1980).

However, several observations indicated that such was not the case. *P. aeruginosa* PAO mutants blocked in catabolic ornithine carbamoyltransferase (Haas et al., 1979), arginine deiminase (Mercenier et al., 1982), or Δ^1-pyrroline 5-carboxylate dehydrogenase still utilize L-arginine effectively as the only carbon and nitrogen source in the presence of air (Haas et al., 1984). It turned out that the oxygen supply has a decisive influence on arginine catabolism in *P. aeruginosa*. During anaerobic conditions or oxygen limitation, the three enzymes of the arginine deiminase pathway are induced strongly and coordinately (Mercenier et al., 1980b); the ATP thus produced from arginine activates motility (Shoesmith and Sherris, 1960) and maintains the membrane potential (Armitage and Evans, 1983). Arginine is converted stoichiometrically to ornithine, which is released into the medium (Vander Wauven et al., 1984). In fact, when terminal electron acceptors (oxygen, nitrate, or nitrite) are not available, *P. aeruginosa* is able to use L-arginine as the only energy source for slow growth, provided that essential cell constituents are supplied by a rich medium. Mutants blocked in arginine deiminase (*arcA*), catabolic ornithine carbamoyltransferase (*arcB*), or carbamate kinase (*arcC*) cannot grow anaerobically on arginine (Vander Wauven et al., 1984). Therefore, the main function of the arginine deiminase pathway in *P. aeruginosa* is to generate energy in the absence of respiration. Since 2 mol of NH_3 is liberated in this pathway, it may also serve to provide nitrogen (Abdelal et al., 1982) or to give protection from acid (Marquis et al., 1987).

In *P. aeruginosa* the aerobic utilization of arginine as a carbon source is independent of the arginine deiminase pathway. A pathway initiated by arginine decarboxylase (enzyme 13 in Fig. 1) operates under aerobic conditions (Mercenier et al., 1980a). Intermediates in this pathway are agmatine and *N*-carbamoylputrescine, and putrescine appears to be an important product (Fig. 1; Kay and

Gronlund, 1969a; Mercenier et al., 1980a). Mutants of strain PAO blocked in the arginine deiminase pathway as well as in agmatine deiminase (*aguA*) or in carbamoylputrescine hydrolase (*aguB*) (enzymes 14 and 15 in Fig. 1) cannot grow on agmatine but are capable of aerobic arginine utilization (Haas et al., 1984). Thus, the arginine decarboxylase pathway does not qualify as a major arginine utilization route in *P. aeruginosa*.

2-Ketoarginine (2-oxo-5-guanidinovalerate) and 4-guanidinobutyrate are good carbon and nitrogen sources for *P. aeruginosa* and inducers of guanidinobutyrase (enzyme 24 in Fig. 1) (Stalon and Mercenier, 1984). In *P. putida*, L-arginine can be catabolized via 2-ketoarginine, 4-guanidinobutyraldehyde, and 4-guanidinobutyrate to 4-aminobutyrate (Fig. 1; Vanderbilt et al., 1975). By analogy, it was postulated that the same pathway existed in *P. aeruginosa* PAO. The problem with this hypothesis was that all attempts to demonstrate an enzyme converting L-arginine to 2-ketoarginine in *P. aeruginosa* were unsuccessful. In particular, neither L-arginine oxidase, an enzyme reported in *P. putida* (Miller and Rodwell, 1971; Vanderbilt et al., 1975), nor L-arginine aminotransferase, an enzyme found in *Arthrobacter simplex* (Tachiki et al., 1980), could be detected in *P. aeruginosa*. However, a specific, D-arginine-inducible D-arginine dehydrogenase was discovered which, in concert with an arginine racemase, could link L-arginine to 2-ketoarginine catabolism (enzymes 20 and 21 in Fig. 1; Jann et al., 1988). To establish the role of this pathway in *P. aeruginosa*, we have isolated mutants defective in 4-guanidinobutyraldehyde dehydrogenase (enzyme 23 in Fig. 1; *kauB*) or guanidinobutyrase (*gbu*). These mutants cannot grow on 2-ketoarginine, but they grow well on L-arginine aerobically. Moreover, mutants blocked in the arginine deiminase, the arginine decarboxylase, and the D-arginine dehydrogenase pathways (*arcAB aguA kauB* or *arcAB aguA gbu*) still utilize L-arginine as the only carbon and nitrogen source (Jann et al., 1988). It follows that in *P. aeruginosa* the bulk of arginine is catabolized via yet another pathway.

This pathway has been elucidated by an analysis of one-step, arginine-nonutilizing (*aru*) mutants of *P. aeruginosa* PAO whose growth is strongly inhibited by L-arginine. These mutants accumulate either N^2-succinylarginine or *N*-succinylglutamate from arginine. In addition, wild-type cells treated with an inhibitor of pyridoxal phosphate-dependent enzymes convert arginine to N^2-succinylornithine (Jann et al., 1986). Enzyme analysis has shown that the succinylated compounds are intermediates of a novel pathway (enzymes 25 through 29 in Fig. 1) which occurs in *P. aeruginosa* (Jann et al., 1986), *Pseudomonas cepacia* (Vander Wauven and Stalon, 1985), and some other bacteria (Stalon et al., 1987). In the first step, arginine succinyltransferase forms N^2-succinylarginine from arginine and succinyl-CoA. When the pathway is blocked after this step, the succinyl-CoA pool is depleted by the reaction with arginine. This presumably disrupts the citric acid cycle and causes the observed arginine sensitivity of *aru* mutants. In the wild type, in contrast, succinate and glutamate are the products of the pathway (Fig. 1). Succinyl-CoA is regenerated from glutamate by the catabolic (NAD-dependent) glutamate dehydrogenase and 2-oxoglutarate dehydrogenase (enzymes 30 and 31 in Fig. 1). This results in a recycling of succinyl-CoA within the pathway. It is interesting that a set of similar

TABLE 1

Enzymes catalyzing more than one reaction in the arginine/ornithine metabolism of *P. aeruginosa*

Enzyme (reaction in Fig. 1)	Other activities of the enzyme (reactions in Fig. 1)	Reference
N^2-Succinylornithine 5-aminotransferase (27)	N^2-Acetylornithine 5-aminotransferase (4); ornithine 5-aminotransferase (33)	Jann et al., 1986 Voellmy and Leisinger, 1975
4-Aminobutyrate aminotransferase (18)	N^2-Acetylornithine 5-aminotransferase (4); ornithine 5-aminotransferase (33); putrescine aminotransferase (16)	Voellmy and Leisinger, 1976
Arginine succinyltransferase (25)	Ornithine succinyltransferase (32)	Vander Wauven et al., 1988
4-Guanidinobutyraldehyde dehydrogenase (23)	4-Aminobutyraldehyde dehydrogenase (17)	Jann et al., 1988

acylated intermediates are found in arginine biosynthesis, but in this case the intermediates are acetylated rather than succinylated and a different type of energy-saving recycling strategy is used for acyl transfer.

In conclusion, *P. aeruginosa* PAO has four different arginine catabolic pathways with specific metabolic roles. From enzyme studies it appears that *P. putida* possesses the same four arginine degradation routes (Stalon et al., 1987). Ornithine, which is a precursor in arginine and putrescine biosynthesis, can be degraded via N^2-succinylornithine (reaction 32 in Fig. 1) or, to a lesser extent, via glutamic 5-semialdehyde (reaction 33) (Vander Wauven et al., 1988).

GENES AND ENZYMES

How many enzymes are involved in the arginine network? About 40 reactions are needed to connect arginine and glutamate metabolism to the citric acid cycle (Fig. 1). From genetic and enzymatic evidence we conclude that four enzymes can perform more than one reaction in arginine metabolism (Table 1). The transamination step in arginine biosynthesis (reaction 4 in Fig. 1) represents a particular case in that it is catalyzed by two inducible, catabolic aminotransferases (Table 1). Overall, however, enzymes with a broad substrate specificity are relatively uncommon and the corresponding savings at the genetic level are not extensive.

If we take into account the genes required for chemotaxis, uptake, and pathway-specific controls, we can expect more than 70 genes to participate in the arginine network. Of these genes, six unlinked arginine biosynthetic loci (*argA*, *-B*, *-C*, *-F*, *-G*, and *-H*) (Haas et al., 1977) and several loci affecting arginine catabolism (Table 2) have been localized on the chromosome map of *P. aeruginosa* PAO. The arginine deiminase pathway genes *arcABC* are organized in an operon; an additional gene, *arcD*, which appears to be required for anaerobic arginine uptake and might code for an arginine:ornithine antiporter, is located upstream of *arcABC* in the same transcriptional unit (Fig. 2). Mutations blocking the succinyltransferase pathway (*aru*) are clustered in the late chromosome region (Table 2). Two genes coding for agmatine breakdown (*aguAB*) are also highly

TABLE 2

Mapped mutations affecting arginine or ornithine catabolism in *P. aeruginosa*

Gene or locus	Map location (min)[a]	Gene product	Reaction in Fig. 1	Reference
arcA	8	Arginine deiminase	10	Mercenier et al., 1982
arcB	8	Catabolic ornithine carbamoyltransferase	11	Haas et al., 1979
arcC	8	Carbamate kinase	12	Vander Wauven et al., 1984
arcD	8	Arginine:ornithine antiporter (?)[b]		Lüthi et al., in press
aguA	18	Agmatine deiminase	14	Haas et al., 1984
aguB	18	*N*-Carbamoylputrescine hydrolase	15	Haas et al., 1984
kauB[c]	11	4-Guanidinobutyraldehyde dehydrogenase	23	Jann et al., 1988
aru-292	66	? (Low levels of all *aru* enzymes)		Jann et al., 1986
aruA[c]	66	Arginine succinyltransferase	25	Vander Wauven et al., 1988
aruB[c]	66	N^2-Succinylarginine dihydrolase	26	Jann et al., 1986
aruE[c]	66	*N*-Succinylglutamate desuccinylase	29	Jann et al., 1986
nirD	60	Positive regulator required for induction of *arc* operon[d]		Van Hartingsveldt et al., 1971; Galimand, unpublished data
oru-310	1	?[e]		Früh et al., 1985
oru-314	40	?[f]		Früh et al., 1985
gln-2020	3	? (Nitrogen metabolism)[g]		Janssen et al., 1982

[a] Map locations are according to Holloway et al. (1987).

[b] See Fig. 2.

[c] Former designations are *ptu* for *kauB* and *oruI* (which includes *argD*) for the *aru* cluster.

[d] The *nirD* mutation has pleiotropic effects (see text).

[e] Catabolic glutamate dehydrogenase (NAD-dependent) noninducible by glutamate; utilization of ornithine blocked (*oruII*).

[f] Anabolic glutamate dehydrogenase (NADP-dependent) nonrepressible by glutamate; utilization of ornithine blocked (*oruIII*).

[g] Glutamine synthetase noninducible by nitrogen limitation; impaired utilization of many nitrogen sources including ornithine.

linked, whereas mutations affecting the control of several pathways are scattered on the chromosome map (Table 2). The picture which emerges from these and other studies is that in *P. aeruginosa* the catabolic genes show a higher degree of clustering than do the anabolic genes (Holloway et al., this volume).

P. aeruginosa has many catabolic pathways that do not occur in *E. coli*; examples in the present context are the D-arginine dehydrogenase, the arginine deiminase, and the succinyltransferase pathways (Cunin et al., 1986). Is the genome of *P. aeruginosa* larger than that of *E. coli*? Recent estimates indicate that the genome size of strain PAO is 5,300 kilobases (Bautsch et al., 1988) to 5,850 kilobases (Holloway et al., this volume), compared to 4,700 kilobases of *E. coli* (Kohara et al., 1987). Thus, in the extra 600 to 1,150 kilobases *P. aeruginosa* could easily accommodate the genetic information for more than 100 catabolic pathways.

SPECIFIC REGULATION

L-Arginine represses one arginine biosynthetic enzyme, anabolic ornithine carbamoyltransferase (the *argF* product, enzyme 6 in Fig. 1; Isaac and Holloway,

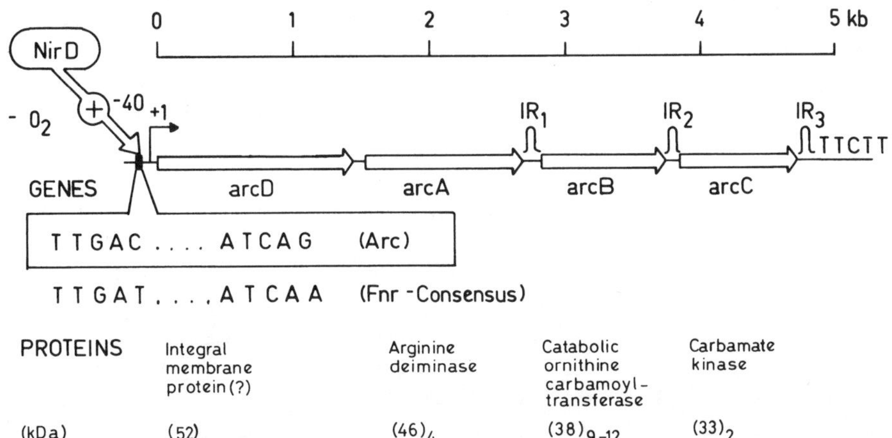

FIGURE 2. Structure and function of the *arc* operon of *P. aeruginosa*. The *arc* genes have been cloned and sequenced, and their functions have been established (Lüthi et al., 1986; Baur et al., 1987, 1989; Lüthi et al., in press). +1, Transcriptional start; IR$_1$, IR$_2$, IR$_3$, inverted repeats. The NirD protein is thought to act as a transcriptional activator in the -40 region of the promoter when oxygen is absent. The ArcD protein might code for an energy-independent arginine:ornithine antiporter similar to the one described in streptococci (Poolman et al., 1987).

1972; Voellmy and Leisinger, 1978), and induces all enzymes of the arginine succinyltransferase pathway as well as arginine decarboxylase (enzymes 25 through 30 and 13; Table 3). Physiological experiments suggest that repression and induction by L-arginine share common regulatory elements (Voellmy and

TABLE 3

Regulation of arginine catabolism in *P. aeruginosa*

Pathway	Growth conditions permitting induction	Enzymes induced (Fig. 1)	Reference
L-Arginine deiminase	Limiting O$_2$ (strong); L-arginine (weak)	10–12	Mercenier et al., 1980b
L-Arginine succinyltransferase	L-Arginine	25–30; 32	Jann et al., 1986
L-Arginine decarboxylase	L-Arginine	13	Mercenier et al., 1980a
	Agmatine, *N*-carbamoyl-putrescine	14–18[a]	
	Putrescine, 4-aminobutyrate	16–18[a]	
D-Arginine dehydrogenase	D-Arginine	21	Jann et al., 1988
	2-Ketoarginine	23[b], 24	
	4-Guanidinobutyrate	18[a], 24	

[a] Succinic semialdehyde dehydrogenase (enzyme 19) has not been tested in *P. aeruginosa*, but is inducible by putrescine and 4-aminobutyrate in a *Pseudomonas* species (Padmanabhan and Tchen, 1969).
[b] 2-Ketoarginine decarboxylase (enzyme 22) has not been tested in *P. aeruginosa*, but is inducible in *P. putida* (Vanderbilt et al., 1975).

Leisinger, 1978). This view is supported by the isolation of regulatory mutants of *P. aeruginosa* with constitutive (high) levels of anabolic ornithine carbamoyltransferase and noninducible (low) levels of succinylornithine 5-aminotransferase (Y. Itoh, personal communication). In other regulatory mutants, the former enzyme is permanently repressed whereas the latter enzyme is expressed at constitutive (high) levels (Voellmy and Leisinger, 1978).

The function of these regulatory elements at the molecular level is unknown. In a heterologous system, the *argF* gene of *P. aeruginosa* is not controlled by the *argR* repressor of *E. coli* (Clarke and Laverack, 1983). The *argR* repressor, with L-arginine, binds to operators (ARG boxes) located upstream of the *E. coli arg* genes and inhibits their transcription (Cunin et al., 1986; Lim et al., 1987). No ARG box can be found in the promoter region of the *P. aeruginosa argF* gene (Itoh et al., 1988), explaining the lack of control of this gene in *E. coli*. A particular sequence, YTTCC . . . (5 to 6 base pairs) . . . YTTCC, occurs three times with regular spacing in the *argF* promoter region and is an operator candidate (Itoh et al., 1988), but further work is needed to elucidate this point.

Both the arginine decarboxylase and the D-arginine dehydrogenase pathways are characterized by a sequential induction pattern involving several intermediates as potential inducers (Table 3); all these compounds are good carbon and nitrogen sources.

GLOBAL CONTROLS

Oxygen limitation and stationary-phase conditions lead to a strong induction of the *arc* operon (Mercenier et al., 1980b). In an induced culture of wild-type *P. aeruginosa* arginine deiminase and catabolic ornithine carbamoyltransferase each constitute several percent of the total cellular protein, and an even higher production of these enzymes is observed in cells carrying an arc^+ recombinant plasmid (Baur et al., 1987). It is therefore pertinent to investigate the mechanisms of *arc* gene expression. A *nirD* mutation, originally shown to affect nitrite reductase expression (Van Hartingsveldt et al., 1971), pleiotropically prevents nitrate respiration, anaerobic arginine degradation, and HCN biosynthesis. In *E. coli* the cloned $nirD^+$ gene permits partial induction of the *Pseudomonas arc* operon, whereas in the absence of $nirD^+$ the *arc* operon is expressed at very low, unregulated levels (Lüthi et al., 1986; M. Galimand, unpublished results). Thus, the *nirD* product may be a *trans*-acting, positive control element, reminiscent of the Fnr protein in enteric bacteria (Jayaraman et al., 1989). A translational *arcA-lacZ* fusion gives induced β-galactosidase levels in *P. aeruginosa*, *Pseudomonas fluorescens*, *P. putida*, *Pseudomonas syringae*, and *Pseudomonas mendocina*, but not in *E. coli* or *P. cepacia* (A. Zimmermann, unpublished data). From this we conclude that a *nirD*-like gene is present in *Pseudomonas* strains of the homology group I (Palleroni, 1986), but absent from *P. cepacia* or *E. coli*.

In the −40 region of the *arc* operon a sequence motif is found that resembles the Fnr consensus sequence in *E. coli* (Fig. 2). A strain with a deletion eliminating the left half of this motif is noninducible for the *arc* enzymes. No *arc* transcripts are detectable in a *nirD* mutant (M. Gamper, unpublished results). Our current model for the induction of the *arc* operon therefore postulates the recognition of the -40 region by a positive transcriptional effector, which might be an activated form of the NirD protein. Whether this activation is directly due to oxygen limitation (i.e., the redox potential), or whether other molecules are involved as signals of energy starvation, remains to be investigated.

The *arc* operon has three inverted repeats (IR_1, IR_2, IR_3) susceptible to forming hairpin structures in the transcript (Fig. 2; Baur et al., 1987, 1989). The IR_3 sequence contains CUUCG in the loop, a sequence known to stabilize RNA hairpins (Tuerk et al., 1988), and is followed by several U's. This structure represents the terminator of the *arc* operon. The role of the other two IRs might be to protect the mRNA from $3' \rightarrow 5'$-exonucleolytic degradation (Baur et al., 1989). In keeping with a stabilizing function of the IRs, we note a very long half-life of ca. 40 min for *arcA* mRNA after induction (Gamper, unpublished data). This mRNA stability may be very important for the high-level expression of the *arc* operon in stationary phase.

Carbon catabolite repression has been demonstrated in many catabolic pathways of *Pseudomonas*. Citric acid cycle intermediates such as succinate are preferred carbon sources and elicit stronger catabolite repression than does glucose. In *P. aeruginosa*, there is no compelling evidence for an involvement of cAMP in this regulation; intracellular cAMP levels do not vary appreciably during growth on different carbon sources and at various growth stages (Phillips and Mulfinger, 1981; Lessie and Phibbs, 1984). In the arginine network, catabolite repression has been shown to act on arginine transport (in *P. putida*; Piggott and Condon, 1982) and on the arginine decarboxylase and succinyltransferase pathways (Voellmy and Leisinger, 1978; Mercenier et al., 1980a; Jann et al., 1986). The catabolite repressor(s) of *Pseudomonas* spp. remains elusive. However, the finding that 2-oxoglutarate mediates cAMP-independent catabolite repression in *E. coli* (Daniel and Danchin, 1986) raises the interesting possibility that 2-oxoglutarate might also be a key compound in catabolite repression of *Pseudomonas* spp.

Nitrogen control, i.e., regulation of enzyme synthesis by NH_4^+ in the growth medium, is well documented in *P. aeruginosa* (van der Drift and Janssen, 1985). NH_4^+ assimilation depends on glutamate synthase and glutamine synthetase (low NH_4^+ pathway; enzymes 37 and 38; Fig. 1) and on anabolic NADP-dependent glutamate dehydrogenase (high NH_4^+ pathway; enzyme 36). Excess NH_4^+ in the medium represses glutamine synthetase and elevates the levels of anabolic glutamate dehydrogenase (van der Drift and Janssen, 1985). Many enzymes involved in the utilization of organic nitrogen sources are under nitrogen control in *Pseudomonas* spp. For example, urease (enzyme 40 in Fig. 1) is repressed by NH_4^+ alone (Janssen et al., 1982), whereas repression of the agmatine-degrading enzymes by NH_4^+ occurs only when succinate is simultaneously present in the medium (Mercenier et al., 1980a). Interestingly, chemotaxis of *P. aeruginosa* towards arginine is also subject to nitrogen control (Craven and Montie, 1985).

Information on the molecular mechanisms of nitrogen control is scanty in *Pseudomonas* spp. It appears likely, however, that the essential features of nitrogen control in enteric bacteria (Gussin et al., 1986) also apply to the pseudomonads: the 2-oxoglutarate/glutamine ratio determines, via a cascade mechanism, the activity of glutamine synthetase (by adenylylation) and the expression of nitrogen assimilation genes (van der Drift and Janssen, 1985; Meyer, 1985). Like *ntrA* mutants of enteric bacteria, an *ntrA* mutant of *P. aeruginosa* is a glutamine auxotroph (Ishimoto and Lory, 1989). A number of *P. aeruginosa* mutants impaired in the utilization of organic nitrogen sources including L-ornithine (Table 2) have been described; some of these mutants might be of the *ntrC* or *ntrB* type.

Nitrogen assimilation in *Pseudomonas* spp. differs from that in enterics in two important aspects. (i) *P. aeruginosa* has an additional enzyme for the conversion of glutamate to 2-oxoglutarate, the catabolic glutamate dehydrogenase (enzyme 30 in Fig. 1). This enzyme is induced by glutamate, ornithine, or arginine (Früh et al., 1985). (ii) Nitrogen starvation leads to a release of 2-oxoglutarate into the medium (von Tigerstrom and Campbell, 1966).

HOW FUTILE CYCLES ARE AVOIDED

Why is biosynthetic arginine not catabolized instantly? An answer lies in the arginine pool size. *P. aeruginosa* growing in minimal medium has an undetectable (<1 μM) intracellular arginine concentration (Kay and Gronlund, 1969b), presumably as the result of an avid arginyl-tRNA synthetase and a very tight feedback inhibition control of the first two arginine biosynthetic enzymes (Haas and Leisinger, 1974, 1975). Extracellular L-arginine at 1 μM is concentrated ~300-fold by active transport (Fan et al., 1972) and thus reaches intracellular concentrations that are sufficient for the induction and the functioning of catabolic enzymes. Another answer may be compartmentation. Arginine decarboxylase of *E. coli* is located in the cell envelope and preferentially converts extracellular arginine to putrescine (Buch and Boyle, 1985). In *P. aeruginosa*, the location of arginine decarboxylase has not been determined, but another catabolic enzyme, *N*-acetylglutamate deacetylase (enzyme 35 in Fig. 1), is a periplasmic enzyme and hence cannot attack the intracellular *N*-acetylglutamate pool (Früh and Leisinger, 1981). A third reason why futile cycles do not occur is regulation of enzyme synthesis and activity. The regulatory mechanisms pertinent to the reactions of carbamoylphosphate, ornithine, and citrulline have been discussed elsewhere (Baur et al., 1989).

ADVANTAGES OF MULTIPLE PATHWAYS

P. aeruginosa is able to adjust to a variety of environmental situations. For example, it thrives in aerobic, aquatic environments with very low nutrient concentrations as well as in anaerobic, nutrient-rich environments such as the human intestine. Arginine metabolism can be adjusted accordingly. In the former situation, a sensitive chemotactic response, potent uptake systems, and multiple degradation pathways ensure optimal utilization of arginine as a nutrient. Even when the major pathway (the succinyltransferase route) is interrupted, arginine can still be degraded via the D-arginine dehydrogenase pathway (Jann et al., 1988). In an anaerobic environment, the utilization of arginine as an energy source becomes an asset. Finally, the extraordinary number of compounds that can be used as carbon and nitrogen sources (Fig. 1) illustrates the contribution of the arginine network to the metabolic versatility of *Pseudomonas*.

ACKNOWLEDGMENTS. D.H. thanks Andrée Lazdunski and Jean-Claude Patte for their hospitality during the time when this review was written. It is a pleasure to acknowledge the long and fruitful collaboration with Victor Stalon and his colleagues in Brussels and Thomas Leisinger in Zürich. We thank Antje Hitz for secretarial assistance and Hélène Paul for help with the figures.

Research in our laboratory was supported by the Schweizerische Nationalfonds and the Eidgenössische Technische Hochschule Zürich. The Cystic Fibrosis Foundation is thanked for travel support.

LITERATURE CITED

Abdelal, A. T., W. F. Bibb, and O. Neinan. 1982. Carbamate kinase from *Pseudomonas aeruginosa*: purification, characterization, physiological role, and regulation. *J. Bacteriol.* **151:**1411–1419.

Armitage, J. P., and M. C. W. Evans. 1983. The motile and tactic behaviour of *Pseudomonas aeruginosa* in anaerobic environments. *FEBS Lett.* **156:**113–118.

Baur, H., E. Lüthi, V. Stalon, A. Mercenier, and D. Haas. 1989. Sequence analysis and expression of the arginine-deiminase and carbamate-kinase genes of *Pseudomonas aeruginosa*. *Eur. J. Biochem.* **179:**53–60.

Baur, H., V. Stalon, P. Falmagne, E. Lüthi, and D. Haas. 1987. Primary and quaternary structure of the catabolic ornithine carbamoyltransferase from *Pseudomonas aeruginosa*. Extensive sequence homology with the anabolic ornithine carbamoyltransferases of *Escherichia coli*. *Eur. J. Biochem.* **166:**111–117.

Bautsch, W., D. Grothues, and B. Tümmler. 1988. Genome fingerprinting of *Pseudomonas aeruginosa* by two-dimensional field inversion gel electrophoresis. *FEMS Microbiol. Lett.* **52:**255–258.

Buch, J. K., and S. M. Boyle. 1985. Biosynthetic arginine decarboxylase in *Escherichia coli* is synthesized as a precursor and located in the cell envelope. *J. Bacteriol.* **163:**522–527.

Clarke, P. H. 1982. The metabolic versatility of pseudomonads. *Antonie van Leeuwenhoek* **48:**105–130.

Clarke, P. H., and P. D. Laverack. 1983. Expression of the *argF* gene of *Pseudomonas aeruginosa* in *Pseudomonas aeruginosa*, *Pseudomonas putida*, and *Escherichia coli*. *J. Bacteriol.* **154:**508–512.

Craven, R., and T. C. Montie. 1985. Regulation of *Pseudomonas aeruginosa* chemotaxis by the nitrogen source. *J. Bacteriol.* **164:**544–549.

Cunin, R., N. Glansdorff, A. Piérard, and V. Stalon. 1986. Biosynthesis and metabolism of arginine in bacteria. *Microbiol. Rev.* **50:**314–352.

Daniel, J., and A. Danchin. 1986. 2-Ketoglutarate as a possible regulatory metabolite involved in cyclic AMP-independent catabolite repression in *Escherichia coli* K12. *Biochimie* **68:**303–310.

Fan, L. G., D. Miller, and V. W. Rodwell. 1972. Metabolism of basic amino acids in *Pseudomonas putida*. Transport of lysine, ornithine, and arginine. *J. Biol. Chem.* **247:**2283–2288.

Frantz, B., and A. M. Chakrabarty. 1986. Degradative plasmids in *Pseudomonas*, p. 295–323. *In* J. R. Sokatch (ed.), *The Bacteria*, vol. X. Academic Press, Inc., Orlando, Fla.

Früh, H., and T. Leisinger. 1981. Properties and localization of N-acetylglutamate deacetylase from *Pseudomonas aeruginosa*. *J. Gen. Microbiol.* **125:**1–10.

Früh, R., D. Haas, and T. Leisinger. 1985. Altered control of glutamate dehydrogenases in ornithine utilization mutants of *Pseudomonas aeruginosa*. *Arch. Microbiol.* **141:**170–176.

Gussin, G. N., C. W. Ronson, and F. M. Ausubel. 1986. Regulation of nitrogen fixation genes. *Annu. Rev. Genet.* **20:**567–591.

Haas, D. 1983. Genetic aspects of biodegradation by pseudomonads. *Experientia* **39:**1199–1213.

Haas, D., R. Evans, A. Mercenier, J.-P. Simon, and V. Stalon. 1979. Genetic and physiological characterization of *Pseudomonas aeruginosa* mutants affected in the catabolic ornithine carbamoyltransferase. *J. Bacteriol.* **139**:713–720.

Haas, D., B. W. Holloway, A. Schamböck, and T. Leisinger. 1977. The genetic organization of arginine biosynthesis in *Pseudomonas aeruginosa*. *Mol. Gen. Genet.* **154**:7–22.

Haas, D., and T. Leisinger. 1974. Multiple control of N-acetylglutamate synthetase from *Pseudomonas aeruginosa*: synergistic inhibition by acetylglutamate and polyamines. *Biochem. Biophys. Res. Commun.* **60**:42–47.

Haas, D., and T. Leisinger. 1975. *N*-Acetylglutamate 5-phosphotransferase of *Pseudomonas aeruginosa*. Catalytic and regulatory properties. *Eur. J. Biochem.* **52**:377–383.

Haas, D., H. Matsumoto, P. Moretti, V. Stalon, and A. Mercenier. 1984. Arginine degradation in *Pseudomonas aeruginosa* mutants blocked in two arginine catabolic pathways. *Mol. Gen. Genet.* **193**:437–444.

Holloway, B. W., K. O'Hoy, and H. Matsumoto. 1987. *Pseudomonas aeruginosa* PAO, p. 213–221. *In* S. J. O'Brien (ed.), *Genetic Maps*, vol. 4. Cold Spring Harbor Laboratory, Cold Spring Harbor, N.Y.

Isaac, J. H., and B. W. Holloway. 1972. Control of arginine biosynthesis in *Pseudomonas aeruginosa*. *J. Gen. Microbiol.* **73**:427–438.

Ishimoto, K. S., and S. Lory. 1989. Formation of pilin in *Pseudomonas aeruginosa* requires the alternative σ factor (RpoN) of RNA polymerase. *Proc. Natl. Acad. Sci. USA* **86**:1954–1957.

Itoh, Y., L. Soldati, V. Stalon, P. Falmagne, Y. Terawaki, T. Leisinger, and D. Haas. 1988. Anabolic ornithine carbamoyltransferase of *Pseudomonas aeruginosa*: nucleotide sequence and transcriptional control of the *argF* structural gene. *J. Bacteriol.* **170**:2725–2734.

Jann, A., H. Matsumoto, and D. Haas. 1988. The fourth arginine catabolic pathway of *Pseudomonas aeruginosa*. *J. Gen. Microbiol.* **134**:1043–1053.

Jann, A., V. Stalon, C. Vander Wauven, T. Leisinger, and D. Haas. 1986. N^2-Succinylated intermediates in an arginine catabolic pathway of *Pseudomonas aeruginosa*. *Proc. Natl. Acad. Sci. USA* **83**:4937–4941.

Janssen, D. B., W. J. A. Habets, J. T. Marugg, and C. van der Drift. 1982. Nitrogen control in *Pseudomonas aeruginosa*: mutants affected in the synthesis of glutamine synthetase, urease, and NADP-dependent glutamate dehydrogenase. *J. Bacteriol.* **151**:22–28.

Jayaraman, P. S., J. A. Cole, and S. J. Busby. 1989. Mutational analysis of the nucleotide sequence at the FNR-dependent *nirB* promoter in *Escherichia coli*. *Nucleic Acids Res.* **17**:135–145.

Kay, W. W., and A. F. Gronlund. 1969a. Amino acid pool formation in *Pseudomonas aeruginosa*. *J. Bacteriol.* **97**:282–291.

Kay, W. W., and A. F. Gronlund. 1969b. Amino acid transport in *Pseudomonas aeruginosa*. *J. Bacteriol.* **97**:273–281.

Kohara, Y., K. Akiyama, and K. Isono. 1987. The physical map of the whole *E. coli* chromosome. Application of a new strategy for rapid analysis and sorting of a large genomic library. *Cell* **50**:495–508.

Leisinger, T., and R. Margraff. 1979. Secondary metabolites of the fluorescent pseudomonads. *Microbiol. Rev.* **43**:422–442.

Lessie, T. G., and P. V. Phibbs, Jr. 1984. Alternative pathways of carbohydrate utilization in pseudomonads. *Annu. Rev. Microbiol.* **38**:359–387.

Lim, D., J. D. Oppenheim, T. Eckhardt, and W. K. Maas. 1987. Nucleotide sequence of the *argR* gene of *Escherichia coli* K-12 and isolation of its product, the arginine repressor. *Proc. Natl. Acad. Sci. USA* **84**:6697–6701.

Lüthi, E., H. Baur, M. Gamper, F. Brunner, D. Villeval, A. Mercenier, and D. Haas. 1990. The *arc* operon for anaerobic arginine catabolism in *Pseudomonas aeruginosa* contains an additional gene, *arcD*, encoding a membrane protein. *Gene*, in press.

Lüthi, E., A. Mercenier, and D. Haas. 1986. The *arcABC* operon required for fermentative growth of *Pseudomonas aeruginosa* on arginine: Tn5-751-assisted cloning and localization of structural genes. *J. Gen. Microbiol.* **132**:2667–2675.

Marquis, R. E., G. R. Bender, D. R. Murray, and A. Wong. 1987. Arginine deiminase system and bacterial adaptation to acid environments. *Appl. Environ. Microbiol.* **53**:198–200.

Meile, L., L. Soldati, and T. Leisinger. 1982. Regulation of proline catabolism in *Pseudomonas aeruginosa* PAO. *Arch. Microbiol.* **132:**189–193.

Mercenier, A., J.-P. Simon, D. Haas, and V. Stalon. 1980a. Catabolism of L-arginine by *Pseudomonas aeruginosa. J. Gen. Microbiol.* **116:**381–389.

Mercenier, A., J.-P. Simon, C. Vander Wauven, D. Haas, and V. Stalon. 1980b. Regulation of enzyme synthesis in the arginine deiminase pathway of *Pseudomonas aeruginosa. J. Bacteriol.* **144:**159–163.

Mercenier, A., V. Stalon, J.-P. Simon, and D. Haas. 1982. Mapping of the arginine deiminase gene in *Pseudomonas aeruginosa. J. Bacteriol.* **149:**787–788.

Meyer, J.-M. 1985. Glutamine synthetase from *Pseudomonas fluorescens*: a tool for studying changes in cell permeability and enzyme regulation. *Curr. Top. Cell. Regul.* **26:**149–161.

Miller, D. L., and V. Rodwell. 1971. Metabolism of basic amino acids in *Pseudomonas putida*. Intermediates in L-arginine catabolism. *J. Biol. Chem.* **246:**5053–5058.

Moench, T. T., and W. A. Konetzka. 1978. Chemotaxis in *Pseudomonas aeruginosa. J. Bacteriol.* **133:**427–429.

Padmanabhan, R., and T. T. Tchen. 1969. Nicotinamide adenine dinucleotide and nicotinamide adenine dinucleotide phosphate-linked succinic semialdehyde dehydrogenases in a *Pseudomonas* species. *J. Bacteriol.* **100:**398–402.

Palleroni, N. J. 1986. Taxonomy of the pseudomonads, p. 3–25. *In* J. R. Sokatch (ed.), *The Bacteria*, vol. X. Academic Press, Inc., Orlando, Fla.

Phillips, A. T., and L. M. Mulfinger. 1981. Cyclic adenosine 3′,5′-monophosphate levels in *Pseudomonas putida* and *Pseudomonas aeruginosa* during induction and carbon catabolite repression of histidase synthesis. *J. Bacteriol.* **145:**1286–1292.

Piggott, R. P., and S. Condon. 1982. Correlation between catabolite repression of arginine transport and repression of anabolic ornithine carbamoyltransferase in *Pseudomonas putida. J. Gen. Microbiol.* **128:**2291–2296.

Poolman, B., A. J. M. Driessen, and W. N. Konings. 1987. Regulation of arginine-ornithine exchange and the arginine deiminase pathway in *Streptococcus lactis. J. Bacteriol.* **169:**5597–5604.

Rahman, M., P. D. Laverack, and P. H. Clarke. 1980. The catabolism of arginine by *Pseudomonas aeruginosa. J. Gen. Microbiol.* **116:**371–380.

Ramos, F., V. Stalon, A. Piérard, and J. M. Wiame. 1967. The specialization of the two ornithine carbamoyltransferases of *Pseudomonas. Biochim. Biophys. Acta* **139:**98–106.

Sherris, J. C., J. G. Shoesmith, M. T. Parker, and D. Breckon. 1959. Tests for the rapid breakdown of arginine by bacteria: their use in the identification of pseudomonads. *J. Gen. Microbiol.* **21:**389–396.

Shoesmith, J. G., and J. C. Sherris. 1960. Studies on the mechanism of arginine-activated motility in a *Pseudomonas* strain. *J. Gen. Microbiol.* **22:**10–24.

Stalon, V., and A. Mercenier. 1984. L-Arginine utilization by *Pseudomonas* species. *J. Gen. Microbiol.* **130:**69–76.

Stalon, V., C. Vander Wauven, P. Momin, and C. Legrain. 1987. Catabolism of arginine, citrulline and ornithine by *Pseudomonas* and related bacteria. *J. Gen. Microbiol.* **133:**2487–2495.

Stolp, H., and D. Gadkari. 1981. Nonpathogenic members of the genus *Pseudomonas*, p. 719–741. *In* M. P. Starr, H. Stolp, H. G. Trüper, A. Balows, and H. G. Schlegel (ed.), *The Prokaryotes*, vol. 1. Springer-Verlag, Berlin.

Tachiki, T., H. Kohno, K. Sugiyama, T. Matsubara, and T. Tochikura. 1980. Purification, properties and formation of arginine-α-ketoglutarate transaminase in *Arthrobacter simplex. Biochim. Biophys. Acta* **615:**79–84.

Thornley, M. J. 1960. The differentiation of *Pseudomonas* from other Gram-negative bacteria on the basis of arginine metabolism. *J. Appl. Bacteriol.* **23:**37–52.

Tuerk, C., P. Gauss, C. Thermes, D. R. Groebe, M. Gayle, N. Guild, G. Stormo, Y. d'Aubenton-Carafa, O. C. Uhlenbeck, I. Tinoco, Jr., E. N. Brody, and L. Gold. 1988. CUUCGG hairpins: extraordinarily stable RNA secondary structures associated with various biochemical processes. *Proc. Natl. Acad. Sci. USA* **85:**1364–1368.

Vanderbilt, A. S., N. S. Gaby, and V. W. Rodwell. 1975. Intermediates and enzymes between α-ketoarginine and γ-guanidinobutyrate in the L-arginine catabolic pathway of *Pseudomonas putida. J. Biol. Chem.* **250:**5322–5329.

Van der Drift, C., and D. B. Janssen. 1985. Regulation of enzymes under nitrogen control in *Pseudomonas aeruginosa. Curr. Top. Cell. Regul.* **26:**485–490.

Vander Wauven, C., A. Jann, D. Haas, T. Leisinger, and V. Stalon. 1988. N^2-Succinylornithine in ornithine catabolism of *Pseudomonas aeruginosa. Arch. Microbiol.* **150:**400–404.

Vander Wauven, C., A. Piérard, M. Kley-Raymann, and D. Haas. 1984. *Pseudomonas aeruginosa* mutants affected in anaerobic growth on arginine: evidence for a four-gene cluster encoding the arginine deiminase pathway. *J. Bacteriol.* **160:**928–934.

Vander Wauven, C., and V. Stalon. 1985. Occurrence of succinyl derivatives in the catabolism of arginine in *Pseudomonas cepacia. J. Bacteriol.* **164:**882–886.

Van Hartingsveldt, J., M. G. Marinus, and A. H. Stouthamer. 1971. Mutants of *Pseudomonas aeruginosa* blocked in nitrate or nitrite dissimilation. *Genetics* **67:**469–482.

Voellmy, R., and T. Leisinger. 1975. Dual role for N^2-acetylornithine 5-aminotransferase from *Pseudomonas aeruginosa* in arginine biosynthesis and arginine catabolism. *J. Bacteriol.* **122:**799–809.

Voellmy, R., and T. Leisinger. 1976. Role of 4-aminobutyrate aminotransferase in the arginine metabolism of *Pseudomonas aeruginosa. J. Bacteriol.* **128:**722–729.

Voellmy, R., and T. Leisinger. 1978. Regulation of enzyme synthesis in the arginine biosynthetic pathway of *Pseudomonas aeruginosa. J. Gen. Microbiol.* **109:**25–35.

Von Tigerstrom, M., and J. J. R. Campbell. 1966. The accumulation of α-ketoglutarate by suspensions of *Pseudomonas aeruginosa. Can. J. Microbiol.* **12:**1005–1013.

Part V

CELL ENVELOPE AND TRANSPORT

Diffusion of Antibiotics via Specific Pathways across the Outer Membrane of *Pseudomonas aeruginosa*

Joaquim Trias and Hiroshi Nikaido

The outer membrane of gram-negative bacteria is a semipermeable membrane that allows the diffusion of small hydrophilic solutes and has very low permeability toward hydrophobic compounds (Nikaido and Vaara, 1987). The permeability properties of this membrane are determined mainly by the properties of the pore-forming proteins and of the specific transport systems that have been described in many gram-negative bacteria (Hancock, 1987). Antibiotics, like nutrients and waste products, may diffuse through the outer membrane. In bacteria, the principal antibiotic targets are located inside the outer membrane, and these compounds have to travel across it in order to be effective. Therefore, the sensitivity of the gram-negative bacteria to an antibiotic is influenced by the permeability properties of the channels present in the outer membrane (Nikaido, 1989).

Low permeability is an efficient way to avoid the action of antibiotics, but it can also be a disadvantage for the cell because it lowers the influx and efflux of nutrients and waste products. Thus, if the cell has a low outer membrane permeability, it will be an advantage to have specific channels in it, since they will allow the passage of nutrients at a faster rate. Also, the presence of a binding site will allow the uptake of nutrients that are found in the medium at low concentrations. Some antibiotics have been designed to take advantage of these systems in order to facilitate transport through the outer membrane. For example, the catechol-cephalosporins mimic siderophores and can be transported through the siderophore uptake system (Curtis et al., 1988). Other antibiotics, such as imipenem, are able to use a specific channel to enter the periplasm of *Pseudomonas aeruginosa* (Trias et al., 1989).

Joaquim Trias and Hiroshi Nikaido ● Department of Microbiology and Immunology, University of California, Berkeley, California 94720.

The intrinsic resistance of *P. aeruginosa* to many antibiotics can be explained by the low permeability of its outer membrane. Using intact-cell experiments, Yoshimura and Nikaido (1982) found that the permeability for cephalothin and cephaloridine was 100- to 500-fold lower than that in *Escherichia coli*. In a similar approach, Angus et al. (1982) showed that the permeability for nitrocefin, a hydrolyzable cepahalosporin, was at least 10- to 100-fold lower than in *E. coli*. This low permeability for hydrophilic compounds is not accompanied by an increase in permeability for hydrophobic antibiotics such as erythromycin and rifampin and indicates that it is the hydrophilic pathway that is more important for *P. aeruginosa* (Nikaido and Hancock, 1986). Outer membrane proteins C, D1, D2, E, F, and P have been reported to produce a channel or pore in *P. aeruginosa* (Benz and Hancock, 1987; Hancock and Carey, 1980; Nikaido and Hancock, 1986; Trias et al., 1988; Yoshihara and Nakae, 1989). Three of these proteins have been demonstrated to be specific channels: protein P, which forms anion-specific channels (Benz and Hancock, 1987); protein D1, which forms glucose-specific channels and is induced when glucose is present in the growth medium (Hancock and Carey, 1980; Trias et al., 1988); and protein D2, which allows the passage of basic amino acids and compounds that mimic their structure (Trias and Nikaido, 1990).

KINETIC BEHAVIOR OF A SPECIFIC CHANNEL

The diffusion kinetics of solutes that travel through the outer membrane via nonspecific pores can be described by Fick's laws of diffusion. Briefly, the velocity of travel (V) is linearly dependent on the difference in solute concentration between the outer medium and the periplasm:

$$V = A \times P \times (C_o - C_i) \tag{1}$$

where P, A, C_o, and C_i are permeability coefficient, area of the membrane, the solute concentration outside, and the solute concentration inside, respectively.

This law assumes that there is no interaction between the pore or channel and the solute. If there is an interaction with a ligand-binding site (e.g., the binding site in protein D1 for glucose and its structural analogs), the diffusion kinetics no longer follow Fick's laws. Several models assuming different degrees of complexity for binding site(s) and for carrier(s) have been proposed (Benz et al., 1987; Stein, 1986). The simplest one would posit a symmetrical channel with a central single binding site, which would be available from either side. The kinetics of solute diffusion is then similar to enzyme kinetics and would obey the following equation (K. B. Gehring, Ph.D. thesis, University of California, Berkeley, 1988):

$$V = V_{max} \times A \times (C_o - C_i)/(C_o + C_i + K_m) \tag{2}$$

We can see that under the binding-site restriction, a particular channel can be described by its K_m and V_{max}. This means that at concentrations close to the K_m, ligand uptake will be much faster than would be expected from simple diffusion following a concentration gradient (equation 1); at high concentrations, the

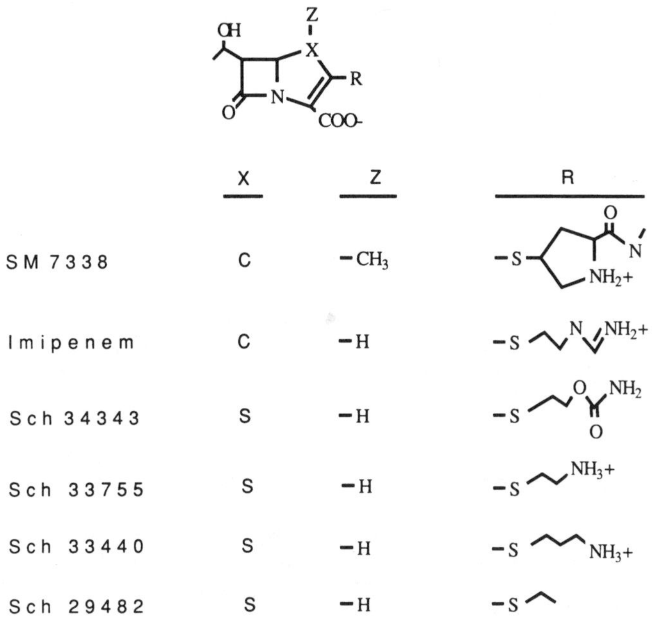

	X	Z	R
S M 7 3 3 8	C	$-CH_3$	
I m i p e n e m	C	$-H$	
S c h 3 4 3 4 3	S	$-H$	
S c h 3 3 7 5 5	S	$-H$	
S c h 3 3 4 4 0	S	$-H$	
S c h 2 9 4 8 2	S	$-H$	

FIGURE 1. Structures of penems and carbapenems.

binding site will be saturated and the velocity of transport will reach a maximum equal to V_{max}. In the latter case, an increase in the concentration gradient will not increase the uptake velocity, as happens in the nonspecific diffusion pathway. When solute concentrations C_o and C_i are much lower than K_m, then the equation simplifies to

$$V = (V_{max}/K_m) \times A \times (C_o - C_i)$$

(3)

which has the form of equation 1, with V_{max}/K_m replacing P.

Antibiotics with a high affinity for a specific channel have the advantage that they will be more effective at low (often physiological) concentrations, since they will be taken up faster. However, resistant strains could arise by shutting down the specific transport system.

PERMEABILITY OF THE OUTER MEMBRANE TO IMIPENEM

The use of imipenem, a carbapenem antibiotic (Fig. 1), led to the isolation of the first imipenem-resistant strains. Some of these strains showed no cross-resistance against other β-lactams, could not hydrolyze or modify the antibiotic, and did not have any apparent change in the penicillin-binding proteins or in their copy number. But the imipenem-resistant strains lacked a major outer membrane protein of molecular weight 45,000 to 49,000, depending of the strain (Quinn et al.,

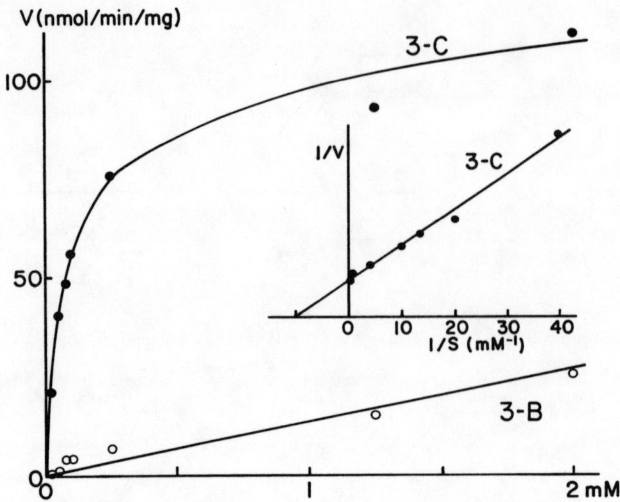

FIGURE 2. Rates of hydrolysis of imipenem by intact cells. Hydrolysis rates were measured at different imipenem concentrations, using intact cells of imipenem-susceptible strain 3-C (●) and resistant strain 3-B (○), both containing pHN4. Hydrolysis rates were corrected for contribution by the leaked-out enzyme (from Trias et al., 1989).

1988). This molecular weight range correspond to the D group of proteins of the outer membrane. These facts suggested that imipenem can travel through the outer membrane of *P. aeruginosa* via a specific channel.

Earlier experiments measuring the MIC of imipenem and other β-lactams, using the hyperpermeable strain from Zimmermann, showed that for imipenem there was only a small difference between the MIC for the hyperpermeable strain Z799/61 and the wild-type strain Z799, suggesting that imipenem could diffuse rapidly through the outer membrane (Williams, 1985). Also, a difference in imipenem permeability between imipenem-resistant and -susceptible strains was demonstrated by Lynch et al. (1987) by measuring imipenem binding to penicillin-binding proteins.

Probably the most accurate way of measuring outer membrane permeability is the Zimmermann-Rosselet method (Nikaido, 1989). Since imipenem is resistant to hydrolysis by the β-lactamases present in *P. aeruginosa*, we constructed, in order to measure the outer membrane permeability with intact cells, a plasmid that carried the *blaS* gene that encodes the L-1 β-lactamase from *Pseudomonas maltophilia* (Dufresne et al., 1988). This enzyme is able to hydrolyze imipenem and other penems and carbapenems. The plasmid (pHN4) was introduced into a set of imipenem-susceptible strains and a set of imipenem-resistant strains. These strains allowed us to monitor the diffusion of imipenem into the periplasm by comparing the hydrolysis rates of intact cells with those obtained from a sonic extract of cells of the same batch.

We found that the resistance of imipenem was due mainly to the low specific permeability to imipenem. Figure 2 shows the kinetics of transport of imipenem at

TABLE 1
Apparent permeability coefficients of outer membranes of imipenem-susceptible strains 3-C and
PAO1 and imipenem-resistant strain 3-B[a]

Substrate	Permeability coefficient (nm/s)		
	3-B	3-C	PAO1
Imipenem[b,c]	6	736	
SM-7338[b]	5.5	73	
Sch 34343[b]	18.5	22.7	
Sch 33755[b]	9	40	
Sch 33440[b]	7.5	24	
Sch 29482[b]	24.5	23.3	
Cephaloridine[c,d]	13	10	10.7
Cephacetrile[d]			7.5

[a] The hydrolysis rates by leaked-out enzymes (measured with supernatants obtained by centrifugation of cell suspensions) were between 10 to 60% of rates measured with intact cells. Rates with intact cells were corrected for these rates of hydrolysis by the leaked-out enzymes.
[b] Substrate concentration was 50 μM (Trias and Nikaido, 1990).
[c] Substrate concentration was 50 μM (Trias et al., 1989).
[d] Substrate concentration was 1 mM (Yoshimura and Nikaido, 1982).

different concentrations. There is a large difference in transport between strains 3-C and 3-B, and imipenem can use a saturable, specific channel with a K_m of approximately 0.1 mM. When we compare the permeabilities of the outer membranes of these strains, we find that at low substrate concentrations, there is a large difference between the susceptible and the resistant strains in permeability of imipenem and some other compounds (Table 1). In the imipenem-resistant strains, since they lack the specific transport system, imipenem permeates mainly through the nonspecific pathways, similar to the case for β-lactams that cannot use any specific transport system; thus, the apparent permeability coefficient of imipenem in the resistant strains is similar to that of cephaloridine in this strain and those of cephaloridine and cephacetrile in PAO1 (Yoshimura and Nikaido, 1982).

Results obtained by using the liposome swelling assay with cell envelopes or outer membrane for assessing the permeability of imipenem can be misleading, since the assay must be performed at a high substrate concentration (about 10 to 40 mM), thus saturating the specific channel. At these concentrations, the permeation observed will come mainly from the activity of the nonspecific pores (Table 2).

Direct measurement of the permeability of purified cell envelopes can also be performed by reconstituting proteoliposomes with the outer membrane, phospholipids, and trapped L-1 β-lactamase. This method allowed us to study the transport of imipenem with purified outer membrane at low, nonsaturating concentrations of imipenem (e.g., 50 μM). Under these conditions, a large difference in permeability between the cell envelopes of the two strains could be seen (Table 3).

TABLE 2

Swelling rates of proteoliposomes with outer membranes of imipenem-susceptible strain 3-C and imipenem-resistant strain 3-B[a]

Source of outer membrane	Relative swelling rate[b] in:		
	Glucose	Imipenem	Cephaloridine
3-C	100	52	42
3-B	105	58	47

[a] Outer membranes (containing about 20 μg of protein) from cells grown in succinate-M63 medium were reconstituted with phospholipids, and the rates of swelling of liposomes were measured after dilution into an isotonic (about 8 mM) solution of glucose, imipenem, or cephaloridine. Results are from Trias et al. (1989).
[b] Percentage of the swelling rate of liposomes containing 3-C outer membrane in glucose.

PERMEABILITY OF THE OUTER MEMBRANE TO OTHER PENEMS AND CARBAPENEMS

If other antibiotics can use the imipenem-specific channel, some cross-resistance would be expected. Cross-resistance between imipenem-resistant *P. aeruginosa* strains and SM-7338, another carbapenem, was found in a multicenter study of the susceptibility to SM-7338 (Jones et al., 1989), suggesting that this channel can be used by more antibiotics. Therefore, we investigated the permeation of other penems and carbapenems with different structures in the R moiety (Fig. 1). These experiments would also give us information about the specificity of the channel. We found that other penems and carbapenems can also travel at higher rates than expected for their molecular weights through the outer membrane of imipenem-susceptible *P. aeruginosa* strains; in the imipenem-resistant strains, the permeability coefficient of all compounds tested was of the same order of magnitude and similar to the values for cephaloridine and cephalothin (Table 1).

It appeared that the velocity of the specific penetration was affected by (i) the presence of a positively charged group in the R moiety and (ii) the distance between the positive charge and the β-lactam ring. The permeabilities of Sch 34343 and Sch 29482, which do not have a positive charge in the R group, were similar between the imipenem-susceptible and -resistant strains. In contrast, imipenem, SM-7338, Sch 33755, and Sch 33440, which have a positive charge in

TABLE 3

Relative permeability toward imipenem measured with vesicles containing L-1 β-lactamase[a]

Strain	Relative rate of permeation in:[b]		
	L broth	M63 + glucose	M63 + sodium succinate
3-C	25	42	100
3-B	5	7	4

[a] Unilamellar liposomes were made with phospholipids and the outer membranes of imipenem-susceptible strain 3-C or imipenem-resistant strain 3-B. The liposomes contained L-1 β-lactamase. Results are from Trias et al. (1989).
[b] Percentage of the coefficient of permeability of imipenem for the outer membrane of susceptible strain 3-C when grown in M63-succinate medium.

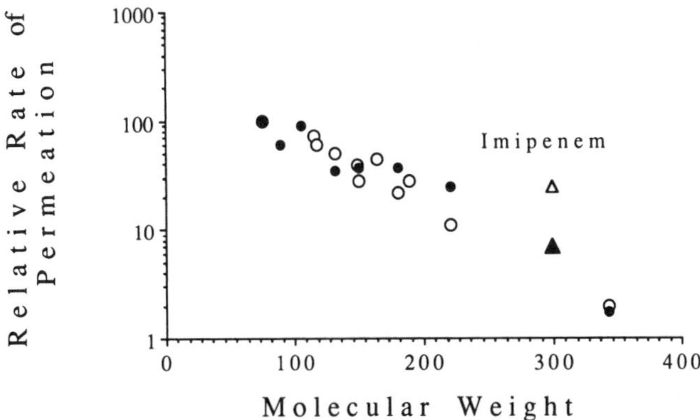

FIGURE 3. Rates of diffusion of solutes of different sizes through the protein D1 (filled symbols) and D2 (open symbols) channels. The rates were determined by measuring the swelling rates of proteoliposomes reconstituted with 10 μg of protein. The rates were normalized to that of glycine, which was taken as 100. Each point represents an average of two to four experiments. (From Trias et al. [1988] and Trias and Nikaido [1990].)

the R moiety, could utilize the channel. Imipenem was the fastest compound at the substrate concentration used, but the difference in permeabilities of the other penems and carbapenems between the two strains could be greater at lower concentrations of substrate if the K_m of the specific transport system is lower for these compounds.

PROTEIN D2

Since Quinn et al. (1988) first noticed that the imipenem-resistant strains lacked a major outer membrane protein in the size range of 45,000 to 49,000 kilodaltons, it has been suggested that the missing outer membrane belongs to the D group of proteins (Lynch et al., 1987). This group is formed by two major proteins: protein D1, which allows the specific permeation of glucose and its structural analogs but also of small hydrophilic compounds (Trias et al., 1988), and protein D2, which also allows the diffusion of small hydrophilic compounds (Yoshihara and Nakae, 1989). Both channels allow the permeation of imipenem, but only protein D2 does so at a higher permeation rate (Fig. 3). Imipenem-resistant strains synthesize D1 but not D2, as shown by Western blots (immunoblots) of electropherograms of the outer membrane with anti-D1 or anti-D2 serum (Trias and Nikaido, 1990).

Protein D2 is therefore responsible for the specific passage of imipenem and other penems and carbapenems, but what is its physiological substrate? We know that penems and carbapenems need a positive charge in the R moiety on C-2 in order to diffuse faster. By measuring the inhibition of imipenem transport by other compounds, we found that this channel also binds basic amino acids such as L-lysine, L-arginine, L-histidine, and L-ornithine, L-lysine being the most effective

TABLE 4

Relative rates of hydrolysis by intact cells of imipenem in the presence of L-lysine and
its structural analogs

Compound	Comment	Relative permeation rate[a]
L-Lysine	Positive charge at C-6	39
L-Norleucine	No NH$_2$ at C-6	100
6-Aminocaproic acid	No NH$_2$ at C-2	105
Caproic acid	No NH$_2$ at C-2 and C-6	102
L-Ornithine	Positive charge at C-5	52
2,5-Diaminobutyric acid	Positive charge at C-4	48
2,3-Diaminopropionic acid	Positive charge at C-3	30

[a] Rates of hydrolysis by intact cells of the D2-synthesizing strain 3-C containing pHN4. The relative intact-cell rates roughly represent the rates of permeation across the outer membrane; 50 μM imipenem and 1 mM tested substrate were used for the intact-cell experiments as previously described (Trias et al., 1989). None of the substrates tested inhibited L-1 β-lactamase. The results were normalized to the hydrolysis of imipenem without any substrate, which was taken as 100.

substrate. Also, small peptides containing basic amino acids such as L-Ala-His and L-Ala-Lys showed inhibition. No inhibition of transport was seen with the following amino acids and peptides used as substrates: L-alanine, glycine, L-valine, L-phenylalanine, L-tryptophan, L-methionine, L-proline, L-cysteine, L-aspartic acid, L-Ala-Leu, L-Pro-Ala, Gly-Gly-Gly, and Gly-Gly-Gly-Gly. L-Lysine was the most effective substrate, as determined by substituting various positions of the molecule and measuring the inhibition (Table 4). Only the presence of a positive charge at a position separated from the carboxyl group appeared to be important for binding to the D2 channel.

It seems likely that imipenem, SM-7338, Sch 33755, and Sch 33440 mimic the structure of these natural substrates, resulting in efficient diffusion through the D2 channel.

ACKNOWLEDGMENTS. This work was supported by Public Health Service research grant AI-09144 from the National Institutes of Health. J.T. was the recipient of a fellowship from Comissió Interdepartamental de Recerca i Innovació Tecnològica de la Generalitat de Catalunya.

We thank John D. Quinn for the gift of the sets of imipenem-resistant and -susceptible *P. aeruginosa* strains.

LITERATURE CITED

Angus, J. H., A. M. Carey, D. A. Caron, A. M. B. Kropinski, and R. E. W. Hancock. 1982. Outer membrane permeability in *Pseudomonas aeruginosa*: comparison of a wild type with an antibiotic-supersusceptible mutant. *Antimicrob. Agents Chemother.* 21:229–309.

Benz, R., and R. E. W. Hancock. 1987. Mechanism of ion transport through the anion-selective channel of the *Pseudomonas aeruginosa* outer membrane. *J. Gen. Physiol.* 89:275–295.

Benz, R., A. Schmid, and G. H. Vos-Scheperkeuter. 1987. Mechanism of sugar transport through the sugar specific LamB channel of *Escherichia coli* outer membrane. *J. Membr. Biol.* 100:21–29.

Curtis, N. A. C., R. L. Eisenstadt, S. J. East, R. J. Cornford, L. A. Walker, and A. J. White. 1988. Iron-regulated outer membrane proteins of *Escherichia coli* K-12 and mechanism of action of catechol-substituted cephalosporins. *Antimicrob. Agents Chemother.* 32:1879–1886.

Dufresne, J., G. Vézina, and R. C. Levesque. 1988. Cloning and expression of the imipenem-hydrolyzing β-lactamase operon from *Pseudomonas maltophilia* in *Escherichia coli*. *Antimicrob. Agents Chemother.* 32:819–826.

Hancock, R. E. W. 1987. Model membrane studies of porin function, p. 187–255. *In* M. Inouye (ed.), *Bacterial Outer Membranes as Model Systems.* John Wiley & Sons, Inc., New York.

Hancock, R. E. W., and A. M. Carey. 1980. Protein D1—a glucose-inducible, pore-forming protein from the outer membrane of *Pseudomonas aeruginosa. FEMS Microbiol. Lett.* **8:**105–109.

Jones, R. N., K. E. Aldridge, S. D. Allen, A. L. Barry, P. C. Fuchs, E. H. Gerlach, and M. A. Pfaller. 1989. Multicenter in vitro evaluation of SM-7338, a new carbapenem. *Antimicrob. Agents Chemother.* **33:**562–565.

Lynch, M. J., G. L. Drusano, and H. L. T. Mobley. 1987. Emergence of resistance to imipenem in *Pseudomonas aeruginosa. Antimicrob. Agents Chemother.* **31:**1892–1896.

Nikaido, H. 1989. Role of the outer membrane of gram-negative bacteria in antimicrobial resistance, p. 1–34. *In* L. E. Bryan (ed.), *Microbial Resistance to Drugs* Springer-Verlag KG, Berlin.

Nikaido, H., and R. E. W. Hancock. 1986. Outer membrane permeability of *Pseudomonas aeruginosa,* p. 145–193. *In* J. R. Sokatch and L. N. Ornston (ed.), *The Bacteria,* vol. 10. *The Biology of Pseudomonas.* Academic Press, Inc., Orlando, Fla.

Nikaido, H., and M. Vaara. 1987. Outer membrane, p. 7–22. *In* F. C. Neidhardt, J. L. Ingraham, B. Magasanik, K. B. Low, M. Schaechter, and H. E. Umbarger (ed.), *Escherichia coli and Salmonella typhimurium: Cellular and Molecular Biology.* American Society for Microbiology, Washington, D.C.

Quinn, J. P., A. E. Studemeister, C. A. DiVincenzo, and S. A. Lerner. 1988. Resistance to imipenem in *Pseudomonas aeruginosa:* clinical experience and biochemical mechanisms. *Rev. Infect. Dis.* **10:**892–898.

Stein, W. D. 1986. *Transport and Diffusion across Cell Membranes.* Academic Press, Inc., Orlando, Fla.

Trias, J., J. Dufresne, R. C. Levesque, and H. Nikaido. 1989. Decreased outer membrane permeability in imipenem-resistant mutants of *Pseudomonas aeruginosa. Antimicrob. Agents Chemother.* **33:**1201–1206.

Trias, J., and H. Nikaido. 1990. Outer membrane D2 catalyzes facilitated diffusion of carbapenems and penems through the outer membrane of *Pseudomonas aeruginosa. Antimicrob. Agents Chemother.* **34:**52–57.

Trias, J., E. Y. Rosenberg, and H. Nikaido. 1988. Specificity of the glucose channel formed by protein D1 of *Pseudomonas aeruginosa. Biochim. Biophys. Acta* **938:**493–496.

Williams, J. R. 1985. Activity of imipenem against *Pseudomonas aeruginosa. Rev. Infect. Dis.* **7:**S411–416.

Yoshihara, E., and T. Nakae. 1989. Identification of porins in the outer membrane of *Pseudomonas aeruginosa* that form small diffusion pores. *J. Biol. Chem* **264:**6297–6301.

Yoshimura, F., and H. Nikaido. 1982. Permeability of *Pseudomonas aeruginosa* outer membrane to hydrophylic solutes. *J. Bacteriol.* **152:**636–642.

Chapter 31

Function and Structure of the Porin Proteins OprF and OprP of *Pseudomonas aeruginosa*

R. J. Siehnel, N. L. Martin, and R. E. W. Hancock

In the outer membranes of gram-negative bacteria like *Pseudomonas aeruginosa*, the channels of porin proteins provide a molecular sieving function for the passage of hydrophilic solutes into the periplasm. Solutes larger than the exclusion limit of the porin channels are unable to cross the outer membrane barrier. There are several excellent reviews of broad scope concerning porins (see Benz [1988] and reviews cited therein). *P. aeruginosa* has four major and two minor outer membrane proteins that have been demonstrated to act as porins (Table 1). These proteins have general properties similar to those of porins from other gram-negative bacteria. The ultimate goal toward understanding the molecular mechanisms involved in the role of porins is a detailed knowledge of the molecular architecture of the porin proteins. In this chapter, we describe our current level of understanding of the functional and structural details of the best-studied porins of *P. aeruginosa*, protein F (OprF) and protein P (OprP) (Table 1).

FUNCTIONAL ASPECTS OF *P. AERUGINOSA* PORIN PROTEINS

Porins of gram-negative bacteria fall into two functional classes. General diffusion porins are chemically nonspecific, although they may be weakly selective, as is the case for the major porins of *Escherichia coli*. Specific porins differ in that they contain saturable binding sites for specific classes of solutes, such as LamB and Tsx of *E. coli* and OprP of *P. aeruginosa* (Benz, 1988). There are also outer membrane proteins, such as OmpA and Braun lipoprotein of *E. coli*, that have been ascribed only structural roles. We review here the current data on the role of OprF of *P. aeruginosa* as both a general diffusion porin and an integral structural protein and the role of OprP as an example of a specific porin in *P. aeruginosa*.

R. J. Siehnel, N. L. Martin, and R. E. W. Hancock • University of British Columbia, Vancouver, British Columbia, Canada V6T 1W5.

TABLE 1
Physical properties of *P. aeruginosa* porin proteins[a]

Porin	Mol wt	Native oligomeric structure	SDS-stable oligomers	Heat-modifiable monomers	Secondary-structure prediction (%)[b]				Conditions favoring production
					H	S	T	C	
OprF	35,250	Trimer	Part	Yes	9	62	20	10	Constitutive
OprP	45,300	Trimer	Yes	No	3	65	26	6	Low phosphate
D2	45,500	—[c]	No	Yes	—	—	—	—	—
D1	46,000	Trimer	No	Yes	—	—	—	—	Glucose as carbon source

[a] Proteins C and E from *P. aeruginosa* have not been described, as we are unsure of their identity. We have not located a major protein banding in the area of protein C on SDS-gels, and two-dimensional gels have shown multiple bands located in the area of protein E (B. L. Angus and R. E. W. Hancock, unpublished results).
[b] H, α helix; S, β sheet; T, β turn; C, random coil. Values were obtained by CD at room temperature in 10 mM Tris–0.1% SDS.
[c] —, Not done.

OprF

As mentioned above, the major outer membrane protein OprF of *P. aeruginosa* is a bifunctional protein, serving both as a porin (Hancock, 1986; Nikaido and Hancock, 1986) and as a protein required for maintaining the structural integrity of *P. aeruginosa* (Gotoh et al., 1989; Woodruff and Hancock, 1988, 1989; see below). OprF purified from *P. aeruginosa* (Benz and Hancock, 1981) or from a clone in *E. coli* (Woodruff et al., 1986) has been shown to form large pores (conductance greater than 4 nS) in addition to smaller pores (0.36 nS) in artificial bilayer experiments. Quantitation of the two sizes of channels revealed the larger pores to be far less prevalent (<1%) than the smaller pores (Woodruff et al., 1986). Recently, there has been some reevaluation of the exclusion limits of *P. aeruginosa* that were previously defined by growth on pentamethionine (Miller and Becker, 1978), susceptibility to large antibiotics (Table 2), liposome swelling assays (Yoshimura et al., 1983), radioactive efflux experiments (Hancock et al., 1979), and the above-mentioned lipid bilayer conductance experiments. These

TABLE 2
Susceptibility of *E. coli* and *P. aeruginosa* to selected antibiotics

Antibiotic	Mol wt	Charge(s)		MIC (µg/ml)		Reference
		+	−	*E. coli*	*P. aeruginosa*	
Piperacillin	516	0	1	2	2	Rolinson, 1986
Ceftazidime	545	1	2	0.12	2	Neu et al., 1988
Cefpiramide	610	0	1	1.1	2.9	Rolinson, 1986
E-1040	636	1	1	0.12	0.25	Neu et al., 1988
Cefsulodin	531	1	2	64	2	Fukasawa et al., 1983
Cefoperazone	644	0	1	0.9	11	Fukasawa et al., 1983
Apalcillin	508	0	1	4	2	Rolinson, 1986
Mureidomycin C	897	1	3	>200	3	Isono et al., 1989

studies are based on plasmolysis experiments (Caulcott et al., 1984; Yoneyama et al., 1986) and liposome swelling assays (Yoshihara et al., 1988; Gotoh et al., 1989) and on the high resistance of *P. aeruginosa* to certain antibiotics (Gotoh et al., 1989). The applicability of these results to the in vivo situation is somewhat controversial, since they predict an exclusion limit of *P. aeruginosa* outer membranes of a molecular weight of approximately 180 (Yoneyama et al., 1986) to 220 (Yoshihara et al., 1988), whereas *P. aeruginosa* is clearly susceptible to antibiotics of much larger molecular weights (Table 2). Conversely, the high resistance of *P. aeruginosa* to certain antibiotics could be accounted for by the small number of large pores (and consequent small area for diffusion of antibiotics) in synergy with a secondary resistance determinant such as periplasmic β-lactamases (see Hancock and Woodruff [1988] for a discussion). It must also be noted that the results of liposome swelling assays of Yoshihara, Nakae, and collaborators are at odds with those previous liposome swelling assays which predict, in agreement with our own data, a larger exclusion limit (Fig. 1). Although we still favor the conclusion that *P. aeruginosa* has a large exclusion limit, there is some doubt as to whether OprF constitutes the large pore (Woodruff and Hancock, 1989). The exact nature of the dual pore size observed with OprF is currently being addressed by genetic manipulations of the four cysteines in OprF that have been hypothesized to be relevant to this phenomenon (Moore et al., 1987) and by investigations of antibiotic-resistant OprF-deficient (Piddock et al., 1987) or OprF-altered (Godfrey and Bryan, 1987) mutants.

OprF has been shown to have homology with OmpA of *E. coli* (see below), and the two proteins show many similarities (Table 3). *P. aeruginosa oprF* mutant strains show many defects similar to those of *E. coli ompA lpp* double mutants, including leakage of periplasmic contents, a rounded morphology, and a need for osmotic stabilization (Woodruff and Hancock, 1989; Gotoh et al., 1989; Sonntag et al., 1978). Furthermore, OprF expressed from the cloned gene could restore elongated morphology to an *E. coli ompA lpp* double mutant (Woodruff and Hancock, 1989), suggesting that the two proteins have interchangeable roles in cell shape determination. Since mutations preventing expression from the *oprF* gene of *P. aeruginosa* are pleiotropic, it is difficult to evaluate the effect of the loss of the porin function even though such mutants arise from a single gene mutation. In the case of constructed insertion mutations in the *oprF* gene, the most overwhelming effects observed were on structural properties and on nonspecific permeability, which could conceivably mask the effect of porin loss (Woodruff and Hancock, 1988, 1989). Nevertheless, such mutants showed a 1.3- to 3.4-fold increase in resistance to a variety of β-lactam antibiotics (Woodruff and Hancock, 1988), thus favoring a role for OprF as porin (although these susceptibility changes are marginal). In contrast, two other groups have published data on OprF-deficient (Piddock et al., 1987) and OprF-altered (Godfrey and Bryan, 1987) mutants with large increases in antibiotic resistance compared with the wild type. However, these mutants require further genetic characterization.

We feel that future studies should rely on point mutations or small insertions or deletions that might disrupt the pore-forming domain without severely affecting the structural domain of OprF. These mutations and their resultant phenotypes

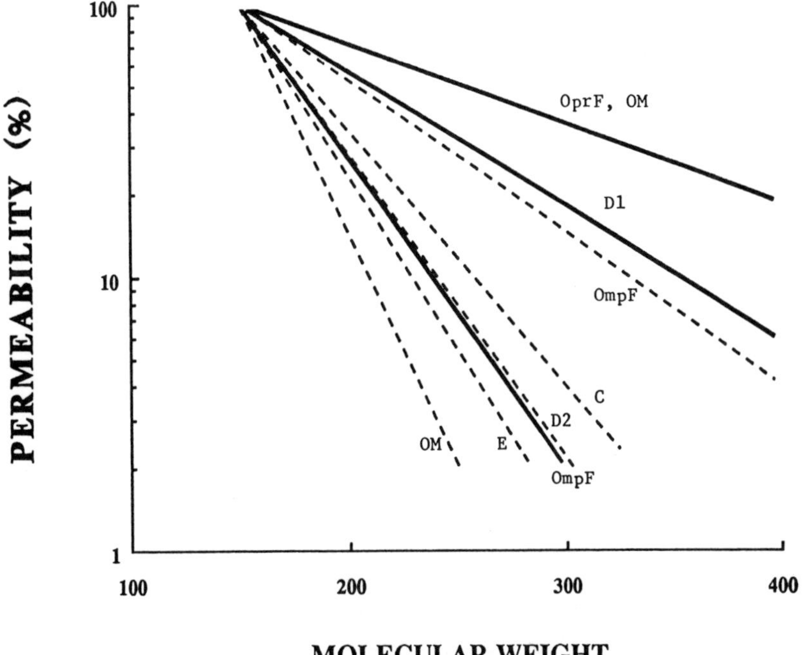

FIGURE 1. Influence of substrate molecular weight on the swelling of liposomes reconstituted with various *P. aeruginosa* porins or outer membrane (OM) preparations or with *E. coli* OmpF porin. For clarity, individual datum points have been omitted and the lines have been adjusted to give 100% swelling with arabinose (molecular weight, 150). The solid lines are data from Nikaido and collaborators as follows: OprF (=F), outer membrane, and D1 (Yoshimura et al., 1983; Trias et al., 1988); and OmpF from *E. coli* (Nikaido and Rosenberg, 1983; Yoshimura et al., 1983). The dashed lines are data from Nakae and collaborators as follows: outer membrane (Yoshihara et al., 1988); C, D2 (=D), and E (Yoshihara and Nakae, 1989); and OmpF from *E. coli* (Yoshihara and Nakae, 1989; a steeper slope was observed by Yoshihara et al. [1988]). Yoshihara and Nakae (1989) observed only weak porin activity for the OprF porin in this assay. Note that major discrepancies were observed in the slopes of the lines observed for both *P. aeruginosa* outer membrane and *E. coli* OmpF. The data for OmpF (solid line), when fit to the Renkin equation, predicted a pore diameter of 1.16 nm, and the data for OprF predicted a 2-nm pore, consistent with other data (Hancock, 1986).

should then be genetically transferred to another strain and their association with antibiotic resistance confirmed. Alternatively, if OmpA from *E. coli* could complement structural defects in *P. aeruginosa oprF* mutants, the effects on antibiotic resistance of the loss of the OprF porin might be more accurately assayed. We consider such manipulations to be absolutely necessary to unequivocally resolve the role of OprF as the major *P. aeruginosa* porin.

OprP

OprP is the porin component of a high-affinity phosphate uptake system that is induced when *P. aeruginosa* is grown in an environment deficient in phosphate

TABLE 3

Comparison of the *E. coli* OmpA protein with the *P. aeruginosa* OprF protein

Protein	Required for growth in low-osmolarity medium	Required for rod-shaped morphology	Immuno-logical cross-reactivity	Sequence related-ness (C terminus)	Mol wt	β structure (β sheet + β turn) (%)	Change in apparent mol wt		Peptido-glycan association	Lipopoly-saccharide association	Products of chemical cross-linking	Role in conjugation	Porin function	No. of cysteines
							Upon heating	Upon trypsin treatment						
OmpA	+[a]	+[a]	+	+	35,159	77	6,000	8,000	+	+	Dimers, trimers	F plasmids	?	2
OprF	+	+	+	+	35,250	82	6,000	8,000	+	+	Dimers, trimers	P1 plasmids	+	4

[a] *lpp* mutant background.

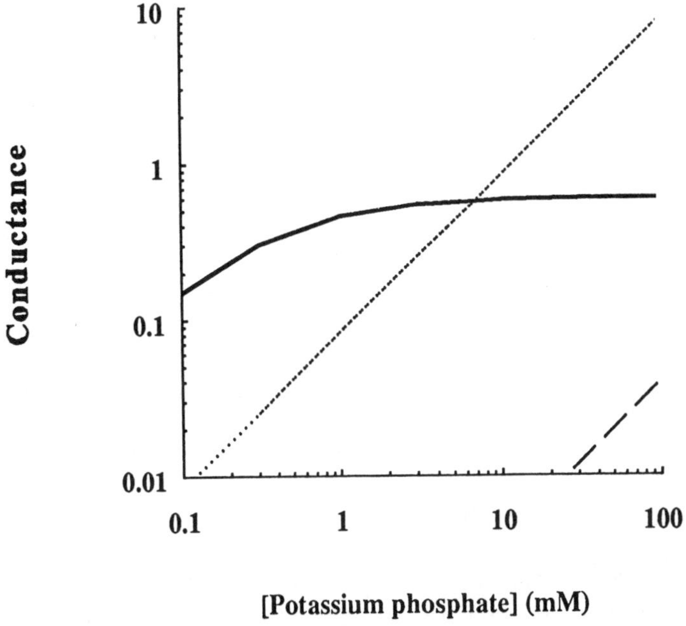

[Potassium phosphate] (mM)

FIGURE 2. Benefit of a specific phosphate channel in the *P. aeruginosa* outer membrane. The total conductances (i.e., transmembrane flux in microsiemens) at various concentrations of potassium phosphate for 10^5 OprP channels (———), 2×10^5 small OprF channels (. . .), and 200 large OprF channels (- - -) were estimated on the basis of published single-channel conductance experiments (Benz and Hancock, 1981; Woodruff et al., 1986; Hancock and Benz, 1986). These numbers of channels represent crude estimates of the numbers of each porin species in a given cell 1 h after induction of OprP by shifting *P. aeruginosa* to phosphate-deficient medium. Note that because OprP contains a phosphate-binding site (K_d of 0.3 mM), it exhibits saturable flux, since association-dissociation at the binding site is rate limiting. At a physiologically relevant phosphate concentration (0.15 mM), at least 20 times more phosphate will pass through OprP than through both OprF channels.

(Hancock et al., 1982). This inducible system also involves a periplasmic phosphate-binding protein (Poole and Hancock, 1983, 1984) and is apparently similar to the high-affinity Pst system induced under similar conditions in *E. coli* (Willsky and Malamy, 1980). The analogous porin in *E. coli* is the PhoE protein. The regulatory mechanism that controls the expression of these regulons appears to have been well conserved. A well-characterized *cis*-acting regulatory sequence of the *pho* regulon (the *pho* box) has been identified preceding the *oprP* gene from *P. aeruginosa* and shown to function in *E. coli* (Siehnel et al., 1988b). In addition, a *phoB*-like gene and a *phoR*-like gene isolated from *P. aeruginosa* have been shown to complement, respectively, the *phoB* and *phoR* regulatory genes of *E. coli* (Filloux et al., 1988). Although this system appears to be conserved, the porins induced show marked differences. PhoE is a general diffusion porin that forms large (1.1 nm), weakly anion selective channels (Benz et al., 1984). In contrast, OprP forms constricted (0.6 nm), anion-specific channels with a saturable phosphate-binding site (Hancock and Benz, 1986; Fig. 2). OprP has been shown to have a K_d of 0.3 mM for phosphate binding at pH 7 (compared with a K_d

of 40 mM for chloride binding [Hancock and Benz, 1986]). It appears to work in conjunction with a periplasmic phosphate-binding protein (K_d of 3.4×10^{-7} M for phosphate) in vivo (Poole and Hancock, 1984; Hancock et al., 1987). Although OprP binds a variety of anions, its affinity for phosphate is at least 60 to 100 times greater than for other anions (Hancock and Benz, 1986), demonstrating its substrate-specific characteristic. Thus, although OprP has a smaller channel than PhoE and the larger OprF channel, it is a much more efficient channel for the transport of phosphate than these general porins at low, physiologically relevant, external phosphate concentrations (e.g., 0.15 mM phosphate; Fig. 2). The low numbers of the large OprF pores per cell and the small channel size of the other OprF pores preclude OprF as an important uptake system for sequestering phosphate under these conditions (Fig. 2). However, OprP is induced at higher phosphate levels in strains lacking OprF (W. A. Woodruff and R. E. W. Hancock, Ph.D. thesis, University of British Columbia, Vancouver, British Columbia, Canada, 1988), indicating that OprF influences the amount of phosphate available to interact with the primary signal controlling the *pho* regulon within the cell and may constitute a secondary phosphate uptake system across the outer membrane.

As suggested above, the saturable nature of OprP makes it amenable to kinetic studies. Since OprP can be expressed in a functional conformation in *E. coli* (Siehnel et al., 1988a), we are now using site-directed mutagenesis to investigate regulatory, functional, and structural aspects of this specific porin (i.e., the identification of the amino acids involved in phosphate binding).

STRUCTURAL ASPECTS OF *P. AERUGINOSA* PORIN PROTEINS

Porin proteins were first isolated from *E. coli*, and the OmpF (matrix protein) was the first porin from which crystals that diffracted to high resolution were grown (Garavito and Rosenbusch, 1980; Garavito et al., 1983). Although many attempts have since been made to elucidate the three-dimensional structure of OmpF and several other bacterial porins by X-ray diffraction and by electron and optical diffraction of specimens prepared for electron microscopy, the actual molecular structure of a porin is yet to be determined. Given that a definitive model of porin structure is not possible until the crystallographic data have been resolved, this section summarizes the structural data available on porins F and P from *P. aeruginosa*, compares these data with information available on other bacterial porins, and presents structural models for these proteins.

OprF

The most prominent constitutively expressed protein in the *P. aeruginosa* outer membrane is OprF. This protein is heat and 2-mercaptoethanol modifiable. Unheated OprF bands at an apparent molecular weight of 36,000, and exhaustively heated (100°C for 60 min) OprF bands at 41,000 in the presence of 2-mercaptoethanol. Without 2-mercaptoethanol, unheated OprF bands at 33,000 and heated OprF bands at 39,000 (Hancock and Carey, 1979). The stability of the protein to boiling in sodium dodecyl sulfate (SDS) might be attributed to the strong association of β strands, since the protein has a high β content, as assessed by circular dichroism (Table 1). The ability of 2-mercaptoethanol to modify the gel mobility of OprF has been ascribed to the possession of two intrachain disulfide bonds (Hancock and Carey, 1979; see below). Small amounts of oligomeric forms of OprF have been observed on Western blots (immunoblots) reacted with monoclonal antibodies specific for OprF (Mutharia and Hancock, 1985). Chemical cross-linking has confirmed that native OprF forms an oligomeric (possibly a trimeric) structure (Angus and Hancock, 1983). Although lipopolysaccharide is normally associated with OprF and can be chemically cross-linked to OprF (Angus and Hancock, 1983), the presence or absence of lipopolysaccharide in protein samples run on SDS-gels does not seem to affect the electrophoretic mobility of OprF (Hancock and Carey, 1979).

Beher et al. (1980) previously described heat-modifiable outer membrane proteins in a large number of enteric and nonenteric bacteria, including *P. aeruginosa* OprF, which were similar to OmpA. The nucleic acid sequence of the *oprF* gene was determined by Duchêne et al. (1988), and they found a short stretch of the deduced amino acid sequence of OprF to be homologous with a 30-amino-acid stretch of OmpA from *E. coli* and from *Enterobacter aerogenes*. Further analysis has shown that the carboxy-terminal half of OprF (from residues 146 to 326) exhibits distinct similarity to the entire carboxy-terminal half (residues 177 to 335) of OmpA from *E. coli* and also to the majority of the amino acid sequence of protein III from *Neisseria gonorrhoeae* (Gotschlich et al., 1987a; Gotschlich et al., 1987b; Woodruff and Hancock, 1989). A number of the OmpA like proteins have been sequenced, and a comparison of their amino acid sequences shows that many of these proteins are much more alike within the carboxy-terminal region than in the amino-terminal region (Klugman et al., 1989; Gotschlich et al., 1987a; Gotschlich et al., 1987b). This relatively constant maintenance of amino acid composition suggests that the carboxy-terminal portion provides an essential functional region of OmpA.

Although there is very little direct amino acid homology in the amino-terminal halves of OmpA and OprF, a comparison of their antigenic indices, which are compiled by summing several weighted measures of secondary structure (hydrophobicity, surface probability, flexibility, and the Chou-Fasman and Garnier-Osguthorpe-Robson predictive methods [Garnier et al., 1978]), shows that the tertiary structures of these proteins are probably quite similar in this region (N. L. Martin and R. E. W. Hancock, in press). Figure 3 consequently predicts OprF, by analogy to OmpA (Klose et al., 1988), to have eight membrane-spanning sequences from residues 1 to 145.

The current predictive model of OmpA from *E. coli* places amino acids 177 to 335 in the periplasm of the cell (Vogel and Jähnig, 1986; Klose et al., 1988), based primarily on the accessibility of a protease cleavage site that releases this carboxy-terminal portion of the protein and on the complete lack of cell surface-exposed areas found in the carboxy-terminal half during extensive mapping studies with spontaneous and genetically engineered mutants resistant to OmpA-specific bacteriophages (Manoil and Rosenbusch, 1982; Morona et al., 1984;

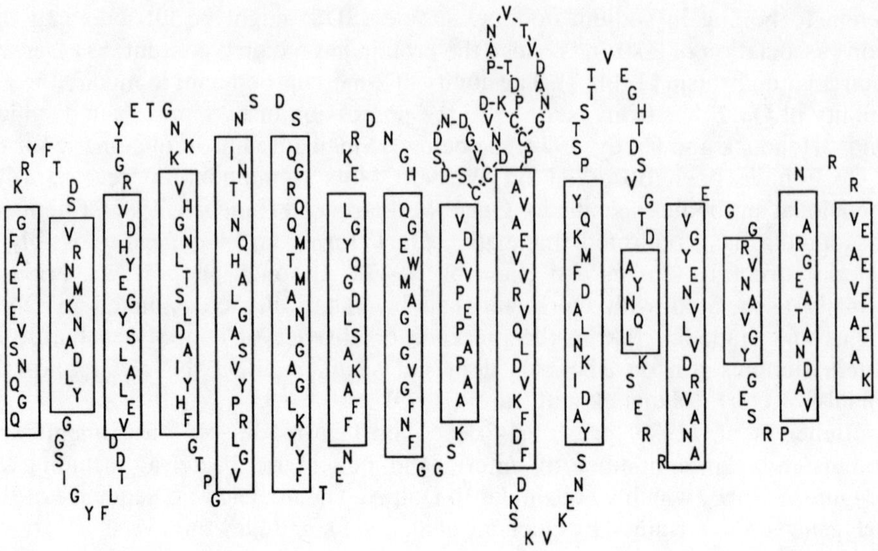

FIGURE 3. Conceptual model of the structure of OprF. Regions predicted (by the method of Paul and Rosenbusch [1985]) to have β structure are boxed and are assumed to sit within the membrane. Positions of the β strands are drawn on the basis of the model of OmpA except that the carboxy-terminal region of OprF is placed in the membrane for reasons discussed in the text, whereas the homologous (Woodruff and Hancock, 1989) region of OmpA has been previously assigned to the periplasm (Morona et al., 1984; Klose et al., 1988).

Klose et al., 1988). In contrast, the carboxy-terminal portion of OprF appears to be surface exposed. Molecular genetic manipulation of the gene for OprF has permitted localization of the surface-exposed epitope of monoclonal antibody MA5-8 to the carboxy-terminal half of the molecule (W. A. Woodruff and R. E. W. Hancock, unpublished data).

Interestingly, in the amino acid comparisons of the second halves of OmpA, protein III, and OprF, the regions that do not match at all are limited to the areas containing cysteine residues in each of these proteins (Woodruff and Hancock, 1989). The four cysteines in OprF are thought to form two disulfide bonds (Hancock and Carey, 1979). In our working model, these disulfides have been placed on the outside surface of the cell, since they may be involved in maintaining the surface-exposed, conformational epitope recognized by monoclonal antibody MA4-4, which is recognized by the antibody only in the unreduced form of OprF (Mutharia and Hancock, 1985).

On a more general level, the large amount of β-sheet structure in outer membrane proteins sets them apart from most other proteins that have been studied in detail. As a result of this predominance of β-sheet content, most existing predictive methods of protein secondary structure greatly underestimate the actual β-sheet content, since these methods were developed for soluble proteins (Garnier et al., 1978) or for membrane proteins with membrane-spanning α helices (Kyte and Doolittle, 1982). Also, these predictive methods do not take

TABLE 4

Comparison of the predicted secondary structure of OprF, using CD and the prediction method
of Garnier et al. (1978)

Structure	Value (% of total)				
	CD, 1–326[a]		Prediction method		
	RT[b]	100 C[c]	1–326	1–161	161–326
α Helix	9	22	30	24	36
β Sheet	62	39	25	25	24
β Turn	20	15	22	23	21
Random coil	10	22	24	29	19

[a] Amino acid residue number.
[b] Room temperature in 10 mM Tris–0.1% SDS.
[c] 100°C for 15 min in 10 mM Tris–0.1% SDS.

into account tertiary and quaternary interactions within the native protein and
between protein oligomers. Table 4 outlines secondary-structure predictions for
OprF, obtained by using circular dichroism (CD) (C. M. Kay, W. D. McCubbin,
E. A. Worobec, N. L. Martin, and R. E. W. Hancock, unpublished data) and the
predictive method of Garnier et al. (1978). The CD values obtained after boiling
the protein in 0.1% SDS most closely resemble the structure predictions from the
amino acid sequence, whereas the CD values for native protein indicate a much
higher β-sheet content and very little α helix. However, it should be noted that the
mild boiling in SDS performed in the CD experiments shown in Table 4 was not
sufficient to cause OprF to alter its migration on SDS-polyacrylamide gels (to its
heat-modified position). Thus, it must retain considerable secondary structure, as
also indicated by CD. We assume that boiling in 0.1% SDS probably destroys
tertiary associations within the protein, rendering it most like a soluble protein
and therefore corresponding more closely to predictions based on the amino acid
sequence alone. The high content of β-sheet structure in native OprF is compatible with much of the protein being inserted in the membrane (Fig. 3).

OprP

The trimeric nature of a functional OprP porin implies that specific molecular
interactions within the monomer and between the monomeric units form the
phosphate-selective pores. To this end, OprP is a very stable protein. Although
trimers are readily dissociated into monomers at 88°C in 2% SDS, dissociations
within the monomer are difficult to induce. CD spectra have indicated a β-sheet
content of 65%, which only drops to 55% after boiling in 0.1% SDS, along with
changes from 3 to 8% for α helix, 26 to 25% for β turn, and 6 to 12% for random
coil (Worobec et al., 1988). OprP trimers, even when they are lipopolysaccharide
free, are also resistant to digestion with several proteases and maintain their
normal SDS-polyacrylamide gel mobility and porin function when attacked by
other proteases. In the latter case, one can observe alterations in gel mobility only
when trimers are dissociated into monomers before electrophoresis (Worobec et
al., 1988).

TABLE 5

Degree of alignment of paired amino acid sequences of bacterial porins

Porins compared	Matches	Conservative substitutions[a]	Gaps introduced
PhoE[b] versus OmpF[b]	230	49	9
PhoE versus OprP[c]	67	59	12
OprP versus P2[d]	52	63	8
OprP versus LamB[b]	76	77	18
P2 versus OmpF	95	94	35

[a] Alignment of sequences was optimized by using the FAST-P algorithm, and conservative substitutions between sequences were assessed by the Dayhoff minimum-mutation matrix (Doolittle, 1986), using a matching score of 0.9 as a cutoff.
[b] From *E. coli*.
[c] From *P. aeruginosa*.
[d] From *H. influenzae*.

Although OprP shows little amino acid sequence homology with OprF (R. J. Siehnel, N. L. Martin, and R. E. W. Hancock, manuscript in preparation), it does exhibit some similarity with porin protein P2 from *Haemophilus influenzae* type B (Vachon et al., 1987) and several regions of homology with LamB and PhoE from *E. coli* (Table 5) which often correspond to cell surface-exposed areas mapped by phage binding and monoclonal antibodies in LamB (Saurin et al., 1989). These regions of homology suggest that these proteins may have evolved from a common ancestral porin protein.

Since OprP contains a phosphate-binding site and is directly involved in the uptake of phosphate, the three-dimensional structure of this protein is expected to be somewhat different from those of the general diffusion porins such as OprF and OmpF. Chemical modification studies aimed at examining the role in ion conductance of charged ε-amino groups of lysine residues are in agreement with this proposal (Hancock and Benz, 1986; Hancock et al., 1986).

Attempts thus far to further define the three-dimensional structure by crystallography have produced crystals too small to allow X-ray analysis (Worobec et al., 1988). It is hoped that combining ongoing studies involving analyses by electron microscopy and optical diffraction with continued efforts at crystallography and analysis by genetic manipulation will provide more information on the molecular structure of OprP in the near future.

SUMMARY

The porin proteins embedded in the outer membrane of *P. aeruginosa* are involved in both nonspecific (e.g., OprF) and specific (e.g., OprP) uptake of molecules across the outer membrane. In artificial membrane systems, OprF preparations demonstrate two distinct pore sizes. Several lines of evidence suggest that OprF is the major porin of *P. aeruginosa*, although this is currently disputed in the literature. In addition to having a permeability function, OprF plays a structural role in maintaining cell shape and in permitting growth in low-osmolarity medium. Indeed, it is both structurally and functionally analogous to the OmpA protein from *E. coli*. OprP, a phosphate-selective porin, is produced only when external phosphate concentrations necessitate a more efficient uptake system for phosphate (in which OprP plays a role). Thus, OprP is part of an adaptation by the cell to allow it to survive under new environmental conditions. Consequently, it can be considered broadly analogous to the *E. coli* LamB maltoporin, with which it demonstrates some sequence relatedness (Table 5). Although the function of porin proteins has been studied for a number of years, it is only recently that the details of the physical structure of these proteins are beginning to be understood. Various techniques have been used quite ingeniously to extract small bits of data, which have then been assembled into models for further, more rigorous testing. By adapting models for the *E. coli* OmpA and LamB proteins, we have now created secondary-structure models of OprF (Fig. 3) and OprP (Siehnel et al., in preparation), respectively. Ultimately, however, crystallographic analysis is the only technique that will provide details on the structure of porins sufficient for a complete understanding of their function. Until the puzzle of porin structure is solved at a molecular resolution, porins will remain only functionally defined as proteins containing water-filled channels that allow compounds into and out of the bacterial cell.

ACKNOWLEDGMENTS. This research was generously supported by the Natural Sciences and Engineering Research Council of Canada and the Canadian Cystic Fibrosis Foundation.

LITERATURE CITED

Angus, B. L., and R. E. W. Hancock. 1983. Outer membrane porin proteins F, P, and D1 of *Pseudomonas aeruginosa* and PhoE of *Escherichia coli*: chemical cross-linking to reveal native oligomers. *J. Bacteriol.* **155**:1042–1051.

Beher, M., C. A. Schnaitman, and A. P. Pugsley. 1980. Major heat-modifiable outer membrane protein in gram-negative bacteria: comparison with the OmpA protein of *Escherichia coli*. *J. Bacteriol.* **143**:906–913.

Benz, R. 1988. Structure and function of porins from gram-negative bacteria. *Annu. Rev. Microbiol.* **42**:359–393.

Benz, R., R. P. Darveau, and R. E. W. Hancock. 1984. Outer membrane protein PhoE from *Escherichia coli* forms anion-selective pores in lipid bilayer membranes. *Eur. J. Biochem.* **140**:319–324.

Benz, R., and R. E. W. Hancock. 1981. Properties of the large ion permeable pores formed from protein F of *Pseudomonas aeruginosa* in lipid bilayer membranes. *Biochim. Biophys. Acta* **646**:298–308.

Caulcott, C. A., M. R. W. Brown, and I. Gonda. 1984. Evidence for small pores in the outer membrane of *Pseudomonas aeruginosa*. *FEMS Microbiol. Lett.* **21**:119–123.

Doolittle, R. F. 1986. *Of URFS and ORFS: a Primer on How To Analyze Derived Amino Acid Sequences*. University Science Books, Mill Valley, Calif.

Duchêne, M., A. Schweizer, F. Lottspeich, G. Krauss, M. Marget, K. Vogel, B.-U. von Specht, and H. Domdey. 1988. Sequence and transcriptional start site of the *Pseudomonas aeruginosa* outer membrane porin protein F gene. *J. Bacteriol.* **170**:155–162.

Filloux, A., M. Bally, C. Soscia, M. Murgier, and A. Lazdunski. 1988. Phosphate regulation in *Pseudomonas aeruginosa*: cloning of the alkaline phosphatase gene and identification of *phoB*- and *phoR*-like genes. *Mol. Gen. Genet.* **212**:510–513.

Fukasawa, M., H. Noguchi, T. Okuda, T. Komatsu, and K. Yano. 1983. In vitro antibacterial activity of SM-1652, a new broad-spectrum cephalosporin with antipseudomonal activity. *Antimicrob. Agents Chemother.* **23**:195–200.

Garavito, R. M., J. Jenkins, J. N. Jansonius, R. Karlsson, and J. P. Rosenbusch. 1983. X-ray diffraction of matrix porin, an integral membrane protein from *E. coli* outer membranes. *J. Mol. Biol.* **164:**313–327.

Garavito, R. M., and J. P. Rosenbusch. 1980. Three-dimensional crystals of an integral membrane protein: an initial X-ray analysis. *J. Cell Biol.* **86:**327–329.

Garnier, J., D. J. Osguthorpe, and B. Robson. 1978. Analysis of the accuracy and implications of simple methods for predicting the secondary structure of globular proteins. *J. Mol. Biol.* **120:**97–120.

Godfrey, A. J., and L. E. Bryan. 1987. Penetration of β-lactams through *Pseudomonas aeruginosa* porin channels. *Antimicrob. Agents Chemother.* **31:**1216–1221.

Gotoh, N., H. Wakebe, E. Yoshihara, T. Nakae, and T. Nishino. 1989. Role of protein F in maintaining structural integrity of the *Pseudomonas aeruginosa* outer membrane. *J. Bacteriol.* **171:**983–990.

Gotschlich, E. C., M. Seiff, and M. S. Blake. 1987a. The DNA sequence of the structural gene of gonococcal protein III and the flanking region containing a repetitive sequence. Homology of protein III with enterobacteria OmpA proteins. *J. Exp. Med.* **165:**471–482.

Gotschlich, E. C., M. E. Sieff, M. S. Blake, and M. Koomey. 1987b. Porin protein of *Neisseria gonorrhoeae*: cloning and gene structure. *Proc. Natl. Acad. Sci. USA* **84:**8135–8139.

Hancock, R. E. W. 1986. Model membrane studies of porin function, p. 187–225. *In* M. Inouye (ed.), *Bacterial Outer Membranes as Model Systems*. John Wiley & Sons, Inc., New York.

Hancock, R. E. W., and R. Benz. 1986. Demonstration and chemical modification of a specific phosphate binding site in the phosphate-starvation inducible outer membrane porin protein P of *Pseudomonas aeruginosa*. *Biochim. Biophys. Acta* **860:**699–707.

Hancock, R. E. W., and A. Carey. 1979. Outer membrane of *Pseudomonas aeruginosa*: heat- and 2-mercaptoethanol-modifiable proteins. *J. Bacteriol.* **140:**902–910.

Hancock, R. E. W., G. M. Decad, and H. Nikaido. 1979. Identification of the protein producing transmembrane diffusion pores in the outer membrane of *Pseudomonas aeruginosa* PAO1. *Biochim. Biophys. Acta* **554:**323–329.

Hancock, R. E. W., K. Poole, and R. Benz. 1982. Outer membrane protein P of *Pseudomonas aeruginosa*: regulation by phosphate deficiency and formation of small anion-specific channels in lipid bilayer membranes. *J. Bacteriol.* **150:**730–738.

Hancock, R. E. W., A. Schmidt, K. Bauer, and R. Benz. 1986. Role of lysines in ion selectivity of bacterial outer membrane porins. *Biochim. Biophys. Acta* **860:**263–267.

Hancock, R. E. W., and W. A. Woodruff. 1988. Roles of porin and β-lactamase in intrinsic antibiotic resistance of *Pseudomonas aeruginosa*. *Rev. Infect. Dis.* **10:**770–755.

Hancock, R. E. W., E. A. Worobec, K. Poole, and R. Benz. 1987. The phosphate binding site of *Pseudomonas aeruginosa* protein P, p. 176–180. *In* A. Torriani-Gorini, S. Silver, F. Rathman, A. Wright, and E. Yagel (ed.), *Phosphate Metabolism and Cellular Regulation in Microorganisms*. American Society for Microbiology, Washington, D.C.

Isono, F., I. Masatoshi, S. Takahashi, and T. Haneish. 1989. Mureidomycins A~D. Novel peptidyl-nucleoside antibiotics with spheroplast forming activity. *J. Antibiot.* **43:**667–679.

Klose, M., H. Schwarz, S. MacIntyre, R. Freudl, M.-L. Eschbach, and U. Henning. 1988. Internal deletions in the gene for an *Escherichia coli* outer membrane protein define an area possibly important for recognition of the outer membrane by this polypeptide. *J. Biol. Chem.* **263:**13291–13296.

Klugman, K. P., E. C. Gotschlich, and M. S. Blake. 1989. Sequence of the structural gene (*rmpM*) for the class 4 outer membrane protein of *Neisseria meningitidis*, homology of the protein to gonococcal protein III and *Escherichia coli* OmpA, and construction of meningococcal strains that lack class 4 protein. *Infect. Immun.* **57:**2066–2071.

Kyte, J., and R. F. Doolittle. 1982. A simple method for displaying the hydropathic character of a protein. *J. Mol. Biol.* **157:**105–132.

Manoil, C., and J. P. Rosenbusch. 1982. Conjugation-deficient mutants of *Escherichia coli* distinguish classes of functions of the outer membrane OmpA protein. *Mol. Gen. Genet.* **187:**148–156.

Miller, R. V., and J. M. Becker. 1978. Peptide utilization in *Pseudomonas aeruginosa*: evidence for a membrane-associated peptidase. *J. Bacteriol.* **133:**165–171.

Moore, R. A., W. A. Woodruff, and R. E. W. Hancock. 1987. Antibiotic uptake pathways across the outer membrane of *Pseudomonas aeruginosa*. *Antibiot. Chemother.* **39:**172–181.

Morona, R., M. Klose, and U. Henning. 1984. *Escherichia coli* K-12 outer membrane protein (OmpA) as a bacteriophage receptor: analysis of mutant genes expressing altered proteins. *J. Bacteriol.* **159:**570–578.

Mutharia, L. M., and R. E. W. Hancock. 1985. Characterization of two surface-localized antigenic sites on porin protein F of *Pseudomonas aeruginosa*. *Can. J. Microbiol.* **31:**381–386.

Neu, H. C., N. Chin, and A. Novelli. 1988. In vitro activity of E-1040, a novel cephalosporin with potent activity against *Pseudomonas aeruginosa*. *Antimicrob. Agents Chemother.* **32:**1666–1675.

Nikaido, H., and R. E. W. Hancock. 1986. Outer membrane permeability of *Pseudomonas aeruginosa*, p. 145–193. *In* J. R. Sokatch and L. N. Ornston (ed.), *The Bacteria*, vol. 10. *The Biology of Pseudomonas*. Academic Press, Inc., Orlando, Fla.

Nikaido, H., and E. Y. Rosenberg. 1983. Porin channels in *Escherichia coli*: studies with liposomes reconstituted from purified proteins. *J. Bacteriol.* **153:**241–252.

Paul, C., and J. P. Rosenbusch. 1985. Folding patterns of porin and bacteriorhodopsin. *EMBO J.* **4:**1593–1597.

Piddock, L. J. V., W. J. A. Winjnards, and R. Wise. 1987. Quinoline/ureidopenicillin cross-resistance. *Lancet* **ii:**907.

Poole, K., and R. E. W. Hancock. 1983. Secretion of alkaline phosphatase and phospholipase C in *Pseudomonas aeruginosa* is specific and does not involve an increase in outer membrane permeability. *FEMS Microbiol. Lett.* **16:**25–29.

Poole, K., and R. E. W. Hancock. 1984. Phosphate transport in *Pseudomonas aeruginosa*. *Eur. J. Biochem.* **144:**607–612.

Rolinson, G. N. 1986. β-Lactam antibiotics. *J. Antimicrob. Chemother.* **17:**5–36.

Saurin, W., E. Francoz, P. Martineau, A. Charbit, E. Dassa, P. Duplay, E. Gilson, A. Molla, G. Ronco, S. Szmelcman, and N. Hofnung. 1989. Periplasmic binding protein dependent transport system for maltose and maltodextrins: some recent studies. *FEMS Microbiol. Rev.* **63:**53–60.

Siehnel, R., E. Worobec, and R. E. W. Hancock. 1988a. Cloning and characterization of the structural gene for the *Pseudomonas aeruginosa* outer membrane phosphate porin protein P. *J. Bacteriol.* **170:**2312–2318.

Siehnel, R., E. Worobec, and R. E. W. Hancock. 1988b. Regulation of components of the *Pseudomonas aeruginosa* phosphate-starvation-inducible regulon in *Escherichia coli*. *Mol. Microbiol.* **2:**347–352.

Sonntag, I., H. Schwarz, Y. Hirota, and U. Henning. 1978. Cell envelope and shape of *Escherichia coli*: multiple mutants missing the outer membrane lipoprotein and other major outer membrane proteins. *J. Bacteriol.* **136:**280–285.

Trias, J., E. Y. Rosenberg, and H. Nikaido. 1988. Specificity of the glucose channel formed by protein D1 of *Pseudomonas aeruginosa*. *Biochim. Biophys. Acta* **938:**493–496.

Vachon, V., D. N. Kristjanson, and J. W. Coulton. 1987. Outer membrane porin protein of *Haemophilus influenzae* type b: pore size and subunit structure. *Can. J. Microbiol.* **34:**134–140.

Vogel, H., and F. Jähnig. 1986. Models for the structure of outer membrane proteins of *Escherichia coli* derived from Raman spectroscopy and prediction methods. *J. Mol. Biol.* **190:**191–199.

Willsky, G. R., and M. H. Malamy. 1980. Characterization of two genetically separable inorganic phosphate transport systems in *Escherichia coli*. *J. Bacteriol.* **144:**356–365.

Woodruff, W. A., and R. E. W. Hancock. 1988. Construction and characterization of *Pseudomonas aeruginosa* porin protein F-deficient mutants after in vivo and in vitro insertion mutagenesis of the cloned gene. *J. Bacteriol.* **170:**2592–2598.

Woodruff, W., and R. E. W. Hancock. 1989. *Pseudomonas aeruginosa* outer membrane protein F: structural role and relationship to the *Escherichia coli* OmpA protein. *J. Bacteriol.* **171:**3304–3309.

Woodruff, W. A., T. R. Parr, R. E. W. Hancock, L. Hanne, T. I. Nicas, and B. Iglewski. 1986. Expression in *Escherichia coli* and function of porin protein F of *Pseudomonas aeruginosa*. *J. Bacteriol.* **167:**473–479.

Worobec, E. A., N. L. Martin, W. D. McCubbin, C. M. Kay, G. D. Bayer, and R. E. W. Hancock. 1988. Large scale purification and biochemical characterization of crystallization-grade porin protein P from *Pseudomonas aeruginosa*. *Biochim. Biophys. Acta* **939:**366–374.

Yoneyama, H., A. Akatsuka, and T. Nakae. 1986. The outer membrane of *Pseudomonas aeruginosa* is a barrier against the penetration of disaccharides. *Biochem. Biophys. Res. Commun.* **134:**106–112.

Yoshihara, E., N. Gotoh, and T. Nakae. 1988. *In vitro* demonstration by the rate assay of the presence of small pore in the outer membrane of *Pseudomonas aeruginosa*. *Biochem. Biophys. Res. Commun.* **156**:470–476.

Yoshihara, E., and T. Nakae. 1989. Identification of porins in the outer membrane of *Pseudomonas aeruginosa* that form small diffusion pores. *J. Biol. Chem.* **264**:6297–6301.

Yoshimura, F., L. S. Zalman, and H. Nikaido. 1983. Purification and properties of *Pseudomonas aeruginosa* porin. *J. Biol. Chem.* **258**:2308–2314.

Chapter 32

Expression, Processing, and Assembly of *Pseudomonas aeruginosa* *N*-Methylphenylalanine Pilin

William Paranchych, Brittan L. Pasloske, and Parimi A. Sastry

Pseudomonas aeruginosa is an opportunistic pathogen that causes local infections in burned tissue or injured corneas and systemic infections in cancer patients or burn victims (Bodey et al., 1983). It is also the major pathogen of nosocomial pneumonias and chronic lung infections in patients with cystic fibrosis (Kohler and White, 1979).

P. aeruginosa produces polar, flexible filaments called pili that have a diameter of 5.2 nm and an average length of 2,500 nm (Bradley, 1972; Folkhard et al., 1981). These pili produce a unique form of locomotion called twitching motility (Henrichsen, 1983) and act as the receptors for a number of pilus-specific bacteriophages (Bradley and Pitt, 1974).

The only detectable subunit of *P. aeruginosa* pili is the 15,000-dalton protein, pilin, which is encoded by a gene found as a single copy in the chromosome (Pasloske et al., 1985). Pilin subunits are assembled in a helical array of five subunits per turn, with a pitch of 4.1 nm (Folkhard et al., 1981; Watts et al., 1983). The pilin of *P. aeruginosa* belongs to a class of pilins characterized by the N-terminal residue, *N*-methylphenylalanine (NMePhe), and by a highly conserved, hydrophobic stretch of 29 amino acids at the N terminus. Such pili have been classified as NMePhe pili (Paranchych and Frost, 1988) and are produced by a number of gram-negative pathogens, including *Neisseria gonorrhoeae*, *Neisseria meningitidis*, *Moraxella bovis*, *Moraxella nonliquefaciens*, and *Bacteroides nodosus*.

This chapter describes studies on the amino acid sequence polymorphism of *Pseudomonas* pilins and the mapping of surface domains of the intact pilus. The effect of several mutations in the N-terminal region of the pilin gene on pilin

---

William Paranchych, Brittan L. Pasloske, and Parimi A. Sastry • Department of Microbiology, University of Alberta, Edmonton, Alberta, Canada T6G 2E9.

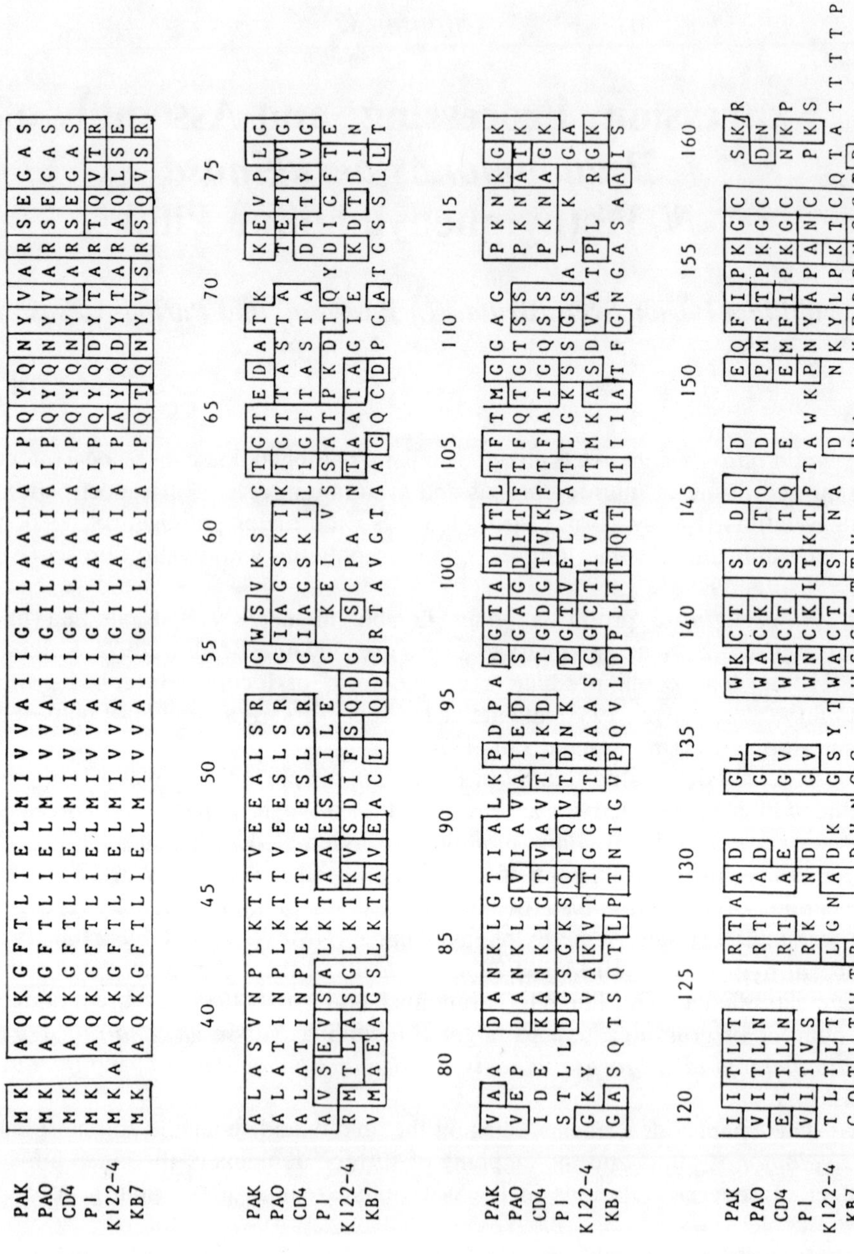
PAK
PAO
CD4
P1
K122-4
KB7
-5
+1
5
10
15
20
25
30
35
40
45
50
55
60
65
70
75
80
85
90
95
100
105
110
115
120
125
130
135
140
145
150
155
160

processing and assembly are also described, as are studies on the regulation of the *P. aeruginosa* pilin promoter by an upstream regulatory DNA sequence.

POLYMORPHISM OF *P. AERUGINOSA* NMePhe PILI

The amino acid sequence of *P. aeruginosa* pilins varies from one strain to another, but the extent of this polymorphism is not yet known. On the basis of nucleotide sequencing studies on the NMePhe pilin genes of numerous strains of *P. aeruginosa*, we have identified six unique pilin types. The predicted amino acid sequences of these six pilin genes, referred to as PAK, PAO, CD, P1, K122-4, and KB7, are shown in Fig. 1. As noted previously (Pasloske et al., 1988c), *P. aeruginosa* pilus proteins are highly homologous from positions 1 to 30 and moderately similar from positions 31 to 55 and from position 105 to the C terminus. The central region, from positions 56 to 104, has few residues that are highly conserved, although certain residues, such as Gly at position 55 and Thr at position 105, are strongly conserved. It is noteworthy that the Cys residues at positions 139 and 157 are highly conserved. In the case of type PAK pilin, these two Cys residues have been shown to be in the oxidized form and connected with a disulfide bridge to form a so-called disulfide loop (Sastry et al., 1985a; Sastry et al., 1985b). It is of interest that P1 pilin is different from the other five types in that it contains the largest putative C-terminal disulfide loop, which has 17 residues rather than the 12 found in the pilins of each other type. The K122-4 pilin has three characteristics that make it unusual: (i) it has seven residues instead of six as a putative leader peptide; (ii) it is the longest NMePhe pilin found in *P. aeruginosa* to date, with 150 residues in its putative mature form; and (iii) it has two additional cysteines at positions 58 and 98.

FREQUENCY DISTRIBUTION OF *P. AERUGINOSA* NMePhe PILIN TYPES AMONG CLINICAL AND ENVIRONMENTAL ISOLATES

To determine the frequency distribution of each of the six pilin types among clinical and environmental isolates, approximately 400 isolates were obtained from a wide range of geographical locations throughout North America. We developed specific probes for each pilus type, using DNA fragments from the hypervariable region of each pilin gene, and carried out slot blot hybridization

---

Figure 1. Comparison of the six predicted amino acid sequences of *P. aeruginosa* PAK (Sastry et al., 1985b), PAO (Sastry et al., 1985a), CD (Pasloske et al., 1988b), P1 (Pasloske et al., 1988c), K122-4 (Pasloske et al., 1988c), and KB7 (this study) pilins. The pilin sequences were aligned to obtain the greatest possible homology by visual examination on the basis of complete identity and by using the amino acid similarity values of Bacon and Anderson (1986). Empty spaces were allowed for best possible alignment; positions occupied by identical amino acids are boxed. Numbering of the amino acids was based on the total number of positions, including spaces, rather than on the numbering of any particular pilin as a standard.

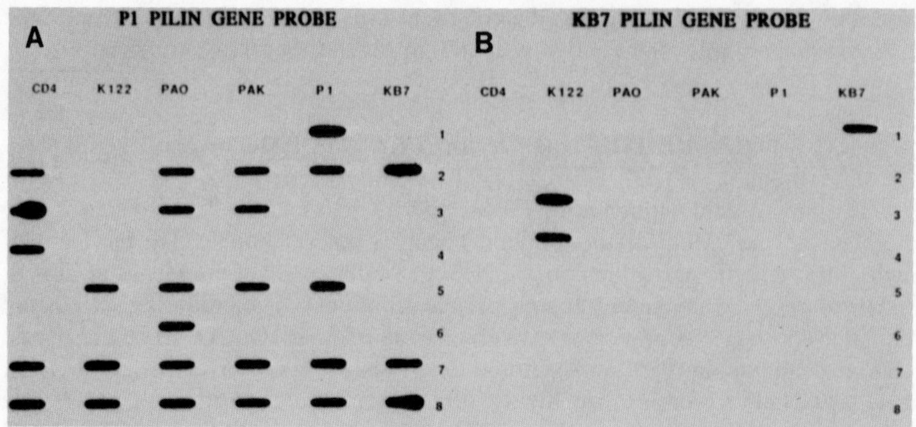

FIGURE 2. DNA slot blot hybridizations using radiolabeled DNA probes specific for the P1 (A) and KB7 (B) pilin genes. Slots in row 1 were loaded with chromosomal DNA of each of the known pilin protypes indicated at the top of each column. Slots in rows 2 to 8 were loaded with chromosomal DNA of 42 separate clinical isolates from cystic fibrosis patients. Hybridizations were carried out under conditions of high stringency.

studies on all of the *P. aeruginosa* isolates. Typical results of such slot blot hybridization studies are shown in Fig. 2. Chromosomal DNAs from 42 different clinical isolates of *P. aeruginosa* were probed under high-stringency conditions with the two probes, P1 and KB7. Only DNA of the P1 prototype was positive with the P1 probe (Fig. 2A, row 1), whereas positive hybridization was seen only with KB7 DNA (Fig. 2B, row 1). The probes for each pilus type were thus highly specific and showed no cross-reactivity with any other pilin types. Of the 42 clinical isolates screened in each of these two panels, 26 or 62%, respectively, were of the P1 type, and 2 or 5% were of the KB7 type. When similar analyses were carried out with probes for all six pilin types on approximately 400 strains, it was confirmed that approximately 60% were of the P1 type. Each of the other types was present at a frequency of about 5%, suggesting that not more than two to three new types are yet to be identified. It is therefore likely that the total number of unique pilin types in *P. aeruginosa* may be eight to nine. This number would be in keeping with results for *B. nodosus* (Anderson et al., 1987) and *M. bovis* (Moore and Rutter, 1987), in which there were fewer than 10 pilus serogroups for each pathogen.

SURFACE DOMAINS OF PAK PILI

Several experimental strategies were used in determining the putative surface domains of PAK pilin indicated in Fig. 3. A variety of native and synthetic peptides representing many different regions of the protein molecule were tested for the ability to interact with antibodies raised against native pili (Sastry et al., 1985b; Lee et al., 1989). Second, antibodies were raised against various synthetic

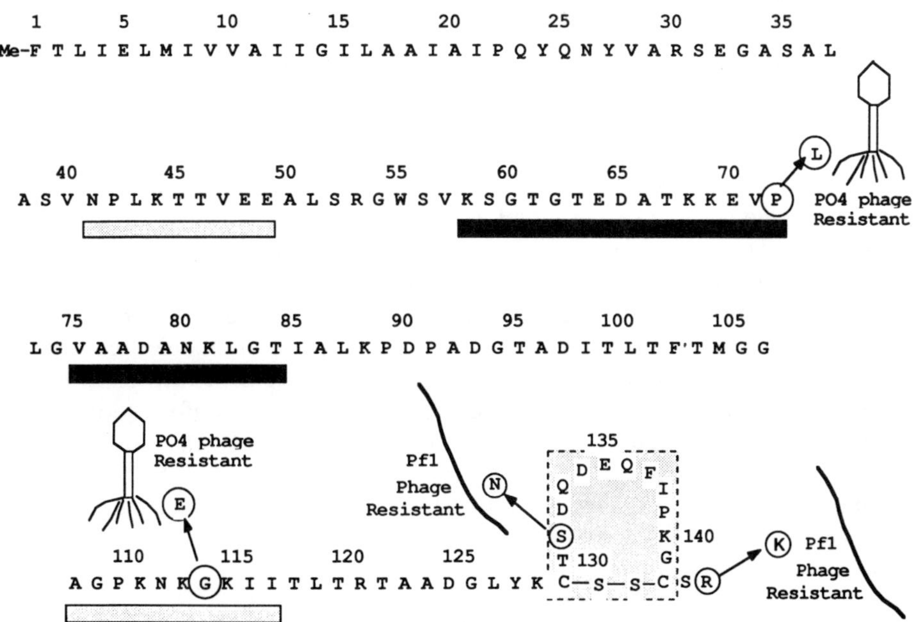

FIGURE 3. Surface domains of PAK pilin in native pili, as determined by immunological studies with native pilin peptides (Sastry et al., 1985b; Paranchych et al., 1986), synthetic peptides (Lee et al., 1989), secondary-structure predictions (Sastry et al., 1985b; Paranchych, 1989), and bacteriophage-resistant mutations (this study). Putative surface domains are indicated by horizontal bars below the sequence and the shaded rectangle encompassing the C-terminal disulfide loop region. Black bars indicate the regions that are strongly immunogenic in native pili (Sastry et al., 1985b).

peptides coupled to carriers such as bovine serum albumin and keyhole limpet hemocyanin and examined for the ability to react with native pili. We also carried out theoretical predictions of surface domains by using a variety of algorithms to predict secondary structure, hydrophilicity, and peptide mobility. Together, these studies indicated that five regions of the pilus protein are situated on the surface of native pili (Fig. 3). Surface domains appear to be located at positions 41 to 49, 58 to 72, 75 to 84, 108 to 116, and 129 to 142. Certain regions are strongly immunogenic when rabbits are immunized with native pili (Fig. 3). Approximately 80 to 85% of antipilus antibodies engendered in rabbits are directed at these two epitopes. Other regions are weakly immunogenic, but antibodies raised against synthetic peptides representing these domains bind to native pili relatively well (Lee et al., 1989; unpublished data).

Finally, we generated mutants resistant to phage PO4, a tailed phage that attaches to the lateral surface of the pilus by wrapping its tail fibers around the pilus (Bradley, 1973a), and Pf1, a filamentous phage that attaches to the tip of the pilus (Bradley, 1973b). The phage-resistant mutations were due to single amino acid substitutions within the putative surface domains (Fig. 3). At residue 72, a Pro-to-Leu replacement rendered the pili unable to interact with the tailed phage PO4, as did a Gly-to-Glu exchange at residue 113. Particularly interesting was the fact that resistance to the tip-binding phage Pf1 involved a Ser-to-Asn exchange within the disulfide loop region and an Arg-to-Lys replacement at the ultimate C-terminal position.

Several recent studies have indicated that the disulfide domain promotes adherence of the pilus to mammalian cell receptors (Paranchych et al., 1986; Irvin et al., 1989). The importance of maintaining the disulfide bridge in the oxidized form was demonstrated recently by Lee et al. (1989). These workers showed that both the oxidized and reduced forms of a 17-residue C-terminal synthetic peptide gave rise to high-titer antibodies against native pili. However, when the Cys residue at position 129 was replaced with an Ala to prevent the possibility of disulfide bridge formation in vivo, the resulting antipeptide antibodies reacted well with the synthetic peptide but not at all with native pili. These observations suggested that the disulfide bridge is important in the conformation of the C-terminal region epitope and provided additional evidence that this region is surface exposed. Because mutations in this region affected binding of the tip-specific phage Pf1, it is possible that the region is exposed at the tip of the pilus.

EFFECT OF PILIN MUTATIONS ON PROCESSING, TRANSPORT, AND ASSEMBLY OF PAK PILIN

Proteins destined for export within procaryotes are usually nascently expressed with an extra 15 to 30 residues at the N terminus (Michaelis and Beckwith, 1982). This extension, known as a signal sequence, contains one or more positively charged residues at the extreme N terminus, followed by a hydrophobic region and then a site of cleavage that is slightly polar (von Heijne, 1985). The first 36-residue region of prepilin is reminiscent of a typical signal sequence except that the cleavage site follows the N-terminal positively charged sequence and the hydrophobic region is not removed. In contrast, other exported proteins in *P. aeruginosa*, such as porin protein F, exotoxin A, and azurin (Duchene et al., 1988; Lory et al., 1988; Canters, 1987), have signal sequences of the conventional length, indicating that NMePhe pilin may follow a different pathway of transport in *P. aeruginosa*. To begin characterizing the relevant amino acids involved in pilin maturation, we created mutations within the conserved N-terminal region of mature pilin (Pasloske et al., 1988a) and observed their effects on leader peptide cleavage and methylation within *P. aeruginosa* (Pasloske and Paranchych, 1988).

A 1.2-kilobase-pair *Hin*dIII DNA fragment containing the PAK pilin gene was subjected to recombinant DNA procedures to generate a deletion mutant in which amino acids 4 to 7 were missing in the mature protein and a missense mutant in which Glu-5 was replaced with Lys (Pasloske et al., 1988a). These mutant genes were introduced into the broad-host-range vector pKT210 and mobilized into a background strain of *P. aeruginosa* PAO (Pasloske and Paranchych, 1988). The resulting bacterial strains were fractionated into inner and outer membranes, separated by sodium dodecyl sulfate-polyacrylamide gel elec-

TABLE 1
Characterization of the N termini of mutant pilins isolated from *P. aeruginosa*
cytoplasmic membrane

Pilus type	Prepilin	Pilin		Pilus assembly
		Unmethylated	Methylated	
Wild type	No	No	Yes	Yes
Glu-5→Lys	No	Yes	No	No
Δ(Ile-4–Met-7)	Yes	Yes	No	No

trophoresis, electroblotted onto polyvinylidene difluoride-paper, and subjected to micro-amino acid sequencing. We also examined each of the strains in the electron microscope to determine whether whole pili were being produced. The results of these studies are summarized in Table 1.

The normal PAK pilin gene produced completely processed pilin, and electron microscopic studies revealed that this pilin was successfully assembled into native pili. The prepilin containing the Glu-5-to-Lys-5 replacement was also completely processed by the leader peptidase, but the subsequent methylation step did not occur. These pilin molecules were not assembled into intact pili. The deletion mutant was partially cleaved by the leader peptidase. However, the cleaved portion was not methylated and did not undergo assembly.

One interpretation of these results is that the Glu residue at position 5 is required for the methylation step and that a methylated phenylalanine is required for pilus assembly. On the other hand, Glu-5 may be required for phenylalanine methylation and pilus assembly. Further studies are in progress to resolve this question.

One interesting aspect of this work was revealed by the electron microscopic studies carried out to determine which of the mutant pilins was assembled into intact pili (Pasloske et al., 1989b). Pilin subunits containing the Glu-to-Lys mutation were incorporated into compound pili together with PAO wild-type subunits. However, the mutant pilins were unable to polymerize as a homopolymer. When wild-type PAK and PAO pilin subunits were expressed in the same bacterial strain, the pilin subunits assembled into homopolymeric pili containing one or the other type of subunit but not both.

EFFECT OF AN UPSTREAM REGULATORY SEQUENCE ON EXPRESSION OF THE PAK PILIN GENE PROMOTER

Johnson et al. (1986) recognized an NtrA-specific consensus sequence in the promoter for the *P. aeruginosa* pilin gene. We subsequently searched the DNA sequence upstream of the pilin gene promoter for regions similar to NifA- or NtrC-binding sites and found a putative regulatory sequence 115 base pairs upstream of the pilin gene transcription start site (Pasloske et al., 1988c). This sequence strongly resembled the NifA-binding sequence of *Klebsiella pneumoniae*, which has the consensus sequence $TGTN_{10}$ ACA (Buck et al., 1986). To determine the functional relevance of this sequence, we compared the levels of pilin expression and quantitatively measured the promoter strengths of DNA fragments with and without the putative recognition sequence. The deletion of a 48-base-pair fragment containing this sequence resulted in much lower pilin and pilus expression and reduced the promoter activity by 90% (Pasloske et al., 1989a). These results indicated that a region of DNA upstream of the Ntr-like pilin promoter operates as a positive regulatory sequence affecting pilin gene expression.

ACKNOWLEDGMENTS. This work was supported by the Medical Research Council of Canada and the Canadian Cystic Fibrosis Foundation. B.L.P. was the recipient of a studentship from the Alberta Heritage Foundation for Medical Research.

We thank Kathy Volpel for technical assistance.

LITERATURE CITED

Anderson, B. J., J. S. Mattick, P. T. Cox, C. L. Kristo, and J. R. Egerton. 1987. Western blot (immunoblot) analysis of the fimbrial antigens of *Bacteroides nodosus*. *J. Bacteriol.* **169**:4018–4023.

Bacon, D. J., and W. F. Anderson. 1986. Multiple sequence alignment. *J. Mol. Biol.* **191**:153–161.

Bodey, B. P., R. Bolivar, V. Fainstein, and L. Jadeja. 1983. Infections caused by *Pseudomonas aeruginosa*. *Rev. Infect. Dis.* **5**:279–313.

Bradley, D. E. 1972. A study on *Pseudomonas aeruginosa*. *Genet. Res.* **19**:39–51.

Bradley, D. E. 1973a. Basic characterization of a *Pseudomonas aeruginosa* pilus-dependent bacteriophage with a long noncontractile tail. *J. Virol.* **12**:1139–1148.

Bradley, D. E. 1973b. The adsorption of the *Pseudomonas aeruginosa* filamentous bacteriophage Pf to its host. *Can. J. Microbiol.* **19**:623–631.

Bradley, D. E., and T. L. Pitt. 1974. Pilus-dependence of four *Pseudomonas aeruginosa* bacteriophages with non-contractile tails. *J. Gen. Virol.* **23**:1–15.

Buck, M., S. Miller, M. Drummond, and R. Dixon. 1986. Upstream activator sequences are present in the promoters of nitrogen fixation genes. *Nature* (London) **320**:374–378.

Canters, G. W. 1987. The azurin gene from *Pseudomonas aeruginosa* codes for a pre-protein with a signal peptide. *FEBS Lett.* **212**:168–172.

Duchene, M., A. Schweizer, F. Lottspeich, G. Krauss, M. Marget, K. Vogel, B. von Specht, and H. Domdey. 1988. Sequence and transcriptional start site of the *Pseudomonas aeruginosa* outer membrane protein F gene. *J. Bacteriol.* **170**:155–162.

Folkhard, W., D. A. Marvin, T. H. Watts, and W. Paranchych. 1981. Structure of polar pili from *Pseudomonas aeruginosa* strains K and O. *J. Mol. Biol.* **149**:79–93.

Henrichsen, J. 1983. Twitching motility. *Annu. Rev. Microbiol.* **37**:81–93.

Irvin, R. T., P. Doig, K. K. Lee, P. A. Sastry, W. Paranchych, T. Todd, and R. S. Hodges. 1989. Characterization of the Pseudomonas aeruginosa pilus adhesin: confirmation that the pilin structural protein subunit contains a human epithelial cell binding dommain. *Infect. Immun.* **57**:3720–3726.

Johnson, K., M. L. Parker, and S. Lory. 1986. Nucleotide sequence and transcriptional initiation site of two *Pseudomonas aeruginosa* pilin genes. *J. Biol. Chem.* **261**:15703–15708.

Kohler, R. B., and A. White. 1979. Miscellaneous *Pseudomonas* disease, p. 446–494. *In* R. G. Doggett (ed.), *Pseudomonas aeruginosa: Clinical Manifestations of Infection and Current Therapy*. Academic Press, Inc., New York.

Lee, K. K., P. A. Sastry, W. Paranchych, and R. S. Hodges. 1989. Immunological studies of the disulfide bridge region of *Pseudomonas aeruginosa* PAK and PAO pilins, using anti-PAK pilus and antipeptide antibodies. *Infect. Immun.* **57**:520–526.

Lory, S., M. S. Strom, and K. Johnson. 1988. Expression and secretion of the cloned *Pseudomonas aeruginosa* exotoxin A by *Escherichia coli*. *J. Bacteriol.* **170**:714–719.

Michaelis, S., and J. Beckwith. 1982. Mechanism of incorporation of cell envelope proteins in *Escherichia coli*. *Annu. Rev. Microbiol.* **36**:435–465.

Moore, L. J., and J. M. Rutter. 1987. Antigenic analysis of fimbrial proteins from *Moraxella bovis*. *J. Clin. Microbiol.* **25**:2063–2070.

Paranchych, W. 1989. Molecular studies on NMePhe pili. *In* B. L. Iglewski and V. L. Clark (ed.), *The Bacteria*. Academic Press, Inc., New York.

Paranchych, W., and L. S. Frost. 1988. The physiology and biochemistry of pili. *Adv. Microb. Physiol.* **29**:53–114.

Paranchych, W., P. A. Sastry, K. Volpel, B. A. Loh, and D. P. Speert. 1986. Fimbriae (pili): molecular basis of *Pseudomonas aeruginosa* adherence. *Clin. Invest. Med.* **9**:113–118.

Pasloske, B. L., M. R. Carpenter, L. S. Frost, B. B. Finlay, and W. Paranchych. 1988a. The expression of *Pseudomonas aeruginosa* PAK pilin gene mutants in *Escherichia coli*. *Mol. Microbiol.* **2**:185–195.

Pasloske, B. L., D. S. Drummond, L. S. Frost, and W. Paranchych. 1989a. The activity of the *Pseudomonas aeruginosa* pilin promoter is enhanced by an upstream regulatory site. *Gene* **81**:25–34.

Pasloske, B. L., B. B. Finlay, and W. Paranchych. 1985. Cloning and sequencing of the *Pseudomonas aeruginosa* PAK pilin gene. *FEBS Lett.* **183**:408–412.

Pasloske, B. L., A. M. Joffe, Q. Sun, K. Volpel, W. Paranchych, F. Eftekhar, and D. P. Speert. 1988b. Serial isolates of *Pseudomonas aeruginosa* from a cystic fibrosis patient have identical pilin sequences. *Infect. Immun.* **56**:665–672.

Pasloske, B. L., and W. Paranchych. 1988. The expression of mutant pilins in *Pseudomonas aeruginosa*: fifth position glutamate affects pilin methylation. *Mol. Microbiol.* **2**:489–495.

Pasloske, B. L., P. A. Sastry, B. B. Finlay, and W. Paranchych. 1988c. Two unusual pilin sequences from different isolates of *Pseudomonas aeruginosa*. *J. Bacteriol.* **170**:3738–3741.

Pasloske, B. L., D. G. Scraba, and W. Paranchych. 1989b. Assembly of mutant pilins in *Pseudomonas aeruginosa*: formation of pili composed of heterologous subunits. *J. Bacteriol.* **171**:2142–2147.

Sastry, P. A., B. B. Finlay, B. L. Pasloske, W. Paranchych, J. R. Pearlstone, and L. B. Smillie. 1985a. Comparative studies of the amino acid and nucleotide sequences of pilin derived from *Pseudomonas aeruginosa* PAK and PAO. *J. Bacteriol.* **164**:571–577.

Sastry, P. A., J. R. Pearlstone, L. B. Smillie, and W. Paranchych. 1985b. Studies on the primary structure and antigenic determinants of pilin isolated from *Pseudomonas aeruginosa* K. *Can. J. Biochem. Cell Biol.* **63**:1006–1011.

von Heijne, G. 1985. Signal sequences: the limits of variation. *J. Mol. Biol.* **184**:99–105.

Watts, T. H., C. M. Kay, and W. Paranchych. 1983. Spectral properties of three quaternary arrangements of *Pseudomonas* pilin. *Biochemistry* **22**:3640–3646.

Chapter 33

Pyocins S1 and S2, Bacteriocins of *Pseudomonas aeruginosa*

Yumiko Sano, Hidenori Matsui, Mieko Kobayashi,
and Makoto Kageyama

Most strains of *Pseudomonas aeruginosa* produce bacteriocins called pyocins. Since the ability to produce pyocins is a stable characteristic, it has been used for typing *P. aeruginosa* strains (Farmer and Herman, 1969; Govan, 1978). We classified pyocins into three groups according to their structures: types R, F, and S (Kageyama, 1975; Kuroda and Kageyama, 1981). R- and F-type pyocins have complex structures similar to those of certain bacteriophage tails, whereas S-type pyocins are sensitive to proteases and have lower molecular weights. S-type pyocins are further differentiated by their action spectra against a set of indicator strains and by their biochemical characteristics. Our unpublished survey for S-type pyocins has shown that pyocins S1, S2, and AP41 are the most frequently found bacteriocins among *Pseudomonas* strains (Table 1). The biochemical characteristics of pyocins S2 and AP41 were studied by us. They were purified to homogeneity, and their mechanisms of killing action were studied. Pyocin S2 interfered with phospholipid synthesis, whereas pyocin AP41 caused DNA breakdown in sensitive strains (Ohkawa et al., 1973; Ohkawa et al., 1975; Sano and Kageyama, 1981).

NATURE OF PYOCIN GENES

A peculiar feature of the pyocins is that their genetic determinants are all located at definite sites on the chromosome. This is in sharp contrast to the case for many other bacteriocins such as colicins, which are of plasmid origin. Thus, the loci of pyocins R1 to R5 and F2 are between *trpCD* and *trpE* (Kageyama, 1975; Shinomiya et al., 1983; K. Kuroda, unpublished data), the locus for pyocin AP41 is between *lys-9015* and *argF* (Sano and Kageyama, 1984), and the locus for

Yumiko Sano, Hidenori Matsui, Mieko Kobayashi, and Makoto Kageyama • Mitsubishi Kasei Institute of Life Sciences, 11, Minamiooya, Machida-shi, Tokyo 194, Japan.

TABLE 1
Classification of S-type pyocins

Producer strain	Indicator strain[a]						Pyocin activity
	NIH 3	PML1516k	PAO3092	NIH 3 S2^r	NIH 3 S1^r	GG B R5^r	
NIH B	S	S	S	S	S	S	AP41 + S1[b]
NIH L	S	S	S	S	S	S	AP41 + S1[b]
SL7	S	S	S	S	S	S	AP41 + S1[b]
NIH 23	S	S	R	S	R	S	S1
NIH H	S	S	R	S	R	S	S1
PML28	S	S	R	S	R	S	S1
QE A	S	S	R	S	R	S	S1
PAO3047	S	S	R	R	S	R	S2
NIH O	S	S	R	R	S	R	S2
NIH 18	S	S	R	R	S	R	S2
PAF41	S	R	S	S	S	R	AP41
GG B	S	R	S	S	S	R	AP41
NIH D	S	R	S	S	S	R	AP41
NIH V	R	S	R	R	R	R	NC[c]
NIH G	R	R	S	R	R	S	NC
NIH C	R	R	R	R	R	S	NC
NCTC 10332	S	S	S	S	R	S	S1 + x[b]
NIH 1	S	S	R	R	S	S	S2 + y[b]

[a] S, Sensitive; R, insensitive to pyocins produced by the strain on the left. References for strains: NIH, Farmer and Herman (1969); GG B, Govan (1978); QE A, Rampling et al. (1975). For other strains, refer to Kageyama (1975).
[b] Produces two S-type pyocins that are separable by gel filtration.
[c] NC, Not characterized.

pyocin S1/S2 is close to *flaY* (M. Kageyama, unpublished data) on the chromosome of the producer strain. To analyze the pyocin genes in more detail, we cloned them on appropriate plasmids. The pyocin AP41 gene had been obtained as an R′68.45 plasmid (Sano and Kageyama, 1984) and sequenced (Y. Sano, unpublished data). Recently, we succeeded in cloning the pyocin S1 and S2 genes. Both genes were isolated from the genomic libraries of NIH H (for pyocin S1) or PAO3012 (for pyocin S2), which were constructed by using the cosmid vector pMMB34. These clones were digested, and the pyocin determinants were recloned as smaller DNA fragments into pUC118 or pUC119. *E. coli* C600 carrying the following plasmids produced pyocin S1 or S2 more abundantly than did the original *Pseudomonas* strains: pUC119-pS1 (2.5-kilobase *Sph*I-*Sst*I fragment of the S1 determinant) and pUC119-pS2 (2.8-kilobase *Pst*I-*Sst*I fragment of the S2 determinant). These plasmids were used to determine DNA sequences and to prepare pyocin proteins.

The genes governing pyocins AP41, S1, and S2 were organized in a similar manner and found to encode two proteins, large and small, transcribed in the same direction; AP41, 83.6 and 10 kilodaltons (kDa); S1, 64.6 and 10 kDa; and S2, 74 and 10 kDa. Striking homology in the amino acid sequences was found among these bacteriocins and colicins. Whereas the N-terminal sequences of the larger components differed considerably from each other, the amino acid sequences of the C-terminal halves of pyocins S1 (377 amino acids) and S2 (378 amino acids)

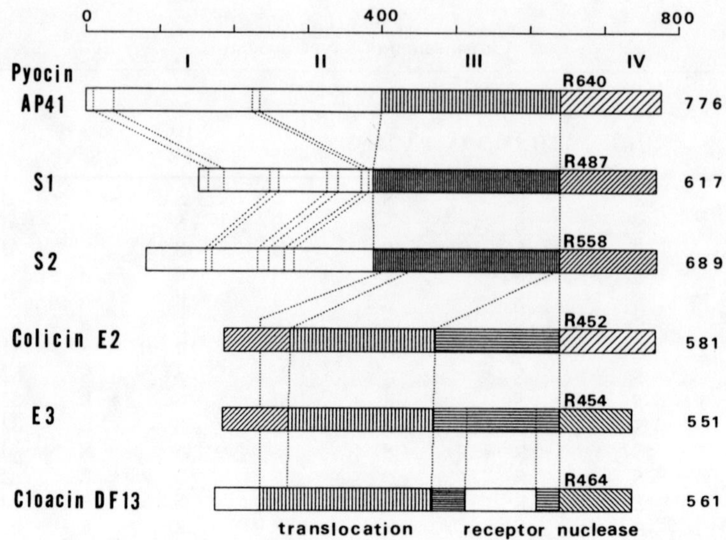

FIGURE 1. Sequence homology in the killer components of pyocins AP41, S1, and S2, colicins E2 and E3, and cloacin DF13. Domains showing homology have the same shading. Lengths are proportional to the number of amino acids of each molecule. An Arg residue near the start point of each nuclease domain is fixed as a reference point (R640 in AP41). The N-terminal Met is lacking in the purified pyocins. Therefore, numbering starts from the second amino acid in these cases. Data are from Cole et al. (1985) (colicin E2), Masaki and Ohta (1985) (colicin E3), and Van den Elzen et al. (1983) (cloacin DF13).

were identical except for one extra Arg insertion in S2 and one replacement (Val→Ile). Furthermore, these regions showed considerable homology to that of pyocin AP41. The C-terminal 130 amino acids showed especially high homology: more than 50% of the amino acids were the same among three pyocins and colicin E2. Central regions of these pyocins showed some homology to the peptides stretching between the N-terminal and the central parts of colicins E2 and E3 and especially cloacin DF13. Comparisons of the structures of the larger components of these bacteriocins are depicted in Fig. 1. The smaller components, which are encoded downstream of the larger components in all cases, were also very similar among these pyocins and colicin E2. Only one amino acid difference was found between the small components of S1 and S2. By analogy with pyocin AP41 and colicins, it is likely that the larger component carries the killing activity and the smaller component confers immunity. No open reading frame was found that corresponds to the lysis gene of colicin.

STRUCTURES OF PYOCIN PROTEINS

Purification of pyocin AP41 has been reported (Sano and Kageyama, 1981). Pyocins S1 and S2 were purified from cloned *Escherichia coli* cells by DEAE-cellulose and carboxymethyl-Sepharose chromatography. The purified preparation of each pyocin was a complex composed of two proteins, as revealed by sodium dodecyl sulfate-polyacrylamide gel electrophoresis. The polypeptide sizes coincided well with those predicted from the DNA sequences. These two protein components were separated by gel filtration in the presence of 7.2 M urea. The N-terminal sequences of these separated components were determined by Edman degradation, and the results were the same as predicted from the DNA sequences. The separated larger component of each pyocin showed essentially the same level of killing activity as did the complex molecule. Thus, the larger components are actually the bacteriocins. The smaller components make cells immune to the pyocins. When the indicator strains were transformed with a cloned DNA for the smaller component, it became insensitive to the respective pyocin. Although all three pyocins are considerably homologous, cross-immunity was found only between pyocins S1 and S2.

BIOLOGICAL ACTIVITIES OF PYOCINS

Previously, we reported that pyocin S2 inhibited phospholipid synthesis (Ohkawa et al., 1975) and that pyocin AP41 caused DNA breakdown in sensitive strains (Sano and Kageyama, 1981). Since the DNA sequences revealed homology among the determinants of these pyocins and colicin E2, and the latter is known to show a DNA endonuclease activity when deprived of its immunity protein (Schaller and Nomura, 1976), we reinvestigated the killing mechanism of pyocins. Both pyocins S1 and S2 promptly and completely inhibited the synthesis of phospholipid, as measured by the incorporation of [2-^{3}H]glycerol into the acid-insoluble fraction. Pyocin AP41 showed no inhibition of lipid synthesis. On the other hand, breakdown of chromosomal DNA was observed not only with pyocin AP41 but also with pyocins S1 and S2. Apparently, this activity was more remarkable with pyocins S1 and S2 than with AP41. DNA breakdown was observable within 10 min after addition of pyocin S1 or S2 to the growing sensitive cultures at 37°C.

DNase activity in vitro was assayed with covalently closed circular DNA as a substrate. The pyocin complex, either AP41, S1, or S2, showed little or no in vitro activity toward covalently closed circular DNA. However, the killer component of either pyocin was able to convert covalently closed circular DNA to open circular, linear and depolymerized forms. This activity was inhibited by the addition of the respective immunity protein. In this case also, the immunity proteins of pyocins S1 and S2 were cross-reactive.

After digestion with proteases, these pyocin complexes lost killing activity and yielded several discrete peptide bands, as revealed by sodium dodecyl sulfate-polyacrylamide gel electrophoresis. These peptides were separated by chromatography in the presence of urea and tested for DNase activity. A 16-kDa peptide from trypsin-treated pyocin AP41, a 15-kDa peptide from thermolysin-digested pyocin S1, and a 17-kDa fraction from V8 protease-digested pyocin S2 showed increase DNase activity. These activities were inhibited by the addition of the corresponding immunity protein. By analysis of the amino acid sequences, the

TABLE 2
Domain structure of pyocins AP41 and S1

Domain type[a]				Killing activity	Receptor specificity	Inhibition of lipid synthesis
I	II	III	IV			
A	A	A	A[b]	+	AP41	−
A		A	A	+	AP41	−
		A	A	−	NT[c]	NT
S		S	S[d]	+	S1	+++
S			S	−	NT	NT
S		S	A	+	S1	+++
S		S		−	S1	+[e]
S		A	A	+	S1	+++

[a] For domains I to IV, see Fig. 1. A, Derived from pyocin AP41; S, derived from pyocin S1.
[b] Original pyocin AP41.
[c] NT, Not tested.
[d] Original pyocin S1.
[e] Partial inhibition by excess amounts.

active AP41-trypsin peptide and the S1-thermolysin peptide were identified as the C-terminal portions of the respective pyocins. These results agree with those obtained with colicin E2 (Yamamoto et al., 1978).

DOMAIN STRUCTURE OF PYOCINS

Killing by a bacteriocin involves the following steps: binding to the receptor, translocation across the membrane, and attack on the target. These functions were assigned to specific domains of the killer protein in the case of several colicins. Comparison of amino acid sequences of three pyocins suggests that they are composed of four (AP41) or three (S1 and S2) domains. To determine the function of each domain, construction of chimeric or deleted proteins was attempted, using restriction sites on cloned DNA. Chimeric proteins between pyocins AP41 and S1 were constructed. The product proteins were partially purified, and their killing activities against a set of indicator strains and effects on lipid synthesis were investigated (Table 2).

Deletion of domain II showed little effect on the killing action of pyocin AP41, whereas the proteins deleting a part of domain I or III lost killing activity. The results with chimeric proteins indicate that domain I determines receptor specificity. Domain I of pyocin S1 also seems to be responsible for the inhibition of lipid synthesis. Domain IV should be responsible for DNase activity since C-terminal peptides showed DNase activity in vitro.

These results indicate that pyocins have a pattern of domain structure different from that of colicins or cloacin. In the latter cases, the domains are arranged (from the N terminus to the C terminus) as follows: translocation, receptor binding, and nuclease (Ohno-Iwashita and Imahori, 1980; Krone et al., 1986). In pyocins, the domains seem to be arranged in the following way: receptor binding (and lipid inhibition), translocation, and nuclease. The nuclease domain is also thought to be the region interacting with the immunity protein in all cases. This hypothesis is consistent with the homology patterns (Fig. 1).

PYOCIN SENSITIVITY AND IRON LIMITATION

The iron concentration in the growth medium affects the susceptibility of an indicator strain to pyocin S2 (Ohkawa et al., 1980). The same situation was found with pyocin S1 but not with AP41. The efficiency of killing as well as the capacity to adsorb pyocin S1 or S2 increased when the cells were grown under iron-limited conditions. Growth under iron limitation was accompanied by the appearance of five new protein bands in the outer membrane, with molecular masses of 75 to 90 kDa. By analogy with the *E. coli* systems, these proteins may act as the receptors for pyocin S1 or S2 and as components of the iron transport system. This point is now under investigation.

CONCLUDING REMARKS

In addition to the previously described pyocin AP41 genes, pyocin S1 and S2 genes were cloned and sequenced. Their protein products were purified and characterized. Striking similarities were found among these pyocins and some colicins in both amino acid sequence and function. These three pyocins caused the breakdown of chromosomal DNA of the sensitive cells. C-terminal peptides of about 15 kDa showed DNA endonuclease activity. In addition, pyocins S1 and S2 showed a unique activity, inhibition of lipid synthesis. The relationship of lipid synthesis inhibition and DNA breakdown in the killing process is not yet clear. Since the killing efficiency of pyocin S1 or S2 is much higher than that of AP41, this relationship may have something to do with efficiency (e.g., better translocation). Another feature of pyocins S1 and S2 is that they require iron limitation for the efficient adsorption to the cells. Iron-regulated outer membrane proteins may be the receptors for these pyocins.

Pyocins and colicins (including cloacin) differ not only in the range of target bacteria but also in the location of their genes, chromosomal or plasmid borne. Yet similarity was found in amino acid sequence and in function. These findings, in combination with further research, should give clues concerning the origin and evolution of bacteriocins.

LITERATURE CITED

Cole, S. T., B. Saint-Joanis, and A. P. Pugsley. 1985. Molecular characterization of the colicin E2 operon and identification of its products. *Mol. Gen. Genet.* **198:**465–472.

Farmer, J. J., and L. G. Herman. 1969. Epidemiological fingerprinting of *Pseudomonas aeruginosa* by the production of and sensitivity to pyocin and bacteriophage. *Appl. Microbiol.* **18:**760–765.

Govan, J. R. W. 1978. Pyocin typing of *Pseudomonas aeruginosa*, p. 61–91. *In* T. Bergan and J. R. Norris (ed.), *Methods in Microbiology*, vol. 10. Academic Press, Inc. (London) Ltd., London.

Kageyama, M. 1975. Bacteriocins and bacteriophages in *Pseudomonas aeruginosa*, p. 291–305. *In* S. Mitsuhashi and H. Hashimoto (ed.), *Microbial Drug Resistance*. University of Tokyo Press, Tokyo.

Krone, W. J. A., P. de Vries, G. Koningstein, A. J. R. de Jong, F. K. de Graaf, and B. Oudega. 1986. Uptake of cloacin DF13 by susceptible cells: removal of immunity protein and fragmentation of cloacin molecules. *J. Bacteriol.* **166**:260–268.

Kuroda, K., and M. Kageyama. 1981. Comparative study on F-type pyocins of *Pseudomonas aeruginosa*. *J. Biochem.* **89**:1721–1736.

Masaki, H., and T. Ohta. 1985. Colicin E3 and its immunity genes. *J. Mol. Biol.* **182**:217–227.

Ohkawa, I., M. Kageyama, and F. Egami. 1973. Purification and properties of pyocin S2. *J. Biochem.* **73**:281–289.

Ohkawa, I., B. Maruo, and M. Kageyama. 1975. Preferential inhibition of lipid synthesis by the bacteriocin pyocin S2. *J. Biochem.* **78**:213–223.

Ohkawa, I., S. Shiga, and M. Kageyama. 1980. Effect of iron concentration in the growth medium on the sensitivity of *Pseudomonas aeruginosa* to pyocin S2. *J. Biochem.* **87**:323–331.

Ohno-Iwashita, Y., and K. Imahori. 1980. Assignment of the functional loci in colicin E2 and E3 molecules by the characterization of their proteolytic fragments. *Biochemistry* **19**:652–659.

Rampling, A., J. L. Whitby, and P. Wildy. 1975. Pyocin-sensitivity testing as a method of typing *Pseudomonas aeruginosa*: use of "phage-free" preparations of pyocin. *J. Med. Microbiol.* **8**:531–541.

Sano, Y., and M. Kageyama. 1981. Purification and properties of an S-type pyocin, pyocin AP41. *J. Bacteriol.* **146**:733–739.

Sano, Y., and M. Kageyama. 1984. Genetic determinant of pyocin AP41 as an insert in the *Pseudomonas aeruginosa* chromosome. *J. Bacteriol.* **158**:562–570.

Schaller, K., and M. Nomura. 1976. Colicin E2 is a DNA endonuclease. *Proc. Natl. Acad. Sci. USA* **73**:3989–3993.

Shinomiya, T., S. Shiga, and M. Kageyama. 1983. Genetic determinant of pyocin R2 in *Pseudomonas aeruginosa* PAO. I. Localization of the pyocin R2 gene cluster between the *trpCD* and *trpE* genes. *Mol. Gen. Genet.* **189**:375–381.

Van den Elzen, P. J. M., H. H. B. Walters, E. Veltkamp, and H. J. J. Nijkamp. 1983. Molecular structure and function of the bacteriocin gene and bacteriocin protein of plasmid Clo DF13. *Nucleic Acids Res.* **11**:2465–2477.

Yamamoto, H., K. Nishida, T. Beppu, and K. Arima. 1978. Tryptic digestion of colicin E2 and its active fragment. *J. Biochem.* **83**:827–834.

Chapter 34

Inorganic Cation and Anion Transport Systems of *Pseudomonas*

Carlos Cervantes and Simon Silver

Little work has been done on the transport of inorganic cations and anions in *Pseudomonas* spp. and closely related organisms. Therefore, this brief review will contain equal parts of what has been done and a plea for important biological understanding that is still terra incognita for *Pseudomonas* physiologists and molecular biologists. If this chapter stimulates new work, then it will justify its place in this symposium volume. Our goal will be similar to that of a dozen years ago, when bacterial cation and anion transport was first reviewed (Silver, 1978). The increase in understanding since that time has been remarkable (Rosen and Silver, 1987).

CATIONS

Potassium

The only published reports of K^+ transport in *Pseudomonas* spp. are those of Thompson and MacLeod (1974) and Hassan and MacLeod (1975) dealing with a marine pseudomonad later reclassified as *Alteromonas haloplanktis*. The kinetic properties were determined for a saturable energy-dependent K^+ transport system, inhibited by Rb^+ and stimulated by Na^+. A ternary complex formed by K^+, Na^+, and a K^+ carrier was proposed (Hassan and MacLeod, 1975).

Walderhaug et al. (1989) recently identified by DNA hybridization sequences homologous to the *Escherichia coli* Kdp K^+ ATPase transport pathway (Walderhaug et al., 1987) in *Pseudomonas aeruginosa* as well as in many species of enterobacteria. Thus, it is likely that pseudomonads possess a K^+ transport system similar to that of Kdp. This system consists of five gene products; KdpA, KdpB, and KdpC are inner membrane proteins that constitute a highly specific

---

Carlos Cervantes • Instituto de Investigaciones Quimico-Biologicas, Universidad Michoacana, 58240 Morelia, Michoacan, Mexico. *Simon Silver* • Department of Microbiology and Immunology, University of Illinois College of Medicine, Chicago, Illinois 60680.

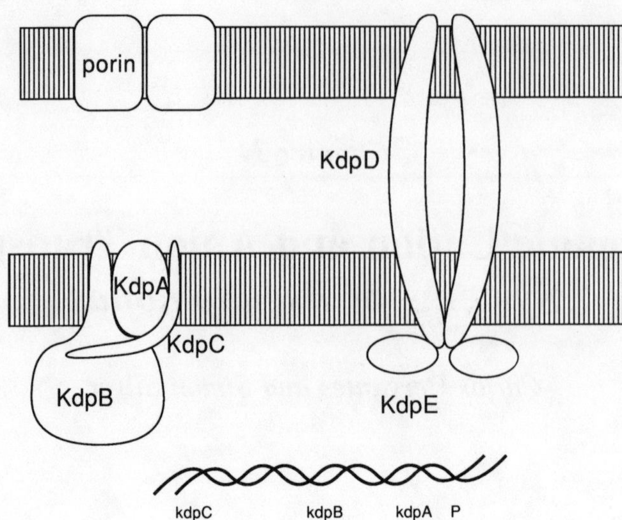

FIGURE 1. Proposed structure of the *E. coli* Kdp ATPase K$^+$ transport system and its regulation (redrawn from Walderhaug et al. [1987]). The sizes and locations of the KdpA, KdpB, and KdpC polypeptides are from sequence modeling.

ATPase transport system (Fig. 1). No specific outer membrane porin has been associated with K$^+$ movement. KdpB is the central ATPase subunit, which is homologous in sequence to other bacterial membrane ATPases and to the P class of eucaryotic ATPases, including the muscle sarcoplasmic reticulum Ca^{2+} ATPase, the animal Na$^+$/K$^+$ ATPase, and others (Walderhaug et al., 1987; Silver et al., 1989). By homology to well-studied ATPases, there is a detailed model of the functioning of this class of transport ATPases (see, for example, Silver et al. [1989]). The roles of the KdpA and KdpC polypeptides are less clear, but the existence of KdpA$^-$ mutants altered in K_m suggests that this subunit is involved in initial recognition of K$^+$ (Walderhaug et al., 1987). The products of two additional genes (KdpD and KdpE) are involved in regulation of Kdp gene function. During conditions of K$^+$ starvation or osmotic upshock (so that increased uptake of K$^+$ is essential), the Kdp system is turned on, perhaps by signal reception by the external segment of KdpD (diagrammed in Fig. 1 as associated with the outer membrane; Walderhaug et al., 1987), followed by transmission of that signal across the membrane to the smaller KdpE protein, which is pictured as interacting directly with the DNA promoter region. The membrane-associated KdpD regulatory protein is shown as cell wall associated (Walderhaug et al., 1987) from detergent solubilization studies, whereas the KdpE regulatory protein is cytoplasmic and thought to associate with the promoter region of the DNA (M. O. Walderhaug, J. Daniel, J. Hesse, and W. Epstein, personal communication). KdpD and KdpE have sequence homologies with other two-component regulatory systems (M. O. Walderhaug et al., manuscript in preparation), including those reported in this volume. Whether the KdpD protein autophosphorylates itself and then *trans*-phosphorylates KdpE has not been tested experimentally. Whether *Pseudomonas* cells also contain a second high-activity but lower-affinity K^+ transport system homologous to the *E. coli* Trk transport system (Walderhaug et al., 1987) is yet to be tested.

Magnesium, Manganese, Zinc, and Nickel

We are not aware of studies on Mg^{2+}, Mn^{2+}, Zn^{2+}, and Ni^{2+} transport in *Pseudomonas* spp. The most related work is that carried out in *Rhodobacter capsulatus* and *Alcaligenes eutrophus*. It is likely that *Pseudomonas* cells possess a Mg^{2+} transport system of the CorA type already found in several gram-negative species (see below). Nies and Silver (1989b) recently described an energy-dependent Mg^{2+} transport system in *A. eutrophus* that shows a broad-substrate range for Mn^{2+}, Co^{2+}, Zn^{2+}, Ni^{2+}, and Cd^{2+}. Uptake of these cations was competitively inhibited by each other and by Mg^{2+} (Nies and Silver, 1989b).

Photosynthetic cells of *R. capsulatus* possess an energy-dependent Mg^{2+} transport system, the rate of which decreases in aerobically grown cells (Jasper and Silver, 1978). This system is competitively inhibited by Mn^{2+}, Co^{2+}, and Fe^{2+} and resembles the *E. coli* CorA transport system (Silver and Lusk, 1987; Snavely et al., 1989). In addition to the CorA magnesium transport system, *E. coli* has an additional and *Salmonella typhimurium* has two other magnesium transport systems (Silver and Lusk, 1987; Snavely et al., 1989). It is hard to imagine that *Pseudomonas* spp. have fewer.

A specific high-affinity Mn^{2+} uptake system was described in *R. capsulatus* (Jasper and Silver, 1978). All bacteria tested have such systems (Silver and Lusk, 1987). Such a specific manganese transport system is likely to occur but has never been demonstrated in *Pseudomonas* spp.

Uptake of Ni^{2+} by Mg^{2+} transport systems has been found in *R. capsulatus* cells (Takakuwa, 1987). Tabillion and Kaltwasser (1977) first described an energy-dependent high-affinity Ni^{2+} transport pathway in *A. eutrophus*. Lohmeyer and Friedrich (1987) found that *A. eutrophus* cells accumulate Ni^{2+} by two different energy-dependent transport systems. Some *A. eutrophus* strains possess plasmids conferring inducible resistance to heavy metals (Mergeay et al., 1985). Energy-dependent efflux of Ni^{2+} (along with Co^{2+}) (Nies and Silver, 1989a; Sensfuss and Schlegel, 1988) or Cd^{2+} (along with Co^{2+} and Zn^{2+}) (Nies and Silver, 1989a) was found as the basis for the resistance phenotype.

Copper

No studies on copper uptake or transport in *Pseudomonas* spp. have been published. Bender and Cooksey (1986) studied the inducible plasmid-mediated copper resistance of the phytopathogen *Pseudomonas syringae*. It is possible that this system is related to a copper resistance system in *E. coli*, in which there are thought to be six genes involved in Cu^{2+} uptake (Rouch et al., 1989; J. Camakaris and B. T. O. Lee, personal communication).

Iron

Most microorganisms have evolved sophisticated mechanisms for the acquisition of iron, involving transport systems consisting of low-molecular-weight carriers called siderophores (Neilands, 1981). *Pseudomonas* strains transport iron through the synthesis of the siderophores pyochelin and pyoverdin (Neilands, 1981). Pseudobactins are siderophores produced by plant root-colonizing *Pseudomonas* strains (see P. J. Weisbeek, W. Bitter, J. Leong, M. Koster, and J. D. Marugg, this volume).

Sodium and Calcium

Little work has been published on Na^{2+} transport in *Pseudomonas* spp. Kodama and Taniguchi (1976) found that *Pseudomonas stutzeri* has an absolute requirement for Na^{2+} for growth. The growth rate of *P. stutzeri* increases as a function of Na^{2+} concentration, but Na^{2+} accumulation was not detected (Kodama and Taniguchi, 1976). The basis for this requirement is probably a required coupling between the Na^+ gradient and solute transport, as was reported in the marine bacterium *Alteromonas haloplanktis* (Hassan and MacLeod, 1975; Niven and MacLeod, 1980).

To our knowledge, no reports on Ca^{2+} transport in *Pseudomonas* spp. have been published. It can be hypothesized that these aerobic nonhalophilic bacteria possess secondary Ca^{2+}/proton antiporters coupled to the proton gradient, as found in *E. coli* (Lynn and Rosen, 1987). Lynn and Rosen (1987) suggested that primary Ca^{2+} ATPase pumps may be limited to bacterial species lacking the ability to generate strong membrane ion gradients.

ANIONS

Phosphate

P. aeruginosa possess two separate pathways for the transport of P_i (Lacoste et al., 1981; Poole and Hancock, 1984). A high-affinity system (K_m of about 1 μM), the synthesis of which is induced by P_i starvation, is competitively inhibited by arsenate (K_i of 0.24 mM) and sensitive to osmotic shock (Lacoste et al., 1981). The properties of this system are comparable to those of the well-studied *E. coli* Pst pathway (Nakata et al., 1987; Rosenberg, 1987) (Fig. 2). The most thoroughly studied component of phosphate transport in *P. aeruginosa* is the P outer membrane protein, which is discussed in detail by R. J. Siehnel, N. L. Martin, and R. E. W. Hancock elsewhere in this volume. The P protein shows substantial differences in pore size and specificity from the analogous outer membrane component of the *E. coli* Pst transport system, which is called PhoE. The P protein, which appears to function as a trimer (Fig. 2), forms a small, highly anion specific pore with a strong phosphate-binding site, quite unlike the larger and only weakly selective pores formed by PhoE. Alkaline phosphatase, which releases P_i, is found in the periplasmic space of *P. aeruginosa* and *E. coli* (Fig. 2).

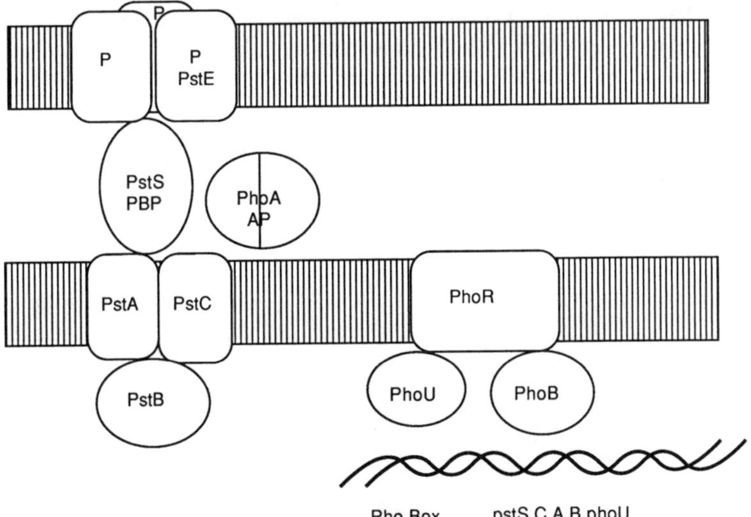

FIGURE 2. Current model for the high-affinity phosphate transport system of *P. aeruginosa* (adapted from Hancock et al. [1987], Nakata et al. [1987], and Rosenberg [1987]). P, Protein P porin of *P. aeruginosa* (or the corresponding PstE protein of *E. coli*); PBP, the PstS periplasmic phosphate-binding protein; AP, alkaline phosphatase, the *phoA* gene product; PstA and PstC, the integral inner membrane proteins; PstB, the peripheral membrane protein of the Pst system. PhoR, PhoB, and PhoU are regulatory proteins governing Pst synthesis (redrawn from Rosenberg [1987] and Nakata et al. [1987]).

The next component of the Pst transport system in *P. aeruginosa* is the phosphate-binding protein (Fig. 2), which is homologous to the similar component of the *E. coli* Pst system. The purified phosphate-binding protein has a submicromolar binding affinity for P_i (Poole and Hancock, 1984) and may be the rate-limiting step determining the overall affinity of the Pst system. The inner membrane components of the highly specific Pst-like phosphate transport system of *Pseudomonas* spp. have not been studied in detail, and therefore the molecular analysis of the system from *E. coli* provides our best model (summarized in Fig. 2). In *E. coli*, two integral inner membrane proteins (PstA and PstC) plus a peripheral inner membrane protein (PstB) constitute the inner membrane transport system. The drawing of one subunit of each in Fig. 2 is for convenience; current thinking more often suggests multiple (two or three) subunits in the active transport complex. Sequence analysis indicates that PstA and PstB are highly hydrophobic (Nakata et al., 1987), whereas the PstB sequence is quite hydrophilic and contains a recognizable ATP-binding "signature." PstB is homologous in amino acid sequence to MalK, OppD, HisP, and comparable components of other multicomponent ATP-dependent transport systems (Nakata et al., 1987; Rosenberg, 1987).

In addition to the five components of the Pst transport system diagrammed in Fig. 2, an additional three proteins are involved in regulation of Pst in *E. coli* (no comparable information is available for *Pseudomonas* spp.). PhoR is an integral membrane protein that is converted from activator to repressor form by PhoU. Another regulatory protein, PhoM, can replace PhoR and is itself sequence homologous to KdpD of the potassium transport system (Waldenhaug et al., in preparation). The reader should be warned that model building based on sequence homologies has run ahead of the hard data both for transport system components and for multiple-component regulatory systems. PhoB is an intracellular polypeptide that interacts with PhoR and with the *pho* box transcriptional promoter for the Pst operon (Fig. 2).

A second P_i transport system in *Pseudomonas* spp. shows lower affinity for P_i (K_m of about 10 μM) and occurs in mutants missing the phosphate-binding protein (Poole and Hancock, 1984). This system is resistant to arsenate and to osmotic shock (Lacoste et al., 1981). Its sensitivity to uncouplers suggested that the low-affinity system might be a proton/phosphate cotransport system and thus similar to the *E. coli* Pit system (Rosenberg, 1987).

Sulfate

Bacterial transport of SO_4^{2-} has been barely studied with the exception of early work done in *S. typhimurium* (Pardee et al., 1966). Ohtake et al. (1987) reported that *Pseudomonas fluorescens* possesses an energy-dependent high-affinity (K_m of 6.4 μM) SO_4^{2-} transport system that was competitively inhibited by CrO_4^{2-} (K_i of 12.7 μM). SO_4^{2-} uptake was repressed by growth on cysteine and derepressed by growth on djenkolic acid (Ohtake et al., 1987), as previously found in *S. typhimurium* (Pardee et al., 1966). A SO_4^{2-} transport pathway with similar properties has been found in *A. eutrophus* (Nies and Silver, 1989b).

Nitrate

In *Pseudomonas* spp. and other bacteria, assimilatory nitrate reductase is a cytoplasmic enzyme. A study with a marine pseudomonad showed a similar concentration for half-saturation of NO_3^- uptake and for the assimilatory nitrate reductase (Brown et al., 1975), indirectly suggesting that no NO_3^- active transport occurred in that organism. However, the need for such a transport pathway was postulated (Silver, 1978). Dissimilatory nitrate reductases of *Pseudomonas* spp. and other bacteria are inner-membrane-associated enzymes, and thus a NO_3^- transport mechanism has also been suggested for this pathway (Stouthamer et al., 1980). NO_3^- (and NO_2^-) transport has been shown to occur via proton symport in anaerobically grown *Pseudomonas denitrificans* and other denitrifying bacteria (Kristjansson et al., 1978).

HEAVY-METAL RESISTANCE SYSTEMS

Among the variety of functions encoded by bacterial plasmids, the ability to confer resistances to toxic heavy metals has received much attention in the last few years (Silver and Misra, 1988). DNA sequence analysis of the resistance

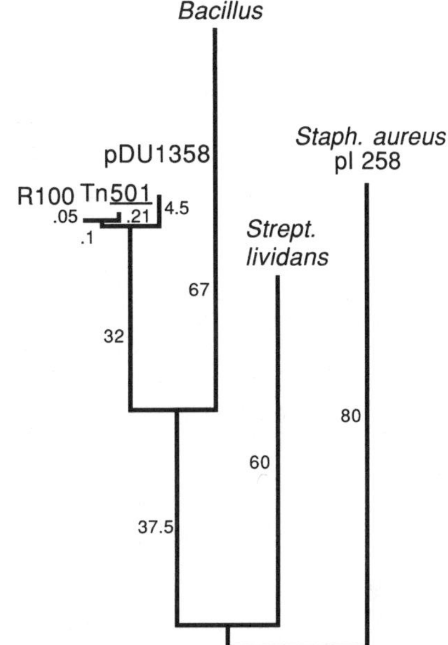

FIGURE 3. Tree of sequence homologies of amino acid sequences of the MerT Hg^{2+} transport proteins from different sources. The sequences from gram-negative bacteria are from *P. aeruginosa* transposon Tn*501*, *Shigella* plasmid R100 (transposon Tn*21*), and *Serratia* plasmid pDU1358. The sequences from gram-positive sources are the *Staphylococcus aureus* plasmid pI258, the chromosomal mercury resistance determinant from *Bacillus* sp., and that from *Streptomyces lividans*. Original references are in Silver and Misra (1988).

determinants has provided detailed understanding of functions, and in some cases, specific transport systems have been demonstrated.

Mercury

Transport of Hg^{2+} has been studied with the *P. aeruginosa* transposon Tn*501*. DNA sequence analysis of the Tn*501* *mer* operon revealed the gene products of the *merP* and *merT* genes, which are involved in Hg^{2+} transport (Silver and Misra, 1988). MerP is a small periplasmic polypeptide whose function appears to be the chelation of Hg^{2+} at the cell surface (Silver and Misra, 1988). Transport of Hg^{2+} to the cytoplasm is then carried out by the MerT protein, which is an inner membrane polypeptide. Once in the cytosol, Hg^{2+} is transferred to, and then reduced by, the mercuric reductase (MerA polypeptide) enzyme to volatile Hg^0 (Silver and Misra, 1988). The MerP and MerT proteins from the *Shigella* plasmid R100 and the *Serratia* plasmid pDU1358 show high amino acid homologies with those from Tn*501* (Fig. 3), suggesting a very similar Hg^{2+} transport mechanism. Recognizable (by sequence homology) but very different MerT transport proteins are found in the mercuric resistance operons of gram-positive bacteria (Fig. 3), which lack periplasmic MerP proteins.

Cadmium

Horitsu and Kato (1980) found that a Cd^{2+}-tolerant *P. aeruginosa* strain transported less Cd^{2+} than did a Cd^{2+}-sensitive derivative. In contrast, a Cd^{2+}-resistant *Pseudomonas putida* strain appeared to actively accumulate Cd^{2+}

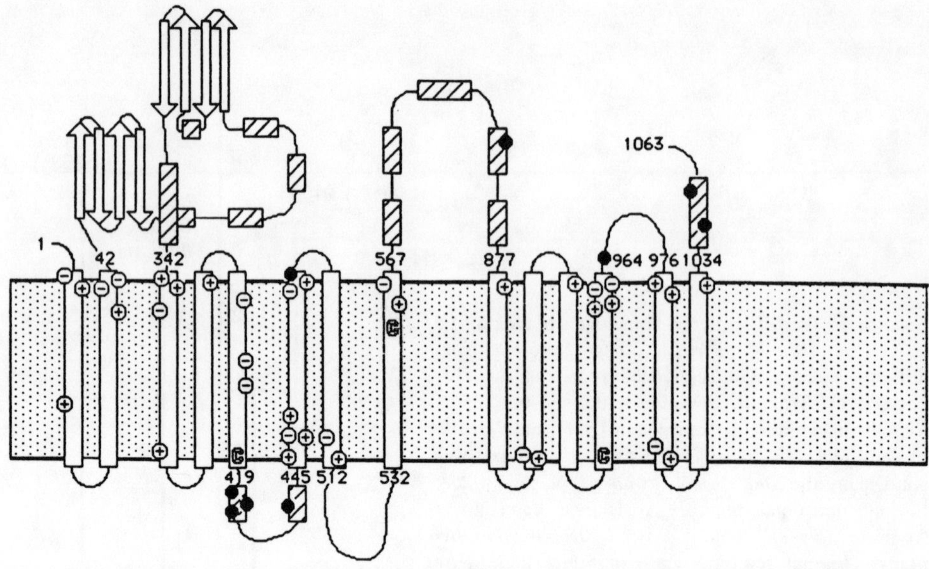

FIGURE 4. Model for the structure of the CzcA protein from the *A. eutrophus* plasmid pMOL30 (D. H. Nies et al., 1989). CzcA is part of the *czc* operon determining resistances to and efflux of Cd^{2+}, Zn^{2+}, and Co^{2+}. Predicted alpha-helical (hatched boxes) and beta-sheet (arrows) segments are indicated. Indicated are cysteine (C), histidines (●), and positively ⊕ and negatively ⊖ charged amino acids. The predicted positions of some residues are represented by numbers (D. H. Nies, personal communication).

(Higham et al., 1984), and the mechanism of resistance was considered to be chelation of Cd^{2+} by polyphosphates or by metallothioneinlike cysteine-rich proteins. However, Higham et al. (1985) found that resistant *P. putida* cells also excluded Cd^{2+} when the metal was at low concentrations. Resistance to Cd^{2+} in *P. putida* GAM-1 was linked to plasmid pGU100, which also conferred Cd^{2+} resistance when transformed into *E. coli* (Horitsu et al., 1986). Decreased uptake of Cd^{2+} was found with plasmid-containing *P. putida* and *E. coli* (Horitsu et al., 1986).

Energy-dependent efflux of Cd^{2+}, Zn^{2+}, and Co^{2+} was demonstrated in *A. eutrophus* cells bearing plasmid pMOL30 (Nies and Silver, 1989a). The cation resistance determinant from this plasmid was sequenced (D. H. Nies et al., 1989). From the DNA sequence and expression studies in *E. coli*, the *czc* operon was found to encode four polypeptides. The CzcA protein (Fig. 4) is essential for the efflux system to function (D. H. Nies et al., 1989). CzcB specifically enhanced Zn^{2+} efflux, and CzcC appeared to be involved in the efflux of Co^{2+} and Cd^{2+}. A regulatory role was proposed from CzcD, which was not necessary for cation resistance of the cloned determinant (D. H. Nies et al., 1989). The Czc system for Cd^{2+}, Zn^{2+}, and Co^{2+} resistance in *Alcaligenes* spp. is now the best-studied cadmium resistance system in gram-negative bacteria related to *Pseudomonas* spp. A very different Cd^{2+} and Zn^{2+} resistance system called CadA (which is based on an efflux ATPase) has been studied in depth in gram-positive bacteria (Silver et al., 1989).

Cobalt and Nickel

In addition to being transported out of *Alcaligenes* cells by the cadmium, zinc, and cobalt (*czc, cobB*) system described above, the same *Alcaligenes* strain harbors a second plasmid with a different cobalt efflux system (*cobA*). This system affords resistance to and effluxes both Co^{2+} and Ni^{2+} from the cells (Sensfuss and Schlegel, 1988; Nies and Silver, 1989a). A single genetic determinant has been cloned and mapped by using restriction nucleases: nickel and cobalt resistances appear to be due to a single system (Siddiqui et al., 1989; A. Nies et al., 1989).

Copper

A plasmid-encoded copper resistance determinant in *P. syringae* was cloned and sequenced (Mellano and Cooksey, 1988). The *Pseudomonas* copper resistance system did not function in *E. coli* and did not hybridize to another plasmid copper resistance determinant that had been cloned from *E. coli* (Bender and Cooksey, 1986). Aside from a repeated small peptide motif suggestive of a copper-binding sequence (Mellano and Cooksey, 1988; described below), there is no direct evidence for a role of copper transport in this resistance mechanism. The copper-resistant *P. syringae* colonies are said to turn bright blue on high-copper agar (D. Cooksey, personal communication), whereas comparable colonies of the *E. coli* copper-resistant strain appear surrounded by a zone clear of visible copper (Camakaris and Lee, personal communication), suggestive of a copper-binding component. Thus, although plasmid-determined copper resistance is well established in *Pseudomonas* spp., any role for transport processes in this resistance remains to be determined.

The copper resistance determinant from the *P. syringae* plasmid was recently sequenced (Mellano and Cooksey, 1988). Again, four open reading frames (ORFs) were identified. The first two ORFs conferred low-level copper resistance. The other two ORFs were required for full copper resistance. The second ORF contained a peptide sequence Asp-His-Ser-X-Met-Gln-Gly-Met repeated five times, and a less conserved but related octapeptide was found four times in the first ORF. These are candidates for a Cu^{2+}-binding motif. From analysis of the predicted amino acid sequences of these four ORFs, the first three started with short membranous segments (potential signal peptides for protein transport) but appeared otherwise to be basically soluble proteins (Mellano and Cooksey, 1988). The remaining ORF has several potential membrane segments, predictive of an integral membrane protein.

Arsenate and Arsenite

Resistance to arsenate is very common in *P. aeruginosa* (Nakahara et al., 1977), yet there is no defined arsenate resistance plasmid, apparently because of the lack of effort to find one. Plasmids conferring resistances to arsenate, arsenite, and antimonate anions were reported in *E. coli*, and the role of transport in these resistances is well understood (Silver and Misra, 1988). Arsenate resistance was shown to be associated with reduced net uptake of arsenate, which enters the cells via both the Pst and the Pit phosphate transport system (see above). Arsenate resistance from the plasmid was additive to the arsenate resistance, determined by chromosomal mutations eliminating the Pit phosphate transport system.

The plasmid determines an arsenate efflux system that functions as an ATPase (Silver and Misra, 1988). The arsenic resistance determinant of one plasmid was cloned and sequenced (Chen et al., 1986). Four gene products are involved. The first is that of the *arsR* gene, a *trans*-acting regulatory protein that responds to arsenate, arsenite, and antimonate [and bismuth(III), toward which the plasmid does not confer resistance]. After a 1-kilobase gap (B. P. Rosen, personal communication), there are the three ORFs sequenced by Chen et al. (1986), *arsA*, *arsB*, and *arsC*. Together, these encode the resistance efflux ATPase. ArsA is the ATPase subunit itself (by homology to other ATP-binding proteins [Chen et al., 1986; Silver et al., 1989] and by direct biochemical determination [Rosen et al., 1988]). The ArsB protein is the integral membrane protein with which ArsA associates (Silver and Misra, 1988; Silver et al., 1989), and ArsC is a specificity-conferring small polypeptide. In the absence of ArsC, the system still confers resistance to (and pumps) arsenite and antimonate, but arsenate resistance and efflux is lost in *arsC* mutants (Chen et al., 1986). The three-component arsenic ATPase shares the efflux mechanism with the cadmium, zinc, and cobalt resistance system as well as with the nickel and cobalt system, but otherwise the amino acid sequences of each of these transport efflux systems are quite different. The arsenic resistance ATPase also shows no similarity in sequence or overall structure to the transport-based chromate resistance system described next.

Chromate

Chromate is a competitive inhibitor of the sulfate transport systems in bacteria, as mentioned above. Decreased uptake of CrO_4^{2-} was shown to be the basis for CrO_4^{2-} resistance conferred by plasmids from *P. fluorescens* (Ohtake et al., 1987) and *P. aeruginosa* (Cervantes and Ohtake, 1988). It is not known whether reduced uptake results from a direct block in cell accumulation or from subsequent efflux.

The CrO_4^{2-} resistance determinant from *P. aeruginosa* plasmid pUM505 was recently cloned and sequenced (Cervantes et al., 1990). A single ORF, encoding the ChrA protein, was found to be necessary and sufficient for expression of CrO_4^{2-} resistance in *P. aeruginosa*. Cervantes et al. (1990) postulated that ChrA was the inner membrane protein responsible for the translocation of CrO_4^{2-}.

CrO_4^{2-} resistance determined by an *A. eutrophus* plasmid was also shown to be due to the reduced accumulation of CrO_4^{2-} (Nies and Silver, 1989a). The nucleotide sequence of this CrO_4^{2-} resistance system was recently completed (A. Nies, D. H. Nies, T. K. Misra, and S. Silver, submitted for publication). The

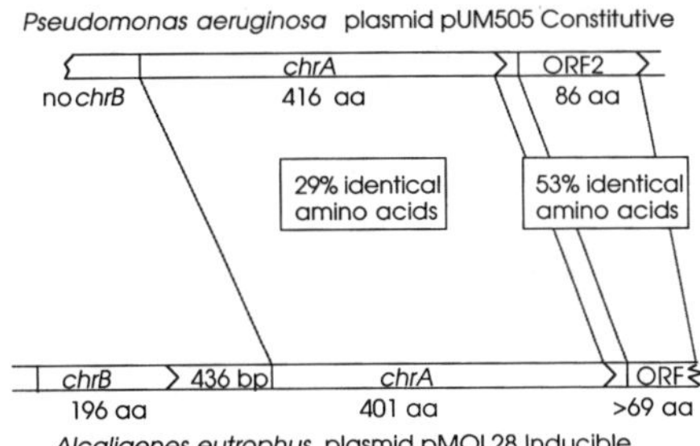

FIGURE 5. Comparison of the chromate resistance determinants from *P. aeruginosa* plasmid pUM505 (Cervantes et al., 1990) and *A. eutrophus* plasmid pMOL30 (Nies et al., submitted).

amino acid sequence of ChrA from the *P. aeruginosa* plasmid system shows a significant homology with the corresponding ChrA sequence from *A. eutrophus* (Fig. 5) even though the DNA determinants are sufficiently dissimilar as not to hybridize in Southern DNA-DNA hybridization tests (Cervantes et al., 1990). The chromate resistance determinant from *A. eutrophus* possesses a second essential ORF (absent in the current sequence from *P. aeruginosa*) encoding the ChrB protein, which may be involved in the inducibility of the chromate resistance determinant (Nies et al., submitted). A third ORF, which is not necessary for expression of CrO_4^{2-} resistance, was found in the derived amino acid sequences of both DNA sequences. Surprisingly, this third ORF is highly homologous in the two sequences (Fig. 5). Thus, it appears that the basic resistance mechanisms of the *P. aeruginosa* and *A. eutrophus* CrO_4^{2-} resistance determinants are similar and involve either a block in chromate uptake or accelerated chromate efflux.

Tellurite

Mutation of the *P. aeruginosa* plasmid RP4 causes expression of a normally cryptic TeO_3^{2-} resistance determinant (Bradley, 1985). Cloning and expression of this determinant revealed a single 40-kilodalton polypeptide that appears to be involved in TeO_3^{2-} resistance (Walter and Taylor, 1989). A different plasmid, pHH1508a, expressed two polypeptides of 23 and 12 kilodaltons from its tellurite resistance determinant, and the RP4 and pHH1508a systems did not hybridize at the DNA level (Walter and Taylor, 1989). The mechanisms of these tellurite resistances are not known.

A more complex TeO_3^{2-} resistance determinant was found on an *Alcaligenes* plasmid and has been sequenced (Jobling and Ritchie, 1988). Five ORFs were identified; three appeared to be for structural genes, whereas the other two ORFs were assigned regulatory roles. Information on the mechanism of this resistance to TeO_3^{2-} is yet to be provided. However, both in *Pseudomonas* and in *Alcaligenes* spp., tellurium reduction is not responsible for resistance. Thus, a transport basis is likely.

ACKNOWLEDGMENTS. The research in our laboratory has been supported by grants from the National Institutes of Health and the National Science Foundation.

Ideas have been generated by free exchanges of information, especially with T. K. Misra, A. Nies, D. H. Nies, G. Nucifora, H. Ohtake, B. P. Rosen, and M. Walderhaug.

LITERATURE CITED

Bender, C. L., and D. A. Cooksey. 1986. Indigenous plasmids in *Pseudomonas syringae* pv. *tomato*: conjugative transfer and role in copper resistance. *J. Bacteriol.* **165:**534–541.

Bradley, D. E. 1985. Detection of tellurite-resistance determinants in IncP plasmids. *J. Gen. Microbiol.* **131:**3135–3137.

Brown, C. M., D. S. MacDonald-Brown, and S. O. Stanley. 1975. Inorganic nitrogen metabolism in marine bacteria: nitrate uptake and reduction in a marine pseudomonad. *Marine Biol.* **31:**7–13.

Cervantes, C., and H. Ohtake. 1988. Plasmid-determined resistance to chromate in *Pseudomonas aeruginosa. FEMS Microbiol. Lett.* **56:**173–176.

Cervantes, C., H. Ohtake, L. Chu, T. K. Misra, and S. Silver. 1990. Cloning, nucleotide sequence, and expression of the chromate resistance determinant of *Pseudomonas aeruginosa* plasmid pUM505. *J. Bacteriol.* **172:**287–291.

Chen, C. M., T. K. Misra, S. Silver, and B. P. Rosen. 1986. Nucleotide sequence of the structural genes for an anion pump. The plasmid-encoded arsenical resistance operon. *J. Biol. Chem.* **261:** 15030–15038.

Hancock, R. E. W., E. A. Worobec, K. Poole, and R. Benz. 1987. Phosphate-binding site of *Pseudomonas aeruginosa* outer membrane protein P, p. 186–190. *In* A. Torriani-Gorini, S. Silver, F. Rothman, A. Wright, and E. Yagil (ed.), *Phosphate Metabolism and Cellular Regulation in Microorganisms.* American Society for Microbiology, Washington, D.C.

Hassan, H. M., and R. A. MacLeod. 1975. Kinetics of Na^+-dependent K^+ ion transport in a marine pseudomonad. *J. Bacteriol.* **121:**160–164.

Higham, D. P., P. J. Sadler, and M. D. Scawen. 1984. Cadmium-resistant *Pseudomonas putida* synthesizes novel cadmium proteins. *Science* **225:**1043–1046.

Higham, D. P., P. J. Sadler, and M. D. Scawen. 1985. Cadmium resistance in *Pseudomonas putida*: growth and uptake of cadmium. *J. Gen. Microbiol.* **131:**2539–2544.

Horitsu, H., and H. Kato. 1980. Comparisons of characteristics of cadmium-tolerant bacterium, *Pseudomonas aeruginosa* G-1 and its cadmium-sensitive mutant strain. *Agric. Biol. Chem.* **44:**777–782.

Horitsu, H., K. Yamamoto, S. Wachi, K. Kawai, and A. Fukuchi. 1986. Plasmid-determined cadmium resistance in *Pseudomonas putida* GAM-1 isolated from soil. *J. Bacteriol.* **165:**334–335.

Jasper, P., and S. Silver. 1978. Divalent cation transport systems of *Rhodopseudomonas capsulata. J. Bacteriol.* **133:**1323–1328.

Jobling, M. G., and D. A. Ritchie. 1988. The nucleotide sequence of a plasmid determinant for resistance to tellurium anions. *Gene* **66:**245–258.

Kodama, T., and S. Taniguchi. 1976. Sodium-dependent growth and respiration of a nonhalophilic bacterium, *Pseudomonas stutzeri. J. Gen. Microbiol.* **96:**17–24.

Kristjansson, J. K., B. Walter, and T. C. Hollocher. 1978. Respiration dependent proton translocation and the transport of nitrate and nitrite in *Paracoccus denitrificans* and other denitrifying bacteria. *Biochemistry* **17:**5014–5019.

Lacoste, A.-M., A. Cassaigne, and E. Neuzil. 1981. Transport of inorganic phosphate in *Pseudomonas aeruginosa. Curr. Microbiol.* **6:**115–120.

Lohmeyer, M., and C. G. Friedrich. 1987. Nickel transport in *Alcaligenes eutrophus. Arch. Microbiol.* **149:**130–135.

Lynn, A. R., and B. P. Rosen. 1987. Calcium transport in prokaryotes, p. 181–201. *In* B. P. Rosen and S. Silver (ed.), *Ion Transport in Prokaryotes.* Academic Press, Inc., San Diego, Calif.

Mellano, M. A., and D. A. Cooksey. 1988. Nucleotide sequence and organization of copper resistance genes from *Pseudomonas syringae* pv. *tomato. J. Bacteriol.* **170:**2879–2883.

Mergeay, M., D. Nies, H. G. Schlegel, J. Gerits, P. Charles, and F. Van Gijsegem. 1985. *Alcaligenes eutrophus* CH34 is a facultative chemolithotroph with plasmid-bound resistance to heavy metals. *J. Bacteriol.* **162:**328–334.

Nakahara, H., T. Ishikawa, Y. Sarai, I. Kondo, H. Kozukue, and S. Silver. 1977. Linkage of mercury, cadmium, and arsenate and drug resistance in clinical isolates of *Pseudomonas aeruginosa*. *Appl. Environ. Microbiol.* **33**:975–976.

Nakata, A., M. Amemura, K. Makino, and H. Shinagawa. 1987. Genetic and biochemical analysis of the phosphate-specific transport system in *Escherichia coli*, p. 150–155. *In* A. Torriani-Gorini, S. Silver, F. Rothman, A. Wright, and E. Yagil (ed.), *Phosphate Metabolism and Cellular Regulation in Microorganisms*. American Society for Microbiology, Washington, D.C.

Neilands, J. B. 1981. Iron absorption and transport in microorganisms. *Annu. Rev. Nutr.* **1**:27–46.

Nies, A., D. H. Nies, and S. Silver. 1989. Cloning and expression of plasmid genes encoding resistances to chromate and cobalt in *Alcaligenes eutrophus*. *J. Bacteriol.* **171**:5065–5070.

Nies, D. H., A. Nies, and S. Silver. 1989. Expression and nucleotide sequence of a plasmid-determined divalent cation efflux system from *Alcaligenes eutrophus*. *Proc. Natl. Acad. Sci. USA* **86**:7351–7355.

Nies, D. H., and S. Silver. 1989a. Plasmid-determined inducible efflux is responsible for resistance to cadmium, zinc, and cobalt in *Alcaligenes eutrophus*. *J. Bacteriol.* **171**:896–900.

Nies, D. H., and S. Silver. 1989b. Metal ion uptake by a plasmid-free metal-sensitive *Alcaligenes eutrophus* strain. *J. Bacteriol.* **171**:4073–4075.

Niven, D. F., and R. A. MacLeod. 1980. Sodium ion substrate symport in a marine bacterium. *J. Bacteriol.* **142**:603–607.

Ohtake, H., C. Cervantes, and S. Silver. 1987. Decreased chromate uptake in *Pseudomonas fluorescens* carrying a chromate resistance plasmid. *J. Bacteriol.* **16**:3853–3856.

Pardee, A. B., L. S. Prestidge, M. B. Whipple, and J. Dreyfuss. 1966. A binding site for sulfate and its relation to sulfate transport into *Salmonella typhimurium*. *J. Biol. Chem.* **241**:3962–3969.

Poole, K., and R. E. W. Hancock. 1984. Phosphate transport in *Pseudomonas aeruginosa*. *Eur. J. Biochem.* **144**:607–612.

Rosen, B. P., and S. Silver (ed.). 1987. *Ion Transport in Prokaryotes*. Academic Press, Inc., San Diego, Calif.

Rosen, B. P., U. Weigel, C. Karkaria, and P. Gangola. 1988. Molecular characterization of an anion pump. The *arsA* gene product is an arsenite (antimonate)-stimulated ATPase. *J. Biol. Chem.* **263**:3067–3070.

Rosenberg, H. 1987. Phosphate transport in prokaryotes, p. 205–248. *In* B. P. Rosen and S. Silver (ed.), *Ion Transport in Prokaryotes*. Academic Press, Inc., San Diego, Calif.

Rouch, D., J. Camakaris, and B. T. O. Lee. 1989. Copper transport in *Escherichia coli*, p. 469–477. *In* D. H. Hamer and D. R. Winge (ed.), *Metal Ion Homeostasis: Molecular Biology and Chemistry*. Alan R. Liss, Inc., New York.

Sensfuss, P., and H. G. Schlegel. 1988. Plasmid pMOL28-encoded resistance to nickel is due to specific efflux. *FEMS Microbiol. Lett.* **55**:295–298.

Siddiqui, R. A., K. Benthin, and H. G. Schlegel. 1989. Cloning of pMOL28-encoded nickel resistance genes and expression in *Alcaligenes eutrophus* and *Pseudomonas* sp. *J. Bacteriol.* **171**:5071–5076.

Silver, S. 1978. Transport of cations and anions, p. 221–324. *In* B. P. Rosen (ed.), *Bacterial Transport*. Marcel Dekker, Inc., New York.

Silver, S., and J. E. Lusk. 1987. Bacterial magnesium, manganese, and zinc transport, p. 165–180. *In* B. P. Rosen and S. Silver (ed.), *Ion Transport in Prokaryotes*. Academic Press, Inc., San Diego, Calif.

Silver, S., and T. K. Misra. 1988. Plasmid-mediated heavy metal resistances. *Annu. Rev. Microbiol.* **42**:717–743.

Silver, S., G. Nucifora, L. Chu, and T. K. Misra. 1989. Bacterial resistance ATPases: primary pumps for exporting toxic cations and anions. *Trends Biochem. Sci.* **14**:76–80.

Snavely, M. D., J. B. Florer, C. G. Miller, and M. E. Maguire. 1989. Magnesium transport in *Salmonella typhimurium*: expression of cloned genes for three distinct Mg^{2+} transport systems. *J. Bacteriol.* **171**:4752–4760.

Stouthamer, A. H., J. van't Riet, and L. F. Oltmann. 1980. Respiration with nitrate as acceptor, p. 19–48. *In* C. J. Knowles (ed.), *Diversity of Bacterial Respiration Systems*. CRC Press, Inc., Boca Raton, Fla.

Tabillion, R., and H. Kaltwasser. 1977. Energy-dependent ^{63}Ni-uptake by *Alcaligenes eutrophus* strains H1 and H16. *Arch Microbiol.* **113:**145–151.

Takakuwa, S. 1987. Nickel uptake in *Rhodopseudomonas capsulata. Arch. Microbiol.* **149:**57–61.

Thompson, J., and R. A. MacLeod. 1974. Potassium transport and the relationship between intracellular potassium concentration and amino acid uptake by cells of a marine pseudomonad. *J. Bacteriol.* **120:**598–603.

Walderhaug, M. O., D. C. Dosch, and W. Epstein. 1987. Potassium transport in bacteria, p. 85–130. *In* B. P. Rosen and S. Silver (ed.), *Ion Transport in Prokaryotes.* Academic Press, Inc., San Diego, Calif.

Walderhaug, M. O., E. D. Litwack, and W. Epstein. 1989. Wide distribution of homologs of *Escherichia coli* Kdp K$^+$-ATPase among gram-negative bacteria. *J. Bacteriol.* **171:**1192–1195.

Walter, E. G., and D. E. Taylor. 1989. Comparison of tellurite resistance determinants from the IncPα plasmid RP4Te^r and the IncHII plasmid pHH1508a. *J. Bacteriol.* **171:**2160–2165.

Part VI

HONORARY PSEUDOMONADS

Genetic Mapping, Cloning, and Expression of Carotenoid and Bacteriochlorophyll Genes of *Rhodobacter*

Robert J. Penfold and John M. Pemberton

Photosynthesis is a biological process of great complexity and importance. Facultatively phototrophic bacteria, such as *Rhodobacter sphaeroides* and *R. capsulatus*, are ideal subjects for the study of this process, since photosynthetic lesions are only conditionally lethal. Accordingly, the biochemical, biophysical, and genetic aspects of photosynthesis have been intensively studied in these bacteria (Scolnik and Marrs, 1987; Kiley and Kaplan, 1988). Photopigments are of central importance in photosynthesis. Bacteriochlorophyll (Bchl) and carotenoid (Crt) molecules are components of the light-harvesting complexes and the photosynthetic reaction center. In addition, Crts are protective agents against photooxidative killing (Siefermann-Harms, 1987).

CHROMOSOME MAPPING

One of the most important discoveries in bacterial photosynthesis during the last 10 to 15 years has been that the photosynthesis genes are clustered on the main chromosome in *Rhodobacter* species (Yen and Marrs, 1976; Marrs, 1981; Pemberton and Bowen, 1981; Bowen and Pemberton, 1985; Willison et al., 1985). Whereas photopigment mutants are easily isolated, being recognized by colony color changes (Cohen-Bazire et al., 1957; Scolnik et al., 1980; Pemberton et al., 1983), mapping by chromosome transfer requires a variety of mutations. The most useful are those in typically chromosomal loci such as amino acid biosynthesis and antibiotic resistance genes. One of the best mutagens for isolating photosynthetic, auxotrophic, and antibiotic-resistant mutants from *Rhodobacter* species is ethyl methanesulfonate. Another mutagen, nitrosoguanidine, typically produces a

Robert J. Penfold and John M. Pemberton • Department of Microbiology, University of Queensland, St. Lucia, Queensland 4067, Australia.

cluster of mutations (Guerola et al., 1971), an undesirable property when one is analyzing an intricately regulated cluster of many genes.

Chromosome transfer in *R. sphaeroides* was first achieved by using R68.45 (Sistrom, 1977), a broad-host-range, multiple-drug resistance (R) plasmid that promotes chromosome transfer in a variety of gram-negative bacteria (Holloway, 1978). R plasmids, carrying mercury transposons with regulated or deficient resolvases, promoted chromosome transfer at a high frequency in *R. sphaeroides*, presumably because of low-level resolution of chromosome::transposon::R plasmid cointegrates. Chromosome maps constructed with the aid of these R plasmid::transposon hybrids showed unequivocally that the photopigment gene cluster was in a single region of the main chromosome (Pemberton and Bowen, 1981; Bowen and Pemberton, 1985). Recently, Willison et al. (1985) produced a circular chromosomal map of *R. capsulatus* that shows a great similarity to the *R. sphaeroides* map in the distribution of markers and their linkage to the photopigment cluster.

BIOCHEMICAL ASPECTS OF CAROTENOGENESIS

The Crt molecule originates from the tail-to-tail condensation of two identical carbon-20 units. It has been suggested that carotenogenic enzymes may distinguish between the halves (Liaaen-Jensen et al., 1961). In *R. sphaeroides* but not *R. capsulatus*, low levels of spirilloxanthin can be formed from hydroxyspheroidene. This occurs via a series of reactions of the same type that convert 7,8,11,12-tetrahydrolycopene into spheroidene (Fig. 1) but occur on the other end of the molecule (Schmidt, 1978). Is this mediated by another set of enzymes, or by the one set of enzymes regulated to act on one end and then the other? Conceivably, regulation of the reaction sequence could be achieved by spatial constraints in a multienzyme complex. Armstrong et al. (1989) postulated that the very hydrophobic *crtK* gene product might act as a membrane attachment point for an enzyme complex.

The Crt pathway (Fig. 1) was constructed from metabolic analyses of Crt mutants. It shows a bifurcated pathway, with the products of *crtD*, *crtF*, and *crtA* having dual substrate activities. This duality may reflect the in vivo situation. However, it may also be artifactual, resulting from slow enzymatic catalysis of a surrogate substrate, allowed by the absence of the normal substrate. Kinetic studies of purified enzymes could clarify this point.

Crts, Bchl phytol side chains, and isoprenoid quinones all stem from the isoprenoid biosynthetic pathway. The ubiquinones found in *R. sphaeroides*, *R. capsulatus*, and *Paracoccus denitrificans* (see next section) all have a carbon-50 isoprenoid side chain (Collins and Jones, 1981). These compounds are essential as part of the electron transport chain and are more polyprenoid than carotenoids. Thus, it would seem that, excluding the use of strictly fermentative growth, mutant analyses could only extend back to the step at which carotenogenesis branches from the isoprenoid pathway, i.e., the synthesis of prephytoene pyrophosphate.

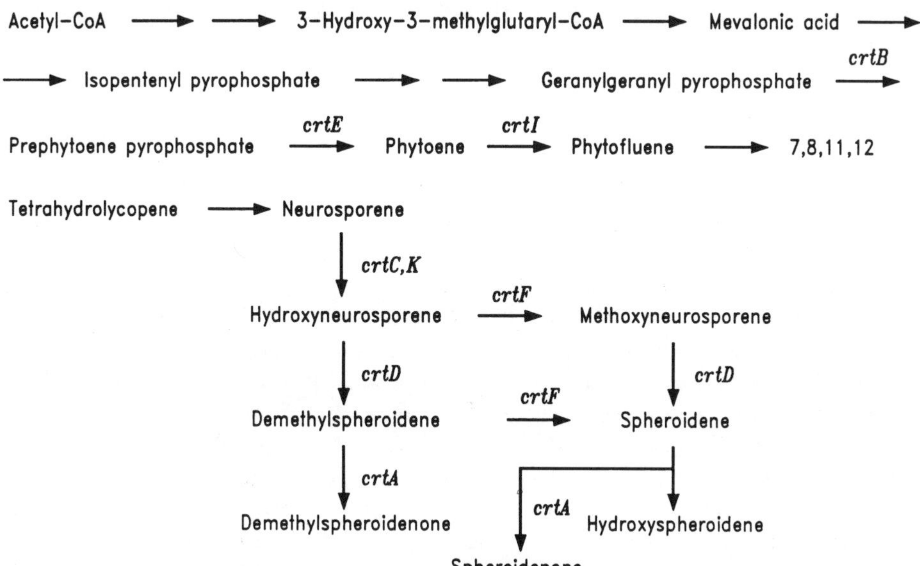

FIGURE 1. Pathway of Crt biosynthesis. Genes assigned to biosynthetic steps are indicated. CoA, Coenzyme A. (Adapted from Giuliano et al. [1988] and Armstrong et al. [1989].)

MAPPING OF Crt GENES

Crt genes were first mapped in *R. capsulatus* via recombinational rescue of point mutations by using a bacteriophagelike gene transfer agent (Yen and Marrs, 1976). Five Crt genes, *crtA* to *-E*, were identified in this way. Similarly, *crtF* and *crtG* were mapped to the cluster by Scolnik et al. (1980), although *crtG* has since been subsumed into the *crtD* gene. Construction of the R-prime plasmid pRPS404, carrying most of the genes for photosynthesis (Marrs, 1981), allowed the alignment of genes *crtA* to *-F* to a physical map by marker rescue (Taylor et al., 1983). Transposon mutagenesis of pRPS404 led Zsebo and Hearst (1984) to map *crtI* to the cluster and *crtJ* approximately 12 kilobases (kb) from the cluster. Sequencing of the 11-kb cluster confirmed the previous mapping and added another gene, *crtK* (Armstrong et al., 1989). Thus, the gene order is *crtJ, -A, -I, -B, -K, -C, -D, -E, -F*. Mutant phenotypes are CrtB, -E, -I, and -J ("blue-green" [white]), CrtC, -K, and -D (green), CrtA (yellow), and CrtF (tan).

In *R. sphaeroides*, chromosome mobilization indicated that genes *crtA* to *-F* were chromosomally located and clustered (Pemberton and Bowen, 1981; Bowen and Pemberton, 1985). After cloning of the cluster (Pemberton and Harding, 1986), the genes were transferred to several nonphotosynthetic relatives of *R. sphaeroides* (Pemberton and Harding, 1987). Every relative synthesized carotenoids, indicating that the 28-kb cloned segment carries all of the genes for Crt biosynthesis. Transposon mutagenesis of this DNA, using *P. denitrificans* as a haploid expression host, suggests that the gene order is similar if not identical to that found in *R. capsulatus* (R. J. Penfold and J. M. Pemberton, unpublished data).

CONTROL OF Crt SYNTHESIS

Both high light intensity and high oxygen tension depress Crt synthesis (Cohen-Bazire et al., 1957). Biel and Marrs (1985) suggested that the effect of oxygen is not direct but occurs via the oxygen-regulated synthesis of Bchl or some other component of the photosynthetic membrane system. However, it is possible that Crts turn over faster in the absence of Crt-binding proteins, which themselves are unstable in the absence of Bchl (Scolnik and Marrs, 1987). Guiliano et al. (1988) found increased steady-state *crtE*, *crtA*, and *crtC* mRNA levels in anaerobic versus aerobic cultures of *R. capsulatus*. An anaerobic-to-aerobic shift induces the conversion of demethylspheroidene and spheroidene into their keto derivatives (Schmidt, 1978). Thus, yellow spheroidene is converted to red spheroidenone by the *crtA* gene product (Scolnik et al., 1980). Interestingly, *P. denitrificans* carrying the Crt genes of *R. sphaeroides* shows the same color change upon exposure to oxygen (Penfold and Pemberton, unpublished observations). Sequencing of the Crt gene cluster has revealed highly conserved palindromic sequences that are homologous to the consensus binding site of a variety of procaryotic DNA-binding regulatory proteins (Armstrong et al., 1989). Undoubtedly, the availability of these sequencing data will stimulate precise analyses of Crt gene regulation by oxygen and light.

MAPPING OF Bchl GENES

Pioneering work by Jones (1978) and Rebiez and Lascelles (1982) led to a proposed pathway for Bchl synthesis (Fig. 2) based on intermediates excreted by mutants. Assaying the pathway has proven particularly difficult; only the product of the *bchH* gene, *S*-adenosylmethionine-Mg-protoporphyrin methyltransferase, has been assayed in vitro (Gibson et al., 1963).

The mapping of *bch* and *crt* genes has proceeded largely in parallel by use of similar methodology. Twelve genes (*bchA*, *-C*, *-I*, *-D*, *-G*, *-J*, *-E*, *-B*, *-F*, *-K*, *-H*, and *-L*, in that order), covering approximately 30 kb, have been mapped in *R. capsulatus* (Yen and Marrs, 1976; Taylor et al., 1983; Zsebo and Hearst, 1984). By using cosmid cloning, 100 kb of the *R. sphaeroides* chromosome has been shown to carry the Crt gene cluster and an undetermined number of Bchl genes (Pemberton and Harding, 1986, 1987; A. H. Ross and J. M. Pemberton, unpublished data). Recently, Coomber and Hunter (1989) isolated smaller overlapping clones covering 45 kb of the photosynthesis region of *R. sphaeroides*. The authors found that the gross organization of photosynthesis genes (*puh*, *bchB*, *bchE*, Crt gene cluster, *bchC*, *bchA*, and *puf*, in that order) was very similar to that found in *R. capsulatus*.

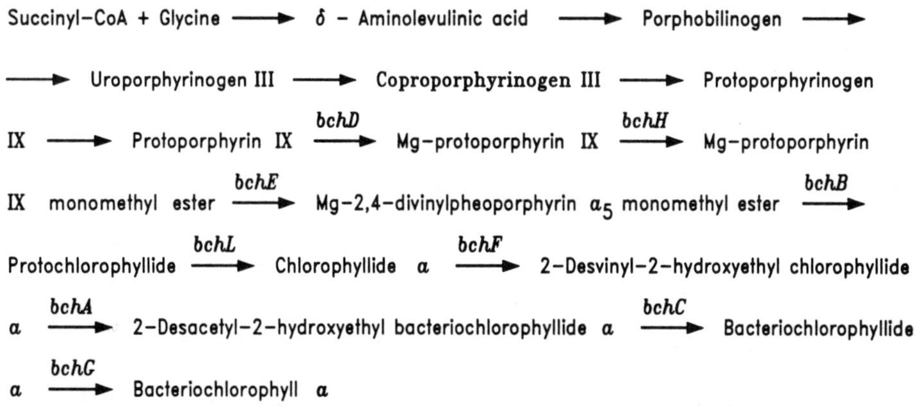

Succinyl–CoA + Glycine ⟶ δ – Aminolevulinic acid ⟶ Porphobilinogen ⟶

⟶ Uroporphyrinogen III ⟶ Coproporphyrinogen III ⟶ Protoporphyrinogen

IX ⟶ Protoporphyrin IX $\xrightarrow{bchD}$ Mg–protoporphyrin IX $\xrightarrow{bchH}$ Mg–protoporphyrin

IX monomethyl ester $\xrightarrow{bchE}$ Mg–2,4–divinylpheoporphyrin a_5 monomethyl ester $\xrightarrow{bchB}$

Protochlorophyllide $\xrightarrow{bchL}$ Chlorophyllide α $\xrightarrow{bchF}$ 2–Desvinyl–2–hydroxyethyl chlorophyllide

α $\xrightarrow{bchA}$ 2–Desacetyl–2–hydroxyethyl bacteriochlorophyllide α $\xrightarrow{bchC}$ Bacteriochlorophyllide

α $\xrightarrow{bchG}$ Bacteriochlorophyll α

FIGURE 2. Pathway of Bchl biosynthesis. Genes assigned to biosynthetic steps are indicated. (Adapted from Jones [1978], Rebeiz and Lascelles [1982], and Hunter and Coomber [1988].)

CONTROL OF Bchl SYNTHESIS

Cohen-Bazire et al. (1957) demonstrated that Bchl synthesis was strongly inhibited by oxygen and to a lesser degree by high light intensities. Subsequent studies of enzymes implicated in the regulation of photopigment production have focused on these variables (Jones, 1978; Rebiez and Lascelles, 1982).

Figure 2 includes a number of reactions critical to the synthesis of tetrapyrroles. The formation of δ-aminolevulinic acid (ALA) by ALA synthase is the first committed step in tetrapyrrole synthesis. ALA synthase activity appears to be controlled through feedback inhibition by hemin or Mg^{2+} protoporphyrin IX (Lascelles, 1978). Two ALA synthases have been isolated from *R. sphaeroides*: a cytoplasmic enzyme presumably associated with chemoheterotrophic growth and a membrane-bound enzyme associated with photosynthetic growth (Fanica-Gaigner and Clement-Metral, 1973). Tai et al. (1988), using an ALA synthase gene probe from *Rhizobium meliloti*, located two distinct genes in *R. sphaeroides* that presumably encode these enzymes.

Under photosynthetic conditions, the differential chelation of metal ions into protoporphyrin IX yields Bchl (Mg), hemes (Fe), and corrinoids (Co). Two chelating enzymes are thought to exist, Mg^{2+} chelatase and ferrochelatase. Mg^{2+} chelatase has yet to be isolated and assayed in vitro, but studies on *R. sphaeroides* suggest that it is membrane bound and inhibited by oxygen (Gorchein, 1973). Ferrochelatase is oxygen sensitive and inserts Fe^{2+}, Co^{2+}, and Zn^{2+} but has little activity towards Mg^{2+} (Rebeiz and Lascelles, 1982). Bauer and Marrs (1988) identified a polypeptide, encoded by *pufQ*, thought to act as a carrier for Bchl intermediates. Such a carrier, proposed by Lascelles (1978), would act as an obligatory membrane-bound cofactor for Bchl synthesis. Control of Bchl levels would thus be achieved by regulating the synthesis and/or activity of a single polypeptide. In addition, the presence of the gene in the *puf* operon potentiates joint regulation for production of Bchl and reaction center/B875 polypeptides.

Finally, the phytol side chain, added to Mg^{2+} bacteriochlorophyllide *a* to give Bchl (Brown and Lascelles, 1972), is derived from geranylgeranyl pyrophosphate (Fig. 1) and thus provides a link between the two photopigment biosynthetic pathways.

CONCLUSION

The question still remains: are all of the genes for photosynthesis clustered in this single region of the chromosome and can they be cloned as a unit and expressed in a nonphotosynthetic bacterium? Mapping, cloning, sequencing, and expression of the Crt genes of *R. sphaeroides* in nonphotosynthetic bacteria is the first step in answering this question. The next step is to use the same techniques for Bchl, cytochrome, *puc*, *puf*, and *puh* gene products and other components of the photosynthetic apparatus.

ACKNOWLEDGMENTS. This work was supported by Australian Research Grants Scheme grant D28315570 from the Australian government and the Mayne Bequest Fund of the University of Queensland. R.J.P. is supported by a Commonwealth postgraduate research award from the Australian government.

We thank Karen Vincent for helpful discussions.

LITERATURE CITED

Armstrong, G. A., M. Alberti, F. Leach, and J. E. Hearst. 1989. Nucleotide sequence, organization, and nature of the protein products of the carotenoid biosynthesis gene cluster of *Rhodobacter capsulatus*. *Mol. Gen. Genet.* **216**:254–268.

Bauer, C. E., and B. L. Marrs. 1988. *Rhodobacter capsulatus puf* operon encodes a regulatory protein (PufQ) for bacteriochlorophyll synthesis. *Proc. Natl. Acad. Sci. USA* **85**:7074–7078.

Biel, A. J., and B. L. Marrs. 1985. Oxygen does not directly regulate carotenoid biosynthesis in *Rhodopseudomonas capsulata*. *J. Bacteriol.* **162**:1320–1321.

Bowen, A. R. St. G., and J. M. Pemberton. 1985. Mercury resistance transposon Tn*813* mediates chromosome transfer in *Rhodopseudomonas sphaeroides* and intergeneric transfer of pBR322, p. 105–115. *In* D. R. Helsinki, S. N. Cohen, D. B. Clewell, D. A. Jackson, and A. Hollaender (ed.), *Plasmids in Bacteria*. Plenum Publishing Corp., New York.

Brown, A. E., and J. Lascelles. 1972. Phytol and bacteriochlorophyll synthesis in *Rhodopseudomonas spheroides*. *Plant Physiol.* **50**:747–749.

Cohen-Bazire, G., W. R. Sistrom, and R. Y. Stanier. 1957. Kinetic studies of pigment synthesis by non-sulfur purple bacteria. *J. Cell. Comp. Physiol.* **49**:25–68.

Collins, M. D. and D. Jones. 1981. Distribution of isoprenoid quinone structural types in bacteria and their taxonomic implications. *Microbiol. Rev.* **45**:316–354.

Coomber, S. A., and C. N. Hunter. 1989. Construction of a physical map of the 45 kb photosynthetic gene cluster of *Rhodobacter sphaeroides*. *Arch. Microbiol.* **151**:454–458.

Fanica-Gaigner, M., and J. Clement-Metral. 1973. Cellular compartmentation of two species of δ-aminolevulinic acid synthetase in a facultative photoheterotrophic bacterium *Rhodopseudomonas sphaeroides*. *Biochem. Biophys. Res. Commun.* **55**:610–615.

Gibson, K. D., A. Neuberger, and G. H. Tait. 1963. Studies on the biosynthesis of porphyrin and bacteriochlorophyll by *Rhodopseudomonas spheroides*. *Biochem. J.* **88**:325–334.

Giuliano, G., D. Pollock, H. Stapp, and P. A. Scolnik. 1988. A genetic-physical map of the *Rhodobacter capsulatus* carotenoid biosynthesis gene cluster. *Mol. Gen. Genet.* **213**:78–83.

Gorchein, A. 1973. Control of magnesium protoporphyrin chelatase activity in *Rhodopseudomonas sphaeroides*. *Biochem. J.* **134**:833–845.

Guerola, N., J. L. Ingraham, and E. Cerda'-Olmedo. 1971. Induction of closely linked multiple mutations by nitrosoguanidine. *Nature* (London) **230**:122–125.

Holloway, B. W. 1978. Plasmids that mobilise bacterial chromosomes. *Plasmid* **2:**1–19.

Hunter, C. N., and S. A. Coomber. 1988. Cloning and oxygen-regulated expression of the bacteriochlorophyll biosynthesis genes *bchE, B, A,* and *C* of *Rhodobacter sphaeroides. J. Gen. Microbiol.* **134:**1491–1497.

Jones, O. T. G. 1978. Biosynthesis of porphyrins, hemes and chlorophylls, p. 751–777. *In* R. K. Clayton and W. R. Sistrom (ed.), *The Photosynthetic Bacteria.* Plenum Publishing Corp., New York.

Kiley, P. J., and S. Kaplan. 1988. Molecular genetics of photosynthetic membrane biosynthesis in *Rhodobacter sphaeroides. Microbiol. Rev.* **52:**50–69.

Lascelles, J. 1978. Regulation of pyrrole synthesis, p. 795–808. *In* R. K. Clayton and W. R. Sistrom (ed.) *The Photosynthetic Bacteria.* Plenum Publishing Corp., New York.

Liaaen-Jensen, S., G. Cohen-Bazire, and R. Y. Stanier. 1961. Biosynthesis of carotenoids in purple bacteria: a re-evaluation based on considerations of chemical structure. *Nature* (London) **192:** 1168–1172.

Marrs, B. 1981. Mobilization of the genes for photosynthesis from *Rhodopseudomonas capsulata* by a promiscuous plasmid. *J. Bacteriol.* **146:**1003–1012.

Pemberton, J. M., and A. R. Bowen. 1981. High frequency chromosome transfer in *Rhodopseudomonas sphaeroides* promoted by the broad-host-range plasmid RP1 carrying the mercury transposon Tn*501. J. Bacteriol.* **147:**110–117.

Pemberton, J. M., S. Cooke, and A. R. St. G. Bowen. 1983. Gene transfer mechanisms among members of the genus *Rhodopseudomonas. Ann. Microbiol.* (Paris) **134b:**195–204.

Pemberton, J. M., and C. M. Harding. 1986. Cloning of carotenoid biosynthesis genes from *Rhodopseudomonas sphaeroides. Curr. Microbiol.* **14:**25–29.

Pemberton, J. M., and C. M. Harding. 1987. Expression of *Rhodopseudomonas sphaeroides* carotenoid photopigment genes in phylogenetically related nonphotosynthetic bacteria. *Curr. Microbiol.* **14:**25–29.

Rebeiz, C. A., and J. Lascelles. 1982. Biosynthesis of pigments in plants and bacteria, p. 699–780. *In* Govindjee (ed.), *Photosynthesis: Energy Conversion by Plants and Bacteria,* vol. 1. Academic Press, Inc., New York.

Schmidt, K. 1978. Biosynthesis of carotenoids, p. 729–750. *In* R. K. Clayton and W. R. Sistrom (ed.), *The Photosynthetic Bacteria.* Plenum Publishing Corp., New York.

Scolnik, P. A., and B. L. Marrs. 1987. Genetic research with photosynthetic bacteria. *Annu. Rev. Microbiol.* **41:**703–726.

Scolnik, P. A., M. A. Walker, and B. L. Marrs. 1980. Biosynthesis of carotenoids from neurosporene in *Rhodopseudomonas capsulata. J. Biol. Chem.* **255:**2427–2432.

Siefermann-Harms, D. 1987. The light-harvesting and protective functions of carotenoids in photosynthetic membranes. *Physiol. Plant.* **69:**561–568.

Sistrom, W. R. 1977. Transfer of chromosomal genes mediated by plasmid R68.45 in *Rhodopseudomonas sphaeroides. J. Bacteriol.* **131:**526–532.

Tai, T., M. D. Moore, and S. Kaplan. 1988. Cloning and characterization of the 5-aminolevulinate synthase gene(s) from *Rhodobacter sphaeroides. Gene* **70:**139–151.

Taylor, D. P., S. N. Cohen, W. G. Clark, and B. L. Marrs. 1983. Alignment of genetic and restriction maps of the photosynthesis region of the *Rhodopseudomonas capsulata* chromosome by a conjugation-mediated marker rescue technique. *J. Bacteriol.* **154:**580–590.

Willison, J. C., G. Ahombo, J. Chabert, J.-P. Magnin, and P. M. Vignais. 1985. Genetic mapping of the *Rhodopseudomonas capsulata* chromosome shows non-clustering of genes involved in nitrogen fixation. *J. Gen. Microbiol.* **131:**3001–3015.

Yen, H., and B. Marrs. 1976. Map of genes for carotenoid and bacteriochlorophyll biosynthesis in *Rhodopseudomonas capsulata. J. Bacteriol.* **126:**619–629.

Zsebo, K. M., and J. E. Hearst. 1984. Genetic-physical mapping of a photosynthetic gene cluster from *R. capsulata. Cell* **37:**937–947.

Chapter 36

Ferric Uptake Regulation (Fur) Repressor: Facts and Fantasies

J. B. Neilands

The purpose of this chapter is not to present new data but rather to review the status of high-affinity, siderophore-microbial iron uptake and to present an overview of the subject. The focus will be on regulation, since this is deemed to be an important feature of iron assimilation in all forms of life. Furthermore, the mode of regulation of iron absorption at the molecular level can now be approached experimentally. As in so many other aspects of experimental biology, work with *Escherichia coli* has led the way. However, research in the field is extending rapidly to other enteric organisms, to gram-negative bacteria generally, and to selected species of gram-positive bacteria and fungi. This seems to be a propitious moment to review the work with *E. coli*.

An important role for iron in biology was established in the early decades of the last century, when the metal was found to be associated with hemoglobin. The research of Keilin (1966) and Warburg (1949) on respiration demonstrated that iron is required for reduction as well as transport of oxygen. In the present context, the studies of McCance and Widdowson (1937) are of seminal importance. Their conclusion that the amount of iron in the animal body "must be regulated by controlled absorption" seems applicable to all species, including microorganisms. For recent reviews, the reader is referred to Braun and Winkelmann (1987), Bagg and Neilands (1987a), Weinberg (1984), and Winkelmann et al. (1987).

IRON IN MICROBIOLOGY

According to present knowledge, the only microbial species that may have zero nutritional need for iron are certain lactobacilli. These species flourish in milk which, like all body secretions, is notoriously low in iron. Archibald (1983) cultured *Lactobacillus plantarum* in media specially treated to remove iron but

---

J. B. Neilands • Biochemistry Department, University of California, Berkeley, California 94720.

still found more than one atom of the metal per bacterial cell. Since the true lactobacilli contain no cytochromes or hydroperoxidases and no heme compounds of any type, and since they have adopted the cobalt-containing rather than the iron-containing form of ribonucleotide reductase, the small amount of iron found probably represented adventitious contamination.

Bacteria and fungi require iron for the synthesis of both heme- and non-heme-containing enzymes, of which there is a considerable variety in most species. It is generally assumed that aerobic growth will elicit a higher demand for iron, since in such circumstances the metal will be diverted into cytochrome synthesis. When iron is limiting, the cell will be switched to a more fermentative mode, and organic acids will be accumulated rather than oxidized through the tricarboxylic acid cycle.

Antibiosis via iron deprivation appears to be a commonly used device to avoid sepsis in animal tissues. Transferrin, the iron-binding protein of serum, is usually only one-third saturated with the metal. Schade and Caroline (1946) were the first to show that the bacteriostatic property of serum could be overcome by the addition of simple iron salts. The lactoferrin found in milk and in tears has a similar antimicrobial role, as does the ovotransferrin of egg white. Among the bacteria, it seems that each species strives to synthesize a specific siderophore and cognate membrane receptor in an attempt to monopolize the iron supply in the immediate vicinity. Since ferric siderophores are generally too large to traverse the small water-filled pores of the outer membrane of gram-negative bacteria, the participation of an outer membrane receptor is required. In the course of evolution, these receptors have become exploited by a range of lethal agents—antibiotics, bacteriophages, and bacteriocins—as a means of gaining entry to the cell.

STRATEGIES FOR MICROBIAL IRON ASSIMILATION

From the foregoing discussion, it is apparent that virtually all microorganisms must have iron to satisfy essential cellular processes such as energy production and replication of DNA. However, the supply is not easily available. In the external environment, the metal is present as insoluble oxy-hydroxide polymers. As an obstacle for pathogenic species, host tissues have the iron tightly seques-tered in heme or proteins. Thus, the options are utilization of chelated iron (protein or nonprotein), reduction to the soluble Fe(II) state, or acidification. The critical role of iron in microbiology appears to have required the employment of all of these devices.

With very few exceptions, microorganisms respond to iron deficiency by excretion of one or more siderophores, which are low-molecular-weight, virtually Fe(III)-specific ligands. The most commonly encountered siderophores are either hydroxamic acids or catechols, with ferrichrome and enterobactin as the proto-typical members of the two classes. Vanoxonin (Kanai et al., 1983), from *Saccharopolyspora hirsuta*, is an example of a simple dipeptide containing both of these functional groups. The alpha-hydroxy acid cluster and the tertiary N of an oxazoline or thiazoline ring are also commonly used to chelate the iron, often as a supplement to hydroxamic acid and catechol ligands. Rhizobactin, from *Rhizobium meliloti* DM4, binds metal ions at a centrally located ethylenediamine moiety surrounded by several carboxylic acid groups (Smith et al., 1985). Maduraferrin, a siderophore from *Actinomadura madurae*, complexes iron via a central hydroxamic acid group and two other chelation centers located at opposite ends of a peptide chain, one a salicylic acid moiety and the other an acid hydrazide group (Keller-Schierlein et al., 1988). Obviously, the structural variety within the siderophore family is expanding rapidly as nuclear magnetic resonance, mass spectroscopy, and crystallography are applied for characterization of new members of the series.

The human pathogens *Neisseria gonorrhoeae* and *N. meningitidis* have dispensed with synthesis of a soluble siderophore but have retained specific surface receptors for iron chelated in the form of transferrin and lactoferrin (Mickelsen and Sparling, 1981).

The common yeast *Saccharomyces cerevisiae* likewise does not form a siderophore, although in minimal medium the organism requires the addition of about 3 μM iron for maximal growth (Neilands, 1987). At low iron levels, the accumulation of organic acids, particularly citrate, may render iron available. In addition, each unit decrease in pH augments the solubility of ferric ion by a factor of 10^3. A recent study shows that *S. cerevisiae*, while not itself synthesizing a siderophore, is able to take up ferrioxamine B via a high-affinity pathway (Lesuisse and Labbe, 1989). This opportunistic strategy is frequently encountered in bacterial species. As in plants, iron starvation resulted in enhanced reductase activity.

Zimmermann et al. (1989) reported a mechanistically novel Fe(III) transport system in *Serratia marcescens*. The system, which is devoid of siderophores and their receptors, could be cloned on a 4.8-kilobase (kb) fragment and expressed in *E. coli*. Chromosomal functions, distinct from the *tonB* and *exbB* genes needed for utilization of siderophore iron, were required for operation of the system in *E. coli*.

THE NEED FOR REGULATION

In the absence of a biological mechanism for excretion of iron, the cellular level is maintained by the rate of absorption. All species have at least some capacity to store the metal, and ferritinlike proteins occur in plants and bacteria. The protein from *E. coli* has recently been sequenced, but it shows little homology to animal ferritin (Andrews et al., 1989). Furthermore, bacterioferritin contains both heme and ferritin iron and displays enzyme activity (cytochome b_1).

Although cytochrome *c* oxidase efficiently adds four electrons to O_2 to form water, a certain level of partially reduced species, such as superoxide and peroxide, must occur in all aerobic tissues. Reactions such as the following, although possibly an oversimplification, demonstrate how tissue-damaging hydroxyl radical can arise from Fe(III) and Fe(II) ions not bound to protein:

$$O_2^{\cdot -} + Fe^{3+} = O_2 + Fe^{2+}$$
$$H_2O_2 + Fe^{2+} = OH^- + OH^{\cdot} + Fe^{3+}$$

The important point to note is that the metal ions act catalytically to generate hydroxyl radicals. Stevens et al. (1988) have reported a higher incidence of cancer in men with elevated body stores of iron.

ORGANIZATION OF THE AEROBACTIN OPERON OF *E. COLI*

It is now about a decade since Laird et al. (1980) and Laird and Young (1980) cloned the enterobactin determinants of *E. coli* and reported the biosynthetic and transport genes for the siderophore to be organized in several transcriptional units and spread over more than 20 kb of DNA. About the same time, Williams (1979) discovered that *E. coli* could synthesize a hydroxamate siderophore coded by pColV-K30, a large conjugative plasmid associated with clinical isolates of the bacterium. After identification of the siderophore as aerobactin (Warner et al., 1981), previously characterized from *Aerobacter aerogenes* I-62 (Gibson and Magrath, 1969), several laboratories participated in elucidation of the molecular genetics of the system. Bindereif and Neilands (1983) obtained two clones from pColV-K30, one about 16 kb and containing the entire regulatory, biosynthetic, and transport genes from the parent plasmid, and the other an 8-kb fragment bearing only the regulatory and biosynthetic determinants. This finding suggested an operon structure, but it was several years before the order and number of the genes could be determined, their products identified, and functions assigned to them. The work has been reviewed by Bagg and Neilands (1987a). The operon contains four genes, designated *iucABCD* (*iuc* for iron uptake chelate), which specify synthesis of aerobactin in four steps from L-lysine and citrate (Fig. 1). The fifth gene, *iutA* (*iut* for iron uptake transport), codes for an outer membrane receptor for ferric aerobactin. A number of additional genes, such as *tonB*, are chromosomally located and are also required for general utilization of siderophore iron.

The aerobactin operon, as a consequence of its presence in *E. coli* and its relative simplicity, is presently the best defined in the siderophore series. Two of the five genes have been sequenced, and three of the four biosynthetic proteins have been isolated in pure form (Neilands, 1987). Biosynthesis of aerobactin is initiated by an oxygenase, the product of *iucD*. The use of *phoA* and *lacZ* fusions proved that the oxygenase is embedded in the cytoplasmic membrane (Herrero et al., 1988). The sequence suggests the presence of an insertionlike element at the N terminus which, however, is not cleaved, and the mature protein retains the element and the initial methionine. The unusual codon usage in *iucD* indicates that it may have the slowest transcriptional rate in the gene cluster and so serve as a pacemaker for aerobactin synthesis. The enzyme is presumed to be a monooxygenase, and it has been obtained in a pure form and shown to require NADPH and FAD as cofactors (Plattner et al., 1989). The second gene, *iucB*, codes for an acetylase transferring the acetyl moiety from acetyl coenzyme A to N^6-hydroxylysine (Coy et al., 1986). The two remaining genes, *iucA* and *iucC*, code for

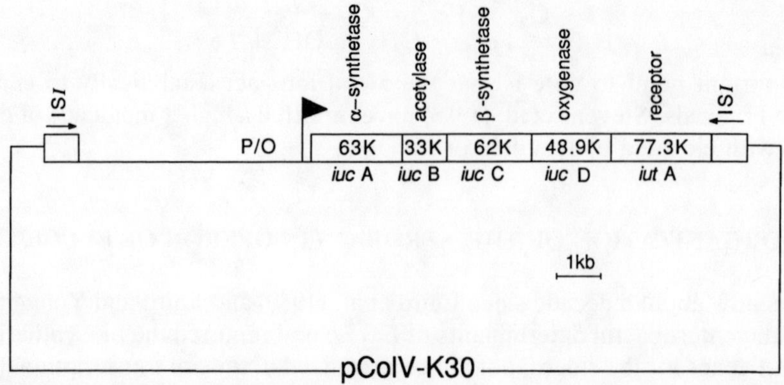

FIGURE 1. Organization of the five-gene aerobactin operon of pColV-K30 containing the biosynthetic (*iuc*) and outer membrane transport (*iut*) genes. Molecular mass values of the corresponding polypeptides given to the nearest 0.1 kilodalton (K) signify that the gene has been sequenced. The flag marks the start of the transcript. Both IS*1* elements engage in cointegrate formation, thus lending a transposonlike character to the cluster (de Lorenzo et al., 1988c). The Fur repressor, when activated by an appropriate divalent metal ion, binds at primary, secondary, and nonspecific sites through the promoter-operator (P/O) region.

subunits of a synthetase which adds, in succession, two residues of N^6-acetyl-N^6-hydroxylysine to the distal carboxyl groups of citrate. The fifth and final gene of the operon, *iutA*, specifies the 74-kilodalton outer membrane protein that serves as a common receptor for ferric aerobactin and cloacin.

Some important work remains to be done in order to clear up all remaining details of the aerobactin operon. Of particular interest would be the discovery of a powerful, nontoxic inhibitor of the monooxygenase that could be used in vivo to block aerobactin synthesis. There is abundant evidence that aerobactin is a virulence factor in bacteria infecting humans and experimental animals (de Lorenzo and Martinez, 1988).

Addition of one side chain of N^6-acetyl-N^6-hydroxylysine to citrate results in the generation of a chiral carbon in the tricarboxylic acid. This product has been isolated, but its absolute configuration has not been determined. Regarding the acetylase, an enzyme of this type should be required for the synthesis of all siderophores containing the hydroxamic acid bond. The enzyme is easily assayed, and, at least from *E. coli*(pColV-K30), is readily isolated by adsorption chromatography on Sepharose CL-6B. Thus, it should be feasible to access at least some of the genes for hydroxamate siderophore synthesis in any microbe by reverse genetics based on the amino acid sequence of the acetylase.

Aerobactin occurs generally, side-by-side with enterobactin, in enteric bacteria. Systems have been described from *Salmonella*, *Shigella*, and *Enterobacter* spp., and in some cases these seem closely homologous to the prototypical one from pColV-K30; in other cases, such as in *Enterobacter cloacae*, the system seems quite unrelated (Crosa et al., 1988). According to a recent report (Valvano and Crosa, 1988), the chromosomally coded aerobactin complex from a K-1 strain of *E. coli* is not regulated in a K-12 background. This finding suggests that the

K-12 repressor does not recognize the K-1 operator, which differs only slightly from that found on pColV-K30.

In view of the prevalence of aerobactin synthesis in clinical isolates of enteric bacteria, it was concluded that the ability to form the siderophore contributes to extracellular pathogenesis and to extracellular stages of growth of intracellular pathogens, such as *Shigella* spp. (de Lorenzo and Martinez, 1988).

FUR-DEPENDENT REGULATION OF GENE EXPRESSION

Ernst et al. (1978) obtained mutants of *Salmonella typhimurium* that constitutively expressed all systems for siderophore synthesis and transport. The mutants were designated *fur* (ferric uptake regulation), and it was considered that they could be defective in formation of a repressor. Hantke (1981) detected the same mutation in *E. coli*, cloned the gene (Hantke, 1984), and together with other researchers sequenced it (Schaffer et al., 1985). The Fur protein was then isolated (Wee et al., 1988) and shown to regulate β-galactosidase synthesis in an in vitro transcription-translation system from *lacZ* fused in the aerobactin operon (Bagg and Neilands, 1987b). Activity was found to be absolutely dependent on the presence of a divalent heavy-metal ion as corepressor, and in the case of iron, strictly reducing conditions were required. From these data, it was reasoned that the biologically active metal species is Fe(II).

Equilibrium dialysis of Fur with radioactive iron in 1% ascorbic acid solution suggests a binding affinity of about 10^5 M, which would be compatible with the metal-binding rather than metalloprotein nature of the repressor (Nakamura et al., 1989). The sites and number of Fe(II) ions bound to Fur are unknown, but since the relatively small protein, 17 kilodaltons, contains 12 histidines, it is probable that imidazole nuclei are involved. In the C-terminal half of the molecule, a pentapeptide, -His-His-His-Asp-His-, is a likely site of attachment of iron. This is followed shortly by a second pentapeptide, -Cys-Leu-Asp-Cys-Gly-, homologous to a common motif in rubredoxins and ferredoxins. Still closer to the C terminus is the order -Cys-X_4-Cys-X_4-His-X-His-, which resembles domains in metal- and DNA-binding proteins. These sequences in Fur are similar to those in several other bacterial proteins which have redox active thiols and which may depend on a change on oxidation state of the coordinated metal ion (Henderson et al., 1989). Two basic mechanisms are possible to account for inactivation of Fur as a *trans*-acting transcriptional regulator of siderophore synthesis (Fig. 2). In mechanism I, the repressor simply dissociates from the operator at low internal levels of Fe(II). In mechanism II, iron starvation results both in a lower concentration of the metal and, for reasons not entirely clear, in a switch to the higher oxidation state. The latter hypothesis has been put forth to explain the regulation of synthesis of manganese superoxide dismutase in *E. coli*, which is known to be iron dependent (Hassan and Moody, 1987). Anaerobically grown *E. coli*, which may have more difficulty in generating Fe(II), are still derepressed in enterobactin synthesis under low iron stress (Lodge and Emery, 1984). Such cells could not make hydroxamate-type siderophore if such synthesis requires (as is believed)

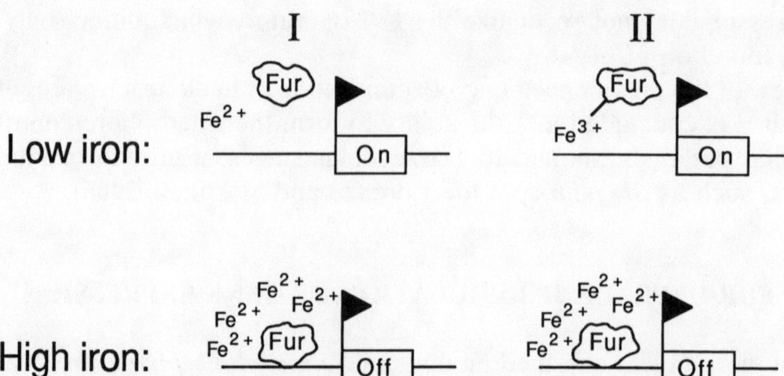

FIGURE 2. Proposed iron associative-dissociative (I) and redox (II) mechanisms for activation-inactivation of the Fur protein of *E. coli* K-12. A redox mechanism involving essential thiols is also possible (see text).

molecular oxygen. Clearly, the functions of the four thiols of Fur require investigation.

Turning to the DNA target, three Fur-regulated genes (Fig. 3), *iuc*, *fur*, and *cir*, have been footprinted, and it is apparent that the repressor, when activated by an appropriate metal ion, recognizes the iron box sequence 5′-GATAATG-ATAATCATTATC, suggested as the primary recognition site (de Lorenzo et al., 1987). A synthetic operator with this sequence placed before *lacZ* as the reporter gene is sufficient for iron regulation in a *fur*+ background (Calderwood and Mekalanos, 1988).

At low nanomolar concentration of Fur, the operator site in the *iuc* promoter is half bound, as estimated by gel shift experiments (Nakamura et al., 1989). Fur initially enters the primary binding site shown in Fig. 3 and at higher levels occupies, in addition, a secondary site displaced toward the operon. Still higher levels of the repressor result in generalized binding through the A+T-rich upstream region. Two factors appear to be involved: site-specific recognition at the iron box, followed by a combination of protein-DNA and protein-protein interactions. The *iuc* promoter is exceptionally strong, and occupation of the two contiguous sites appears necessary for complete repression of the system (de Lorenzo et al., 1988a). Application of the hydroxyl radical footprinting technique indicates that the metal-laden repressor binds around the DNA helix.

An iron box array, with only one more mismatch from the consensus than *iuc*, occurs also in the promoter for the *fur* gene (Fig. 3). The affinity of Fur for its own operator was estimated to be some 40-fold lower than the affinity of the repressor for the *iuc* operator (de Lorenzo et al., 1988b). In this case, no secondary site was occupied. A further difference was the detection of an upstream catabolite gene activator protein (CAP) site that differed in only two mismatches from the consensus CAP sequence. Use of *cya* and *crp* mutants proved the site to be functional. The *fur* gene is thus negatively regulated by its own product, which requires heavy-metal activation, and is positively regulated

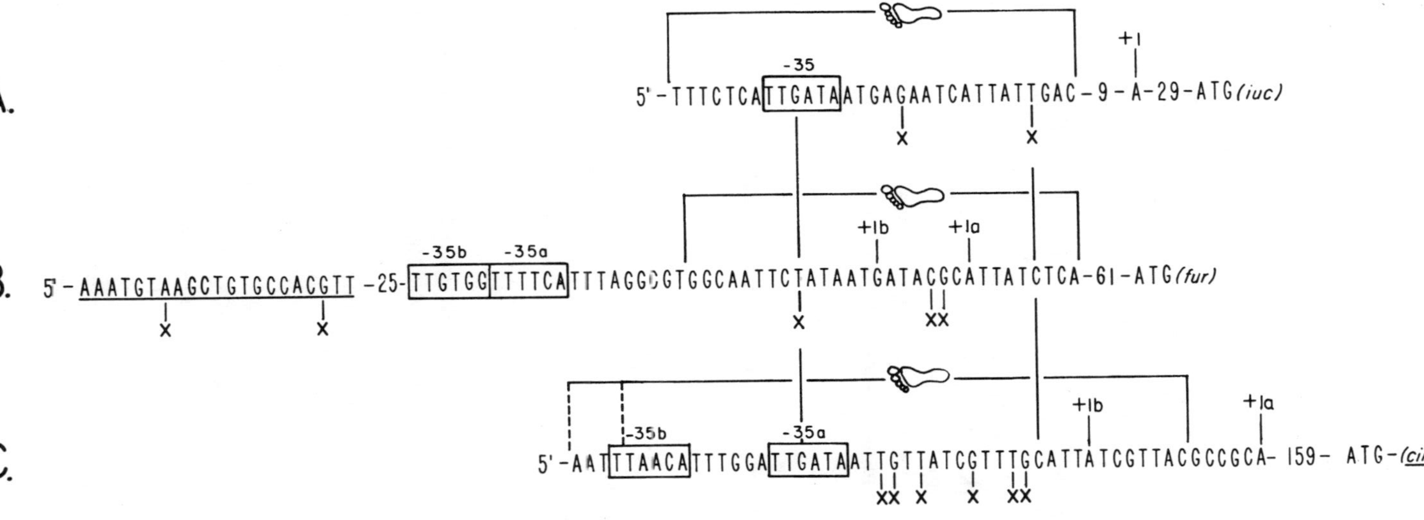

FIGURE 3. Comparison of the operator sites of the aerobactin operon (A), the *fur* gene (B), and the colicin I receptor (C). The footprint symbol indicates the sequences protected by Fur repressor. In sequence A, only the primary binding site is illustrated; in sequence C, the left extremity is uncertain and is indicated by two dashed vertical lines. The iron box consensus sequence, 5'-GATAATGATAAT-CATTATC, is contained within the vertical lines connecting B to A and C. An x indicates a mismatch from the consensus. Numbers refer to the numbers of intervening bases. In sequence B, the CAP sequence is underlined. See de Lorenzo et al. (1988a, 1988b) and Griggs and Konisky (1989).

by the CAP system. This ties iron assimilation into the general metabolic status of the cell.

The third gene that has been footprinted by Fur, *cir*, codes for an outer membrane receptor protein that has long been known to be induced at low iron concentrations. Recent evidence suggests that this receptor may be required for the uptake of ferric monocatechol-type siderophores (Curtis et al., 1988). Footprinting experiments show that the *cir* operator has a relatively high affinity for Fur despite only 68% homology to the consensus iron box (Griggs and Konisky, 1989). As with the *fur* operator, only one site is occupied. Curiously, the *cir* gene is preceded by a short open reading frame, the significance of which for iron assimilation is not understood.

An iron box with varying degrees of homology to the consensus occurs in the upstream regions of a few dozen other iron-regulated genes from *E. coli* (J. B. Neilands, *in* G. Eichhorn, ed., *Advances in Inorganic Chemistry*, in press), from other gram-negative bacteria, such as *Cornyebacterium diphtheriae* (Tai and Holmes, 1988), and even from a cyanobacterial species (Reddy et al., 1988). In the absence of work with reporter genes and footprinting analysis, the role of Fur-like proteins in these species remains somewhat speculative.

THE *ent-fep* GENE CLUSTER

Considerable progress has recently been achieved in deciphering the organization and regulation of the *ent-fep* region at min 13 of the *E. coli* chromosome, encoding genes for biosynthesis of enterobactin and transport of its ferric complex (Earhart, 1987; Pettis et al., 1988; Ozenberger et al., 1989; Nahlik et al., 1989). The general organization of the cluster is $entD \leftarrow fepA \leftarrow P/O \rightarrow fes \rightarrow entF \rightarrow fepE//fepC \leftarrow fepG \leftarrow fepD \leftarrow fepB \leftarrow P/O \rightarrow entC \rightarrow entE \rightarrow entB \rightarrow entA$. In this array, P/O represents bidirectional promoter-operators specifying transcripts from opposite strands. Each of the four putative operators carried at least one iron box sequence. The genes *entC*, *-E*, *-B*, and *-A* comprise an operon. Three soluble enzymes, the products of *entC*, *entB*, and *entA*, convert chorismate to 2,3-dihydroxybenzoic acid. The remaining *ent* genes are required for condensation of this acid with L-serine and conversion of the product via a multienzyme complex to its cyclic trimer, enterobactin. The six *fep* genes code for outer membrane, periplasmic, and cytoplasmic proteins required for ferric enterobactin uptake. Of these, the product of *fepA*, the ferric enterobactin receptor, has been isolated and crystallized (Jalal and van der Helm, 1989). Cells defective in *fes* accumulate ferric enterobactin and become visibly pink in color. Whereas *fes* is thought to code for an esterase needed for hydrolysis of ferric enterobactin and concomitant release of the iron, carbocyclic and aromatic analogs of the siderophore without ester bonds are effective sources of iron for *E. coli* (Hollifield and Neilands, 1978). The mechanism of action of the Fes protein remains unknown.

Table 1

Phenotypes of the *fur* mutation in *E. coli* K-12[a]

System	Effect	Reference

Siderophores
  Enterobactin
  Aerobactin
  Ferrichrome
  Coprogen
  Rhodotorulic acid
  Ferric citrate
	Constitutive biosynthesis of ligands
	  and receptors for ferric
	  complexes	

Ferrous iron transport	Enhanced Fe(II) uptake	Hantke, 1987a
Lethal agents	Constitutive biosynthesis of outer membrane receptors	Staudenmaier et al., 1989
Dicarboxylic acids, acetate	Poor growth	
Manganese resistance	Increased	Hantke, 1987b
Shiga-like toxin	Constitutive synthesis	Calderwood and Mekalanos, 1987
Superoxide dismutase B	Not expressed	Neiderhoffer et al., 1989
Hemolysin	Constitutive biosynthesis (some)	Grunig and Lebek, 1988

[a] For a general reference, see Bagg and Neilands (1987a).

THE ANGUIBACTIN SYSTEM OF *V. ANGUILLARUM* (pJM1)

Vibrio anguillarum, the causative agent of an economically important septicemic infection of fish, is dependent for its virulence on the presence of a 65-kb plasmid (Tolmasky et al., 1988). Some 25 kb of this plasmid, pJM1, encodes the biosynthetic and transport genes for a siderophore, anguibactin. This compound has now been analyzed by X-ray diffraction, and its structure (Jalal et al., 1989) has been shown to be an elaborated form of pyochelin, from *Pseudomonas aeruginosa* (Ankenbauer et al., 1989). As in the case with enterobactin, biosynthetic and transport genes are interspersed, and the cluster is organized into several transcriptional units. The system is controlled by both positive and negative elements. Negative regulation is at the transcriptional level and requires iron.

PERSPECTIVE

It is now a well-established fact that the Fur protein can act as a classical transcriptional repressor. The detection of an extremely high affinity of the Fur protein for the *iuc* operator in vitro created the momentary illusion that the repressor had a single, simple function, namely, reversible binding of Fe(II) and subsequent association with the iron box sequence of siderophore-related genes in *E. coli* K-12. In fact, Fur is part of a global regulon (Table 1). Some of these effects, such as derepression of receptors for lethal agents and sensitivity to

Mn^{2+}, are readily explicable, since they are directly tied to siderophore expression. Others, like regulation of *sodB* and utilization of small carbon substrates, are completely unexplained at present. Furthermore, it is entirely possible that Fur, like other repressors, will be found to play an activator role.

Answers to some of these questions might be sought by application of a systematic two-dimensional gel analysis of proteins in isogenic wild-type and *fur* mutants. In addition, study of *fur* mutants in bacteria both closely and more distinctly related to *E. coli* may afford valuable insights to the structural requirements for activity.

The model for repression by Fur postulates a fluctuating level of Fe^{2+} inside the cell. This remains to be demonstrated, as does the role of the CAP system in stimulating the formation of Fur.

Some obvious additional questions that need to be posed regarding Fur relate to its standard protein chemistry. Does it exist in solution as a dimer, and what is the effect of divalent metal ions on its oligomerization? How many metal ions are bound per monomer, and what is the site of binding? What is the stoichiometry of binding of metallo-Fur to the operator?

With respect to DNA, we need to ask whether there is more than the iron box operator determining the level of expression of iron-regulated genes. For example, are there secondary structures, such as stem-loops, that affect read-out from the transcript?

The Fur system of *E. coli* K-12 is the best defined, in molecular terms, for regulation of assimilation of any nutritious metal ion in any living cell. Be that as it may, we still have much to learn about the manifold changes wrought by the *fur* mutation and about the chemistry and mode of action of Fur.

LITERATURE CITED

Andrews, S. C., J. M. A. Smith, J. R. Guest, and P. M. Harrison. 1989. Amino acid sequence of the bacterioferritin (cytochrome b$_1$) of *Escherichia coli* K-12. *Biochem. Biophys. Res. Commun.* **158**:489–496.

Ankenbauer, R. G., T. Toyokuni, A. Staley, K. L. Rinehart, and C. D. Cox. 1989. Synthesis and biological activity of pyochelin, a siderophore of *Pseudomonas aeruginosa*. *J. Bacteriol.* **170**:5344–5351.

Archibald, F. 1983. *Lactobacillus plantarum*, an organism not requiring iron. *FEMS Microbiol. Lett.* **19**:29–32.

Bagg, A., and J. B. Neilands. 1987a. Molecular mechanism of regulation of siderophore-mediated iron assimilation. *Microbiol. Rev.* **51**:509–518.

Bagg, A., and J. B. Neilands. 1987b. Ferric uptake regulation protein acts as repressor, employing iron (II) as co-factor to bind the operator of an iron transport operon in *Escherichia coli*. *Biochemistry* **26**:5471–5477.

Bindereif, A., and J. B. Neilands. 1983. Cloning of the aerobactin mediated iron assimilation system of plasmid ColV. *J. Bacteriol.* **153**:1111–1113.

Braun, V., and G. Winkelmann. 1987. Microbial iron transport: structure and function of siderophores. *Prog. Clin. Biochem. Med.* **5**:67–99.

Calderwood, S. B., and J. J. Mekalanos. 1987. Iron regulation of Shiga-like toxin expression in *Escherichia coli* is mediated by the *fur* locus. *J. Bacteriol.* **169**:4759–4764.

Calderwood, S. B., and J. J. Mekalanos. 1988. Confirmation of the Fur operator site by insertion of a synthetic oligonucleotide into an operon fusion plasmid. *J. Bacteriol.* **170**:1015–1017.

Coy, M., B. H. Paw, A. Bindereif, and J. B. Neilands. 1986. Isolation and properties of N^ϵ-hydroxylysine-acetylcoenzyme A-N^ϵ transacetylase from *Escherichia coli* pABN11. *Biochemistry* **25**:2485–2489.

Crosa, L. M., M. K. Wolf, L. A. Actis, J. Sanders-Loehr, and J. H. Crosa. 1988. New aerobactin mediated iron uptake system in a septicemia-causing strain of *Enterobacter cloacae*. *J. Bacteriol.* **170**:5539–5544.

Curtis, N. A. C., R. L. Eisenstadt, S. J. East, R. J. Cornford, L. A. Walker, and A. J. White. 1988. Iron regulated outer membrane proteins of *Escherichia coli* K-12 and mechanism of action of catechol-substituted cephalosporins. *Antimicrob. Agents Chemother.* **32**:1879–1886.

de Lorenzo, V., F. Giovannini, M. Herero, and J. B. Neilands. 1988a. Metal ion regulation of gene expression. *J. Mol. Biol.* **203**:875–884.

de Lorenzo, V., M. Herrero, F. Giovannini, and J. B. Neilands. 1988b. Fur (*ferric uptake regulation*) protein and CAP (catabolite-activator protein) modulate transcription of *fur* gene in *Escherichia coli*. *Eur. J. Biochem.* **173**:537–546.

de Lorenzo, V., M. Herrero, and J. B. Neilands. 1988c. IS1-mediated mobility of the aerobactin system of pColV-K30 in *Escherichia coli*. *Mol. Gen. Genet.* **213**:487–490.

de Lorenzo, V., and J. L. Martinez. 1988. Aerobactin production as virulence factor: a re-evaluation. *Eur. J. Clin. Microbiol. Infect. Dis.* **7**:621–629.

de Lorenzo, V., S. Wee, M. Herrero, and J. B. Neilands. 1987. Operator sequences of the aerobactin operon of plasmid ColV-K30 binding the ferric uptake regulation (*fur*) repressor. *J. Bacteriol.* **169**:2624–2630.

Earhart, C. F. 1987. Ferri-enterobactin transport in *Escherichia coli*, p. 67–84. *In* G. Winkelmann, D. van der Helm, and J. B. Neilands (ed.), *Iron Transport in Microbes, Plants and Animals*. VCH Publishers, Weinheim, Federal Republic of Germany.

Ernst, J. F., R. L. Bennett, and L. I. Rothfield. 1978. Constitutive expression of the iron enterochelin and ferrichrome uptake systems in a mutant strain of *Salmonella typhimurium*. *J. Bacteriol.* **135**:928–934.

Gibson, F., and D. J. Magrath. 1969. The isolation and characterization of a hydroxamic acid (aerobactin) formed by *Aerobacter aerogenes* 62-I. *Biochim. Biophys. Acta* **192**:175–184.

Griggs, D. W., and J. Konisky. 1989. Mechanism for iron-regulated transcription of the *Escherichia coli cir* gene. *J. Bacteriol.* **171**:1048–1054.

Grunig, H. M., and G. Lebek. 1988. Haemolytic activity and characteristics of plasmid and chromosomally borne genes from *E. coli* of different origin. *Zentralbl. Bakteriol. Parasitenkd. Infektionskr. Hyg. Abt. 1 Orig. Reihe A* **267**:485–494.

Hantke, K. 1981. Regulation of ferric iron transport in *E. coli*: isolation of a constitutive mutant. *Mol. Gen. Genet.* **182**:288–292.

Hantke, K. 1984. Cloning of the repressor protein gene of iron regulated system in *E. coli* K-12. *Mol. Gen. Genet.* **197**:337–341.

Hantke, K. 1987a. Ferrous iron transport mutants in *Escherichia coli* K-12. *FEMS Microbiol. Lett.* **44**:53–57.

Hantke, K. 1987b. Selection procedure for deregulated iron transport mutants (*fur*) in *Escherichia coli* K-12: *fur* not only affects iron metabolism. *Mol. Gen. Genet.* **210**:135–139.

Hassan, H. M., and C. S. Moody. 1987. Regulation of manganese-containing superoxide dismutase in *Escherichia coli*. *J. Biol. Chem.* **262**:17173–17177.

Henderson, N., S. Austin, and R. A. Dixon. 1989. Role of metal ions in negative regulation of nitrogen fixation by the *nifL* gene product from *Klebsiella pneumoniae*. *Mol. Gen. Genet.* **216**:484–491.

Herrero, M., V. de Lorenzo, and J. B. Neilands. 1988. Nucleotide sequence of the *iucD* gene of the pColV-K30 aerobactin operon and topology of its product studied with *phoA* and *lacZ* fusions. *J. Bacteriol.* **170**:56–64.

Hollifield, W. C., and J. B. Neilands. 1978. Ferric enterobactin transport system in *Escherichia coli* K-12. *Biochemistry* **17**:1922–1928.

Jalal, M. A., M. B. Hossain, D. van der Helm, J. Sanders-Loehr, L. A. Actis, and J. H. Crosa. 1989. Structure of anguibactin, a unique plasmid-related bacterial siderophore from the fish pathogen *Vibrio anguillarum*. *J. Am. Chem. Soc.* **111**:292–296.

Jalal, M. A., and D. van der Helm. 1989. Purification and crystallization of ferric enterobactin receptor protein, FepA, from the outer membranes of *Escherichia coli* UT5600/pBB2. *FEBS Lett.* **243:** 366–370.

Kanai, F., T. Sawa, M. Hamada, H. Naganawa, T. Takeuchi, and H. Umezawa. 1983. Vanoxonin, a new inhibitor of thymidylate synthetase. *J. Antibiot.* **36:**656–660.

Keilin, D. 1966. The history of cell respiration and cytochrome. Cambridge University Press, Cambridge.

Keller-Schierlein, W., L. Hagmann, H. Zahner, and W. Huhn. 1988. Maduraferrin, a new siderophore from *Actinomadura madurae*. *Helv. Chim. Acta* **71:**1528–1540.

Laird, A. J., D. W. Ribbons, G. C. Woodrow, and I. G. Young. 1980. Bacteriophage µ mediated gene transposition and *in vitro* cloning of the enterochelin gene cluster of *Escherichia coli*. *Gene* **11:**347–357.

Laird, A. J., and I. G. Young. 1980. Tn*5* mutagenesis of the enterochelin gene cluster of *Escherichia coli*. *Gene* **11:**359–366.

Lesuisse, E., and P. Labbe. 1989. Reductive and non-reductive mechanisms of iron assimilation by the yeast *Saccharomyces cerevisiae*. *J. Gen. Microbiol.* **135:**257–263.

Lodge, J. S., and T. Emery. 1984. Anaerobic iron uptake by *Escherichia coli*. *J. Bacteriol.* **160:**801–804.

McCance, R. A., and E. M. Widdowson. 1937. Absorption and excretion of iron. *Lancet* **ii:**680–684.

Mickelsen, P. A., and P. F. Sparling. 1981. Ability of *Neisseria gonorrhoeae*, *Neisseria meningitidis*, and commensal *Neisseria* species to obtain iron from transferrin and iron compounds. *Infect. Immun.* **33:**555–564.

Nahlik, M. S., T. J. Brickman, B. A. Ozenberger, and M. A. McIntosh. 1989. Nucleotide sequence and transcriptional organization of the *Escherichia coli* enterobactin biosynthesis cistrons *entB* and *entA*. *J. Bacteriol.* **171:**784–790.

Nakamura, K., V. de Lorenzo, and J. B. Neilands. 1989. *In* T. D. Tullius (ed.), *Metal-DNA Chemistry*. Symposium Series no. 402. American Chemical Society, Washington, D.C.

Neilands, J. B. 1987. Comparative biochemistry of microbial iron assimilation, p. 3–33. *In* G. Winkelmann, D. van der Helm, and J. B. Neilands (ed.), *Iron Transport in Microbes, Plants and Animals*. VCH Publishers, Weinheim, Federal Republic of Germany.

Niederhoffer, E., C. M. Naranjo, and J. A. Fee. 1989. Relationship of the superoxide dismutase genes, *sodA* and *sodB*, to the iron uptake regulon in *E. coli*, p. 149–158. *In* D. Winge and D. Hamer (ed.), *Metal Ion Homeostasis*. Alan R. Liss, Inc., New York.

Ozenberger, B. A., T. J. Brickman, and M. A. McIntosh. 1989. Nucleotide sequence of the *Escherichia coli* isochorismate synthetase gene *entC* and evolutionary relationship to other chorismate-utilizing enzymes. *J. Bacteriol.* **171:**775–783.

Pettis, G. S., T. J. Brickman, and M. A. McIntosh. 1988. Transcriptional mapping and nucleotide sequence of the *Escherichia coli fepA-fes* enterobactin region. *J. Biol. Chem.* **263:**18857–18863.

Plattner, H.-J., P. Pfefferle, A. Romaguera, S. Waschutza, and H. Diekmann. 1989. Isolation and some properties of lysine N^6-hydroxylase from *Escherichia coli* strain EN222. *Biol. Metals* **2:**1–5.

Reddy, K. J., G. S. Bullerjahn, D. M. Sherman, and L. A. Sherman. 1988. Cloning, nucleotide sequence and mutagenesis of a gene (*irpA*) involved in iron-deficient growth of the cyanobacterium *Synechococcus* sp. strain PCC79421. *J. Bacteriol.* **170:**4466–4476.

Schade, A. L., and L. Caroline. 1946. An iron binding component in human blood plasma. *Science* **104:**340–341.

Schaffer, S., K. Hantke, and V. Braun. 1985. Nucleotide sequence of the iron regulatory gene *fur*. *Mol. Gen. Genet.* **201:**204–212.

Smith, M. J., J. N. Shoolery, B. Schwyn, I. Holden, and J. B. Neilands. 1985. Rhizobactin, a structurally novel siderophore from *Rhizobium meliloti*. *J. Am. Chem. Soc.* **107:**1739–1743.

Staudenmaier, H., B. Von Hove, Z. Yaraghi, and V. Braun. 1989. Nucleotide sequences of the *fecBCDE* genes and locations of the proteins suggest a periplasmic binding protein dependent transport mechanism for iron (III) dicitrate in *Escherichia coli*. *J. Bacteriol.* **171:**2626–2633.

Stevens, R. G., D. Y. Jones, M. Smicozzi, and P. R. Taylor. 1988. Body stores and the risk of cancer. *N. Engl. J. Med.* **319:**1047–1052.

Tai, S. S., and R. K. Holmes. 1988. Iron regulation of the cloned diphtheria promoter in *Escherichia coli*. *Infect. Immun.* **56:**2430–2436.

Tolmasky, M. E., L. A. Actis, and J. H. Crosa. 1988. Genetic analysis of the iron uptake region of the *Vibrio anguillarum* plasmid pJM1. *J. Bacteriol.* **170:**1913–1919.

Valvano, M. A., and J. H. Crosa. 1988. Molecular cloning, expression and regulation in *Escherichia coli* K-12 of a chromosome-mediated aerobactin iron transport system from a human invasive strain of *E. coli*. *J. Bacteriol.* **170:**5529–5538.

Warburg, O. 1949. *Heavy Metal Prosthetic Groups*. Clarendon Press, Oxford.

Warner, P. J., P. H. Williams, A. Bindereif, and J. B. Neilands. 1981. ColV plasmid specified aerobactin synthesis by invasive strains of *Escherichia coli*. *Infect. Immun.* **33:**540–545.

Wee, S., J. B. Neilands, M. L. Bittner, B. C. Hemming, B. L. Haymore, and R. Seethram. 1988. Expression, isolation and properties of Fur (*f*erric *u*ptake *r*egulation) protein of *Escherichia coli* K-12. *Biol. Metals* **1:**62–68.

Weinberg, E. D. 1984. Iron withholding: a defense against infection and disease. *Physiol. Rev.* **64:**65–102.

Williams, P. H. 1979. Novel iron uptake system specified by ColV plasmids. *Infect. Immun.* **26:**925–932.

Winkelmann, G., D. van der Helm, and J. B. Neilands (ed.). 1987. *Iron Transport in Microbes, Plants and Animals*. VCH Publishers, Weinheim, Federal Republic of Germany.

Zimmermann, L., A.-M. Angerer, and V. Braun. 1989. Mechanistically novel iron(III) transport system in *Serratia marcescens*. *J. Bacteriol.* **171:**238–243.

Chapter 37

Gene Control of Photosynthetic Membrane Assembly: the Chromosomes of *Rhodobacter sphaeroides*

Samuel Kaplan and Antonius Suwanto

Rhodobacter sphaeroides is a purple, nonsulfur photosynthetic eubacterium able to grow aerobically as a chemoheterotroph and possessing a typical gram-negative morphology. When grown anaerobically in the light, *R. sphaeroides* undergoes an extensive morphological transformation in which the cell membrane undergoes a series of localized differentiations giving rise to the intracytoplasmic membrane system comprising the photosynthetic apparatus and possessing those structural components associated with the entrapment of light energy, electron transport, and the bioenergetics of photosynthesis (Kiley and Kaplan, 1988).

Critical features of these light reactions include the presence of the spectral complexes associated with photosynthesis such as the B875 (B875-α and -β polypeptides) and B800-850 (B800-850-α and -β polypeptides) light-harvesting complexes that function to absorb light energy and transfer this energy to the reaction center (RC; H, L, and M polypeptides) (Meinhardt et al., 1985). These three spectral complexes made up of seven unique polypeptides are encoded by *pufBALM* (B875-β/α; RC-L,M), *puhA* (RC-H), and *pucBA* (B800-850-β/α) (Kiley and Kaplan, 1988). Within the RC, an electron ejected from one of a special pair of bacteriochlorophylls is used to generate a transmembrane potential, with the electrons being cycled back to the oxidized RC after passage through the cytochrome b/c_1 complex encoded by the *fbc* operon (Gabellini et al., 1985) via the mobile electron carrier cytochrome c_2 encoded by *cycA* (Donohue et al., 1986).

Syntheses of bacteriochlorophyll, heme, and vitamin B_{12} involve 5-aminolevulinic acid as the first committed step in the biosynthetic pathway. In *R. sphaeroides*, two duplicate genes, *hemA* and *hemT*, appear to encode this

---

Samuel Kaplan and Antonius Suwanto • Department of Microbiology, The University of Texas Medical School at Houston, 6431 Fannin, P.O. Box 20708, Houston, Texas 77225.

function (Tai et al., 1988). Carbon dioxide fixation involves an operational Calvin cycle including at least two unique enzymes. The first is phosphoribulokinase, encoded by *prkA* and *prkB*, since *R. sphaeroides* possesses two unique genes for this enzyme. The second enzyme is ribulose-1,5-bisphosphate carboxylase/oxygenase, encoded by *rbcL* and *rbcS* for the large- and small-subunit form of the enzyme (form I) and *rbcR* for the large-subunit form (form II) (Hallenbeck and Kaplan, 1988; Tabita, 1988).

Although we have focused on gene-protein relationships and mechanisms of regulation that involve the photosynthetic activities of *R. sphaeroides*, we have been impressed by the remarkable metabolic diversity (e.g., N_2 fixation and anaerobic respiration) of this organism as well as the ability of this organism to regain photosynthetic growth in mutants possessing seemingly lethal genetic blocks involving critical photosynthetic activities. Further, the presence of extensively duplicated genetic regions coding for activities involved in CO_2 fixation and 5-aminolevulinic acid biosynthesis have brought into sharp focus the need for a more thorough understanding of the overall genetic organization of *R. sphaeroides*. Lacking the facile genetic analyses associated with various well-studied experimental systems, we elected to determine the physical structure of the *R. sphaeroides* genome and to place within this physical context the genetic markers now available as well as to provide a framework for those that will become available. We have reasoned that our ability to understand photosynthetic membrane assembly could be enhanced by a more detailed knowledge of the molecular genetics of *R. sphaeroides*.

RESTRICTION ENDONUCLEASE ANALYSIS

Recent advances in the preparation and separation of large DNA fragments have made it possible for us to construct a physical map of the *R. sphaeroides* genome. As an initial approach, it was necessary to determine what restriction endonucleases would be appropriate for such an analysis and then to determine which DNA fragments of the total genomic DNA are of chromosomal origin and which are of plasmid origin (Suwanto and Kaplan, 1989a, 1989b). We had previously shown that *R. sphaeroides* contains five cryptic, endogenous plasmids (Fornari et al., 1984).

In a Beckman TAFE apparatus, *Ase*I digested total genomic DNA from *R. sphaeroides* into 17 resolvable DNA fragments ranging in size from 3 to 1,105 kilobases (kb). Using a range of pulse times, we could resolve the large, mid-size, and small *Ase*I-generated fragments into a series of unique bands (Fig. 1). The 3-, 4-, and 5-kb *Ase*I fragments are too diffuse to be seen, but their existence has been independently established. The restriction endonucleases *Spe*I, *Dra*I, and *Sna*BI also yielded restriction patterns that were easily resolvable. Each of these enzymes has as its recognition sites, DNA sequences that are more A+T rich, reflecting their usefulness because of the high G+C content of *R. sphaeroides*. However, *Ssp*I (5'-AATATT) digests *R. sphaeroides* genomic DNA into more than 200 fragments, and *Ase*I (5'-ATTAAT) yields only 17 fragments. Thus,

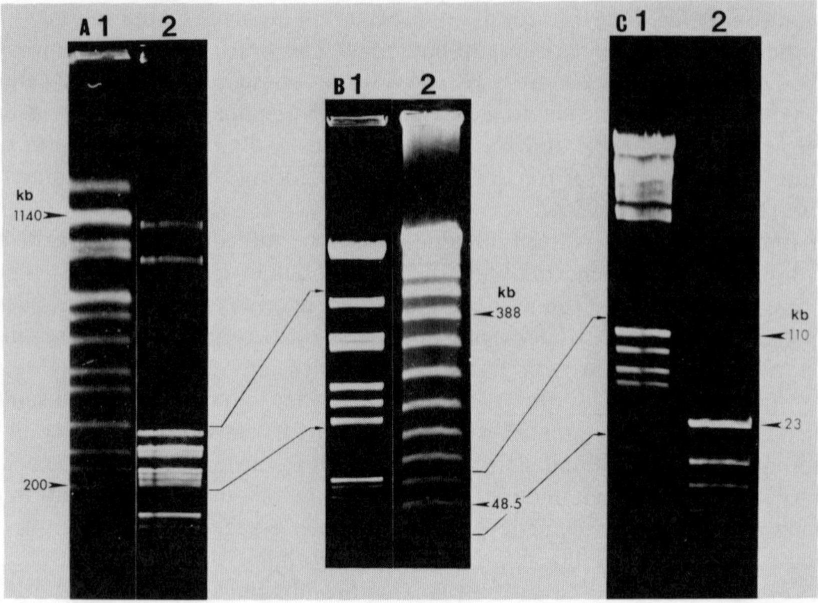

FIGURE 1. Pulsed-field agarose gel electrophoresis of *R. sphaeroides* 2.4.1 genomic DNA digested with *Ase*I. (A) Optimal separation of the largest DNA fragments; 55-s pulse, 18-h run. Lanes: 1, yeast chromosome standards; 2, *Ase*I digest. (B) Optimal separation of the medium-sized DNA fragments; 23-s pulse, 18-h run. Lanes: 1, *Ase*I digest; 2, lambda ladder standards. (C) Optimal separation of small DNA fragments; 9-s pulse, 16-h run. Lanes: 1, *Ase*I digest; 2, lambda *Hin*dIII standards. (From Suwanto and Kaplan, 1989a.)

although the usefulness of a group of restriction enzymes may be indicated by the G+C content of the DNA to be digested, any given specific enzyme may or may not be useful.

The total genomic DNA as determined from *Ase*I digestions is 4,262 ± 108 kb (Table 1). This estimate does not include the two undigested plasmid DNAs of 105 and 42 kb, for a total genome size of 4,412 kb. With *Spe*I there are 17 resolvable DNA fragments (4,419 kb of total genomic DNA), with *Dra*I there are 24 resolvable fragments (4,117 kb), and with *Sna*BI there are 10 resolvable fragments (4,194 kb) (Table 2). The results for total genomic DNA obtained with *Dra*I and *Sna*BI appear to be lower than those obtained with *Spe*I and *Ase*I. In the former case, several of the endogenous plasmids remained undigested and thus are not included in the totals. However, when allowances are made, the total genome size in all cases is approximately 4,400 kb.

ORIGIN OF RESTRICTION FRAGMENTS

Because it is impossible to display all of the results related to these studies, we will discuss only those that exemplify certain principles of experimental

TABLE 1
*Ase*I fragment sizes of *R. sphaeroides* 2.4.1 total genomic DNA[a]

Total genomic DNA (kb)	Endogenous plasmids (kb)
1,150 ± 42	110
910 ± 24	105 (uncut)
410 ± 5.3	97
360 ± 4.7	63
340 ± 5.6	42 (uncut)
270 ± 5.7	31
244 ± 3.1	448
214 ± 3.7	
110 ± 0.3[b]	
97 ± 1.6[b]	
73 ± 1.7	
63 ± 2.2[b]	
31 ± 2.9[b]	
18 ± 2.6	
5 ± 1.1	
4 ± 1.0	
3 ± 0.7	
4,265 ± 108.2	

[a] From Suwanto and Kaplan, 1989a.
[b] Of plasmid origin; see right-hand column.

TABLE 2
R. sphaeroides 2.4.1 fragment sizes as determined by pulsed-field
gel electrophoresis[a]

Fragment size (kb) after digestion with:		
*Spe*I	*Dra*I	*Sna*BI
1,645	800	1,225[b]
735	675[b]	1,200[b]
710	660[b]	784
575	635[b]	370
110 (2)[c]	245 (2)	300
105	110	130
90	105	100
73	85 (2)	55
65	65	18
52	60 (3)	12
40	50 (2)	4,194
32	35	
31	31	
17 (2)	18	
12	12	
4,419	10	
	8	
	7	
	6	
	4,117	

[a] From Suwanto and Kaplan, 1989a.
[b] Seen as a single broad band.
[c] Numbers in parentheses indicate the number of DNA fragments in that size class.

approach. For example, how were the *Ase*I fragments derived from total genomic DNA determined to be of plasmid origin? Plasmid DNA was isolated and digested with *Ase*I and electrophoresed alongside *Ase*I-digested total genomic DNA. The 110-, 97-, 63-, and 31-kb *Ase*I bands are plasmid derived. Using either the 31- or 63-kb *Ase*I fragment as a probe against a digestion of total genomic DNA, these hybridized to their homologous counterparts in the *Ase*I digest of bulk plasmid DNA as well as to the 110-kb *Ase*I fragment. We know from earlier studies that many of the endogenous plasmids share sequence homology and that the 31- and 63-kb *Ase*I fragments are contained within a single plasmid. Two plasmids, 105 and 42 kb, that were undigested by *Ase*I were observed in both the linear and supercoiled forms.

Another general approach to providing specific assignments of each of the *Ase*I fragments to either chromosomal or plasmid DNA has been to show that specific Tn*5* insertions into plasmid DNA can be correlated with a shift in mobility of specific *Ase*I-generated DNA fragments. Upon insertion of Tn*5* into the 97-kb fragment, the fragment was shifted to 102 kb, and it specifically probed with Tn*5*. Similarly, the 110-kb fragment was displaced by the insertion of Tn*5* to a mobility of 115 kb. Each of these Tn*5* insertions was shown to be of plasmid origin when undigested DNA was analyzed. Furthermore, the ethidium bromide staining intensity of the 110-kb fragment is always substantially brighter than all of the other *Ase*I-generated fragments and has led us to conclude that this plasmid is probably multicopy.

If we lyse our cells in the agarose plug and subject the undigested DNA to electrophoresis, the plasmids in either the linear (pulse-dependent) or supercoiled (pulse-independent) form can be separated. Nicked plasmid DNA will not move from the well. Three regions of DNA, designated A, B and C, can be observed after ethidium bromide staining. Region B represents the cluster of four plasmids between 95 and 110 kb, and region C corresponds to the 42-kb plasmid, all in their supercoiled form. A Tn*5* probe hybridizes to one of the plasmid DNAs (original 97 kb). The supercoiled form of the 42-kb plasmid has been shifted and probes with Tn*5* after insertion of Tn*5*. Likewise, the 110-kb plasmid is shifted in its mobility and probes with Tn*5*.

ANALYSIS OF MULTIPLE FRAGMENTS

Another difficulty in designating the origin and number(s) of each of the DNA fragments shown earlier pertains to the presence of more than a single fragment in a particular region of the digestion pattern of the DNA. For example, for the *Dra*I digest of total genomic DNA, the region designated 650 kb consists of more than a single DNA fragment. Thus, the question is, How many fragments are in this region and what are their precise sizes?

Strain PRKB⁻ contains a spectinomycin and streptomycin resistance cartridge that has two *Dra*I sites inserted into *prkB*; therefore, digestion with *Dra*I should cut any DNA fragment in which the cartridge exists into two new DNA fragments (the 2-kb cartridge is too small to be observed). Using a series of single

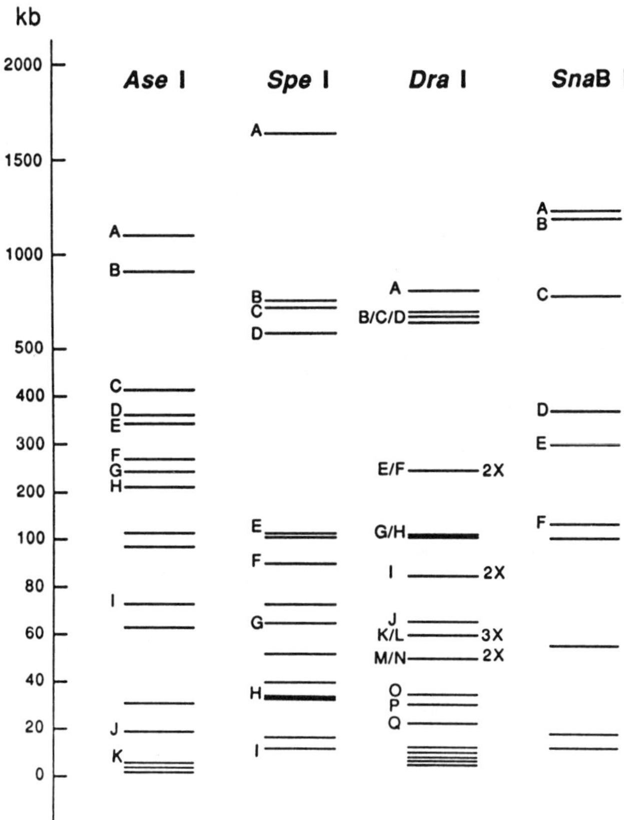

FIGURE 2. Idealized gel band plot of the *R. sphaeroides* 2.4.1 genomic DNA restriction fragments, with estimated sizes. Enzyme digests are listed at the top. Bands without designation are derived from endogenous plasmids.

and double restriction enzyme digests of the wild-type and PRKB⁻ strains, we were able to demonstrate that the broad band at 650 kb actually consisted of three unique *Dra*I restriction fragments.

With these kinds of analyses, the specific banding pattern for total genomic DNA has been resolved by using the restriction endonucleases *Ase*I, *Spe*I, *Dra*I, and *Sna*BI (Fig. 2). In each digest, bands designated by a letter are derived from chromosomal DNA, and those lacking such a designation are of plasmid origin. Similarly, doublet and triplet bands are also designated. By using a large variety of specific probes, we have managed to localize a substantial number of specific genes or markers to almost all of the DNA fragments, as shown for an *Ase*I digest of total genomic DNA (Fig. 3; not all of the available markers are presented).

CHROMOSOMAL MAPPING

Having determined which of the DNA fragments derived from the digestion of total genomic DNA of *R. sphaeroides* are of plasmid origin and having

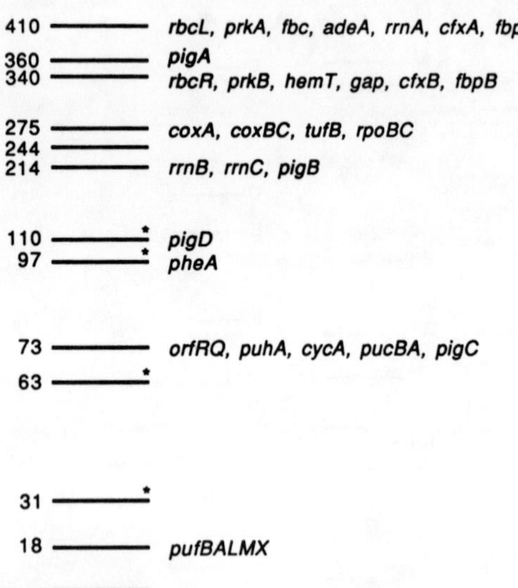

FIGURE 3. Assignment of genes, operons, and other markers to the restriction fragments derived from the *Ase*I digest of the *R. sphaeroides* 2.4.1 genome. Bands with an asterisk are derived from endogenous plasmids. Circles represent the endogenous (uncut) plasmids that have no *Ase*I site. (From Suwanto and Kaplan, 1989a.)

enumerated and identified each fragment, we are able to reconstruct the chromosomal complement of this organism. One approach to linking the separable restriction endonuclease-generated DNA fragments is to identify specific DNA fragments that contain junction regions between two known fragments.

We screened our cosmid libraries in a search for specific junction fragments. One such example is derived from Cos 662. When this cosmid was used as a probe of the *Ase*I digest of total genomic DNA, it could identify the 244- and 18-kb *Ase*I fragments as forming a junction. When only a small piece of the cosmid DNA insert was used as a probe, it uniquely identified the 244-kb *Ase*I fragment. Similarly, a second cosmid, Cos 440, was able to join the 910- and 73-kb *Ase*I fragments. Previous experiments (mapping of the photosynthetic gene cluster) showed that the 18- and 73-kb *Ase*I fragments were linked and therefore that the cluster of 244-, 18-, 73-, and 910-kb fragments are all linked to one another.

A second approach that we used to link the individual *Ase*I fragments was the application of double and triple restriction endonuclease digestions coupled with the use of Southern hybridizations using specific gene probes. *Spe*I-digested total genomic DNA revealed a single, large (1,645-kb) DNA fragment. Southern hybridizations showed that *pufBA*, *nifHDK*, and Cos 662 (244- and 18-kb *Ase*I fragments) were all contained within the 1,645-kb *Spe*I fragment. Digestion of *Spe*I-generated DNA fragments with *Ase*I revealed the presence of the 244-, 18-, 73-, and 910-kb *Ase*I fragments; therefore, these *Ase*I fragments do not contain an *Spe*I site and are all within the 1,645-kb *Spe*I fragment. Further, using *rbcL* as a probe, we were able to show that *rbcL* was localized within the 1,645-kb *Spe*I fragment. Since *rbcL* is a unique marker for the 410-kb *Ase*I fragment, this fragment must be linked to one end of the cluster of 244-, 18-, 73-, and 910-kb fragments. The question is where—to the 910-kb or to the 244-kb *Ase*I fragment? When genomic DNA is double digested with *Spe*I and *Ase*I, a unique 370-kb fragment that probes with *rbcL* is generated. This 370-kb fragment must be derived from the 410-kb *Ase*I fragment, since none of the 244-, 18-, 73-, or 910-kb *Ase*I fragments contains an *Spe*I site, and therefore one end of the 1,645-kb *Spe*I fragment has within it the 370-kb *Ase*I-*Spe*I fragment. Next, *rbcL* was used to probe *Dra*I, *Dra*I-*Spe*I, and *Dra*I-*Ase*I digestions of total genomic DNA. We observed hybridization of *rbcL* to the 800-kb *Dra*I and *Dra*I-*Spe*I DNA fragment as well as to the 150-kb *Dra*I-*Ase*I fragment. We have also shown that the 635-kb *Dra*I fragment encompasses the 244-, 18-, and 73-kb *Ase*I fragments as well as a 290-kb portion of the 910-kb *Ase*I fragment and that this 635-kb *Dra*I fragment was intact after *Dra*I-*Spe*I double digestion. Therefore, the 635-kb *Dra*I fragment lies within the 1,645-kb *Spe*I fragment and contains *nifHDK* and *pufBA*. As described above, the 800-kb *Dra*I fragment is not digested with *Spe*I; therefore, this 800-kb fragment must also lie within the 1,645-kb *Spe*I fragment, since the 1,645-kb *Spe*I fragment is absent in the *Dra*I-*Spe*I double digest. The presence of *rbcL* in a 150-kb *Dra*I-*Ase*I fragment means that this *Ase*I site must reside toward one end of the 800-kb *Dra*I fragment that is opposite the 635-kb *Dra*I fragment containing *puf*, *nifHDK*. Therefore, the 370-kb *Spe*I-*Ase*I fragment that probes with *rbcL* must be linked to the 910-kb *Ase*I fragment, with the 40-kb *Spe*I-*Ase*I fragment derived from the 410-kb *Ase*I fragment away from the junction of the 910- and 410-kb *Ase*I fragments.

By using the above-described approaches, we arrived at the intermediate situation shown in Fig. 4, where all of the *Ase*I fragments fall into one of two contiguous segments, as is also the case for the *Spe*I fragments. The *Dra*I fragments are in the innermost circle, and the two largest *Sna*BI fragments are shown between the *Ase*I and *Spe*I fragments. If the D-E-H segments are linked to the remaining *Ase*I fragments, then the *Sna*BI overlap should link *Ase*I G to either *Ase*I D-E-H or H-E-D.

We also know that the *Sna*BI fragment of 784 kb resides entirely within *Ase*I D-E-H segment, whose total size is 914 kb; therefore, where is the 130-kb of DNA containing a *Sna*BI site that remains unaccounted for? It could only be part of the large 1,225-kb *Sna*BI fragment, since this is the only region of either large *Sna*BI fragment for which an assignment has not been made. But this is impossible, since the 900-kb *Sna*BI-*Spe*I fragment must border a 300-kb DNA fragment to yield a 1,225-kb *Sna*BI fragment. Something is, therefore, wrong! This was the first

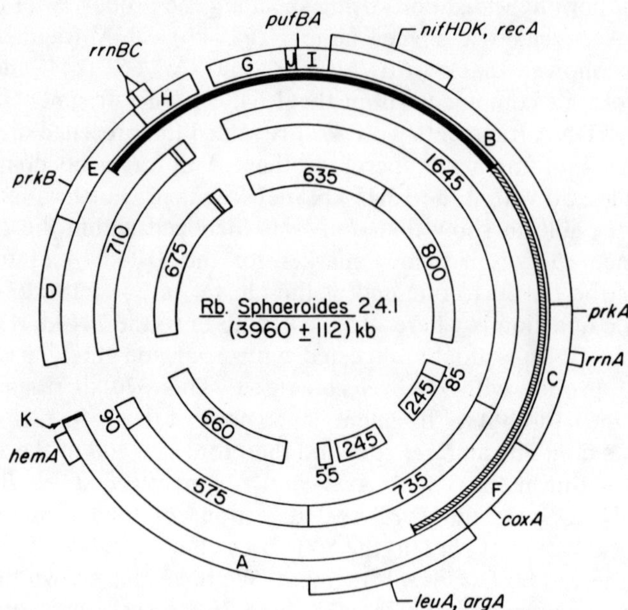

FIGURE 4. Intermediate physical map of *R. sphaeroides* chromosomes showing the only possible location of the *Ase*I D-E-H fragments relative to the other *Ase*I chromosomal fragments. The outer circle represents *Ase*I, and the middle circle represents *Spe*I; the inner circle is for *Dra*I-generated restriction maps. The thickened line between the *Ase*I and *Spe*I restriction maps represents the position of the two largest *Sna*BI fragments. (From Suwanto and Kaplan, 1989b.)

indication that the *Ase*I D-E-H segment could not be joined to the other contiguous set of *Ase*I fragments.

Using *hemA* as a probe of a series of single and multiple digestions of total genomic DNA, we were able to demonstrate that *Ase*I fragments G-J-I-B-C-F-A-K were circular, with a size of 3,046 ± 95 kb. In a *Sna*BI digest of total genomic DNA, *hemA* probed to the large 1,225-kb *Sna*BI fragment as well as to a 90-kb *Spe*I fragment generated from a *Sna*BI-*Spe*I double digest; therefore, *hemA* has to be closely linked to *pufBA*, and we can circularize the eight contiguous *Ase*I fragments G through K.

What is the nature of *Ase*I fragments D-E-H, since they are neither part of chromosome I nor of known plasmid origin? If we electrophorese undigested total genomic DNA derived from two independent strains of *R. sphaeroides* containing single Tn5 insertions (Fig. 5), we can readily observe regions A, B, C, and D, where C and D are the intact supercoiled plasmids occupying size ranges of 100 and 42 kb, respectively. Region A is the linearized chromosome I, composed of the eight contiguous circularized *Ase*I fragments described above, and region B is chromosome II, composed of the three contiguous *Ase*I fragments. Note that Tn5 hybridizes uniquely to either region A or region B but not both, nor does Tn5 hybridize to region C or D, eliminating the possibility that regions A and B are some form of cointegrate structure composed of the smaller plasmids.

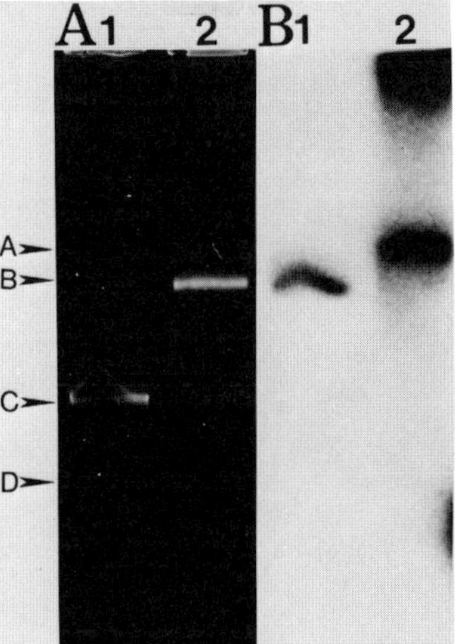

FIGURE 5. Southern hybridization analysis of electrophoresed, undigested total genomic DNA. (A) Ethidium bromide-stained gel; TAFE run at 50 s, 21 h. Lanes: 1, strain MS2-II6; 2, strain MS2-R. (B) Autoradiogram of panel A, using Tn5 as a probe. Region A is the linearized form of chromosome I, region B is the linearized form of chromosome II, region C is the four endogenous plasmids with sizes between 95 and 110 kb, and region D is the 42-kb plasmid. (From Suwanto and Kaplan, 1989b.)

Similarly, when *hemT* and the spectinomycin-streptomycin resistance cartridge in PRKB⁻ were used as probes of the undigested DNAs derived from the wild type in the former case and a *prkB* mutation in the latter, we observed the following. Each is a specific probe to region B or chromosome II, consisting of *Ase*I fragment D-H-E. When *hemA*, a probe specific for chromosome I, was used, only region A or chromosome I was hybridized. Therefore, regions A and B are unique and correspond to chromosomes I and II, respectively. In another approach, a specific junction fragment unambiguously linked *Ase*I fragments D and E and showed that D-H-E had to exist as a circular structure. Finally, we can show in yet another way that chromosome II exists as a closed circle, by demonstrating unequivocally that it does not exist in a linear form.

SUMMARY

We summarize all of these results in Fig. 6, where both chromosomes I and II, having sizes of approximately 3,050 and 914 kb, respectively, are shown with some of their appropriate markers. Each has been designated a chromosome because each contains *rrn* operons, *rrnA* on chromosome I and *rrnB* and *rrnC* on chromosome II. Other data, although not firmly established, indicate that *rrnA* is absolutely essential for growth of *R. sphaeroides* under all known growth conditions. Similarly, at least one copy of either *rrnB* or *rrnC* appears to be essential for cell survival. The chromosomes are present in a 1:1 ratio.

Thus, we define the chromosome complement of an organism as collectively consisting of the minimal number of DNA molecules required to effect the whole of the central dogma, i.e., DNA, RNA, and protein synthesis. To our knowledge, *R. sphaeroides* 2.4.1 is the first bacterium determined to possess two unique chromosomes. We suspect that it will not be the last. Furthermore, the genomic organization of *R. sphaeroides* represents one of only a few of the procaryotic

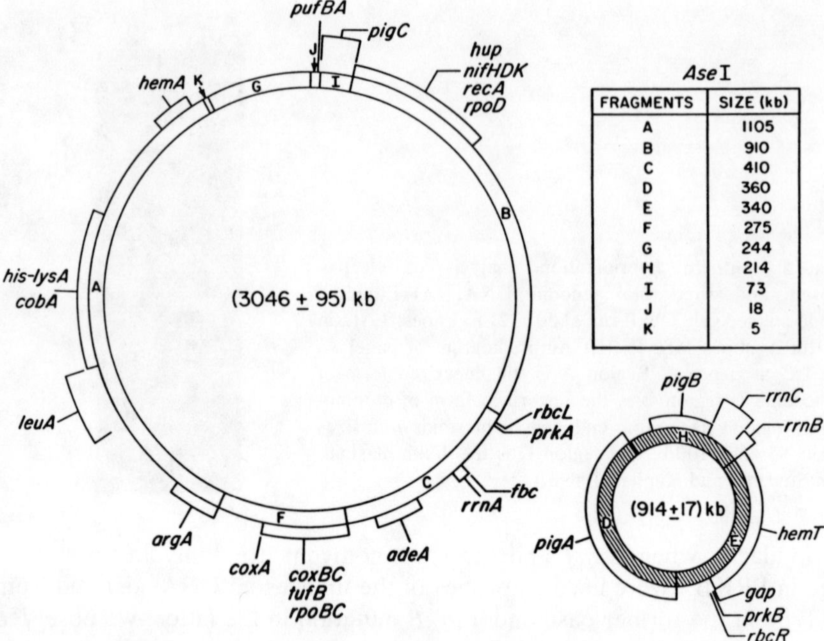

FRAGMENTS	SIZE (kb)
A	1105
B	910
C	410
D	360
E	340
F	275
G	244
H	214
I	73
J	18
K	5

FIGURE 6. Entire physical and limited genetic maps of the two *R. sphaeroides* chromosomes. The physical maps only show the *Ase*I restriction map. Notation: *pufBA*, *puf* operon; *pigC*, pigment mutant; *hup*, hydrogenase; *nifHDK*, nitrogen fixation; *recA*, recombination deficient; *rpoD*, σ^{70}-like gene; *rbcL*, form I region; *fbc*, for cytochrome b/c_1 genes; *rrnA*, *-B*, and *-C*, rRNA; *adeA*, adenine; *coxBC*, cytochrome oxidase; *tufB*, elongation factor; *rpoBC*, RNA polymerase subunits; *coxA*, cytochrome oxidase subunit; *argA*, arginine; *leuA*, leucine; *cobA*, vitamin B_{12} synthesis; *his-lysA*, auxotrophic marker; *hemA* and *hemT*, 5-aminolevulinic acid synthase; *pigA* and *pigB*, pigment mutants; *gapB*, *prkB*, and *rbcB*, form II region.

genomes that have been physically organized, and it is by far the most complex, consisting of 4,400 kb of DNA and seven replicons. Although the data are still sparse, it is already apparent that the number of *rrn* cistrons can vary widely. Also, the relative locations of specific genes should be considered among the various genomes so constructed. It is likely that the availability of the physical maps of the different procaryotes is likely to accelerate.

ACKNOWLEDGMENT. We acknowledge the very generous support of Public Health Service research grant GM 31667 from the National Institutes of Health.

LITERATURE CITED

Donohue, T. J., A. G. McEwan, and S. Kaplan. 1986. Cloning, DNA sequence, and expression of the *Rhodobacter sphaeroides* cytochrome c_2 gene. *J. Bacteriol.* **168**:962–972.

Fornari, C. S., M. Watkins, and S. Kaplan. 1984. Plasmid distribution and analysis in *Rhodopseudomonas sphaeroides*. *Plasmid* **11**:39–47.

Gabellini, N., U. Harnisch, J. E. G. McCarthy, G. Hauska, and W. Sebald. 1985. Cloning and expression of the *fbc* operon encoding FeS protein, cytochrome b and cytochrome c1 from the *Rhodopseudomonas sphaeroides* b/c1 complex. *EMBO J.* **4**:549–553.

Hallenbeck, P. L., and S. Kaplan. 1988. Structural gene regions of *Rhodobacter sphaeroides* involved in CO₂ fixation. *Photosyn. Res.* **19:**63–71.

Kiley, P. J., and S. Kaplan. 1988. Molecular genetics of photosynthetic membrane biosynthesis in *Rhodobacter sphaeroides. Microb. Rev.* **52:**50–69.

Meinhardt, S. W., P. J. Kiley, S. Kaplan, A. R. Crofts, and S. Harayama. 1985. Characterization of light-harvesting mutants of *Rhodopseudomonas sphaeroides.* I. Measurement of the efficiency of energy transfer from light-harvesting complexes to the reaction center. *Arch. Biochem. Biophys.* **236:**130–139.

Suwanto, A., and S. Kaplan. 1989a. Physical and genetic mapping of the *Rhodobacter sphaeroides* 2.4.1 genome: genome size, fragment identification, and gene localization. *J. Bacteriol.* **171:** 5840–5849.

Suwanto, A., and S. Kaplan. 1989b. Physical and genetic mapping of the *Rhodobacter sphaeroides* 2.4.1 genome: presence of two unique circular chromosomes. *J. Bacteriol.* **171:**5850–5859.

Tabita, F. R. 1988. Molecular and cellular regulation of autotrophic carbon dioxide fixation in microorganisms. *Microbiol. Rev.* **52:**155–189.

Tai, T.-N., M. D. Moore, and S. Kaplan. 1988. Cloning and characterization of the 5-aminolevulinate synthase gene(s) from *Rhodobacter sphaeroides. Gene* **70:**139–151.

Chapter 38

Genes for Hydrogen Oxidation and Denitrification Form Two Clusters on Megaplasmid pHG1 of *Alcaligenes eutrophus*

*Bärbel Friedrich, Christian Böcker, Günther Eberz,
Thomas Eitinger, Karin Horstmann, Christiane Kortlüke,
Detlef Römermann, Edward Schwartz, Andrea Tran-Betcke,
Ute Warnecke, and Jürgen Warrelmann*

ALTERNATIVE METABOLIC ACTIVITIES IN *A. EUTROPHUS*

Alcaligenes eutrophus has important features in common with the pseudomonads: a strict respiratory metabolism and the ability to decompose an enormous range of organic substances, including sugars, organic acids, and aromatic compounds. The most remarkable characteristics of *A. eutrophus*, however, are its facultative metabolic activities. In addition to using organic carbon sources heterotrophically, *A. eutrophus* can utilize inorganic carbon by autotrophic CO_2 fixation. The energy for this process is derived from the oxidation of molecular hydrogen. Oxygen is nonessential for heterotrophic growth, provided that nitrate or nitrite is present as a terminal electron acceptor in the denitrification pathway (reviewed by Bowien and Schlegel [1981]).

Plasmids that encode complex physiological pathways such as the degradation of aromatic compounds are found predominantly in the pseudomonads and related organisms. *A. eutrophus* adds two interesting physiological capabilities to the list of plasmid-encoded functions: hydrogen-dependent autotrophy and denitrification. The genes coding for autotrophic CO_2 fixation (*cfx*) are present in one chromosomal and one plasmid-borne copy (reviewed by Friedrich [1989]).

This chapter focuses on the organization and expression of genes of the hydrogen-oxidizing enzyme (Hox) system; present knowledge of the plasmid-

Bärbel Friedrich, Christian Böcker, Günther Eberz, Thomas Eitinger, Karin Horstmann, Christiane Kortlüke, Detlef Römermann, Edward Schwartz, Andrea Tran-Betcke, Ute Warnecke, and Jürgen Warrelmann ● Institut für Pflanzenphysiologie und Mikrobiologie der Freien Universität Berlin, D-1000 Berlin 33, Federal Republic of Germany.

TABLE 1
Biochemical properties of the two hydrogenases of *A. eutrophus*[a]

Protein	Cellular location	Molecular mass (kilodaltons)	Subunit composition (molecular mass [kilodaltons])	Metal and cofactor content	Electron acceptor
HoxS	Cytoplasm	205	α (63) β (56) γ (30) δ (26)	2 Ni, 16 Fe, 1 FMN	NAD
HoxP	Membrane	95	L (62) S (31)	0.65 Ni, 7–9 Fe	ND, MV[b]

[a] From reviews by Schlegel (1989) and Friedrich (1989).
[b] ND, No data on the physiological acceptor; MV, methylene blue.

encoded determinants for denitrification (Nar/Nir) by *A. eutrophus* is only briefly summarized.

BIOCHEMISTRY AND PHYSIOLOGY OF THE TWO HYDROGENASES IN *A. EUTROPHUS*

Hydrogenases are iron-sulfur proteins catalyzing either the consumption or the production of H_2 according to the equation $H_2 \leftrightarrow 2H^+ + 2e^-$. Theoretically, the reaction is bidirectional; in vivo, however, the reaction is directed by the physiological context. Hydrogenases can be classified on the basis of metal content into three groups: [Fe], [NiFe], and [NiFeSe] hydrogenases (reviewed by Fauque et al. [1988]). The two hydrogenases present in *A. eutrophus* belong to the largest class of [NiFe] hydrogenases and differ in cellular location, subunit composition, and cofactor content (Table 1).

The soluble, tetrameric, NAD-reducing hydrogenase (HoxS) supplies the cells with reducing equivalents that are either consumed directly in biosynthetic processes or converted into high-energy bonds via the respiratory chain (Fig. 1). The membrane-bound, heterodimeric hydrogenase (HoxP) does not react with NAD but is linked to the electron transport chain (via an unknown acceptor molecule), generating ATP. HoxP activity can be assayed by the hydrogen-dependent methylene blue reduction.

Whereas most lithoautotrophic bacteria contain HoxP-like enzymes, HoxS-like enzymes have been found only in strains of *Alcaligenes* spp. and in the gram-positive actinomycete *Nocardia opaca* (reviewed by Schlegel [1989]). The acquisition of an additional NAD-reducing enzyme appears to be beneficial for *A. eutrophus*, since the loss of HoxS activity in *hoxS* mutants significantly reduced the rate of growth on H_2, whereas mutants deficient in HoxP function were only slightly affected in H_2-dependent autotrophic growth (Table 2). In addition, introduction of a *hoxS*-carrying recombinant plasmid into the hydrogen bacterium

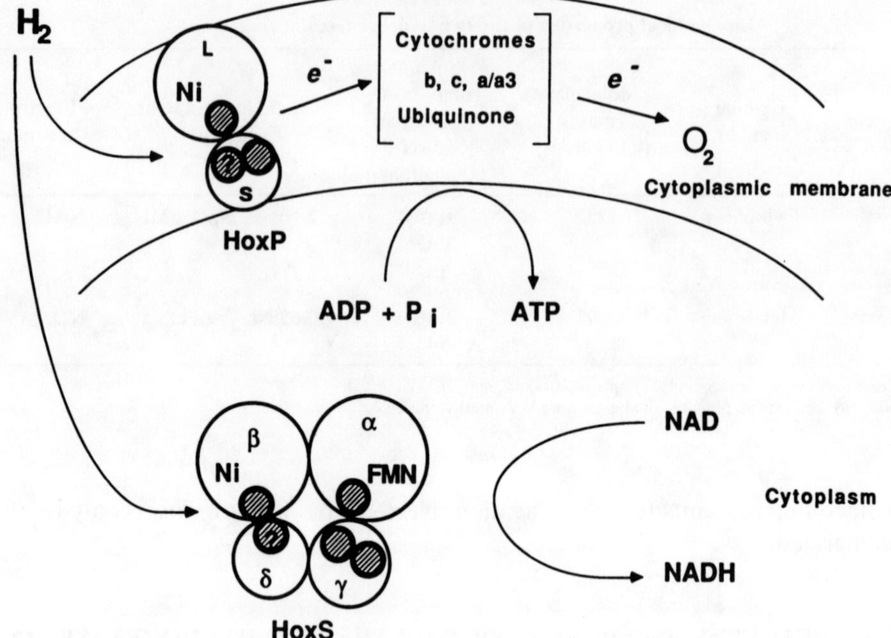

FIGURE 1. Model for the physiological function of HoxS and HoxP in *A. eutrophus*, modified as described by Schlegel (1989). The hydrogenase subunits are indicated by circles; shaded circles represent the presumptive positions of iron-sulfur clusters deduced from the nucleotide sequence of the structural genes.

Pseudomonas facilis, which possesses only HoxP activity, enhanced the rate of growth of H_2 (Table 2).

According to a model deduced for the *N. opaca* hydrogenase (Schneider et al., 1984), the β and δ subunits of the HoxS enzyme form a dimer that appears to be functionally equivalent to the large (L) and small (S) subunits of HoxP. Thus, it constitutes the prototypic hydrogenase, with nickel presumably in the catalytic center (Fig. 1). A second and larger dimer, composed of the α and γ subunits, is

TABLE 2
Contribution of HoxS to lithoautotrophic growth[a]

Strain	Phenotype	Doubling time (h) on H_2-CO_2-O_2
A. eutrophus H16	HoxS⁺ HoxP⁺	3.6
A. eutrophus HF15	HoxS⁻ HoxP⁺	12
A. eutrophus HF08	HoxS⁺ HoxP⁻	4.2
P. facilis DSM 620	HoxS⁻ HoxP⁺	11.4
P. facilis(pGE15)	HoxS⁺ HoxP⁺	8.8

[a] From Warnecke and Friedrich (unpublished results).

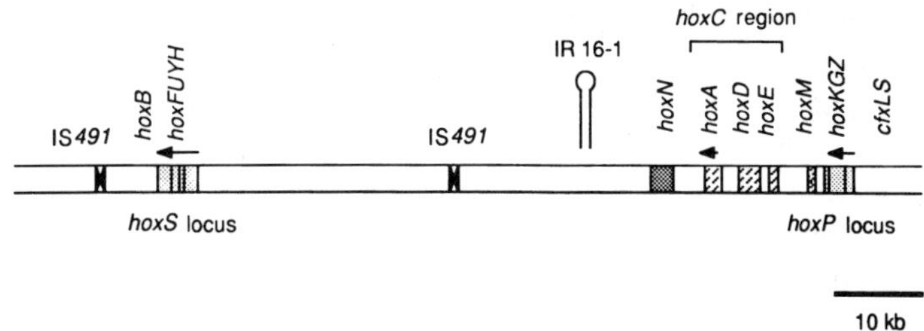

FIGURE 2. Structure of the *hox* gene cluster of megaplasmid pHG1 of *A. eutrophus*. Arrows indicate direction of transcription. See text for details.

associated with FMN. A role in electron transfer to NAD has been proposed for the αγ moiety, since this aggregate exhibits NADH-oxidizing activity.

STRUCTURE OF THE PLASMID-ENCODED HYDROGENASE GENE CLUSTER

The first evidence for involvement of megaplasmids in hydrogen metabolism of *A. eutrophus* came from the phenotype of plasmid-free mutants. Plasmid-free strains irreversibly lost the ability to grow autotrophically on H_2. The capacity to oxidize hydrogen (Hox) could be restored only by reintroduction of the plasmid. The 450-kilobase (kb) plasmid pHG1 of *A. eutrophus* H16 was found to be self-transmissible in conjugation at frequencies of up to 10^{-2} per donor. Mating experiments with various Hox mutants defective in the structure or regulation of HoxS or HoxP as donors and plasmid-free strains as recipients yielded transconjugants that displayed the donor phenotype (reviewed by Friedrich [1989]). The results suggested that plasmid pHG1 carried not merely a minor component of Hox metabolism but a whole set of hydrogenase-specifying genes (*hox*).

This conclusion was substantiated by analyses of *hox* insertion and deletion mutants, gene exchange experiments, and molecular cloning of the structural and regulatory *hox* genes. *A. eutrophus* proved to be an ideal system for these studies, since the availability of pure megaplasmid DNA permitted precise restriction nuclease analysis, a straightforward search for structural alterations in the plasmid, and the construction of a megaplasmid specific gene library. The genetic map shown in Fig. 2 summarizes the results of these studies.

At least five independent *hox* loci are distributed in a region of approximately 100 kb of plasmid pHG1. This so-called *hox* gene cluster is flanked by the two structural gene complexes, *hoxS* and *hoxP*. The *hoxS* locus codes for the four subunits of the NAD-reducing hydrogenase (HoxS), and the *hoxP* locus encodes the large and the small subunits of the membrane-bound hydrogenase (HoxP). These loci were initially isolated from a gene library by mutant complementation (Eberz et al., 1986).

The nucleotide sequences of the *hoxS* and *hoxP* loci have now been determined in our laboratory. The predicted amino acid sequences exhibit extensive homology with conserved DNA regions of related hydrogenases, presumably representing sites that are important for the catalytic reaction. Although data on transcription start sites, promoter activities, and transcription terminators are still limited, the results suggest that the genes of the *hoxS* and *hoxP* loci constitute two operons (Fig. 2). The six structural genes are tightly linked and separated by relatively short intergenic regions. The sequence of the small subunit predicts a leader peptide of 43 amino acids. With respect to evolution, it is interesting that the primary amino acid sequence of the HoxP protein is highly homologous (80% overall homology) to that of membrane-bound hydrogenases from *Bradyrhizobium japonicum* (Sayavedra-Soto et al., 1988) and *Rhodobacter capsulatus* (Leclerc et al., 1988). The Ni^{2+}-containing β subunit of HoxS contains conserved domains but appears more closely related to the corresponding subunit of the methyl viologen-reducing hydrogenase from *Methanobacterium thermoautotrophicum* (Reeve et al., 1989) than to its *Alcaligenes* cellular counterpart, HoxP.

Two other loci, *hoxB* and *hoxM* (Fig. 2), lie downstream of *hoxS* and *hoxP*, respectively. The nucleotide sequences of these regions have not yet been determined. On the basis of complementation studies, we conclude that *hoxB* encodes a small dimeric protein consisting of 18.8-kilodalton subunits. Similar proteins have been found in all HoxS-containing organisms studied to date. The molar ratio of the *hoxB* and *hoxS* gene products is approximately 4:1 (Kärst et al., 1987). HoxB may be involved in the assembly of the HoxS holoenzyme.

The *hoxM* locus, which lies downstream of *hoxP*, appears to participate in the attachment of HoxP to the membrane. This is suggested by the observation that the transfer of a *hoxM*-containing recombinant plasmid into a strain in which HoxP is either soluble or only loosely attached to the membrane (Friedrich et al., 1986) yielded transconjugants with HoxP tightly bound to the membrane (C. Kortlüke, M. Rohde, and B. Friedrich, unpublished results).

The internal region of the *hox* gene cluster contains an array of genes assigned to the *hoxC* and *hoxN* regions. The products of these genes are required for the synthesis or activation of the two hydrogenases of *A. eutrophus*. The role of these functions in H_2 metabolism is discussed below.

The observation that spontaneous deletions and insertions frequently occurred in the *hox* gene cluster (reviewed by Friedrich [1989]) prompted a search for *A. eutrophus*-specific insertion elements. Analysis of HoxP⁻ mutants revealed in two cases the presence of a 1.3-kb insertion. This element, designated IS*491*, has features typical of procaryotic insertion sequences: the termini are marked by (imperfect) inverted repeats, and an 8-base-pair duplication of target sequence flanks the insertion. At least four copies of IS*491* are present in *A. eutrophus* H16. Interestingly two of these copies map in the *hox* gene cluster of plasmid pHG1 (Fig. 2; E. Schwartz and B. Friedrich, unpublished results). Previous electron microscopic studies revealed two extensive palindromic regions on plasmid pHG1. One of these elements, IR 16-1, was shown to be approximately 7.4 kb in size and located between the *hoxS* and *hoxN* loci (Fig. 2; Rohde et al., 1986). The structures and functions of these elements are unknown.

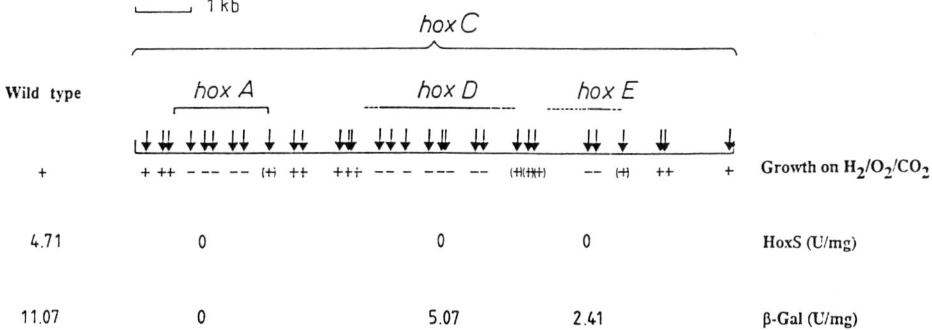

FIGURE 3. Phenotypes of random Tn5 insertions in the *hoxC* region of plasmid pHG1. Symbols and abbreviations: ↓, sites of insertion; +, wild-type like; (+), leaky; −, no growth on H_2-CO_2-O_2; HoxS, activity of NAD-reducing hydrogenase; β-Gal, activity of β-galactosidase tested with a *hoxS-lacZ* fusion.

REGULATORY AND ACCESSORY GENES REQUIRED FOR THE SYNTHESIS OF CATALYTICALLY ACTIVE HYDROGENASES

Expression of the structural genes coding for HoxS and HoxP is coordinate and strictly dependent on expression of the products of two other genes, *hno* and *hoxA*. *hno*, which is homologous to the *ntrA* gene of enteric bacteria, maps on the chromosome (see below). The *hoxA* locus, formerly designated *hoxC* (Eberz et al., 1986), is located on the megaplasmid. *hoxA* encodes a hydrogenase-specific regulator that responds to the redox status of the cell and to temperature. This conclusion is based on the following physiological and genetic evidence. (i) Synthesis of hydrogenase in *A. eutrophus* is derepressed at low redox potentials and is independent of H_2 (Friedrich, 1982). The transfer of plasmid pHG1 or the cloned *hoxA* gene into the H_2-inducible strain *Alcaligenes hydrogenophilus* confers the donor-specific phenotype on the transconjugants. Synthesis of hydrogenase is rendered H_2 independent (G. Eberz and B. Friedrich, unpublished results). (ii) *A. eutrophus* can grow heterotrophically at temperatures of up to 40°C. Growth on H_2-CO_2-O_2 ceases at 33°C because of a shutoff of hydrogenase synthesis (reviewed by Friedrich [1989]). Temperature-resistant mutants were found to carry mutations in the *hoxA* gene.

The *hoxA* gene has now been expressed in *Escherichia coli* as a 49-kilodalton polypeptide. Nucleotide sequence analysis of the *hoxA* gene indicates similarities between the hypothetical gene product and positive regulatory proteins of other organisms. Alignment of the predicted amino acid sequence of HoxA with the amino acid sequences of transcriptional activators revealed extensive homology to NtrC and NifA of *Klebsiella pneumoniae*. Both of these proteins are involved in the regulation of nitrogen metabolism (reviewed by Ausubel [1984]).

The 10.6-kb *hoxC* locus (Fig. 2) contains, in addition to *hoxA*, at least two other *hox* determinants, designated *hoxD* and *hoxE* (Fig. 3). Random insertions in the *hoxC* region generated by mutagenesis with transposon Tn5 resulted in mutants that had lost the ability to grow autotrophically on H_2. Assay of enzyme activity confirmed that the mutants were devoid of catalytically active hydrogenase, as shown for HoxS in Fig. 3. Immunological assays for hydrogenase (data not shown) and experiments with a *hoxS-lacZ* gene fusion permitted phenotypic differentiation of the various *hoxC* mutations. As expected, HoxA$^-$ mutants were entirely devoid of HoxS activity (Fig. 3) and were antigenically HoxS$^-$ (data not shown). Furthermore, when the *hoxS-lacZ* gene fusion was introduced into the mutants in *trans*, they failed to express β-galactosidase activity. Mutations in *hoxE* and *hoxD* resulted in low levels of hydrogenase-specific antigen (data not shown) and reduced levels of β-galactosidase activity (50% of the wild-type level for *hoxD* and 20% for *hoxE*) when tested for this effect on the gene fusion (Fig. 3). On the basis of these results, we conclude that *hoxD* and *hoxE* are essential for the formation of enzymatically active HoxS and HoxP, possibly by mediating the incorporation of nickel ions into the catalytic centers of these proteins. It was previously shown that nickel incorporation occurs during hydrogenase synthesis and not at subsequent stages (Friedrich et al., 1984). Our data on *hoxD* and *hoxE* indicate that their products not only dramatically affect the activity of the hydrogenases but also affect to some extent the rate of synthesis of these enzymes. The latter effect could be explained by the assumption that the *hoxD* and *hoxE* gene products modulate not only hydrogenase activity but also the activity of the regulator HoxA. Moreover, active hydrogenase itself may be involved in the control mechanism.

A plasmid locus involved in Ni metabolism (*hoxN*) was identified adjacent to *hoxA* (Fig. 2). Mutants with deletions in the *hoxN* region were shown to require the addition of nickel chloride for autotrophic growth on H_2, whereas the wild type grew well on media containing only traces of nickel present as contaminants. The symptoms of nickel deficiency in HoxN$^-$ mutants were enhanced by increasing the concentration of magnesium ions in the medium and alleviated by transfer of the *hoxN*-containing recombinant plasmid pCH125 (Eberz et al., 1989). Lohmeyer and Friedrich (1987) had previously demonstrated that nickel uptake is mediated by two nickel transport systems: a magnesium transporter and a nickel-specific high-affinity carrier. The latter appears to be encoded by *hoxN* (Eberz et al., 1989). A subclone carrying 2.2 kb of the *hoxN* region efficiently complements *hoxN* mutants. Expression studies in *E. coli* have identified two proteins encoded on the subcloned segment (T. Eitinger and B. Friedrich, unpublished results).

THE CHROMOSOMAL GENE *hno* (*rpoN*) CONTROLS HYDROGEN OXIDATION AND DENITRIFICATION

In one class of hydrogenase mutants from *A. eutrophus*, both nitrate and hydrogen metabolism were affected. This mutation was found to map on the chromosome (reviewed by Friedrich [1989]). The genetic locus defined by these mutations was designated *hno* (hydrogen, nitrate, and others). More recently, it has become apparent that disruption of the *hno* locus has extremely pleiotropic physiological effects. Hno$^-$ mutants were impaired in at least eight physiological

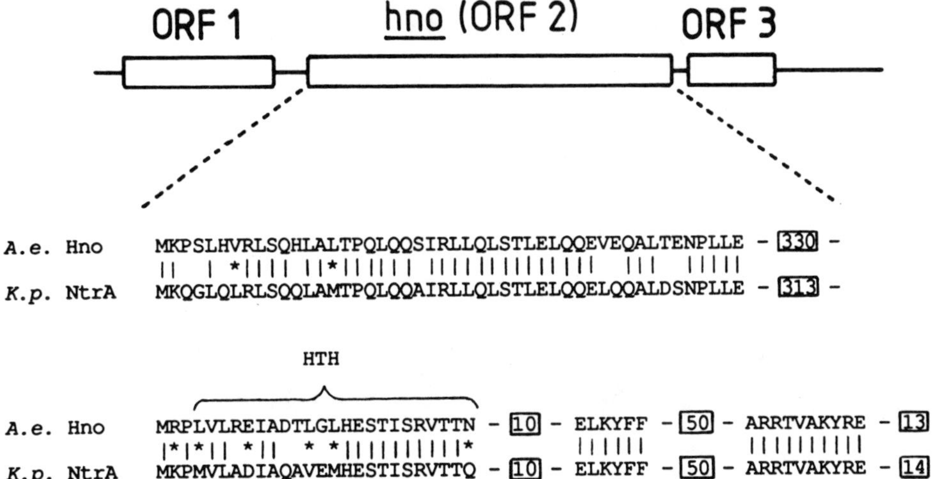

FIGURE 4. Schematic diagram of the ORFs flanking the *hno* gene and comparison of conserved regions of the deduced amino acid sequences of the *A. eutrophus* (*A.e.*) *hno* gene product (J. Warrelmann and B. Friedrich, unpublished results) and the *K. pneumoniae* (*K.p.*) *ntrA* gene product (Merrick and Gibbins, 1985). Symbols: |, identical residues; *, chemically similar residues. Numbers of intragenic amino acids are boxed.

functions, including H_2 oxidation, expression of enzymes catalyzing CO_2 fixation, utilization of nitrate and urea as nitrogen sources, nitrate respiration, and the uptake of C_4 dicarboxylic acids (Römermann et al., 1988). Similar pleiotropic mutants have subsequently been isolated from the hydrogen bacterium *P. facilis*. The cloned *hno* gene from *A. eutrophus* was found to complement the *hno* mutations in both *A. eutrophus* and *P. facilis*. Surprisingly, it also restored glutamine auxotrophy in NtrA⁻ mutants of enteric bacteria (Römermann et al., 1989). NtrA⁻ (or RpoN⁻) mutants are defective in a sigma factor (σ^{54}) that confers altered promoter specificity on the core enzyme of RNA polymerase (reviewed by Helmann and Chamberlin [1988]). The results of the complementation studies strongly suggested that the *hno* loci of *A. eutrophus* and *P. facilis* encode a sigma factor functionally related to σ^{54}. This conclusion was substantiated by comparisons of the nucleotide and deduced amino acid sequences: the *hno* gene is clearly related to *ntrA* (*rpoN*) of *Rhizobium meliloti* and *K. pneumoniae*. The highly conserved regions are shown in Fig. 4.

It is interesting that *hno* of *A. eutrophus* is preceded at a distance of 134 bp by another open reading frame (ORF), designated ORF1. This ORF could code for a protein of 260 amino acids. It has 57% overall homology with the ORF1 adjacent to the *ntrA* gene in *R. meliloti*. There is also evidence for the presence of a conserved ORF upstream of the *ntrA* gene in both *K. pneumoniae* and *Salmonella typhimurium*. It has been noted that ORF1 shows homology to members of a superfamily of ATP-binding proteins (Albright et al., 1989). A third ORF lies downstream of the *hno* gene in *A. eutrophus* (Fig. 4).

Although the transcription start sites of *hoxS*, *hoxP*, and *hoxA* have not been

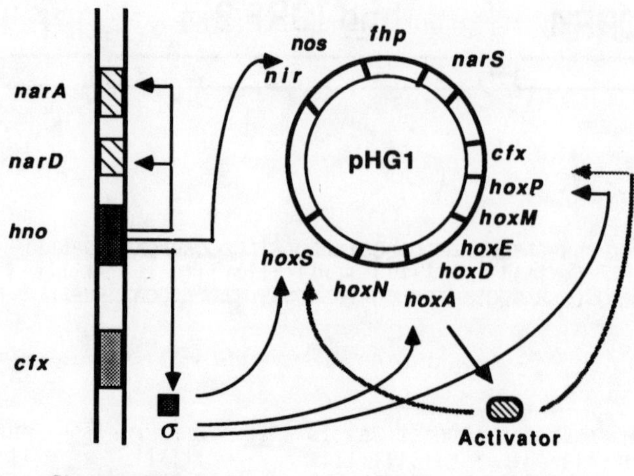

FIGURE 5. Hypothetical arrangement of genes involved in hydrogen oxidation (*hox*), autotrophic CO_2 fixation (*cfx*), reduction of nitrate (*narA*, -*D*, and -*S*), and dissimilation of nitrite (*nir*) and N_2O (*nos*). *fhp* codes for a flavohemoprotein of unknown physiological function (Weihs et al., 1989). The *hno* product is thought to be a minor sigma factor of RNA polymerase.

determined, nucleotide sequence analysis of the respective control regions revealed in all three cases the presence of -12 and -24 consensus motifs very similar to those of the *nif* and *ntrA* promoters of enteric bacteria (Beynon et al., 1983). Thus, the *hox* gene cluster provides a unique opportunity to study the function of a group of promoters presumably controlled by the minor sigma factor σ^{54} acting in concert with activator proteins such as HoxA.

CONCLUSIONS AND OUTLOOK

Our knowledge of the other metabolic loci, *nir*, *nos*, and *narS*, of plasmid pHG1 is still very limited and not nearly as detailed as that on *hox*. Therefore, the experimental results on these functions are only schematically summarized in a general model (Fig. 5). The loss of plasmid pHG1 in *A. eutrophus* was shown to be associated with the loss of the ability to grow anaerobically on nitrate. Plasmid-free mutants retained the capacity for low-level reduction of nitrate to nitrite. Conversion of the resulting nitrite to the gaseous products N_2O and N_2 was, however, abolished (Römermann and Friedrich, 1985). Recent results obtained from studies on mutants and biochemical investigations indicate that *A. eutrophus* has three nitrate reductase activities, two that are chromosomally encoded (*narD* and *narA*) and one that originates from the plasmid (*narS*). NarA appears to be involved in the assimilation of nitrate as a nitrogen source, and NarD seems to be associated with nitrate dissimilation. Both activities are impaired in Hno$^-$ mutants. Thus, we postulate that an alternative sigma factor encoded by *hno* is involved in the expression of *narA* and *narD* genes. The physiological role of the Hno-independent NarS activity is not yet clear. NarS is formed under conditions of energy limitation and does not require nitrate for induction (U. Warnecke and B. Friedrich, unpublished results).

A cosmid clone with a large (approximately 32 kb) fragment of pHG1 was shown to restore nitrite dissimilatory functions (*nir/nos*) in a plasmid-free mutant of *A. eutrophus*. Southern analyses with the structural gene of the N_2O reductase from *Pseudomonas stutzeri* (Viebrock and Zumft, 1988) as the probe gave a positive hybridization signal with an internal fragment of the cosmid insert. Moreover, biochemical evidence suggests that the cosmid carries the structural gene(s) for a cytochrome *cd*-type nitrite reductase (B. Schneider, R. Sann, and B. Friedrich, unpublished results). Future studies will concentrate on analysis of the structure and regulation of *nir/nos* functions, characterization of NarS activity, and elucidation of the contribution of NarS to denitrification.

Our future work on the *hox* gene cluster will be organized in two major projects: (i) structural analysis of the *hox* genes and (ii) studies on the regulation of *hox* gene expression. The first area of investigation entails identification of the catalytic sites in the hydrogenase proteins. These presumably incorporate the cysteine residues that supposedly form complexes with the iron-nickel ligands. Several questions raised in this chapter relate to the function of the accessory genes *hoxB*, *hoxM*, *hoxD*, *hoxE*, and *hoxN*. By analyzing appropriate mutants, we hope to obtain information on the assembly of HoxS and HoxP and the transport of these enzymes to their sites of action in the cell. Furthermore, we will investigate how the cofactors, especially nickel ions, are incorporated into the hydrogenase proteins. The first step in this process is probably catalyzed by the product(s) of *hoxN*, which appears to specifically mediate nickel transport across the cytoplasmic membrane.

Regulation of the *hox* genes appears to be extremely complex. The alternative sigma factor Hno (RpoN) and the activator HoxA represent two major components in this control circuitry. Our future experimental work will be aimed at an understanding of the regulation of *hno* and *hoxA*. It is unknown whether *hoxA* is part of a two-component system like the *ntrC/ntrB* system. It will be crucial for an understanding of *hox* regulation to determine how the environmental redox signal is transmitted to *hoxA*. Prerequisites to answering these questions are purification of the regulatory proteins and construction of appropriate subclones harboring their respective target sites.

Finally, we must keep in mind certain aspects of DNA topology and RNA stability. The latter appears to be of particular importance, since evidence is accumulating that the *hoxS* mRNA is extremely stable; this transcript has a half-life of more than 1 h (U. Oelmüller and C. G. Friedrich, personal communication), which is very unusual for procaryotic mRNA. Preliminary analyses of the structure of the DNA of the *hox* region has revealed some intriguing features such as inverted repeats and large hairpin-forming units. Further studies may eventually contribute to our understanding of the regulation of the *hox* genes and the distribution of hydrogen-oxidizing ability among phylogenetically diverse microorganisms.

418   Friedrich et al.

ACKNOWLEDGMENTS. The excellent technical assistance of Anke Nies and Marita Feldotte is gratefully acknowledged. We thank Doris Matzkuhn for preparing the manuscript.

The research reported here was supported by grants from the Deutsche Forschungs-gemeinschaft.

LITERATURE CITED

Albright, L. M., C. W. Ronson, B. T. Nixon, and F. M. Ausubel. 1989. Identification of a gene linked to *Rhizobium meliloti ntrA* whose product is homologous to a family to ATP-binding proteins. *J. Bacteriol.* **171:**1932–1941.

Ausubel, F. M. 1984. Regulation of nitrogen fixation genes. *Cell* **37:**5–6.

Beynon, J., M. Cannon, V. Buchanon-Wollaston, and J. Cannon. 1983. The *nif* promoters of *Klebsiella pneumoniae* have a characteristic primary structure. *Cell* **34:**665–671.

Bowien, B., and H. G. Schlegel. 1981. Physiology and biochemistry of aerobic hydrogen-oxidizing bacteria. *Annu. Rev. Microbiol.* **35:**405–452.

Eberz, G., T. Eitinger, and B. Friedrich. 1989. Genetic determinants of a nickel-specific transport system are part of the plasmid-encoded hydrogenase gene cluster in *Alcaligenes eutrophus. J. Bacteriol.* **171:**1340–1345.

Eberz, G., C. Hogrefe, C. Kortlüke, A. Kamienski, and B. Friedrich. 1986. Molecular cloning of structural and regulatory hydrogenase (*hox*) genes of *Alcaligenes eutrophus* H16. *J. Bacteriol.* **168:**636–641.

Fauque, G., H. D. Peck, Jr., J. G. Moura, B. H. Huynh, Y. Berlier, D. V. DerVartanian, M. Teixeira, A. E. Przybyla, P. A. Lespinat, I. Moura, and J. LeGall. 1988. The three classes of hydrogenases from sulfate-reducing bacteria of the genus *Desulfovibrio. FEMS Microbiol. Rev.* **54:**299–344.

Friedrich, B. 1989. Genetics of energy converting systems in aerobic chemolithotrophs, p. 415–436. *In* H. G. Schlegel and B. Bowien (ed.), *Autotrophic Bacteria.* Brock/Springer Series in Contemporary Biosciences. Science Technology Publishers, Madison Wis., and Springer-Verlag KG, Heidelberg, Federal Republic of Germany.

Friedrich, B., C. Kortlüke, C. Hogrefe, G. Eberz, B. Silber, and J. Warrelmann. 1986. Genetics of hydrogenase from aerobic lithoautotrophic bacteria. *Biochimie* **68:**133–145.

Friedrich, C. G. 1982. Derepression of hydrogenase during limitation of electron donors and derepression of ribulosebisphosphate carboxylase during carbon limitation of *Alcaligenes eutrophus. J. Bacteriol.* **149:**203–210.

Friedrich, C. G., S. Suetin, and M. Lohmeyer. 1984. Nickel and iron incorporation into soluble hydrogenase of *Alcaligenes eutrophus. Arch. Microbiol.* **140:**206–211.

Helmann, J. D., and M. J. Chamberlin. 1988. Structure and function of bacterial sigma factors. *Annu. Rev. Biochem.* **57:**839–872.

Kärst, U., S. Suetin, and C. G. Friedrich. 1987. Purification and properties of a protein linked to the soluble hydrogenase of hydrogen-oxidizing bacteria. *J. Bacteriol.* **169:**2079–2085.

Leclerc, M., A. Colbeau, B. Cauvin, and P. M. Vignais. 1988. Cloning and sequencing of the genes encoding the large and the small subunits of the H_2 uptake hydrogenase *hup* of *Rhodobacter capsulatus. Mol. Gen. Genet.* **214:**97–107. (Erratum, **215:**368, 1989.)

Lohmeyer, M., and C. G. Friedrich. 1987. Nickel transport in *Alcaligenes eutrophus. Arch. Microbiol.* **149:**130–135.

Merrick, M. J., and J. R. Gibbins. 1985. The nucleotide sequence of the nitrogen regulation gene *ntrA* of *Klebsiella pneumoniae* and comparison with conserved features in bacterial sigma factors. *Nucleic Acids Res.* **13:**7607–7620.

Reeve, J. N., G. S. Beckler, D. S. Cram, P. T. Hamilton, J. W. Brown, J. A. Krzycki, A. F. Kolodziej, L. Alex, W. H. Orme-Johnson, and C. C. Walsh. 1989. A hydrogenase linked gene in *Methanobacterium thermoautotrophicum* ΔH encodes a poly-ferredoxin. *Proc. Natl. Acad. Sci. USA* **86:** 3031–3035.

Rohde, C., W. Johanssen, and F. Mayer. 1986. Electron microscopic localization of hydrogenase genes on the megaplasmid pHG1 in *Alcaligenes eutrophus. Mol. Gen. Genet.* **202:**476–480.

Römermann, D., and B. Friedrich. 1985. Denitrification by *Alcaligenes eutrophus* is plasmid dependent. *J. Bacteriol.* **162:**852–854.

Römermann, D., M. Lohmeyer, C. G. Friedrich, and B. Friedrich. 1988. Pleiotropic mutants from *Alcaligenes eutrophus* defective in the metabolism of hydrogen, nitrate, urea and fumarate. *Arch. Microbiol.* **149**:471–475.

Römermann, D., J. Warrelmann, R. A. Bender, and B. Friedrich. 1989. An *rpoN*-like gene of *Alcaligenes eutrophus* and *Pseudomonas facilis* controls the expression of diverse metabolic pathways. *J. Bacteriol.* **171**:1093–1099.

Sayavedra-Soto, L. A., G. K. Powell, H. J. Evans, and R. O. Morris. 1988. Nucleotide sequence of the genetic loci encoding subunits of *Bradyrhizobium japonicum* uptake hydrogenase. *Proc. Natl. Acad. Sci. USA* **85**:8395–8399.

Schlegel, H. G. 1989. Aerobic hydrogen-oxidizing (Knallgas) bacteria, p. 305–329. *In* H. G. Schlegel and B. Bowien (ed.), *Autotrophic Bacteria*. Brock/Springer Series in Contempory Biosciences. Science Technology Publishers, Madison, Wis., and Springer-Verlag KG, Heidelberg, Federal Republic of Germany.

Schneider, K., R. Cammack, and H. G. Schlegel. 1984. Content and localization of FMN, Fe-S clusters and nickel in the NAD-linked hydrogenase of *Nocardia opaca* 1b. *Eur. J. Biochem.* **142**:75–84.

Viebrock, A., and W. G. Zumft. 1988. Molecular cloning, heterologous expression, and primary structure of the structural gene for the copper enzyme nitrous oxide reductase from denitrifying *Pseudomonas stutzeri*. *J. Bacteriol.* **170**:4658–4668.

Weihs, V., K. Schmidt, B. Schneider, and B. Friedrich. 1989. The formation of an oxygen-binding flavohemoprotein in *Alcaligenes eutrophus* is plasmid-determined. *Arch. Microbiol.* **151**:546–550.

Index